Get Connected!

http://connection.LWW.com

Connect to a one-of-a-kind resource for students!

connection

Access everything you need at connection

- **E-mail updates** notify you of recent changes on the site and of content updates to the texts.

- **Chat rooms** enable on-line discussions for you to efficiently discuss specific topics with your peers and professor.

- **Message boards** make communication a snap.

- **Create-your-own-website**, using **connection's** easy-to-use format, stores the syllabus, notes, and schedule.

And just for the student...

- **Calendar of events** to keep up with the latest in the field of practical and vocational nursing.

- **Internet links** direct you to online resources for additional information on nursing fundamentals.

Register in 3 easy steps...

1. Simply log on to the **connection** website and access the Resource Center for practical and vocational nursing.

2. Enter your name and e-mail address, and set-up a user name and password.

3. Now you have immediate access to all the benefits of **connection**.

Connect today.
http://connection.LWW.com/go/lpnresources

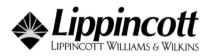

Lippincott
LIPPINCOTT WILLIAMS & WILKINS

For additional information about connection, visit
www.LWW.com/promo/connection

G452-01-P   N1NXG452

Introductory Pediatric Nursing

SIXTH EDITION

BROADRIBB'S

Introductory Pediatric Nursing

SIXTH EDITION

Nancy T. Hatfield, MA, BSN, RN
Director/Department Chairperson
Practical Nursing/Health Occupations
Albuquerque Public Schools
Career Enrichment Center
Albuquerque, New Mexico

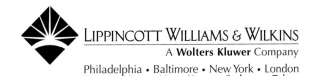

LIPPINCOTT WILLIAMS & WILKINS
A **Wolters Kluwer** Company

Philadelphia • Baltimore • New York • London
Buenos Aires • Hong Kong • Sydney • Tokyo

LIPPINCOTT COPYRIGHT STATEMENT FOR NURSING BOOKS

Acquisitions Editor: Lisa Stead
Editorial Assistant: Susan Barta Rainey
Senior Production Manager: Helen Ewan
Design: BJ Crim
Indexer: Angie Wiley
Printer: Quebecor

Managing Editor: Joe Morita
Senior Project Editor: Tom Gibbons
Art Director: Carolyn O'Brien
Manufacturing Manager: William Alberti
Compositor: Peirce Graphics

6th Edition

9 8 7 6 5 4 3 2

Library of Congress Cataloging-in-Publication Data
Hatfield, Nancy.
    Broadribb's Introductory pediatric nursing.—6th ed. / Nancy Hatfield.
        p. cm.
    Fifth ed. by Margaret G. Marks.
    Includes bibliographical references and index.
    ISBN 0-7817-3778-8 (pbk. : alk. paper)
    1. Pediatric nursing. I. Title: Introductory pediatric nursing. II. Broadribb, Violet.
Introductory pediatric nursing. III. Title.

RJ245 .B764 2003
610.73'62—dc21
                                                    2002190724

Care has been taken to confirm the accuracy of the information presented and to describe generally accepted practices. However, the authors, editors, and publisher are not responsible for errors or omissions or for any consequences from application of the information in this book and make no warranty, express or implied, with respect to the content of the publication.

The authors, editors, and publisher have exerted every effort to ensure that drug selection and dosage set forth in this text are in accordance with the current recommendations and practice at the time of publication. However, in view of ongoing research, changes in government regulations, and the constant flow of information relating to drug therapy and drug reactions, the reader is urged to check the package insert for each drug for any change in indications and dosage and for added warnings and precautions. This is particularly important when the recommended agent is a new or infrequently employed drug.

Some drugs and medical devices presented in this publication have Food and Drug Administration (FDA) clearance for limited use in restricted research settings. It is the responsibility of the health care provider to ascertain the FDA status of each drug or device planned for use in his or her clinical practice.

Dedication

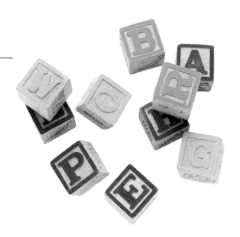

To John

My partner, my best friend; you are the light and love of my life

To Mikayla and Jeff

You taught me about children, caring, and happiness; my greatest joy in life is being your Mom

To Mom and Dad

Your unconditional love allowed me to be the child I was and the adult I am

Nancy T. Hatfield

Reviewers

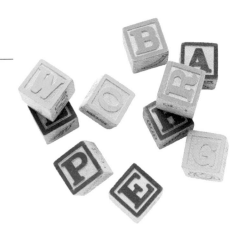

Susan Beggs, RN, MSN
Associate Professor
Vocational and Registered Nursing
Austin Community College
Austin, Texas

Pattie Garrett Clark, RN, MSN
Associate Professor of Nursing
Nursing Department
Abraham Baldwin College
Tifton, Georgia

Rosalinda H. Giffard, MSN, RNC, CS, FNP
Assistant Program Director
Vocational Nursing
UTB/TSC
Brownsville, Texas

Karen Kathryn Haagensen, RNC
Faculty
Vocational Nursing
Howard College
San Angelo, Texas

Barbara J. Kish, RN, BSN
Assistant Professor of Nursing
Health Technologies (LPN Program)
Belmont Technical College
St. Clairsville, Ohio

Frances E. Roebuck, RN, BSN
Nursing Instructor
Practical Nursing Department
Miami Valley Career Technology Center
Clayton, Ohio

Russlyn A. St. John, RN, MSN
Associate Professor
Practical Nursing
St. Charles County Community College
Florissant, Missouri

Debbie Theysohn, RN, BSN, MS
LPN Instructor
Nursing Department
Sullivan County Board of Cooperative Educational
  Services
Damascus, Pennsylvania

Darlyn DeHart Weikel, RN, MS
Associate Professor
Nursing Department
North Central State College
Galion, Ohio

Preface

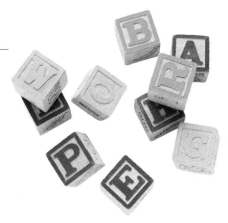

The sixth edition of *Broadribb's Introductory Pediatric Nursing* reflects the underlying philosophy of love and caring for children evident in earlier editions. The content has been updated and revised according to the most current information available, while maintaining the organization and integrity of the previous editions. In this edition we have continued the use of family caregivers to recognize that many children live in families other than traditional two-parent family homes. We recognize that cultural sensitivity and awareness are important aspects of caring for children and we have broadened the cultural viewpoints in this edition.

Pediatric health care has seen a shift from the hospital setting into community and home settings. More responsibility has fallen on the family caregivers to care for the ill child, so in this edition we continue to stress teaching the child and the family, with an emphasis on prevention. The nursing process has been used as the foundation for presenting nursing care. Implementation is presented in a narrative format to enable the discussion from which planning, goal setting, and implementation can be put into action. The newest and most current NANDA terminology has been used to update the possible nursing diagnosis for health care concerns.

We continue to strive to keep the readability of the text at a level with which the student can be comfortable. In recognition of the limited time that the student has and the frustration that can result from having to turn to a dictionary or glossary for words that are unfamiliar, we have attempted to identify all possible unfamiliar terms and define them within the text. This increases the reading ease for the student, decreasing the time necessary to complete the assigned reading and enhancing the understanding of the information. A four-color format, updated photos, drawings, tables, and diagrams will further aid the student in using this edition.

This edition offers the instructor and student of pediatric nursing a user-friendly, comprehensive quick reference to features in the text. Nursing programs using a body systems approach to teaching pediatrics will find the table of contents according to body systems a valuable resource for use in their curriculum. This text allows the student to study growth and development according to ages; the body systems table of contents further directs the use of this text to help the student learn about diseases and disorders in each of the body systems. Additionally, the quick reference to the Family Teaching Tips, Nursing Care Plans, Personal Glimpses, and Communication Boxes offers easy and efficient access to these features.

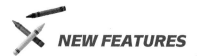

NEW FEATURES

In an effort to provide the instructor and student with a text that is informative, exciting, and easy to use, we have incorporated a number of new features throughout the text, many of which are included in each chapter. In this edition, we have added websites and Internet resources as well as activities to increase the student's use of the expanding opportunities the Internet offers. The new features include:

Internet Activity. Each chapter includes an Internet activity, which helps the student explore the Internet. Each activity takes the student step by step into a site where they can access new and updated information, resources to share with children and families, and fun activities to use with pediatric patients. Some of the activities require the use of Acrobat Reader. This can be downloaded free of charge for the student to readily view the site.

Websites. Included in the bibliography of every chapter are websites the student can refer to regarding topics included in that chapter. These sites also offer resource information the student can share with family caregivers. Throughout the text, websites are included as resources for the student to access available sites discussing certain diseases and disorders as well as offering support and information for families.

Learning Opportunities. To further enhance the student's critical thinking experiences, a learning opportunity has been added to each of the Personal Glimpses, which had a positive response in the previous edition.

Workbook Section. At the end of each chapter a workbook section has been added. The workbook includes:

- **NCLEX-Style Review Questions** written to test the student's ability to apply the material from the chapter. These questions use the client-nurse format to encourage the student to critically think about patient situations as well as the nurse response or action.
- **Study Activities** include interactive activities requiring the student to participate in the learning process. Important material from the chapter has been incorporated into this section to help the student review and synthesize the chapter content. The instructor will find many of the activities appropriate for individual or class assignments.
- **Critical Thinking** questions provide the student opportunities to problem solve and think about his or her own ideas and feelings. Critical thinking situations encourage the student to think about the chapter content in practical terms. These situations require the student to incorporate knowledge gained from the chapter and apply it to real-life problems. The instructor can also use them as a tool to stimulate class discussion.
- **Dosage Calculations** are found in each workbook chapter where diseases and disorders are covered. This section offers the student practice in pediatric dosage calculations that can be directly applied in a clinical setting.

SPECIAL FEATURES

Key Terms. A list of terms that may be unfamiliar to students and that are considered essential to the chapter's understanding appears at the beginning of each chapter. The first appearance in the chapter of each of these terms is in boldface type, with the definition included in the text. All key terms also are included in a glossary at the end of the text.

Student Objectives. Measurable student-oriented objectives are included at the beginning of each chapter. These help to guide the student in recognizing the focus of the chapter and provide the instructor with guidance for evaluating the student's understanding of the information presented in the chapter.

Nursing Process. The nursing process serves as an organizing structure for the discussion of nursing care for many of the health problems covered in the text. These provide the student with a foundation from which individualized nursing care plans can be developed. Each Nursing Process section includes nursing assessment, relevant nursing diagnoses, outcome identification and planning, implementation, outcome criteria, and evaluation. Emphasis is placed on the importance of involving the child and family caregivers in the assessment process. In the Nursing Process sections we have used updated and current NANDA-approved nursing diagnoses, many of which have been newly named. These are used to represent appropriate concerns for a particular condition, but we do not attempt to include all diagnoses that could be identified. Outcome identification focuses on setting goals for the child and family caregiver. The student will find the goals more specific, measurable, and realistic and will be able to relate the goals to patient situations and care plan development. Outcome criteria and evaluation provide a goal for each nursing diagnosis and criteria to measure the successful accomplishment of that goal.

Nursing Care Plans. Throughout the text Nursing Care Plans are presented to provide the student with a model to follow in using the information from the nursing process to develop specific nursing care plans. To make the care plans more meaningful, a scenario has been constructed for each one.

Family Teaching Tips. Information that the student can use in teaching family caregivers and children is presented in highlighted boxes ready for use.

Personal Glimpses. Personal Glimpses are presented in every chapter. These are actual first-person narratives, unedited, just as the individual wrote them. The Glimpses help the student have a view of an experience a child or caregiver had in a given situation and their feelings about or during the incident. These are presented to enhance the student's understanding and appreciation of the feelings of others. Following each Personal Glimpse is a Learning Opportunity, which encourages students to think of how they might react or respond in the situation presented.

Communication Boxes. We feel communication is an important aspect of the foundation of caring for others. In a number of the nursing care chapters we have placed communication situations, with examples of more effective and less effective communications and the mechanisms that help or hinder in the given illustration.

Tables, Drawings, and Photographs. These important aspects of the text have been updated and clarified with the addition of new material and color photographs.

Key Points. We have selected key points from each chapter to help the student focus on the important aspects. This provides a quick review of essential elements of the chapter.

Bibliography. Each Bibliography contains references that the student can readily turn to for additional information on conditions discussed in the chapter. Websites are also included in each chapter to offer the student access to additional information.

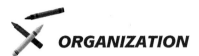

ORGANIZATION

The text is divided into four units to provide an orderly approach to the content. The first unit helps build a foundation for the student beginning the study of pediatric nursing. This unit introduces the student to caring for the child in various settings. The basic approach to the study of health problems of children is organized within a framework of growth and development. Growth and development is presented for an age group, and the specific health problems that commonly affect that age group are discussed in the following chapter. This approach has been well received by nursing students and continues to provide a user-friendly approach to the study of nursing care of children.

Unit 1, Foundations of Pediatric and Family Health Care, introduces the student in Chapter 1 to a brief history of pediatrics and pediatric nursing and the nursing process. Communicating with children and families is also included. Chapter 2 follows with a discussion of the family, its structure, and family factors that influence the growth and development of children. Concepts of growth and development are presented to provide a foundation for discussion in later chapters on growth and development. Chapter 3, Community-Based Care of the Child, introduces community-based health care and discusses the various settings in the community through which health care is provided for the child. Chapter 4, Care of the Hospitalized Child, presents the pediatric unit, infection control in the pediatric setting, admission and discharge, the child undergoing surgery, pain management, the hospital play program, and safety in the hospital. Chapter 5, Assessment of the Child (Data Collection), includes collecting subjective and objective data from the child and the family. The chapter also includes interviewing and obtaining a history, general physical assessments and exams, and assisting with diagnostic tests. Chapter 6, Procedures and Treatments, covers specific procedures for the pediatric patient as well as the role of the nurse in assisting with procedures and treatments. Chapter 7, Medication Administration and IV Therapy, includes

dosage calculation, administration of medications by various routes, and intravenous therapy.

Unit 2, Care of the Newborn, presents the characteristics of the normal newborn, newborn feeding, and family interaction and adjustment. Chapter 9 addresses the health problems of the newborn, including congenital anomalies and congenital disorders.

Unit 3, Care of the Child, is organized by developmental stages, from infancy through adolescence. The even-numbered chapters cover growth and development of the designated age group, and the odd-numbered chapters follow with health problems common to that age. Although many conditions are not limited to a specific age, they are included in the age group in which they most often occur. The nursing process and nursing care plans are integrated through this unit, as well as Personal Glimpses and Communication Boxes.

Unit 4, Care of the At-Risk Child, focuses on several societal problems and their effect on children. Chapter 20 explores the impact that substance abuse in the family has on the child. The issues of child abuse, runaway children, latchkey children, children of divorces, and homeless children and families are also examined. Chapter 21 discusses the concerns that face the family of a child with a chronic illness. The impact on the family of caring for a child with a chronic illness and the nurse's role in assisting and supporting these families is presented. Chapter 22 concludes with the dying child. Included in this chapter is a teaching aid to help the nurse perform a self-examination of personal attitudes about death and dying, as well as concrete guidelines to use when interacting with a grieving child or adult.

Throughout the text, family-centered care is stressed. Developmental enrichment and stimulation are stressed in the sections on nursing process. The basic premise of each child's self worth is fundamental in all of the nursing care presented.

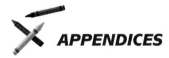

APPENDICES

Five appendices are included at the back of the text and contain important information for the nursing student in pediatrics:

- **Appendix A** Growth Charts
- **Appendix B** Pulse, Respiration, and Blood Pressure Values for Children
- **Appendix C** Conversion Chart: Fahrenheit to Celsius
- **Appendix D** Good Sources of Essential Nutrients
- **Appendix E** Standard Precautions

Acknowledgments

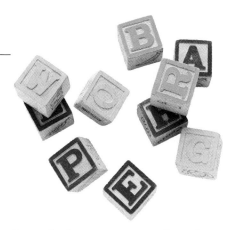

From the day I said "yes" to the challenge of updating and revising this sixth edition of *Broadribb's Introductory Pediatric Nursing*, I have felt supported by my "team" at Lippincott Williams & Willkins. Although the faces of the team have changed from the beginning to the completion, I sincerely appreciate and have enjoyed working with each person along the path. My thanks and heartfeld gratitude to:

Danielle DiPalma for being the anchor and lifeline for me in this project. Her hard work in the previous edition and her knowledge of the content made her assistance invaluable. The time she took in helping me build a foundation for this edition proved to be the key to the success of this revision.

Joe Morita for his encouragement, understanding, and expertise in the day-by-day management of the project after coming aboard midstream.

Lisa Stead for supporting a revision of the text and her belief that I could successfully do the job. She was always in the background with an answer whenever there was a question.

Michael Porter for his willingness, precision, and sense of humor in stepping in and helping fine-tune and complete the task at hand.

Karin McAndrews for her assurance and confidence that I could do the project and her gentle persuasion until I said yes.

Lisa Popeck for her calm, clear manner in helping get the project off the ground.

Margaret G. Marks for her hours of hard work and commitment on the previous editions.

All the others who have been involved in the project and who worked diligently to complete this revision, many of whose names I don't even know.

I would like to thank my husband, John, for his never-ending confidence, patience, and encouragement as well as the hours of household responsibilities he took on, all with a smile and a quiet, sincere support of my project. I appreciate and thank my children Mikayla and Jeff and my parents Edgar and Lucy Thomas for encouraging me to accept the challenge, being my cheering section and for the phone calls, positive words and memorable quotes, always just when I needed them. It was their belief in me that helped me recognize that my dream of writing could be a reality. My sisters, brothers, extended family, and special friends listened to me, gave me insight and advice, took pictures, and helped me affirm that this project could be accomplished. Thank you all for loving and supporting me.

Contents

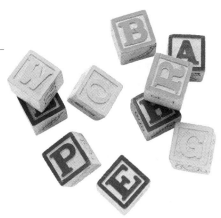

Table of Contents for the Body Systems–Based Pediatric Curriculum

Nursing programs using a body systems approach to teaching pediatrics will find this table of contents according to body systems a valuable resource for use in their curriculum. The student and instructor can use the table of contents as a guide to help them find the specific pages, which present the diseases and disorders in each of the body systems.

Quick Reference to Features

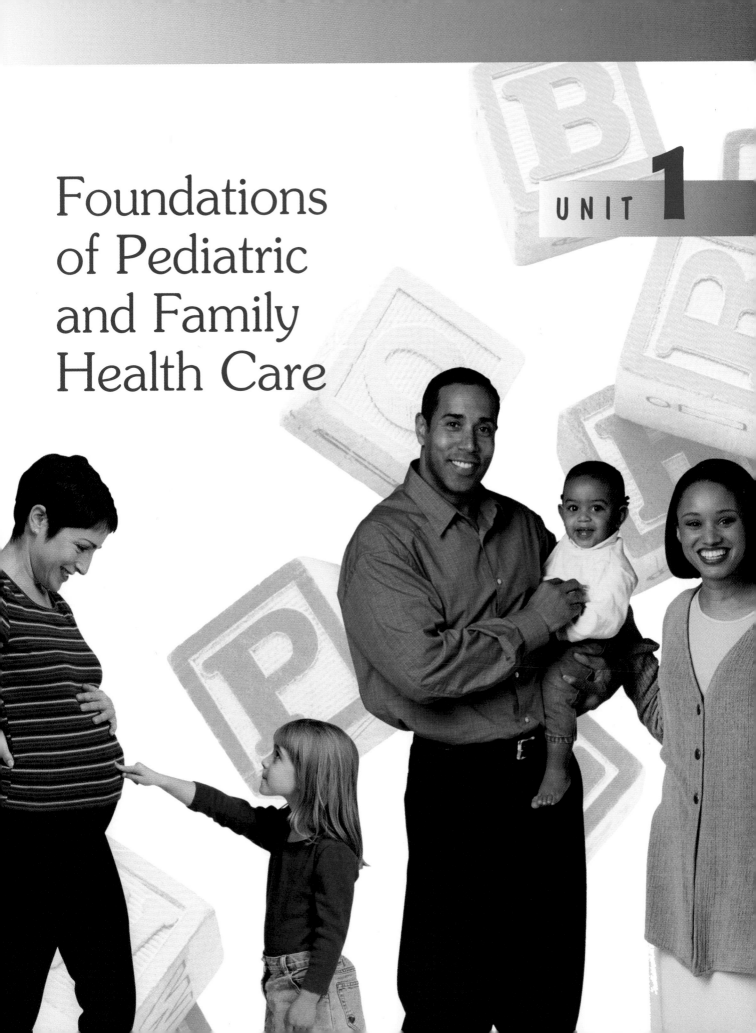

Foundations of Pediatric and Family Health Care

The Nurse's Role in a Changing Child Health Care Environment

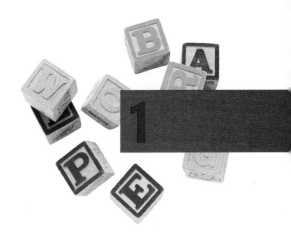

STUDENT OBJECTIVES

On completion of this chapter, the student will be able to

1. State where the United States ranks compared with other developed countries in terms of infant mortality rate.
2. State two causes of the high rate of infant mortality in the United States.
3. Describe the post–World War I atmosphere in the care of children and its effect on those children.
4. List the five steps of the nursing process.
5. Name the people involved in setting goals or outcomes for the child.
6. Explain the importance of complete and accurate documentation.
7. Discuss one of the most important aspects of communication.
8. State the purpose of using reflective statements when communicating with a caregiver or child.
9. List four categories of cultural attitudes that influence planning of care for the child.

KEY TERMS

actual nursing diagnoses
critical pathways
dependent nursing actions
independent nursing actions
interdependent nursing actions
nursing process
objective data
outcomes
pediatric nurse practitioner
primary nursing
risk nursing diagnoses
subjective data
wellness nursing diagnoses

The nurse preparing to care for today's and tomorrow's children and families faces vastly different responsibilities and challenges than did the pediatric nurse of even a decade ago. Nurses and other health professionals are becoming increasingly concerned with much more than the care of sick children. Health teaching; preventing illness; and promoting optimal (most desirable or satisfactory) physical, developmental, and emotional health have become a significant part of contemporary nursing.

Scientific and technologic advances have reduced the incidence of communicable disease and have helped to control metabolic disorders such as diabetes. As a result, more health care is provided outside the hospital. Patients now receive health care in the home, at schools and clinics, and from their primary care provider. Prenatal diagnosis of birth defects, transfusions, other treatments for the unborn fetus, and improved life-support systems for premature infants are but a few examples of the rapid progress in child care.

Controversy continues to rage about choices in family planning. In January 1973, a Supreme Court decision declared abortion legal anywhere in the United States. In 1981, efforts were made to convince Congress that legislation should be passed to make all abortions illegal on the alleged grounds that the fetus is a person and, therefore, has the right to life. In the 1990s, bitter debate between "pro-life" and "pro-choice" groups raged and seems likely to continue for many years.

Tremendous sociologic changes have affected attitudes toward and concepts in child health. American society is largely suburban with a population of highly mobile persons and families. The women's movement has focused new attention on the needs of families in which the mother works outside the home. Escalating divorce rates, changes in attitudes toward sexual roles, and general acceptance of unmarried mothers have increased the number of single-parent families. Many people have come to regard health care as a right, not a privilege, and expect to receive fair value for their investment. In addition, the demand for financial responsibility in health care has contributed to shortened hospital stays and alternative methods of health care delivery.

The reduction in the incidence of communicable and infectious diseases has made it possible to devote more attention to such critical problems as child abuse, learning and behavior disorders, developmental disabilities, and chronic illness. Research in these areas continues; as these findings become available, nurses will be among the practitioners who will help translate this research into improved health care for children and families.

Nurses' ability to translate the relevant medical research into practice, however, is based on their understanding of the predictable but variable phases of a child's growth and development and their understanding of and sensitivity to the importance of family interactions.

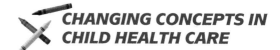

CHANGING CONCEPTS IN CHILD HEALTH CARE

Child health care has evolved from a sideline of internal medicine to a specialty that focuses on the child and the child's family in health and illness through all phases of development. Technologic advances account for many changes in the last 50 years, but sociologic changes, particularly society's view of the child and the child's needs, have been just as important.

Institutional Care

Pediatrics is a relatively new medical specialty, developing only in the mid-1800s. In colonial times, epidemics were common and many children died in infancy or childhood. Families were large because so many children did not live to adulthood. Children were viewed as additional hands to help with the family farm chores. Children often were cared for by the adults in the family or by a neighbor with a reputation of being able to care for the sick. In some cases, disease wiped out entire families. Native American children, usually cared for by medicine men, were exposed to new and fatal diseases. Children of slaves received only the care their slave owner cared to provide.

The first children's hospital opened in Philadelphia in 1855. Until that point in Western civilization, children were not considered important except as contributors to family income. Hospitalized children were cared for in hospitals as adults were, often in the same bed.

Unfortunately early institutions for children were notorious for their unsanitary conditions, neglect, and lack of proper infant nutrition. Well into the 19th century, mortality rates were commonly 50% to 100% among institutionalized children in asylums or hospitals.

Arthur Jacobi, a Prussian-born physician, has been recognized as the father of pediatrics. Under his direction, several New York hospitals opened pediatric units. He helped found the American Pediatric Society in 1888. During the early 1900s, intractable diarrhea was a primary cause of death in children's institutions. Initiation of the simple practices of boiling milk and isolating children with septic conditions lowered the incidence of diarrhea. This practice of pasteurizing milk was instrumental in decreasing the rate of death in children.

After World War I, a period of strict asepsis began. Babies were placed in individual cubicles, and the nurses were strictly forbidden to pick up the children except when necessary. Crib sides were draped with clean sheets, leaving infants with nothing to do but stare at the ceiling. The importance of toys in a child's environment appears not to have been recognized; besides, it was thought that such objects could transmit infection. Parents were allowed to visit for half an hour or perhaps 1 hour each week and they were forbidden to pick up their children under penalty of having their visiting privileges revoked.

Despite these precautions, high infant mortality rates continued. One of the first people to suspect the cause was Joseph Brennaman, a physician at Children's Memorial Hospital, Chicago. In 1932, he suggested that the infants suffered from a lack of stimulation; other concerned child specialists became interested. In the 1940s, Ren Spitz published the results of studies that supported his contention that deprivation of maternal care caused a state of dazed stupor in an infant. He believed this condition could become irreversible if the child were not returned to the mother promptly. He termed this state "anaclitic depression." He also coined the term *hospitalism*, which he defined as "a vitiated condition of the body due to long confinement in the hospital" (*vitiated* means feeble or weak). Later the term came to be used almost entirely to denote the harmful effects of institutional care on infants. Another physician, Bakwin, found that infants hospitalized for a long time actually developed physical symptoms that he attributed to a lack of emotional stimulation and a lack of feeding satisfaction.

Working under the auspices of the World Health Organization, John Bowlby of London explored the subject of maternal deprivation thoroughly. His 1951 study, which received worldwide attention, revealed the negative results of the separation of child and mother due to hospitalization. Bowlby's work, together with that of associate John Robertson, led to a reevaluation and liberalization of hospital visiting policies for children.

In the 1970s and 1980s, Marshall Klaus and John Kennell, physicians at Rainbow Babies and Children's Hospital, Cleveland, carried out important studies on the effect of the separation of newborns and parents. They established that this early separation may have long-term effects on family relationships and that offering the new family an opportunity to be together at birth and for a significant period after birth may

provide benefits that last well into early childhood (Fig. 1–1). These findings also have helped to modify hospital policies.

Hospital regulations changed slowly, but gradually they began to reflect the needs of children and their families. Isolation practices have been relaxed for children who do not have infectious diseases; children are encouraged to ambulate as early as possible and to visit the playroom where they can be with other children. Nurses at all levels who work with children are prepared to understand, value, and use play as a therapeutic tool in the daily care of children.

Family-Centered Care

Family-centered nursing is a new and broadened concept in the health care system of the United States. No longer are children treated merely as clinical cases with attention given exclusively to their medical problems. Instead health care providers recognize that children belong to a family, a community, and a particular way of life or culture and that their health is influenced by these and other factors (Fig. 1–2). Separating children from their backgrounds means that their needs are met only in a superficial manner, if at all. Even if nursing takes place entirely inside hospital walls, family-centered care pays attention to each child's unique emotional, developmental, social, and scholastic needs as well as physical ones. Family-centered nursing care also strives to help family members alleviate their fears and anxieties, cope and function normally, and understand the child's condition and their role in the healing process.

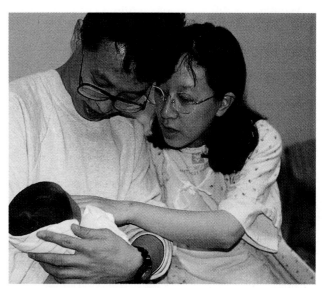

● *Figure 1.1* The mother, father, and infant son soon after birth.

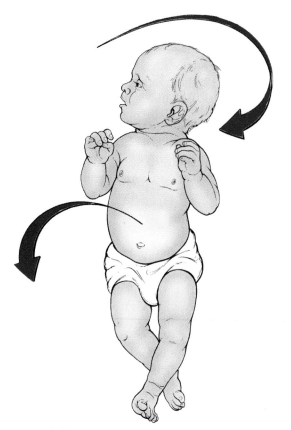

● *Figure 1.2* Internal and external factors that influence the health and illness patterns of the child.

Regionalized Care

During the past several decades there has been a definite trend toward centralization and regionalization of pediatric services. Providing high-quality medical care in pediatrics necessitated moving the child to medical teaching centers with the best resources for diagnosis and treatment. To contribute to economic responsibility by avoiding duplication of services and equipment, the most intricate and expensive services and the most highly specialized personnel were made available in the centralized location: pediatric neurologists, adolescent allergy specialists, pediatric oncologists, nurse play therapists, child psychiatrists, pediatric nurse practitioners, and clinical nurse specialists. Here are found geneticists, neonatal intensive care units, computed tomography scanners, burn care units, and other highly specialized equipment and units.

Regionalized care often takes the pediatric patient far from home. The family caregivers must travel a longer distance to visit than if the child were at the local suburban hospital. Family-centered care becomes even more important under these circumstances. Measures are always taken to keep the child's hospitalization as brief as possible, the child as ambulatory as possible, and the family as close as possible.

For the child, separation from the family is traumatic and may actually retard recovery. Many of these regionalized centers (tertiary care hospitals) have accommodations where families may stay while their children are hospitalized.

Other Innovative Child Health Care Programs

Many pediatric hospitals have home care programs for children with chronic illness such as leukemia, hemophilia, and cystic fibrosis. Between hospitalizations, the hospital's home health nurses monitor the child's condition in the home, thus providing continuity of care.

Some pediatric heath care providers use **primary nursing,** a system whereby one nurse plans the total care for a child and directs the efforts of nurses on the other two shifts. The primary nurse is responsible for the child's care at all times and often makes home visits to the child after discharge and before readmission. In facilities where primary nursing is not practiced, a good procedure is to assign the same nurse to a child to provide stability in the child's care.

Case management is an approach somewhat similar to primary nursing but with more concern and involvement with cost effectiveness and quality of care. Case management plans are multidisciplinary plans that include all aspects of and participants in the child's care. A nursing case manager is assigned to a child or group of children with similar conditions. Outcomes within specific time lines are established. These time lines have various names but are often called **critical pathways.** Regular documentation of care provides the opportunity for daily evaluation to determine where delays may be occurring so that appropriate adjustments in care can be made. Case management plans also can include the child's home care. Case management results in better coordination of care and less fragmentation and has led to increased family satisfaction.

Many children now are being cared for in health maintenance organizations (HMOs). HMOs are professional groups of physicians, laboratory service personnel, nurse practitioners, nurses, and consultants who care for the family's health on a continuing basis; HMOs are geared toward health care and disease prevention. The family pays a set fee for total care including any necessary hospitalization. The emphasis is on health and prevention in contrast to the acute care, cure-oriented pediatric medical center.

In some private practices and in many clinic settings, the child is cared for by a **pediatric nurse practitioner,** a professional nurse prepared at the postbaccalaureate level to give primary health care to children and families. Pediatric nurse practitioners use pediatricians or family physicians as consultants but offer day-to-day assessment and care.

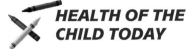

HEALTH OF THE CHILD TODAY

In the first half of the 20th century, many children died during or after childbirth or in early childhood as a result of disease, infections, or injuries. Technologic and socioeconomic changes have influenced the health care provided to children and also the health problems that confront today's children. Communicable diseases of childhood and their complications are no longer a serious threat to the health of children. As the 21st century begins, health problems for children focus much more on social concerns (Table 1–1). These issues are summarized below and will be discussed throughout the text.

Infants

Despite remarkable advances in many areas of maternal and child health, the maternal and infant mortality statistics are still grim. Infant mortality declined steadily in the 1960s and 1970s, but the 1980s and 1990s saw a stall in that decline. In 2001, the United States ranked 19th and Canada ranked 12th in the rate of infant deaths among developed countries (Fig. 1–3). Of even greater concern is the fact some U.S. cities had twice the national infant mortality rate.

Many factors may be associated with infants' high mortality rate and poor health. Low birth weight and late or nonexistent prenatal care are main factors in the poor rankings in infant mortality.[1] Other major factors that compromise infants' health include congenital anomalies, sudden infant death syndrome, respiratory distress syndrome, and increasing rates of human immunodeficiency virus (HIV). Low birth weight and other causes of infant death and chronic illness are often linked to maternal factors such as lack of prenatal care, smoking, use of alcohol and illicit drugs, pregnancy before age 18 or after age 40, poor nutrition, lower socioeconomic status, lower

TABLE 1.1	Every Day in America the Following Occurrences Take Place					
	All U.S. Children	Black Children	White Children	Latino Children	Asian American Children	Native American Children
Children and youths under 25 die from HIV infection	3	2	1	—	—	—
Children and youths under 20 commit suicide	6	1	5	—	—	—
Children and youths under 20 are homicide victims	13	6	5	—	—	—
Children and youths under 20 are killed by guns	15	5	7	—	—	—
Children and youths under 20 die from accidental injuries	34	6	28	—	—	—
Babies die before their first birthday	78	24	51	11	2	1
Babies are born at very low birth weight (<3 lb 4 oz)	156	49	92	21	5	1
Babies are born at low birth weight (<5.5 lb)	817	212	536	121	32	7
Babies are born to teenage mothers	1,354	372	959	334	24	22
Babies are born to mothers who had late or no prenatal care	410	114	275	124	18	9
Babies are born into poverty	1,951	723	13,231	679	—	—
Children and youths under 18 are arrested for drug offenses	351	143	270	—	4	3
Children and youths under 18 are arrested for violent crimes	186	105	126	—	4	2
Students drop out of high school each school day	2,911	500	2,144	672	—	—

Source: Children's Defense Fund, 2001.

(Note: not all totals equal 100%.)

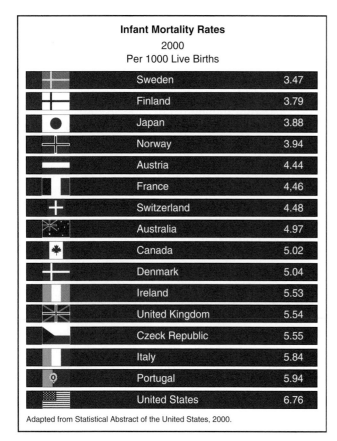

Infant Mortality Rates
2000
Per 1000 Live Births

Sweden	3.47
Finland	3.79
Japan	3.88
Norway	3.94
Austria	4.44
France	4,46
Switzerland	4.48
Australia	4.97
Canada	5.02
Denmark	5.04
Ireland	5.53
United Kingdom	5.54
Czeck Republic	5.55
Italy	5.84
Portugal	5.94
United States	6.76

Adapted from Statistical Abstract of the United States, 2000.

● *Figure 1.3* 2001 infant mortality rates per 1000 live births. (Adapted from Statistical Abstract of the United States, 2000.)

educational levels, and environmental hazards. Both infant and maternal mortality rates are much higher among nonwhite populations; studies repeatedly attribute high mortality rates to lack of adequate prenatal care and an increased birth rate among the high-risk group of women 15 to 19 years of age. The lack of adequate financial resources, insurance, and education regarding birth control and health care in general contributes to this situation.

National Commission to Prevent
Infant Mortality

In 1986, Congress established the National Commission to Prevent Infant Mortality and charged it with the responsibility of creating a national strategic plan to reduce infant mortality and morbidity rates in the United States. The Commission's first report in 1988, *Death Before Life: The Tragedy of Infant Mortality*, listed two primary objectives: to make the health of mothers and babies a national priority and to provide universal access to care for all pregnant women and children. The Commission concluded that educating the nation about the health needs of mothers and babies would cause a national response to the problem and that women would have to be given

information and motivation to reduce infant mortality and morbidity rates. The Commission also stated that barriers of finances, geography, education, social position, behavior, and program administration problems must be eliminated to provide universal access to health care. In February 1990, the Commission published *Troubling Trends: The Health of the Next Generation*, which concluded that early prenatal care along with smoking cessation, pregnancy planning, and nutrition counseling and food supplementation, would result in heavier and healthier infants. The Commission has been successful in its objective of decreasing infant mortality. There was a significant decline in infant mortality between 1995 to 1996.[2] The hope is that the decline will continue.

Children and Adolescents

Infectious diseases such as polio, diphtheria, scarlet fever, measles, and whooping cough once posed the greatest threat to children. However, today the largest risk to all children and adolescents is unintentional injury, frequently the result of motor vehicle accidents. Other unintentional injuries include drowning, falls, poisonings, and fires. Families, communities, and government agencies are minimizing the risks of injury-related death through protection and safety measures.

Developmental problems related to socioeconomic factors are on the rise, including mental retardation, learning disorders, emotional and behavioral problems, and speech and vision impairments. Lead poisoning appears to be a major threat to the child's developmental well being. Although strict laws have minimized the amount of lead in gas, air, food, and industrial emissions, many children live and play in substandard housing areas where they are exposed to chipped lead-based paint, dust, and soil.

Other prevalent factors that affect children's health include respiratory illness, violence toward children in the form of child abuse and neglect, homicide, suicide, cigarette smoking, alcohol and illicit drug use, risky sexual behavior, obesity, and lack of exercise.

Healthy living habits are established early in childhood. Many schools educate students about the hazards of tobacco, drugs, and the importance of exercise, nutrition, and safe sex. Many also provide immunization and screening programs. However, there is still a need for improvements and increases in the number of educational and support programs available to children, families, and communities. The program goals should be to alleviate many child health problems and provide children with adequate tools to make healthy living choices well into adulthood.

Healthy People 2010

In 1990, a national consortium of more than 300 organizations developed a set of objectives for the year 2000, *Healthy People 2000*. Prevention of illness, or health promotion, was the underlying goal of these objectives. States were encouraged to set their own objectives. Priority areas specifically affecting children were identified. These objectives were reviewed mid-decade; although there had been progress in some goals, much remained to be accomplished. The initiative has continued and *Healthy People 2010* outlines two basic goals for health promotion and disease prevention. Goal one is to increase quality and years of healthy life; goal two is to eliminate health disparities.[3] These goals are divided further into focus areas and attainment objectives. Many of the focus areas and objectives directly relate to children and their health care (Table 1–2). Nurses caring for children use these objectives as underlying guidelines in planning care.

INTERNET EXERCISE 1-1

http://web.health.gov/healthypeople/

Healthy People—Leading Health Indicators
Click on What are the Leading Health Indicators?

TABLE 1.2 | *Healthy People 2010:* **Focus Areas Related to Children**

Focus Area: Access to Quality Health Services
Goal: Improve access to comprehensive, high-quality health care services.
  Single toll-free number for poison control centers
  Special needs for children
Focus Area: Educational and Community-Based Programs
Goal: Increase the quality, availability, and effectiveness of education and community-based programs designed to prevent disease and improve health and quality of life.
  School health education
  School nurse-to-student ratio
  Community health promotion programs
Focus Area: Environmental Health
Goal: Promote health for all through a healthy environment.
  Elevated blood lead levels in children
  School policies to protect against environmental hazards
Focus Area: Family Planning
Goal: Improve pregnancy planning and spacing and prevent unintended pregnancy.
  Adolescent pregnancy
  Abstinence before age 15 and among adolescents age 15 to 17 years
Focus Area: HIV
Goal: Prevent HIV infection and its related illness and death.
  Perinatally acquired HIV infection
Focus Area: Immunization and Infectious Diseases
Goal: Prevent disease, disability, and death from infectious disease including vaccine-preventable diseases.
  Hepatitis B and bacterial meningitis in infants and young children
  Antibiotics prescribed for ear infections
  Vaccination coverage and strategies
Focus Area: Injury and Violence Prevention
Goal: Reduce injuries, disabilities, and deaths due to unintentional injuries and violence.
  Child fatality review
  Deaths from firearms, poisoning, suffocation, motor vehicle crashes
  Child restraints

  Drownings
  Maltreatment and maltreatment fatalities of children
Focus Area: Maternal, Infant, and Child Health
Goal: Improve the health and well-being of women, infants, children, and families.
  Fetal, infant, child, adolescent deaths
  Low birth weight and very low birth weight, pre-term births
  Developmental disabilities
Focus Area: Nutrition and Overweight
Goal: Promote health and reduce chronic disease associated with diet and weight.
  Overweight or obesity in children and adolescents
Focus Area: Physical Fitness and Activity
Goal: Improve health, fitness, and quality of life through daily physical activity.
  Physical activity in children and adolescents
Focus Area: Sexually Transmitted Diseases
Goal: Promote responsible sexual behaviors, increase access to quality services to prevent STDs and their complications.
  Responsible adolescent sexual behavior
Focus Area: Substance Abuse
Goal: Reduce substance abuse to protect the health, safety and quality of life for all especially children.
  Adverse consequences of substance use and abuse
  Substance use and abuse
Focus Area: Tobacco Use
Goal: Reduce illness, disability, and death related to tobacco use and exposure to secondhand smoke.
  Adolescent tobacco use, age, and initiation of tobacco use
  Smoking cessation by adolescents
  Exposure to tobacco smoke at home among children
Focus Area: Vision and Hearing
Goal: Improve the visual and hearing health of the nation.
  Vision screening for children
  Impairment in children and adolescents
  Newborn hearing screening, evaluation, and intervention
  Otitis media
  Noise-induced hearing loss in children

Adapted from National Center for Health Statistics, *Healthy People 2010*, Hyattsville, MD, 2001.

1. Make a list of the leading health indicators.
   Hit the back arrow and return to Leading Health Indicators.
   Click on Resources for Individual Action.

2. What is a resource site you could share with a family caregiver regarding health care access?

3. What is a resource site you could share with someone needing information on injury or violence?

THE NURSE'S CHANGING ROLE IN CHILD HEALTH CARE

The image of nursing has changed and the horizons and responsibilities have broadened tremendously in recent years. The primary thrust of health care is toward prevention. In addition to the treatment of disease and physical problems, modern-day child care addresses growth and development and anticipatory guidance on maturational and common health problems. Teaching is also an important aspect of caring for the child; clients are educated on a variety of topics from follow-up of immunizations to other, more traditional aspects of health.

Nurses at all levels are legally accountable for their actions and assume new responsibilities and accountability with every advance in education. Nurses practicing in any pediatric setting at all levels must keep up to date with education and information on how to help their young patients and where to direct families for help when other resources are needed. When the nurse functions as a teacher, adviser, and resource person, it is important that the information and advice provided be correct, pertinent, and useful to the person in need.

As mentioned earlier, pediatric nurse practitioners have taken a significant place in caring for children. Some of these nurses specialize in school nursing or oncology among other areas. In addition, clinical nurse specialists are nurses with advanced education prepared to provide care at any stage of illness or wellness.

In many settings, nurses can provide health education to both children and their families. Such teaching may be concerned with safety, nutrition, health habits, immunizations, dental care, healthy development, and discipline. Some of these settings include schools, home, and ambulatory settings. In schools, nurses have become much more than Band-Aid dispensers: they monitor well children including their immunizations and their growth and development. School nurses often present or are consultants in classroom health education programs

and often serve on committees that evaluate children with educational and social adjustment problems. For children with long-term or chronic illnesses, nurses can help provide care in the home. This home care often is part of a collaboration with other health care professionals. Ambulatory care settings help avoid separating the child from the family and provide a less costly means of administering health care to children. The pediatric nurse plays an important role in ambulatory settings.

In addition, nurses are contributing to health care research that will help lead to more improvements in the care of children and their families.

Health teaching is one of the most important aspects of promoting wellness. Nurses are often in a position to do incidental teaching as well as more organized formal teaching. Nurses also must be aware that they serve as role models to others in practicing good health habits. Some examples of possible teaching opportunities include those in a work environment such as helping the child and family understand a diagnosis or proposed treatment, understanding medications, and providing teaching materials to children and families. In the community, the nurse can be an advocate for healthy living practices and policies or can serve as a volunteer in community organizations to promote healthy growth and development and anticipatory guidance. Nurses can become involved with their schools to offer knowledge and expertise in wellness practices. They should use every opportunity to contribute to and encourage healthy living practices.

Throughout this text, teaching opportunities are identified and teaching suggestions supplied. Nurses are encouraged to use these suggestions as a foundation for further teaching. During any teaching, however, the nurse must be alert to the abilities of the child and the family to understand the material being presented. By using methods of feedback, questions and answers, and demonstrations when appropriate, the nurse can confirm that the information is understood. This also gives the nurse the opportunity to reinforce any areas of weak information. With experience, nurses can become very competent teachers.

THE NURSING PROCESS

The **nursing process** is a proven form of problem solving based on the scientific method. The nursing process consists of five components:

- Assessment
- Nursing diagnosis

- Outcome identification and planning
- Implementation
- Evaluation

Based on the data collected during the assessment, nursing diagnoses are determined, nursing care is planned and implemented, and the results are evaluated. The process does not end here but continues through reassessment, establishment of new diagnoses, additional plans, implementation, and evaluation until all the child's nursing problems are identified and dealt with (Fig. 1–4).

Assessment

Nursing assessment is a skill that must be practiced and perfected through study and experience. The practical nurse collects data and contributes to the child's assessment. The nurse must be skilled in understanding the concepts of verbal and nonverbal communication; concepts of growth and development; anatomy, physiology, and pathophysiology; and the influence of cultural heritage and family social structure. The data collected during the assessment of the child and family form the basis of all the child's nursing care.

Assessment and data collection begin with the admission interview and physical exam. During this phase, a relationship of trust begins to build between the nurse, the child, and the family caregivers. This relationship forms more quickly when the nurse is sensitive to the family's cultural background. Careful listening and recording of **subjective data** (data spoken by the child or family) and careful observation and recording of **objective data** (observable by the nurse) are essential to obtain a complete picture.

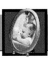

A PERSONAL GLIMPSE

My Grandpa's eyes gave me my first vision of nursing. A Licensed Practical Nurse, he filled my head with hospital stories and my belly with chocolate milk. He saw people hurt by pain and fear, and he made them feel better. I wasn't much bigger than the children I saw, but I knew I wanted to make them feel better too. So I went to nursing school in the same hospital where I shared chocolate milk with Grandpa.

My pediatric nursing career started at graduation 25 years ago. Back then, the community pediatric unit was always filled to capacity. Outpatient and critical care services for children were minimal, so disorders ranged from the mild to the severe. Newborns through teens were treated for everything from mild diarrhea to significant trauma. But two things remained constant regardless of age or diagnosis: the pain and the fear.

Soon, helping sick children feel better was no longer enough. I realized early in my career that the best way to help was to prevent children from getting sick in the first place. So I went back to school through baccalaureate and masters' degrees to become a Pediatric Nurse Practitioner. Seventeen years later, I still practice as a PNP in a rural community.

Changes in health care have put more emphasis on the various nonhospital settings, where most children receive care. Healthy children are less likely to become ill and more likely to become healthy adults. Prevention and health promotion are essential. They should be part of the care of all children (and adults!) including those who are hospitalized. I always take the time to teach the importance of immunizations, proper nutrition, growth, and development. A little goes a long way, and there is tremendous satisfaction in knowing that I've helped to ease pain and fear before they have a chance to get started.

Mary

> ▶ **LEARNING OPPORTUNITY:** What are the challenges for the nurse caring for the child in a community health setting? Describe the priorities of the pediatric nurse in health promotion and disease prevention.

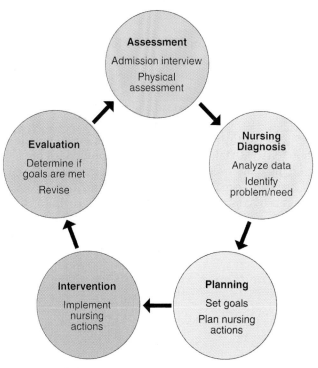

● *Figure 1.4* Diagram of the nursing process.

Nursing Diagnosis

The process of determining a nursing diagnosis begins with the analysis of information (data) gathered during the assessment. Along with the registered nurse or other healthcare professional, the practical nurse participates in the development of a nursing diagnosis based on actual or potential health problems that fall within the range of nursing practice. These diagnoses are not medical diagnoses but are based on the individual response to a disease process, condition, or situation. Nursing diagnoses change as the patient's responses change; therefore, diagnoses are in a continual state of reevaluation and modification.

Nursing diagnoses are subdivided into three types: actual, risk, and wellness diagnoses. **Actual nursing diagnoses** identify existing health problems. For example, a child who has asthma may have an actual diagnosis stated as *Ineffective Airway Clearance related to increased mucous production as evidenced by dyspnea and wheezing.* This statement identifies a health problem the child actually has (ineffective airway clearance), the factor that contributes to its cause (increased mucous production), and the signs and symptoms. This is an actual nursing diagnosis because of the presence of signs and symptoms and the child's inability to clear the airway effectively.

Risk nursing diagnoses identify health problems to which the patient is especially vulnerable. These identify patients at high risk for a particular problem. An example of a risk nursing diagnosis is *Risk for Injury related to uncontrolled muscular activity secondary to seizure.*

Wellness nursing diagnoses identify the potential of a person, family, or community to move from one level of wellness to a higher level. For example, a wellness diagnosis for a family adapting well to the birth of a second child might be *Readiness for Enhanced Family Coping.*

The North American Nursing Diagnosis Association (NANDA) first published an approved list of nursing diagnoses in 1973; since then the list has been revised and expanded periodically. Nursing diagnoses continue to be developed and revised to keep them current and useful in describing what nurses contribute to health care.

Outcome Identification and Planning

To plan nursing care for the child, data must be collected (assessment) and analyzed (nursing diagnosis) and outcomes identified in cooperation with the child and family caregiver. These **outcomes** (goals) should be specific, stated in measurable terms, and include a time frame. For example, a short-term expected outcome for a child with asthma could be "The child will demonstrate use of metered-dose inhaler within 2 days." The goal must be realistic, child-focused, and attainable. After mutual goal setting has been accomplished, nursing actions are proposed. Although a number of possible diagnoses may be identified, the nurse must review them, rank them by urgency, and select those that require the most immediate attention.

After selecting the first goals to accomplish, the nurse must propose nursing interventions to achieve them. This is the planning aspect of the nursing process. These nursing interventions may be based on clinical experience, knowledge of the health problem, standards of care, standard care plans, or other resources. The interventions should be discussed with the child and family caregiver to determine if they are practical and workable. Proposed interventions are modified to fit the individual child. If standardized care plans are used, they must be individualized to reflect the child's age and developmental level, cognitive level, and family, economic, and cultural influences. Expected outcomes are set with specific measurable criteria and time lines.

Implementation

Implementation is the process of putting the nursing care plan into action. These actions may be independent, dependent, or interdependent. **Independent nursing actions** are actions that may be performed based on the nurse's own clinical judgment, for example, initiating protective skin care for an area that might break down. **Dependent nursing actions,** such as administering analgesics for pain, are actions that the nurse performs as a result of a physician's order. **Interdependent nursing actions** are actions that the nurse must accomplish in conjunction with other health team members such as meal planning with the dietary therapist and teaching breathing exercises with the respiratory therapist.

Evaluation

Evaluation is a vital part of the nursing process. The practical nurse participates with other members of the health care team in the child's evaluation. Evaluation measures the success or failure of the nursing plan of care. Like assessment, evaluation is an ongoing process. Evaluation is achieved by determining if the identified outcomes have been met. The criteria of the nursing outcomes determine if the interventions were effective. If the goals have not been met in the specified time, or if implementation is unsuccessful, a particular intervention may need to be reassessed and revised. Possibly the outcome criterion is unrealistic and needs to be discarded or adjusted. The child and the family must be assessed to determine progress adequately. Both objective data (measurable) and subjective data (based on responses from the child and family) are used in the evaluation.

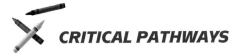

CRITICAL PATHWAYS

Concerns about cost containment, quality improvement, and managed care have led to a system of standard guidelines termed **critical pathways** in many facilities. Critical pathways are standard plans of care used to organize and monitor the care provided. They include all aspects of care such as diagnostic tests, consultations, treatments, activities, procedures, teaching, and discharge planning. Other names for clinical pathways are CareMap, collaborative care plans, case management plans, clinical paths, and multidisciplinary plans. To ensure success,

the critical pathways must be a collaborative effort of all disciplines involved; all members of the health team must follow them.

The nursing process is part of the underlying framework of critical pathways. Nursing diagnoses and intermediate and discharge outcomes are necessary to avoid fragmenting care. Documentation of nursing interventions and outcomes is essential to the overall process. The nurse must thoroughly understand the nursing process to achieve accountability when providing care in a setting where critical pathways are used (Table 1–3).

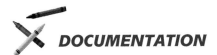

DOCUMENTATION

One of the most important parts of nursing care is recording information about the patient on the permanent record. This record, the patient's chart, is a legal document and must be accurate and complete. Nursing care provided and responses to care are

TABLE 1.3	Critical Path for School-ager With Long-Leg Cast Postfracture	
A Critical Pathway is an abbreviated form of care plan used by the entire multidisciplinary team. It provides outcome-based guidelines for goal achievement within a designated length of stay.		
	Day One	**Day Two**
Diagnostic Tests	CBC X-ray left leg.	
Assessments	Establish baseline neurovascular status, then neurovascular checks every 2 hours. Inspect cast. Head, chest, and abdominal assessment for other injuries Assess skin integrity.	Neurovascular checks every 4 hours Teach family neurovascular checks. Inspect cast. Teach family cast inspection. Assess skin integrity. Teach family skin integrity assessment.
Diet	Diet as tolerated	Diet as tolerated Instruct on adding foods rich in protein.
Activity	Elevate leg when lying or sitting. Start non–weight-bearing crutch walking. Initiate safety precautions.	Elevate leg when lying or sitting. Assess ability to use non–weight-bearing crutch walking for discharge. Maintain safety precautions.
Medications	Tylenol with codeine for pain as ordered	Tylenol with codeine for pain as ordered Tylenol for pain as ordered
Psychosocial	Assess developmental status. Promote self-care (bathing, dressing, grooming, etc.) Provide diversional activities. Assist in continuing school work. Safety teaching	Instruct on diversional activities for home. Instruct family on how to promote self-care. Reinforce safety teaching.
Discharge Planning	Teach cast care. Teach crutch walking. Arrange for home tutoring.	Provide written instructions and obtain feedback on cast care. Provide written instructions and obtain feedback on crutch walking. Provide written instructions for home tutoring. Include family and child in teaching. Arrange for follow-up appointment.

included. In pediatric settings, documentation is extremely important because those records can be used in legal situations many years after they are written. These records include the nurse's observations and findings and they help explain and justify the actions taken.

Documentation may be done in various forms including admission assessments, nurse's or progress notes, graphic sheets, checklists, medication records, and discharge teaching or summaries. Many health care settings use computerized or bedside documentation records. Whatever the system or form used, concise, factual information is charted. Everything written must be legible and clear and include the date and time. Nursing actions such as medication administration must be documented as soon as possible following the intervention to ensure the action is communicated, especially in the care of children.

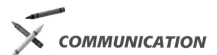

COMMUNICATION

Although most people think of communication as an oral or written exchange of words, communication also includes the body language, facial expressions, voice intonations, and emotions behind the words exchanged between two or more people. One of the most important aspects of communication is listening to the other person. Listening is more than hearing. It includes "tuning in" to the other person, being sensitive to feelings, and concentrating on what the other person is trying to express. The nurse must be aware of underlying emotions and recognize their effects on the communication process. It is also important to clarify statements and feelings expressed by the child or caregiver. A reflective statement may indicate what the nurse believed was expressed. For instance, the nurse might say, "You seem worried about Maria's loss of appetite." In this way the speaker may confirm or deny that the nurse has interpreted correctly. To communicate successfully with children and caregivers, the pediatric nurse must be especially skilled in listening.

Listening

Listening to another person involves more than simply hearing words. *Attending* (giving the other person physical signs that you are listening) indicates to the speaker that you are listening. Eye contact, a posture of attention, and avoiding distractions are essential to attending. All may be lost if the speaker feels the listener is not paying attention.

Following, the next step, means encouraging the speaker by staying out of his or her way. Do not stop the speaker by making judgmental statements, giving advice, or reassuring him or her. For instance, "Don't be so down in the dumps" is a judgmental statement that may cause the person to withdraw. "Get up and move around; things are bound to get better" is an example of advice that most often will turn the speaker off. "You're going to be fine before you know it" is an example of reassuring that does not help the person with the problem. A positive response that would be helpful instead of judgmental might be, "You look as though something is bothering you." This gives the person an opportunity to open up and indicates that the listener is tuned in. "Can you tell me what you see as your biggest problem?" gives the speaker encouragement to share his or her worries. "You look as though you feel that things are not going very well" is a description of what the person's body language message means to the listener and offers an invitation for the speaker to share what is on his or her mind.

On the other hand, remember that the speaker may not want to talk at that particular time. Respect those feelings.

In listening to another person, there may be times when the best response is silence to allow the speaker to have room to think and slowly express him or herself. Observe the other person's body language and expressions and think about what they are communicating. Think about what the other person is saying instead of worrying about what response to give. Focus on the speaker and reflect what he or she has said. "You sound concerned about the pain you are having" appropriately reflects a speaker who has related that the pain comes and goes and radiates from here to there. This helps clarify that both people are talking about the same thing. "You are frustrated about the pace of your recovery" may help the speaker put his or her feelings into words. At the very least, the speaker can deny or agree that this is an accurate assessment of his or her feelings.

With children, it is often helpful to talk about how a doll, a teddy bear, or another toy is feeling. This enables the child to talk about the toy's fears, which accurately reflect the child's feelings. When the speaker (caregiver or child) uses a "feeling" word, it is helpful for the listener to rephrase what he or she believes the person is saying so that both are using the same frame of reference. For example if the caregiver says "I'm scared," the nurse could respond, "You're worried about the outcome of your child's surgery." This gives the person an opportunity to affirm that the nurse understands or to clarify further what the concerns are.

Communicating With Children

Nurses are constantly communicating with patients, even though they may be unable to understand the words or respond. Infants evaluate actions, not realizing that nurses who handle them abruptly and hurriedly may be rushed or insecure; these small patients feel only that these nurses are frightening and unloving.

The child who is old enough to distinguish between people (generally after 6 months of age) tends to be frightened of strangers. Sudden, abrupt, or noisy approaches are almost certain to signal danger to the child. The child needs time to evaluate the situation while still secure in the familiar arms of the caregiver. The nurse should not rush the situation but allow time for the child to initiate the relationship. Often the conversation may be started through the child's doll or stuffed animal. The nurse may ask the toy's name and address the toy, or just call it "Dolly," "Teddy," "Puppy," or "Kitty" if the child will not reveal the name. The nurse also may ask the toy how it feels, referring to the part of the body that is the child's problem. For example, "Are you having trouble breathing today, Dolly?"

Distrust of strangers may last through the first 3 or 4 years of life. A casual approach with reluctant children is usually more effective. Children who show rejecting or aggressive behavior are putting up a defense against their own fears, and the behavior should be ignored unless it threatens the child's well-being or that of someone else.

Some nurses have difficulty accepting their own feelings while working with children. Each nurse brings personal feelings, fears, and conflicts to a new situation. Many nurses feel inadequate when beginning relationships with children. Nurses need to be willing to accept the fact that they are also human. A good nurse is self-accepting and self-confident but does not necessarily begin that way; this comes with maturity and insight.

When speaking with small or young children, the nurse should not stand over them and talk down to them but should get down on eye level with them (Fig. 1–5). The best plan is to speak in a slow, clear, positive voice, and use simple words. Sentences should be short, and statements or questions should be expressed positively. Choices should be simple and offered only if a choice actually exists. Do not say, "Do you want to take your medicine now?" if there is no other option. Listen to the child's fears and worries; be honest in your answers.

The perceptions of young children are literal. For instance, if the nurse says, "This will only be a little bee sting," children actually visualize being stung by a bee, which may be traumatic. As a result of this

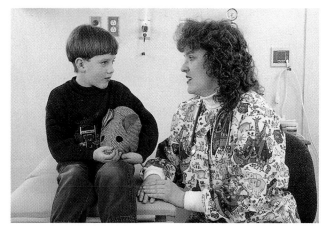

● **Figure 1.5** During a conversation with the child, the nurse gets down on eye level and uses easy, positive language. She also may include a favorite toy or doll in the conversation. (© B. Proud.)

literal perception, the nurse must be careful to use positive explanations in terms that are familiar and non-threatening to the child.

School-age children are interested in knowing what and why. Explanations that help them understand how equipment works are important to them. These children do not need a complex or detailed explanation; a simple response is best. Children of this age will ask more questions if their curiosity is not satisfied.

It may be challenging to communicate with adolescents. Young teenagers frequently waver between thinking like a child and thinking like an adult. Sometimes the adolescent does not want to reveal much if a parent is present. Teens may need to relate information that they do not wish others to know. A discussion about confidentiality may set the adolescent's concerns at ease. The adolescent needs to know that the nurse will listen attentively in an open-minded, nonjudgmental way.

The adolescent and the family may not view a problem in the same way. If this is the case, the problem may need to be defined more clearly so that an agreement may be reached, if possible. The nurse may be instrumental in assisting with the resolution of disagreements between the family and the adolescent.

Communicating With Family Caregivers

Routine conferences among the nursing staff, physicians, child-life workers, physical therapists, and other personnel concerned with children in the health care facility are helpful in gaining an understanding of child patients. The individuals who care for the child in the home setting are known as family caregivers. These people are usually the child's parents or other family members. Because living and family situations are so varied, it is important for the nurse to identify who the child's family caregivers are so they can participate in providing information relevant to the child's care and help with planning for the child's health care needs. Conferring with the family caregivers and other members of the health care team helps form a clearer picture of the child, promotes better understanding of his or her behavior, and presents an opportunity to consider differing types of treatment and relationships. The outcomes of routine conferences are rewarding to both patient and nursing staff. When the family caregivers attend they gain valuable insights and understanding. Some health care facilities prefer to hold parent group sessions. In either instance, it is most important that family caregivers are kept well informed about what is going on and what is being planned for their sick child (Fig. 1–6).

Much may be done to make the caregivers feel welcome and important. When a procedure is planned, the caregiver may be told what is going to happen and be invited to help, if practical. However, no caregiver who is reluctant to help with or observe a procedure should be urged to stay or made to feel that involvement is a duty that should be fulfilled. Some caregivers are so anxious and apprehensive that they communicate their concern to the child rather than provide support. Attitudes from the caregiver may easily be conveyed to the child, which sometimes causes negative reactions from the child. The nurse must be alert for any negative attitudes. Listening and communication skills are extremely important when working with the caregiver. Giving the caregiver time to discuss anxieties and concerns, exploring these problems with the caregiver, and demonstrating genuine caring and concern help ease these feelings. The nurse must remember that part of the nursing role is to be an ambassador of good will to the child and the family.

An older child may feel self-sufficient and may view the family caregiver's presence as being treated "like a baby." However, it is normal to regress during illness, and most children of any age appreciate the presence of a reassuring, self-controlled person during trying, uncomfortable times. The child needs to be able to trust the environment. If, as often happens, the child regresses in handling the overwhelming distress, the presence of a family caregiver may offer support.

Influences on Communication

Verbal and nonverbal communication styles may be influenced by several factors such as family, culture, community, religion, personality, and age. Varying styles of communication may cause conflict and misunderstanding among people. For example, one person may come from a family in which loud yelling is a loving form of self-expression. A second person may come from a family in which issues are calmly or stoically discussed. To the first person, the second person's lack of emotion about issues may seem uncaring. To the second person, the first person's emotional outbursts may seem aggressive and unkind. Another person may handle feelings by becoming quiet and uncommunicative; this too is a communication style.

These are just a few of the many different styles of communication. The nurse does not need to know all these communication styles but should remember that differences exist. The nurse must first understand his or her own communication style. This helps the nurse realize his or her communication expectations and gain a sense of how he or she may be perceived by others. Only after self-understanding can the nurse distinguish differences in communication styles and understand the ways in which others attempt to communicate.

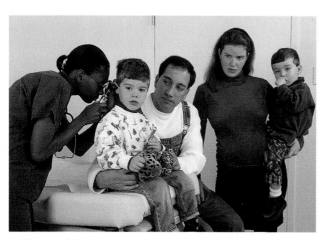

● **Figure 1.6** During a routine assessment or a more involved procedure, caregivers often find comfort in remaining close to the child and being well informed. (© B. Proud.)

KEY POINTS

◗ Many changes have taken place in the care of children in the past century. Until the early part of the 20th century, children were treated as miniature adults and were expected to behave that way.

◗ Progress in medical science has advanced so rapidly and become so sophisticated that many children with chronic or serious conditions are cared for in regionalized centers, creating a need for caring for the family in a "home away from home" atmosphere.

◗ *Healthy People 2010* sets goals for health care with a

focus on health promotion and prevention of illness as the nation approaches the year 2010.

▶ The role of the nurse has changed to include responsibilities of teacher, adviser, resource person, and researcher as well as caretaker.

▶ Although its infant mortality rate is improving, the United States still remains behind most other industrialized countries. Lack of or inadequate prenatal care is believed to be major cause of this problem.

▶ Pediatric nursing consists of preventive care of the well child as much as or more than care of the ill child.

▶ Nurses are caring for the health of children in many nontraditional settings including schools, home, and ambulatory care units.

▶ The nursing process is essential in the problem-solving process necessary to plan nursing care.

▶ Documentation is one of the most important responsibilities in caring for the pediatric patient.

▶ Listening includes really focusing on the speaker to determine what the speaker is trying to communicate.

▶ Communication with children and their families is a continuous process. The nurse must work to become a skilled communicator to meet the needs of children and their families.

REFERENCES

1. National Center for Health Statistics, Centers for Disease Control Prevention, Fact Sheet, 2001.
2. Alden, ER. (1999) The field of pediatrics. In *Oski's pediatrics: Principles and practice* (3rd ed). Philadelphia: Lippincott Williams & Wilkins.
3. Healthy People 2010, A Systematic Approach to Health Improvement, 2001, *www.health.gov/healthypeople*.

BIBLIOGRAPHY

Cone TE Jr. (1980) *History of American pediatrics*. Boston: Little Brown.

Craven RF, Hirnle CJ. (1999) *Fundamentals of nursing* (3rd ed). Philadelphia: Lippincott Williams & Wilkins.

Douglas CY. (2001) Child health policy: Health insurance programs for children. *Journal of Pediatric Nursing*, 16(1), 63–5.

Ekegren K. (2001) The advocate: Resources for child advocacy. *Journal of the Society of Pediatric Nurses*, 6(2), 95–6.

Herrman JW. (2001) Updates & kidbits: Pediatric nursing and Healthy People 2010: A call to action. *Pediatric Nursing*, 27(1), 82–86.

Kleinpell R. (2000) Healthy people 2010:The nation's new health agenda. *Nursing Spectrum*. Available at: *http://community.nursingspectrum.com/MagazineArticles*.

Meier E. (2000) Legislative and policy update: Children and international human rights abuses. *Pediatric Nursing*, 26(5), 545–6.

NANDA Nursing Diagnoses: Definitions and Classification 2001–2002. (2001) Philadelphia: North American Nursing Diagnosis Association.

Pillitteri A. (1999) *Maternal and child health nursing* (3rd ed). Philadelphia: Lippincott Williams & Wilkins.

Wong DL. (1998) *Whaley and Wong's nursing care of infants and children* (6th ed). St. Louis: Mosby.

Wong DL, Perry S, Hockenberry M. (2002) *Maternal child nursing care* (2nd ed). St. Louis: Mosby.

Websites
www.childstats.gov
www.health.gov/healthypeople
www.dhhs.gov

Workbook

NCLEX-STYLE REVIEW QUESTIONS

1. The nursing process is a scientific method and proven form of

   a. Cost containment

   b. Problem solving

   c. Oral communication

   d. Health teaching

2. The nurse collects data and begins to develop a trust relationship with the patient in which step of the nursing process?

   a. Assessment

   b. Planning

   c. Implementation

   d. Evaluation

3. The nurse carries out the nursing care for the patient in which step of the nursing process?

   a. Assessment

   b. Planning

   c. Implementation

   d. Evaluation

4. When a nurse is working with patients, the MOST important aspect of communication is for the nurse to

   a. Observe facial expressions.

   b. Listen to what is being said.

   c. Restate the words heard.

   d. Clarify the statements made.

5. In caring for patients, a healthcare team often uses critical pathways. Which of the following is the MOST important to ensure success when using a critical pathway? The critical pathway

   a. Decreases cost for the patient and hospital

   b. Is followed by all members of the health team

   c. Provides organization for the care of the patient

   d. Includes all treatments and procedures

STUDY ACTIVITIES

1. Choose the three social issues you think have the highest impact on health care concerns of children (use Table 1–1). Using these issues, complete the following table.

Social Issue	How Does This Issue Impact Children's Health Care?	What Is the Nurse's Role in Dealing With This Issue?

2. Kathi, a 5-year-old, has just returned from surgery. Her mother is nervously watching the IV line and asks you, "Is that IV running all right?"

   a. Write a response that is an example of reflective listening.

   b. Explain how reflective listening helps facilitate communication.

3. Vincent is trying to be a "tough" teenager after his football injury. He is scheduled for knee surgery. On entering his room, you notice his eyes are red.

   a. Describe what you would say to establish effective communication with Vincent.

   b. Write a scenario of how the conversation with Vincent might go.

CRITICAL THINKING

1. Describe sociologic changes that have affected child health concepts and attitudes.
2. Discuss how children were cared for in institutions in the 19th and early 20th centuries. Describe the hospital care of infants and children in the period immediately after World War I.
3. While working, you overhear an older nurse complaining about family caregivers "being underfoot so much and interfering with patient care." Describe how you would defend open visiting for family caregivers to this person.

The Family and Child

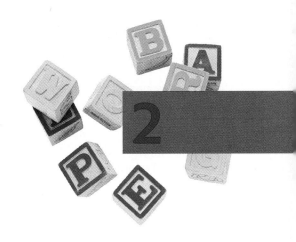

2

THE FAMILY AS A SOCIAL UNIT
Family Function
Family Structure
Family Factors That Influence Children

CONCEPTS OF CHILD DEVELOPMENT
Sigmund Freud
Erik Erikson
Jean Piaget
Lawrence Kohlberg
Other Theorists

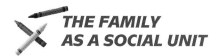

THE FAMILY AS A SOCIAL UNIT

The arrival of a baby alters forever the relationship of a couple and establishes a new social unit—a family—in which all members influence and are influenced by each other. Each subsequent child joining that family continues the process of reshaping the individual members and the family unit. In addition, the community affects family members as individuals and as a family unit.

Nursing care of children demands a solid understanding of normal patterns of growth and development—physical, psychological, social, and intellectual (cognitive)—and an awareness of the many factors that influence those patterns. It also demands an appreciation for the uniqueness of each child and each family. For nursing care to be complete and as effective as possible, a child must be considered as a member of a family and a larger community.

Throughout history, family structure has evolved in response to ongoing social and economic changes. Today's families may only faintly resemble the nuclear families of 30 or 40 years ago in which the father worked outside the home and the mother cared for the children. However, nuclear families in the 1950s and 1960s were far different from the farming families of centuries ago. It is estimated that in 60% to 70% of today's families with school-age children, only one parent lives at home. More than 50% of American women with a child younger than age 1 year work outside the home. Changes such as these create bigger demands on parents and have contributed to the growing demands on public institutions to fill the gaps. "Blended" families or stepfamilies have created other major changes in family structure and interactions within the family. Divorce, abandonment, and delayed childbearing are all contributing factors.

Family Function

The family is civilization's oldest and most basic social unit. The family's primary purpose is to ensure survival of the unit and its individual members and to continue the society and its knowledge, customs, values, and beliefs. It establishes a primary connection with a group responsible for a person until that person becomes independent. Although family structure varies among different cultures, its functions related to children are similar: providing physical care, educating and training children, and protecting children's psychological and emotional health.

Physical Care

The family is responsible for meeting each child's basic needs for food, clothing, shelter, and protection from harm including illness. The work necessary to meet these needs was once clearly divided between mother and father, with the mother providing total care for the child and the father providing the resources to make care possible. These attitudes have changed so that in a two-parent family, each parent has an opportunity to share in the joys and trials of child care and other aspects of family living. In the **single-parent family,** one person must assume all these responsibilities.

Education and Training

Within the family, a child learns the rules of the society and the culture in which the family lives: its language, values, ethics, and acceptable behaviors. This process, called **socialization,** is accomplished by training and education. The family teaches children acceptable ways of meeting physical needs, such as eating and elimination, and certain skills such as dressing oneself. The family educates children about relationships with other people inside and outside the family. Children learn what is permitted and approved within their society and what is forbidden.

Psychological and Emotional Health

Research studies continue to support the importance of early parent-child relationships to emotional adjustment in later life. Even a few hours may constitute a critical period in the emotional bond between parent and child. Although the results of these studies are controversial, it is generally agreed that young children are highly sensitive to psychological influences, and those influences may have long-range positive or negative effects.

Within the family, children learn who they are and how their behavior affects other family members. Children observe and imitate the behavior of family members, learning quickly which behaviors are rewarded and which are punished. Participation in a family is a child's only rehearsal for parenthood. How parents treat the child has a powerful influence on how the child will treat future children. Studies show that many abusive parents were abused by their parents as children.

Family Structure

Various traditional and nontraditional family structures exist. The traditional structures that occur in many cultures are the nuclear family and the extended family. Nontraditional variations include the single-parent family, the communal family, the stepfamily, and the gay or lesbian family.

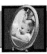

Nuclear Family

The **nuclear family** is composed of a man, a woman, and their children (either biologic or adopted) who share a common household (Fig. 2–1). This was once the typical American family structure; now fewer than one-third of families in the United States fit this pattern. The nuclear family is a more mobile and independent unit than an extended family but is often part of a network of related nuclear families within close geographic proximity.

Extended Family

Typical of agricultural societies, the **extended family** consists of one or more nuclear families plus other relatives, often crossing generations to include grandparents, aunts, uncles, and cousins. The needs of individual members are subordinate to the needs of the group, and children are considered an economic asset. Grandparents aid in childrearing, and children learn respect for their elders by observing their parents' behavior toward the older generation.

Single-Parent Family

Rising divorce rates, the women's movement, increasing acceptance of children born out of wedlock, and changes in adoption laws reflecting a more liberal attitude toward adoption have combined to produce a growing number of **single-parent families.** About 23% of households in the United States are included in this category, and most are headed by women.[1] Although this family situation places a heavy burden on the parent, no conclusive evidence is available to show its effects on children. At some time in their

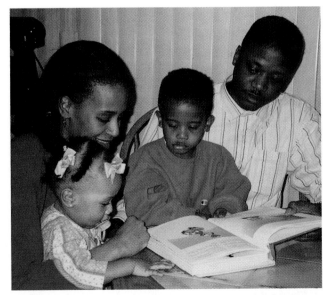

● **Figure 2.1** The nuclear family is an important and prominent type of family structure in American society. This nuclear family enjoys reading together.

A PERSONAL GLIMPSE

Living with both my mother and grandmother definitely has its advantages. Even though I had a male figure around me while I was growing up, it wasn't really the same as having a father who would always be there. I lived with my aunt and her family along with my mother and my grandmother. I had my uncle or cousin to turn to if I needed advice that my mother or my grandmother couldn't give me. However, my uncle wasn't always around, neither was my cousin, so a lot of my questions were left unanswered. Questions that I didn't think anybody else other than a man could answer. I learned a lot of things on my own, whether it was by experience or by asking somebody else.

Things are different now. It's only my mother, my grandmother, and myself. As I grow older, I'm finding that I can open up to the both of them a lot more. There is no reason to keep secrets. I can tell them anything and they understand. Actually they are a lot more understanding than I thought they would be about certain things. Everyday I'm realizing that I can tell them anything.

People often ask me what it is like not knowing about my father. They ask me if I'm curious about my father. And I say, "Of course I'm curious. Who wouldn't be?" I also tell them that love is a lot stronger than curiosity. I love and care about my mother and grandmother more than anything in this world. No one father could ever give me as much love and devotion as the two of them give me. And I wouldn't give that up for anything.

Juan, age 15 years

▶ **LEARNING OPPORTUNITY:** Where would you direct this mother in your community to go to find opportunities for her son to interact with male adults who could be positive role models for him? What are the reasons it would be important for this child to have appropriate adult male role models? If someone other than their biological parent has raised a child, what are some of the reasons these individuals seek out their biological parents?

lives, more than 50% of children in the United States may be part of a single-parent family.

Communal Family

During the early 1960s, increasing numbers of young adults began to challenge the values and traditions of the American social system. One result of that challenge was the establishing of communal groups and collectives, or **communal families.** This alternative structure occurs in many settings and may favor either a primitive or a modern lifestyle. Members of a communal family share responsibility for homemaking and childrearing; all children are the collective responsibility of adult members. Not actually a new family structure, the communal family is a variation of the extended family. The number of communal family units has decreased in recent years.

Gay or Lesbian Family

In the gay or lesbian family, two people of the same sex live together, bound by formal or informal commitment, with or without children. Children may be the result of a prior heterosexual mating or a product of the foster-child system, adoption, artificial insemination, or surrogacy. Although these families often face complex issues including discrimination, studies of children in such families show that they are not harmed by membership in this type of family.[2] The children of a gay or lesbian family are no more likely to become homosexual than are children of heterosexual families.

Stepfamily or Blended Family

The **stepfamily** is made up of the custodial parent and children and a new spouse. As the divorce rate has climbed, the number of stepfamilies has increased. If both partners in the marriage bring children from a previous marriage into the household, the family is usually termed a **blended family.** The stress that remarriage of the custodial parent places on a child seems to depend in part on the child's age. Initially there is an increase in the number of problems in children of all ages. However, younger children apparently can form an attachment to the new parent and accept that person in the parenting role better than adolescents do. Adolescents, already engaged in searching for identity and exploring their own sexuality, may view the presence of a nonbiological parent as an intrusion. When children from each partner's former marriage are brought into the family, the incidence of problems increases. Second marriages often produce children of that union, which contributes to the adjustment problems of the family members. However, remarriage may provide the stability of a two-parent family, which may offer additional resources for the child. Each family is unique and has its own set of challenges and advantages.

Cohabitation Family

In the nuclear family, the parents are married; in the **cohabitation family,** couples live together but are not married. The children in this family may be children of earlier unions or they may be a result of this union. These families may be long-lasting or lead to marriage but are sometimes less stable because the

relationships may be temporary. In any family situation with frequent changes in the adult relationships, children may feel a sense of insecurity.

Family Factors That Influence Children

Family Size

The number of children in the family has a significant impact on family interactions. The smaller the family, the more time there is for individual attention to each child. Children in small families, particularly only children, often spend more time with adults and, therefore, relate better with adults than with peers. Only children tend to be more advanced in language development and intellectual achievement.

Understandably a large family emphasizes the group more than the child. Less time is available for parental attention to each child. There is greater interdependence among these children and less dependence on the parents (Fig. 2–2).

Sibling Order and Sex

Whether a child is the firstborn, a middle child, or the youngest also makes a difference in the child's relationships and behavior. Firstborn children command a great deal of attention from parents and grandparents and also are affected by their parents' inexperience, anxieties, and uncertainties. Often the parents' expectations for the oldest child are greater than for subsequent children. Generally firstborn children are greater achievers than their siblings are.

With second and subsequent children, parents tend to be more relaxed and permissive. These children are likely to be more relaxed and are slower to develop language skills. They often identify more with peers than with parents.

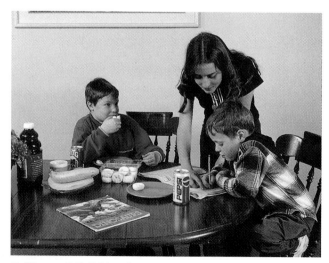

● **Figure 2.2** Children from large families learn to care for one another. Many older children are expected to help with homework and prepare after-school snacks. (© B. Proud.)

Sexual identity in relation to siblings also affects a child's development. Girls raised with older brothers tend to have more male-associated interests than girls raised with older sisters. Boys raised with older brothers tend to be more aggressive than are boys with older sisters.[3]

Parental Behavior

Many factors have contributed to the change in the traditional mother-at-home, father-at-work image of the American family (Fig. 2–3). Sixty-five percent of American mothers of children younger than age 18 years work outside the home. Some mothers work because they are the family's only source of income, others because the family's economic status demands a second income, and still others because the woman's career is highly valued. More than half of all children between ages 3 and 5 years spend part of their day being cared for by someone other than their parents.

Many factors contribute to the trend for families to spend less time together. Both parents may work; the children participate in many school activities; family members watch television rather than talking together at mealtime or eat fast food or individual meals without sitting down together as a family; there is an emphasis on the acquisition of material goods rather than the development of relationships. All these factors contribute to a breakdown in family communication, and they are typical of many families. Their impact on today's children, the parents of tomorrow, is unknown.

Divorce

From 1970 to 1990, the number of divorces increased every year. Although there has been a slight decrease in this number in recent years, more than 1 million children younger than age 18 years have been involved in a divorce each year. Although obviously these children are affected, it is difficult to determine the exact extent of the damage. Children whose lives were seriously disrupted before a divorce may feel relieved, at least initially, when the situation is resolved. Others who were unaware of parental conflict and felt that their lives were happy may feel frightened and abandoned. All these emotions depend on the children involved, their ages, and the kind of care and relationships they experience with their parents after the divorce.

Children may go through many emotions when a divorce occurs. Feelings of grief, anger, rejection, and self-worthlessness are common. These emotions may follow the children for years, even into adulthood, even though children may understand the reason for the divorce. In addition, the parents, either custodial or noncustodial, may try to influence the child's thinking about the other parent, placing the child in an emotional trap. If the noncustodial parent does not keep in regular contact with the child, feelings of rejection may be overwhelming. The child often desperately wants a sign of that parent's continuing love.

Culture

Each child is the product of a family, a culture, and a community. In some cultures, family life is gentle, permissive, and loving; in others, unquestioning obedience is demanded and pain and hardship are to be stoically endured. The child may be from a cultural group that places a high value on children, giving them lots of attention from many relatives and friends, or the child may be from a group that has taught the child from early childhood to fend for oneself.

Culture also determines the family's health beliefs and practices. Respect for a child's cultural heritage and individuality is an essential part of nursing care. To plan culturally appropriate and acceptable care, nurses need to understand the health practices and lifestyle of families from various cultures. Rather than memorizing a list of generalized facts regarding different cultures, it is more useful for the nurse to develop **cultural competency,** the capacity to work effectively with people by integrating the elements of their culture into nursing care.[4] To develop cultural competency, the nurse must first understand cultural influences on his or her life. The nurse must recognize surface cultural influences (e.g., language, food, clothing) as well as hidden cultural influences (e.g., communication styles, beliefs, attitudes, values, perceptions). Then the nurse may recognize and accept the different attitudes, behaviors, and values of another person's culture.

Integrating cultural attitudes toward food, cleanliness, respect, and freedom are of utmost importance. The nurse must be especially sensitive to the fears of the child who is separated from his or her own culture

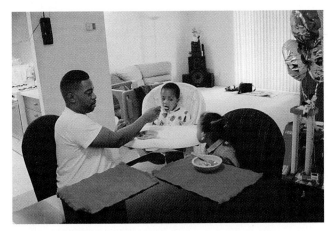

● **Figure 2.3** In some American families, traditional roles are being reversed. The father cares for the children while the mother is at work.

for the first time and finds the food, language, people, and surroundings of the health care facility totally alien. Cultural competency promotes cooperation from the child and family and minimizes frustration. These factors are essential in restoring health so that the child may once again be a functioning part of the family and the community, whatever the cultural background.

INTERNET EXERCISE 2-1

http://www.culturediversity.org

Transcultural Nursing
Click on Cultural Competency.

1. What is the definition of cultural competence?

2. What are the five essential elements necessary for an organization to become culturally competent?

3. What are the four major challenges to attaining cultural competency?

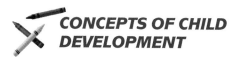

CONCEPTS OF CHILD DEVELOPMENT

Growth and development refers to the total growth of the child from birth toward maturity. **Growth** is

the physical increase in the body's size and appearance caused by increasing numbers of new cells. **Development** is the progressive change in the child's maturation. **Developmental tasks** are basic achievements associated with each stage of development. These tasks must be mastered to move successfully to the next developmental stage. Developmental tasks must be completed successfully at each stage for a person to achieve maturity.

How a helpless infant grows and develops into a fully functioning independent adult has fascinated scientists for years. Four pioneering researchers whose theories in this area are widely accepted are Sigmund Freud, Erik Erikson, Jean Piaget, and Lawrence Kohlberg (Table 2–1). Their theories present human development as a series of overlapping stages that occur in predictable patterns. These stages are only approximations of what is likely to happen in children at various ages, and each child's development may differ from these stages.

Sigmund Freud

Most modern psychologists base their understanding of children at least partly on the work of Sigmund Freud. His theories are concerned primarily with the **libido** (sexual drive or development). Although Freud did not study children, his work focused on

TABLE 2.1	Comparative Summary of Theories of Freud, Erikson, Piaget, and Kohlberg				
Age (years)	Stage	Freud (Psychosexual Development)	Erikson (Psychosocial Development)	Piaget (Intellectual Development)	Kohlberg (Moral Development)
1	Infancy	Oral Stage	Trust vs. Mistrust	Sensorimotor Phase	Stage 0—Do what pleases me
2–3	Toddlerhood	Anal Stage	Autonomy vs. Shame		Preconventional Level Stage I—Avoid punishment
4–6	Preschool (early childhood)	Phallic (infant genital) Oedipal Stage	Initiative vs. Guilt	Preoperational Phase	Preconventional Level Stage 2—Do what benefits me
7–12	School-age (middle childhood)	Latency Stage	Industry vs. Inferiority	Concrete Operational Phase	Conventional Level Stage 3 (Age 7–10)— Avoid disapproval Stage 4 (Age 10–12)— Do duty, obey laws
13–18	Adolescence	Genital Stage (puberty)	Identity vs. Identity Confusion	Formal Operational Phase	Postconventional Level Stage 5 (Age 13)— Maintain respect of others Stage 6 (Age 15)— Implement personal principles

childhood development as a cause of later conflict. Freud believed that a child who did not adequately resolve a particular stage of development would have a fixation (compulsion) that correlated with that stage. Freud described three levels of consciousness: the **id,** which controls physical need and instincts of the body; the **ego,** the conscious self, which controls the pleasure principle of the id by delaying the instincts until an appropriate time; and the **superego,** the conscience or parental value system. These consciousness levels interact to check behavior and balance each other. The psychosexual stages in Freud's theory are the oral, anal, phallic, latency, and genital stages of development.

Oral Stage (Ages 0–2 Years)

The newborn first relates almost entirely to the mother (or someone taking a motherly role), and the first experiences with body satisfaction come through the mouth. This is true not only of sucking but also of making noises, crying, and breathing. It is through the mouth that the baby expresses needs and finds satisfaction and begins to make sense of the world.

Anal Stage (Ages 2–3 Years)

This stage is the child's first encounter with the serious need to learn self-control and to take responsibility. Toilet training looms large in the minds of many people as an important phase in childhood. Because elimination is one of the child's first experiences of creativity, it represents the beginnings of the desire to mold and control the environment; this is the "mudpie period" in the child's life.

The child has pride in the product created. Cleanliness and this natural pride do not always go together, so it may be necessary to help direct this pride and interest into more acceptable behaviors. Playing with such materials as modeling clay, crayons, and dough helps put the child's natural interests to good use, a process called **sublimation.**

Phallic (Infant Genital) Stage (Ages 3–6 Years)

It is only natural that interest moves to the genital area as a source of pride and curiosity. To the child's mind, this area constitutes the difference between boys and girls, a difference that the child is beginning to be aware of socially. The superego begins to develop during this stage; by 10 years of age (the end of the latency stage), superego is well established.

At about this time, a boy begins to take pride in being a male and a girl in being a female. In many families, a new brother or sister also arrives, arousing the child's natural interest in human origins.

This stage is when the child begins to understand what it means to be a boy or a girl. The parents' reaction to the child's genital exploration may determine whether the child learns to feel satisfied with himself or herself as a sexual being or is laden with feelings of guilt and dissatisfaction throughout life.

Freud hypothesized that this awareness of genital differences leads to a time of conflict in the child's emotional relationships with parents. The conflict occurs between attachment to and imitation of the parent of the same sex and the appeal of the other parent. The boy who for years has depended on his mother for all his emotional and physical needs now is confronted by his desire to be a man (Oedipus complex). The girl, who has imitated her mother, now finds her father a real attraction (Electra complex). This is not only social but also sexual; it is through contact with parents that the child learns to relate to the opposite sex. The child learns the interests, attitudes, concerns, and wishes of the opposite sex.

Latency Stage (Ages 6–10 Years)

The latency stage is the time of primary schooling, when the child is preparing for adult life but must await maturity to exercise initiative in adult living. It is the time when the child's sense of moral responsibility (the superego) is built, based on what has been taught through the parents' words and actions.

When placed in an unfamiliar setting, children in this stage may become confused because they do not know what is expected of them. They need the sense of security that comes from approval and praise and usually respond favorably to a brief explanation of "how we do things here."

Genital Stage (Ages 11–13 Years)

Physical puberty is occurring at an increasingly early age, and social puberty occurs even earlier largely due to the influence of sexual frankness on television and in movies and the print media. At puberty, all the child's earlier learning is concentrated on the powerful biological drive of finding and relating to a mate. In earlier societies, mating and forming a family occurred at a young age. Our society delays mating for many years after puberty, creating a time of confusion and turmoil during which biologic readiness must take second place to educational and economic goals. This is a sensitive period when privacy is important and great uncertainty exists about relating to any members of the opposite sex.

Erik Erikson

Building on Freud's theories, Erikson described human psychosocial development as a series of tasks or crises. This development depends on a self-healing process within the person that helps counterbalance the stresses created by natural and accidental crises. The self-healing process is delayed by any major crisis, such as hospitalization, that interrupts normal development. Interruptions may cause regression to an earlier stage such as the older child who begins to wet the bed when hospitalized. Erikson commented that "children 'fall apart' repeatedly, and unlike Humpty Dumpty, grow together again," if they are given time and sympathy and are not interfered with.[5]

Erikson formulated a series of eight **developmental tasks** or crises; the first five pertain to children and youth. To present a complete view of Erikson's theory, all eight tasks are presented. In each task, the person must master the central problem before moving on to the next one. Each task holds positive and negative counterparts, and each of the first five implies new developmental tasks for parents (Table 2–2).

Trust Versus Mistrust (Ages 0–1 Year)

The infant has no way to control the world other than crying for help and hoping for rescue. During the first year, the child learns whether the world can be trusted to give love and concern or only frustration, fear, and despair. The infant who is fed on demand learns to trust that cries communicating need will be answered. The baby fed according to the nurse or caregiver's schedule does not understand the importance of routine but only that these cries may go unanswered.

Autonomy Versus Doubt and Shame (Ages 1–3 Years)

Even the smallest child wants to feel in control and needs to learn to perform tasks independently, even when this takes a long time or makes a mess. The toddler gains reassurance from self-feeding, from crawling or walking alone where it is safe, and from being free to handle materials and learn about things in the environment.

A toddler exploring the environment begins to explore and learn about his or her body too. If caregivers react appropriately to this normal behavior, the child will gain self-respect and pride. If, however, caregivers shame the child for responding to this natural curiosity, the child may develop and sustain the belief that somehow the body is dirty, nasty, and bad.

Initiative Versus Guilt (Ages 3–6 Years)

During this period, the child engages in active, assertive play. Steadily improving physical coordination and expanding social skills encourage "showing off" to gain adult attention and, the child hopes, approval. The preschool child, still self-centered, plays alone, although in the company of other children; interaction comes later. These children want to know what the rules are and enjoy "being good" and the adult approval that action gains. During this time, the child develops a conscience and accepts punishment for doing wrong because it relieves feelings of guilt.

TABLE 2.2	Child and Parent Developmental Tasks According to Erikson

Developmental Level	Basic Task	Stage of Parental Development	Parental Task
Infant	Trust	Learning to recognize and interpret infant's cues	To interpret cues and respond positively to the infant's needs; hold, cuddle, and talk to infant
Toddler	Autonomy	Learning to accept child's need for self-mastery	To accept child's growing need for freedom while setting consistent, realistic limits; offer support and understanding when separation anxiety occurs
Preschooler	Initiative	Learning to allow child to explore surrounding environment	To allow independent development while modeling necessary standards; generously praise child's endeavors to build child's self-esteem
School-Age	Industry	Learning to accept rejection without deserting	To accept child's successes and defeats, assuring child of acceptance to be there when needed without intruding unnecessarily
Adolescent	Identity	Learning to build a new life, supporting the emergence of the adolescent as an individual	To be available when adolescent feels need; provide examples of positive moral values; keep communication channels open; adjust to changing family roles and relationships during and after the adolescent's struggle to establish an identity

Children in this phase of development generally do not have a concept of time and the changes it imposes on nursing shifts. Explaining that it is time for a nurse to go home to his or her own family may help an unhappy child realize that the nurse is not leaving because of any negative behavior of the child's. The child needs a familiar frame of reference to understand when something is going to happen. For example, the parent or caregiver may say, "I will be back when your lunch comes" or "I will be back when the cartoons come on TV."

Industry Versus Inferiority (Ages 6–12 Years)

Children begin to seek achievement in this phase. They learn to interact with others and sometimes to compete with them. They like activities they can follow through to completion and tangible results.

Competition is healthy as long as the standards are not so high that the child feels there is no chance of winning. Praise, not criticism, helps the child to build self-esteem and avoid feelings of inferiority. It is important to emphasize that everyone is a unique person and deserves to be appreciated for his or her own special qualities.

Identity Versus Identity Confusion (Ages 12–18 Years)

Adolescents are confronted by marked physical and emotional changes and the knowledge that soon they will be responsible for their own lives. The adolescent develops a sense of being an independent person with unique ideals and goals and may feel that parents, caregivers, and other adults refuse to grant that independence. Adolescents may break rules just to prove that they can. Stress, anxiety, and mood swings are typical of this phase. Relationships with peers are more important than ever.

Intimacy Versus Isolation (Early Adulthood)

This is the period during which the person tries to establish intimate personal relationships with friends and an intimate love relationship with one person. Difficulty in establishing intimacy results in feelings of isolation.

Generativity Versus Self-Absorption (Young and Middle Adulthood)

For many people, this phase means marriage and family, but for others it may mean fulfillment in some other way—a profession, a business career, or a religious vocation. The person who does not find this fulfillment becomes self-absorbed and ceases to develop socially.

Ego Integrity Versus Despair (Old Age)

This final phase is the least understood of all, for it means finding satisfaction with oneself, one's achievements, and one's present condition without regret for the past or fear for the future.

Jean Piaget

Freud and Erikson studied psychosexual and psychosocial development; Piaget brought new insight into **cognitive** (intellectual) **development**—how a child learns and develops that quality called intelligence. He described intellectual development as a sequence of four principal stages, each made up of several substages.[6] All children move through these stages in the same order, but each moves at his or her own pace.

Sensorimotor Phase (Ages 0–2 Years)

The newborn behaves at a sensorimotor level linked entirely to desires for physical satisfaction. The newborn feels, hears, sees, tastes, and smells countless new things and moves in an apparently random way. Purposeful activities are controlled by reflexive responses to the environment. For example, while nursing, the newborn gazes intently at the mother's face, grasps her finger, smells the nipple, and tastes the milk, thus involving all senses.

As the infant grows, an understanding of cause and effect develops. When random arm motions strike the string of bells stretched across the crib, the newborn hears the sound made and eventually can manipulate the arms deliberately to make the bells ring.

In the same way, newborns cannot understand words or even the tone of voice; only through hearing conversation directed to them can they pick out sounds and begin to understand. As the infant produces verbal noises, the responses of those nearby are encouraging and eventually help the infant learn to talk.

Preoperational Phase (Ages 2–7 Years)

The child in this phase of development is **egocentric;** that is he or she cannot look at something from another's point of view. The child's interpretation of the world is from a self-centered point of view and in terms of what is seen, heard, or otherwise experienced directly.

This child has no concept of quantity; if it looks like more, it *is* more. Four ounces of juice poured into two glasses looks like more than four ounces in one glass. A sense of time is not yet developed; thus the preschooler or early school-age child cannot always tell if something happened a day ago, a week ago, or a year ago.

Concrete Operations (Ages 7–11 Years)

During this stage, children develop the ability to begin problem solving in a concrete, systematic way. They can classify and organize information about their environment. Unlike in the preoperational stage, children begin to understand that volume or weight may remain the same even though the appearance changes. These children can consider another's point of view and can deal simultaneously with more than one aspect of a situation.

Formal Operations (Ages 12–15 Years)

The adolescent is capable of dealing with ideas, abstract concepts described only in words or symbols. The person of this age begins to understand jokes based on double meanings and enjoys reading and discussing theories and philosophies. Adolescents can observe then draw logical conclusions from their observations.

Lawrence Kohlberg

Each of the theorists focuses on one element in the development of children. Kohlberg's theory is about the development of moral reasoning in children. Moral development closely follows **cognitive development** because reasoning and abstract thinking (the ability to conceptualize an idea without physical representation) are necessary to make moral judgments. Kohlberg's theory is divided into three levels with two or three stages in each level.

Preconventional Level (Premoral Level)

During the first 2 years (stage 0), there is no moral sensitivity. This is a time of egocentricity; decisions are made with regard only to what pleases the child or makes him or her feel good and what displeases or hurts the child. The child is not aware of how his or her behavior may affect others. The child simply reacts to pleasure with love and to hurtful experiences with anger.

In stage 1, punishment and obedience orientation (ages 2 to 3 years), the child determines right or wrong by the physical consequence of a particular act. The child simply obeys the person in power with no understanding of the underlying moral principle. For children of this age, if they get punished for doing something, then it is wrong; if they do not get punished, it is right.

In stage 2, naive instrumental self-indulgence (ages 4 to 7 years), the child views a specific act as right if it satisfies his or her needs. Children follow the rules to benefit themselves. They think, "I'll do something for you if you'll do something for me" and, on the other hand, "If you do something bad to me, I'll do something bad to you." This is basically the attitude of "an eye for an eye."

Conventional Level

As concrete operational thought develops, children can engage in moral reasoning. School-age children

become aware of the feelings of others. Living up to expectations is a primary concern regardless of the consequences.

In stage 3, "good-boy" orientation (ages 7 to 10 years), being "nice" is very important. Children want to avoid a guilty conscience. Pleasing others is very important.

In stage 4, law and order orientation (ages 10 to 12 years), showing respect to others, obeying the rules, and maintaining social order is the desired behavior. "Right" is defined as something that finds favor with family, teachers, and friends. "Wrong" is symbolized by broken relationships.

Postconventional Level (Principled Level)

By adolescence, the child usually achieves Piaget's formal operational stage. To achieve the postconventional level, the adolescent must have attained the formal operational stage. As a result, many persons do not reach this level.

In stage 5, social contract orientation (ages 13 to 18 years), personal standards, and personal rights are defined by culturally accepted values. A person's rights must not be violated for the welfare of the group. The end no longer justifies the means. Laws are for mutual good, cooperation, and development.

Stage 6, personal principles, is not attained very frequently. The person who reaches this level does what he or she thinks is right without regard for legal restrictions, the cost to self, or the views of others. Because of this person's deep respect for life, he or she would not do anything that would intentionally harm him or herself or another.

Other Theorists

Freud, Erikson, Piaget, and Kohlberg are only four of the many researchers who have studied the development of children and families. During the 1940s and 1950s, Arnold Gesell studied many infants and talked with their parents concerning children's behavior. From his studies emerged a series of developmental landmarks that are still considered valid and the observation that children progress through a series of "easy" and "difficult" phases as they develop. For example, he labeled one period the "terrible twos," the time when a toddler begins to assert new mobility and coordination to gain parental attention, even if the attention is unfavorable. Knowing that these cycles are normal makes it easier for parents to cope.

Carl Jung's contribution to the study of child growth and development focused on the inner sequence of events that shape the personality. He emphasized that human development follows predetermined patterns called **archetypes.** These archetypes replace the instinctive behavior present in other animals. Interaction of the archetypes with the outside environment is evident throughout human life. For example, a normal child learns to suck, crawl, walk, and talk without any instruction, but the details of how the child does these things come from observation and imitation of others.

Jung believed that the first 3 years of a child's life are spent coordinating experiences and learning to make a conscious personality, a distinct person who is separate from the rest of the environment. In the following years, the child learns to make sense of the environment by associating new discoveries to a general approach to the world. Dreams and nightmares help express personality developments that for some reason do not find a conscious outlet.

Jung points out that what happens to a child is not so critical to the child's development as the responses to these happenings. A hospital experience may permanently scar a child's personality if the child's natural feeling of terror is overlooked. Hospitalization may be accepted and even become a point of pride, however, if carried out in an atmosphere of assurance and support of the child's emotional concern and the need for love and acceptance.

The interaction between inner development and the environment is particularly clear in studies of young children who have been deprived in some way. John Bowlby's studies of children who were not held or loved and Bruno Bettelheim's studies of children given good physical care but little or no emotional satisfaction indicate how vital psychological interaction is.

In recent years, the theories of Erikson, Piaget, and Kohlberg have been criticized for being gender specific to males and culturally specific to Caucasians. In response, several theorists have conducted research on the growth and development of females and varying ethnic groups. Most notably, Carol Gilligan researched the moral development of males and females, and Patricia Green sought to construct a "truly universal theory of development through the empirical and theoretical understanding of cultural diversity."[7]

KEY POINTS

▶ The family is the basic social unit. It provides for survival and teaches the knowledge, customs, values, and beliefs of the family's culture.

▶ Mobility, changing attitudes about children born out of wedlock and about divorce, women working outside the home, and changes in adoption laws all have contributed to an increase in single-parent families.

▶ Family size and the child's birth position in the family affect the child's development.

▶ A child's growth and development follows a pattern similar for all children.

▶ Erikson's theory of psychosocial development sets out sequential tasks that the child must successfully complete before going on to the next stage.

▶ Cognitive and moral development flow along together because reasoning is necessary for more advanced moral development.

REFERENCES

1. United States Bureau of Census. *Statistical abstract of the United States: 2000.* Washington DC: Superintendent of Documents, 2000.
2. Gottman J. (1990) Children of gay and lesbian parents. In Bozett FW, Sussman M, eds. *Homosexuality and family relations.* New York: Harrington Park
3. Craig G. (1992) *Human development* (6th ed). Englewood Cliffs, NJ: Prentice-Hall.
4. Snow C. (1996) *Cultural sensitivity workshop.* Philadelphia: Nationality Service Council, United Way.
5. Erikson EH, Senn MJE. (1958) *Symposium on the healthy personality.* New York: Macy Foundation.
6. Piaget J. (1967) *The language and thought of the child.* Cleveland: World Publishing.
7. Cocking RR, Greenfield PM, eds. (1994) *Cross-cultural roots of minority child development.* Hillside, NJ: Lawrence Erlbaum Associates.

BIBLIOGRAPHY

Ahmann E, Johnson BH. (2001) Family matters: New guidance materials promote family-centered change in health care institutions. *Pediatric Nursing,* 27(2), 173–5.

Barry P. (2001) *Mental health and mental illness* (7th ed). Philadelphia: Lippincott Williams & Wilkins.

Bowlby J. (1969) *Attachment.* New York: Basic Books.

Clayton M. (2000) Health and social policy: Influences on family-centered care. *Pediatric Nursing,* 12(8), 31–3.

Erikson EH. (1963) *Childhood and society* (2nd ed). New York: Norton.

Fuller Q. (2000) Cultural competence in pediatric nursing. *Nursing Spectrum.* Available at: *http://community.nursingspectrum.com/MagazineArticles.*

Gilligan C. (1982) *In a different voice.* Cambridge, MA: Howard University Press.

Monsen RB. (2001) Raising kids, grandparents bear a burden. *Journal of Pediatric Nursing,* 16(2), 130–1.

Newton MS. (2000) Family-centered care: Current realities in parent participation. *Pediatric Nursing,* 26(2), 164–8.

Patterson GJ. (1996) Lesbian and gay parenthood, *Handbook of Parenting.* Hillsdale, NJ: Lawrence Erlbaum Associates.

Schuster C, Ashburn S. (1992) *The process of human development* (3rd ed). Philadelphia: JB Lippincott.

Shives L, Isaacs A. (2001) *Basic concepts of psychiatric-mental health* (5th ed). Philadelphia: Lippincott Williams & Wilkins.

Sperhac AM, Strodtbeck F. (2001) Advanced practice in

pediatric nursing: Blending roles. *Journal of Pediatric Nursing*, 16(2), 120–6.

Wadsworth BJ. (1984) *Piaget's theory of cognitive and affective development.* New York: Longman.

Wegner G, Alexander R. (1999) *Readings in family nursing.* Philadelphia: Lippincott Williams & Wilkins.

Woodring BC. (2000) Family matters: If you have taught, have the child and family learned? *Pediatric Nursing,* 26(5), 505–9.

Websites

Cultural Competence. Available at: *www.air.org/cecp/cultural.*

Minority Health. Available at: *www.omhrc.gov/omhhome.htm.*

Ethnic and Racial Health Disparities. Available at: *http://raceandhealth.hhs.gov.*

Workbook

NCLEX-STYLE REVIEW QUESTIONS

1. The nurse observes that during feeding the newborn looks at the mother's face and holds her finger. According to Piaget, these observations indicate the child is in which phase of development?

   a. Sensorimotor

   b. Preoperational

   c. Concrete operations

   d. Formal operations

2. The nurse is caring for a toddler who has recently turned 2 years old. Of the following behaviors by the toddler, which would indicate the toddler is attempting to become autonomous? The toddler

   a. Cries when the caregiver leaves

   b. Walks alone around the room

   c. "Shows off" to get attention

   d. Competes when playing games

3. In working with a preschool age child, which of the following statements made by the child's caregiver would indicated an understanding of this child's stage of growth and development?

   a. "My child always wants her own way."

   b. "Why won't my child play with other children?"

   c. "I will tell my child I will be back after lunch."

   d. "She doesn't know when she has done something wrong."

4. In an interview, a 9-year-old child makes the following statement to the nurse, "I like to play basketball, especially when we win." This statement indicates this child is developing which basic task of child development?

   a. Trust

   b. Autonomy

   c. Initiative

   d. Industry

5. In discussing needs of adolescents with family caregivers, the nurse explains that to support the adolescent in developing her or his own identity, it would be MOST important for the adolescent caregiver to

   a. Respond to physical needs.

   b. Praise the child's actions.

   c. Accept the child's defeats.

   d. Maintain open communication.

STUDY ACTIVITIES

1. Using the following table, compare the theories of Freud, Erickson, Piaget, and Kohlberg regarding children who are in the early elementary school years.

	Name of Theorist	Main Ideas and Similarities Between Theorists' Ideas
Latency stage Industry stage Concrete operational stage Conventional level		

2. Ask your classmates how many children there were in their family as they grew up, the sex of their siblings, and where they ranked in birth order. Ask them how they believe these factors affected their development and academic success. Ask for concrete examples of why they feel this way.

3. From your classmate's answers to question 2, what are your conclusions about the effects of sibling number, birth order, and sex in relationship to development?

CRITICAL THINKING

1. Describe changes in family structure that have occurred since the middle of the 20th century.
2. What effects will the various family structures, traditional and non-traditional, have on children in the 21st century?
3. Erikson identified trust as the development task for the first stage of life. Discuss why successful accomplishment of this task is essential to the person's future happiness and adjustment.

Community-Based Care of the Child

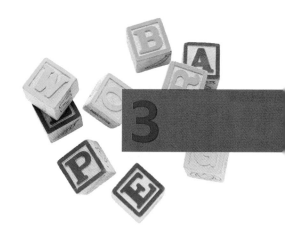

3

HEALTH CARE SHIFT: FROM HOSPITAL TO COMMUNITY
Community-Based Nursing
Community Care Settings for the Child
SKILLS OF THE COMMUNITY-BASED NURSE
The Nursing Process
Communication
Teaching
Case Management
Client Advocacy
THE CHALLENGE OF COMMUNITY-BASED NURSING
Unique Aspects
Issues Facing Children and Families
Rewards of Community-Based Nursing

STUDENT OBJECTIVES

On completion of this chapter, the student will be able to

1. Identify the focus of community-based nursing.
2. Describe advantages of community-based health care for the child and family.
3. Identify community settings where children are cared for.
4. List conditions of infants or children that may be treated in home care settings.
5. Differentiate between primary, secondary, and tertiary prevention. Give an example of each.
6. Describe at least five community-based nursing settings.
7. Discuss what information a nurse needs to successfully teach a group of children.
8. Describe how child advocacy helps children in community-based health care.
9. Identify and explain the unique characteristics of community-based nursing.

KEY TERMS

case management
child advocacy
community-based nursing
primary prevention
secondary prevention
tertiary prevention

HEALTH CARE SHIFT: FROM HOSPITAL TO COMMUNITY

In the last century, health care has gone through a number of changes. The sophisticated health care currently available is extremely expensive and has strained health care funding to a point where other health care approaches have become necessary. This need for change has led to the emergence of community-based health care and an emphasis on wellness and preventive health care. Children, especially those with serious or extensive health care needs, are cared for in hospital settings as well. Care of the hospitalized child will be discussed in Chapter 4.

The shift to community-based health care has been a positive factor in children's care. The child is no longer viewed simply as a person with an illness, but rather as a child who is a member of a family from a certain community with deep-seated cultural values, social customs, and preferences (Fig. 3–1). Learning about the child's community then using that knowledge improves the level of care the child receives. In the community, the child can also receive preventive care and wellness teaching not usually available unless one is ill in the hospital setting.

Community-Based Nursing

Community-based nursing focuses on prevention and is directed toward persons and families within a community. The goals are to help persons meet their health care needs and to maintain continuity of care as they move through the various health care settings available to them. The role of the nurse who works in the community is different from that of the hospital nurse. Generally the nurse in the community focuses on **primary prevention** (the level of prevention that includes teaching regarding safety, diet, rest, exercise, and disease prevention through immunizations), which emphasizes the role of teacher and client advocate. Examples of primary prevention are a school nurse giving a drug education program to a fourth-grade class and a nurse in a well-baby clinic giving family health teaching about home safety practices for a toddler.

In some community settings, the nurse's role focuses on **secondary prevention** (the level of prevention that focuses on early diagnosis and initiation of treatment). Such settings are clinics, home care nursing, and schools. The nurse participates in screening measures such as height, weight, hearing, and vision. During child assessments and follow-up, the nurse compiles a health history and conducts other assessments including vital signs, blood work, and other diagnostic tests as ordered by the health care practitioner. One example of secondary prevention is when the school nurse identifies a child with pediculosis (head lice). The school nurse would contact the child's family caregivers and provide instructions on the care of the child and other family members to eliminate the infestation.

Another example of secondary prevention is a community clinic nurse's identification of a child who is underweight and possibly anemic. The nurse works with the family caregiver to review the family's dietary habits and nutritional state. This would help determine if the problem is limited to this child or if other family members are also malnourished and if there is lack of knowledge or inadequate means. After finding these answers, the nurse can help the family caregiver provide better nutrition for the child and other family members as needed.

Tertiary prevention (prevention focusing on rehabilitation and teaching to prevent further injury or illness) occurs in special settings for high-risk infants and children, special intervention programs, group homes, and selected outpatient settings focusing on rehabilitation such as orthopedic clinics. Tertiary prevention is illustrated by the example of a young rural family with a child who has spina bifida and needs to be catheterized several times a day. The child is seen regularly at a specialized clinic at a major medical center. The family has no insurance, and the cost of catheters has become just one more item they feel they cannot handle. The nurse helps the family explore additional resources for financial help such as an organization that will help fund their trips to the clinic for regular appointments and also finds a source to cover the costs of catheters and other incidental expenses.

Such a broad selection of settings and roles places the nurse in a remarkable situation. Children are seen in settings familiar to them (homes, schools,

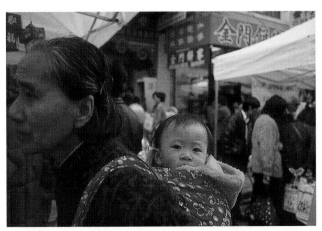

● *Figure 3.1* Many cultural preferences are seen in families. In some cultures, extended family members such as grandparents participate in raising children.

or community centers). In the community setting, the child's caregivers can more freely make choices, for instance, welcoming the nurse into their home following a medication regimen rather than in the hospital, which may be perceived as a strange territory. Although involved in direct care, the nurse in the community spends a great part of his or her time as a communicator, teacher, administrator, and manager.

Community Care Settings for the Child

Care for a child is provided in a wide variety of community settings. Some settings provide primarily wellness care; others provide specialized care for children with a particular diagnosis or condition. These include outpatient settings, home care, schools, camps, community centers, parishes, intervention programs, and group homes.

Outpatient Settings

Outpatient settings for children are varied; as the health care delivery system continues to move into the community, more settings will be developed. Outpatient settings are organized according to who offers the services and who pays for them. Public (tax-supported) outpatient clinics may be an extension of a hospital's services or may be sponsored by a regional, county, or city health department. Private (based on fees charged) clinics are owned and operated by corporations or individuals and operate for a profit. A third system is the growing network of health maintenance organizations (HMOs). Some HMO plans charge a small co-payment for each visit. However under the HMO system, the family is not free to choose the specialty care the child may receive. The child's primary care provider determines what, if any, specialized care is needed and who will administer that care.

Clinic services are based on community needs. Examples include a well-baby clinic offered by the county health department, an orthopedic clinic offered by a regional children's hospital, or a pediatric clinic of an HMO. Infants, children, and caregivers use the clinics for education, anticipatory guidance, immunizations, diagnosis, treatment, and rehabilitation.

A specialty clinic focuses on one aspect of an infant or child's well-being, for instance, dentistry, oncology, sickle cell anemia, or HIV/AIDS. Some health department clinics specialize in high-risk infants born to drug-addicted mothers, children of parents with a history of child abuse, or low-birth weight infants. Nurses in these clinics devote much of their efforts to parental education and guidance as well as follow-up services for the child.

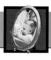

A PERSONAL GLIMPSE

The clinic is where you go when you're on the public access card and cannot afford real insurance. You hardly see the same doctor twice. A lot are interns working out their internship.

My baby was about 2 months old when he developed a bumpy rash on the crown of this head. I took him to the clinic because it was spreading and I didn't know what it could be. A doctor, who I could hardly understand, was on duty. This was the same doctor that told me I had chickenpox when I was pregnant (I didn't). He looked at the rash and looked at me very strange, then said, "This looks similar to a rash connected to HIV." He requested a test for AIDS! You cannot know the thoughts that go through your head. How? Where? Who? Why? Then I remembered that I had been tested when I first found out I was pregnant and it was negative. Since Jack, the baby's father, and I had not been with anyone else, I knew there must be another reason for this rash.

That doctor never took a sample to test or asked another doctor to come in and look at the rash. I took little Tommy home and started to use an ointment I'd heard about on his head every day for about a month. The rash went away and I've changed clinics since—like they're not all really the same. You get what you pay for.

Michelle

> **LEARNING OPPORTUNITY:** What feelings do you think this mother might have been experiencing in this situation? What specific things could the nurse do to be of support and help to this mother?

Home Health Care

Infants, children, and their families make up a significant proportion of the home health care population. Shortened acute care stays have contributed to the increasing number of children cared for by home nurses. Children are often more comfortable in familiar home surroundings (Fig. 3–2). Children and infants can be successfully treated for many conditions at home where they and their caregivers are more comfortable and they can receive the love and attention of family members. The child's caregivers feel more confident about performing treatments and procedures when they have the guidance of the home nurse. Common conditions for which an infant or child may receive home care services include

• Phototherapy for elevated bilirubin levels

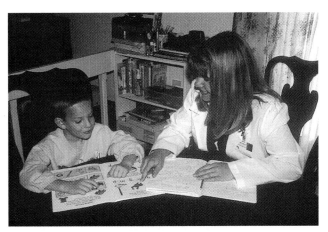

● **Figure 3.2** During a visit by the nurse, the child is comforted by the familiar surroundings of his home.

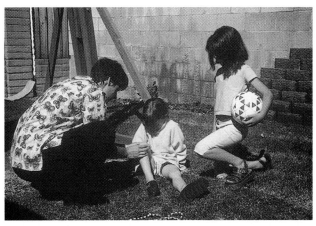

● **Figure 3.3** The school nurse cares for a young girl who injured her knee on the playground. In addition to first aid, the school nurse's duties include counseling, health education, and health promotion.

- Intravenous antibiotic therapy for systemic infections
- Postoperative care
- Chronic conditions such as asthma, sickle cell anemia, cystic fibrosis, HIV/AIDS, and leukemia and other cancers
- Respirator-dependent children
- Reconstructive or corrective surgery for congenital malformations
- Corrective orthopedic surgery.

Other home health care team members may include a physical therapist, speech therapist, occupational therapist, home schooling teacher, home health aide, primary health care provider (physician or nurse practitioner), and social worker. Members of the team vary with the child's health needs.

Schools and Camps

Health care has been practiced for many years in schools and camps, but the role of health care professionals in these settings has expanded (Fig. 3–3). The school nurse may be responsible for classroom teaching, health screenings, immunizations, first aid for injured children, care of ill children, administering medication, assisting with sports physicals, and identifying children with problems and recommending programs for them. Classroom teaching geared for each grade level can cover personal hygiene, sex education, substance abuse, safety, and emotional health. Many mainstreamed children have chronic health problems that need daily supervision or care—for example, a child with spina bifida who needs to be catheterized several times during the day or a diabetic child who needs to perform glucose monitoring and administer insulin during school hours.

Health records are maintained on each child. Some schools have clinics that provide routine dental care, physicals, screening for vision, hearing, scoliosis, tuberculosis, and follow-up on immunizations.

Children learn to know the school nurse over a number of years and usually establish a comfortable, friendly relationship that often aids the nurse in helping the child solve his or her health problems.

The camp nurse knows the child for a much briefer time, but many camp nurses establish warm relationships with the children in their care. Camp nurses provide first aid for campers and staff, maintain health records, teach first aid and cardiopulmonary resuscitation, offer relevant health education, maintain an infirmary for ill campers, and dispense tender loving care to homesick children.

At camps for children with special needs, the campers' health care needs determine the type of nursing care required. For example at a camp for diabetic children, the nurse may teach self-administration of insulin and the many aspects of diabetic care. Other camps may cater to children with developmental delays, physical challenges, or chronic illness such as asthma or cystic fibrosis. Others have specific purposes such as weight control or behavior management. In each of these settings, the nurse provides basic health care with individualized health teaching based on the camp population. Each type of camping brings its own challenges and rewards; the benefits to the children and their families are often exceptional.

INTERNET EXERCISE 3-1

http://www.faculty.fairfield.edu/fleitas/contents.html

Bandaides & Blackboards
Click on Kids.
Go to Lots of stories and click on the star.

1. In working with school age children what are some of the stories in this site you would encourage the children to read?

2. List the topics and diseases included in the stories that you could share with school age children.

Community Centers, Parishes, and Intervention Programs

Community centers and parishes provide care relevant to a particular community. Parish centers may sponsor outreach programs in a church, synagogue, or other religious setting. The services offered by these centers are designed to meet community needs. For example, in areas with many homeless persons, centers may provide basic health care and nutrition. These centers may also provide food, clothing, money, or other resources. Other centers may provide childcare classes for new mothers or young families.

Some communities offer walk-in or residential clinics for special purposes such as teen pregnancy, alcohol and drug abuse, nutritional guidance, and family violence. Other specialized clinics offer programs on HIV/AIDS, cancer, and mental health; provide maternal and well-baby care; and offer day care services for children or the elderly.

Many communities also have services provided by volunteer service organizations such as the Lions, Rotary Club, Shriners, or Kiwanis. Some of these organizations have specific goals. For example, the Shriners sponsor clinics for children with orthopedic problems.

In any community center, there are people who can benefit from the services of health care professionals. Often the health services focus on education and other primary prevention practices. Nurses can help design safety, exercise, and nutrition programs; provide basic immunization services; conduct parenting classes; organize crisis intervention programs for youth and teens; and help organize health fairs. The health care staff may be paid or may work on a volunteer basis, or there may be a combination of paid and volunteer staff.

Many services can be provided to smaller groups of infants and children with special needs. Such intervention programs may be supported by federal or state funds and offered through the school district or private associations for developmentally delayed, physically challenged, or emotionally disturbed children. The interventions are often multidisciplinary, consisting of a team of professionals who work together to meet the multiple needs of the child.

Professional teams may consist of a teacher, psychologist, neurologist, physical therapist, social worker, physician, and nurse. The most important team members are the family caregivers and the child, and it is essential to include them in planning meetings and program intervention development. The nurse's role as a team member involves interpreting diagnoses or medical orders to other team members and the family, teaching the family how to manage a medically fragile child, and integrating the family into intervention programs effectively.

Residential Programs

Residential programs, often called group homes, provide services for a number of health needs. Those geared primarily to children include chemical dependency treatment centers and homes for children with mental or emotional health needs, pregnant adolescents, and abused children. These homes vary in size and setup according to the children's needs.

Depending on the number of children a home serves, the nurse may be contracted to provide specific services. The nurse may work for the local health department or for a corporation that owns several group homes. For example, in a home with six children with minimal disabilities, the nurse may visit every 2 weeks to meet with and educate the staff, update health records, and provide immunizations. This may be all the health care service the home requires to maintain its group home license.

Homes that serve many children or that serve children with very complex needs may need to have nurses 24 hours a day. Often licensing standards require this complete coverage in addition to meeting the health care needs of the children. Some homes hire a multidisciplinary team of health care practitioners that may include nurses, medical social workers, psychologists, physical, speech, or occupational therapists, special education teachers, home health aides or attendants, and physicians. Not all the team members provide services to group homes on a full-time basis.

SKILLS OF THE COMMUNITY-BASED NURSE

The nursing process serves as the foundation of nursing care for the child in the community just as it does for the child in a health care facility. Communication with the child and family is essential. Teaching is a fundamental part of community-based care because of the emphasis on health promotion and preventive health care. Case management is necessary to direct the child's care and determine that care's progress through the health care system.

The Nursing Process

Although the family of the child in a health care facility is important, in the community setting the family takes on even greater importance. Understanding the family structure and the roles and functions of family members is vital to caring for the child in the community (for a review of the nursing process, see Chap. 1).

In the initial family assessment interview, the nurse determines how various family members affect the child and his or her condition. The nurse may obtain additional information by picking up on cues in the child's environment. After collecting the data and completing the assessment, the registered nurse and the health care team analyze the information and identify the family's needs and strengths. They determine nursing diagnoses and proceed with the plan based on the development of expected outcomes related specifically to the child. The expected outcomes are mutually set with the family to encourage family interaction and cooperation. In the community setting, the family is much more directly involved in providing care for the child; thus, their compliance is essential to the success of that care. Interventions are initiated based on the expected outcomes. Family teaching is vital. As the interventions are performed, the results are documented and evaluated, and the ongoing cycle of the nursing process continues.

Communication

Positive, effective communication is fundamental to the nursing process and the care of the child in the community. The principles of communication, verbal

COMMUNICATIONS BOX 3-1

At a neighborhood clinic, a mother rushes in with her young child in her arms. She is upset and unsure of herself. A nurse is at the desk.

LESS EFFECTIVE COMMUNICATION	MORE EFFECTIVE COMMUNICATION

LESS EFFECTIVE COMMUNICATION

Nurse: Can I help you?
Mother: (Anxiously) My baby is sick.
Nurse: Just have a seat in the waiting area and we'll call you. (Hands her a clipboard with papers attached.) Fill this out while you wait.
Mother: (Nervously goes to seat. Cradles baby in arms.)
After 45 minutes, the nurse calls the mother.
Nurse: Have a seat here while we go over your information. (Looking at clipboard) You haven't filled any of this out.
Mother: No, I . . . I was busy with the baby.
Nurse: I don't have time to fill all of these out with everyone. Can you read this?
Mother: (Very softly) I left my glasses at home.
Nurse: Oh, all right, but you better remember your glasses after this. You need to do these papers yourself.

> *During this interview, the nurse has been centered on his/her own concerns and does not read any of the mother's concerns or clues. The nurse does not ask what is wrong with the baby, so the nurse has no real idea if the baby can safely wait or not. The nurse hands the mother the clipboard to fill out without trying to find out if that is something the mother can do. When the mother came back with the unanswered question- naire, the nurse was abrupt and was not sensitive to the mother's possible inability to read. The nurse was not tuned in to the mother's needs*

MORE EFFECTIVE COMMUNICATION

Nurse: Can I help you?
Mother: (Anxiously) My baby is sick
Nurse: How has the baby been acting?
Mother: She's been really fussy. She hasn't been able to sleep at night and she has been spitting up a lot.
Nurse: Has she had any fever?
Mother: I don't know. I don't have a thermometer.
Nurse: Have a seat in the waiting area and I'll call you as soon as possible. Do you think you will be able to fill out these information papers?
Mother: I don't know if I can with the baby and all.
Nurse: No problem. I'll call you as soon as possible to help you fill out these papers.
Mother: Thank you.

> *The nurse in this instance initially gave the mother an opportunity to tell how her baby is. This helps the nurse decide if they can wait for attention. After hearing the mother's response about the thermometer, the nurse suspects she may not be able to read. For this reason she gives the mother a non-threatening reason to say that she wouldn't be able to fill out the papers. When the mother accepts that offer, the nurse reassures her that this is fine. The mother's self-respect remains intact and she is grateful. The nurse throughout this interview has picked up on clues of behavior and responses to determine this mother's circumstances.*

and nonverbal, are covered in Chapter 1. Establishing rapport with the child and the family, understanding and appropriately responding to cultural practices, and being sensitive to the needs of the child and family all require good communication skills.

Teaching

Teaching is one of the most important facets of nursing care. Health education is very important in community-based care. In many settings, child health care involves teaching of small groups—the child, family caregivers, older siblings, and members of the extended family. However, teaching need not be limited to family members or the child's immediate surroundings. Depending on the setting and the child's age, the nurse may teach large groups of children and families on various topics that focus on primary prevention (Fig. 3–4).

To teach a group successfully, the nurse must know the needs of the target population and have the appropriate teaching skills, strategies, and resources. If the nurse is familiar with the children, he or she already has some important information such as their age, educational level, ethnic and gender mix, language barriers, and any previous teaching the group has had on the subject. When teaching an unfamiliar group, the nurse can ask the group leader for this information to help develop an appropriate teaching plan. The nurse should review growth and developmental principles to identify the appropriate level of information, learning activities, and average attention span. Additional information includes any available teaching resources, group size, seating arrangements, and other advantages or restrictions of the environment. For instance, the nurse may want to find out

- Are the chairs movable for small-group discussions?
- Is there a VCR to show a video?

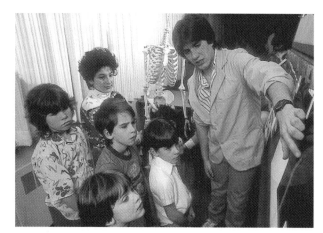

● *Figure 3.4* Teaching plays a major role in community-based nursing. Here a nurse is teaching a group of children.

- Can the children go outside?
- Will a lot of noise disturb others in the building?
- Will the classroom teacher or teacher's aide be in attendance?

Being prepared makes all the difference between a successful and an unsuccessful group teaching experience.

Case Management

Case management (a systematic process that ensures that a client's multiple health and service needs are met) may be a formal or an informal process. In some community-based agencies, case management is formalized. In these systems, the agency or insurer who pays for the health care services predetermines the contact with the client. In other settings, the nurse may determine the needed follow-up and either provide the needed services or assist with referrals to obtain services.

If case management is formalized, the insurer pays for nursing services. The case manager's role is clearly outlined with care plans, protocols, and limits to service determined by the insurer. In community agencies where nursing services are part of the overall services (for instance, schools or group homes), the intensity of follow-up is determined by the agency's philosophy, available resources, and the nurse's perception of the role and his or her individual skills.

Client Advocacy

Client advocacy is speaking or acting on behalf of others to help them gain greater independence and to make the health care delivery system more responsive and relevant to their needs. The nurse working in a community setting often can develop longer relationships with children and their families because of the continuous nature of client contact in outpatient, school, or other settings. This additional contact time allows the nurse to discover broader health and welfare issues. Example of interventions include

- Teaching a family about the services for which their child is eligible
- Identifying inexpensive or free transportation services to medical appointments
- Making the several phone calls necessary to establish eligibility for and to acquire special equipment needed by a physically challenged child.

Examples of **child advocacy** are limitless and include health and social welfare services that intertwine in ways that families cannot manage alone. One example is assistance with referrals and acquisition of needed resources. As a member of a team of health

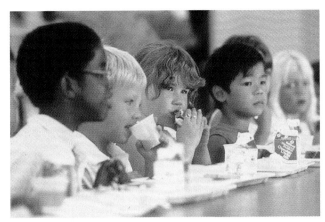

● *Figure 3.5* A nurse advocate can help the child enter a school lunch program so that nutritional needs are met.

care professionals, the nurse assists with the referral process. This process focuses on getting the child to the services needed or obtaining the resources needed. Actions taken are geared toward improving the child's health or quality of life. The nurse must be knowledgeable about community resources, contact persons, and details of appropriate applications, and other required documentation (Fig. 3–5).

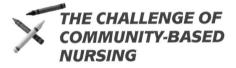

THE CHALLENGE OF COMMUNITY-BASED NURSING

There are several differences between caring for children in a hospital or clinic and caring for children in community settings. Community-based work requires a different set of skills.

The Unique Aspects of Community-Based Nursing

Community-based nursing practice is autonomous. The nurse must be self-reliant to be successful. There may not be many other health care practitioners; those available may be physically distant. To provide children and families with high-quality care, the nurse must have well-developed assessment and decision-making skills.

Community practice also tends to be more holistic. The child is viewed as an integrated whole mind, body, and spirit interacting with the environment. The effects of the child's health on family functioning, the impact on the child's educational progress, the multiple services the family and child need to improve the quality of life—all are considered by the community nurse.

A final difference is the focus on wellness. Some community settings have a population of children

with an illness or diagnosis in common such as cerebral palsy or diabetes. Working with these children involves managing their disease or limitations with a wellness focus. For instance, the focus might be on how the child with cerebral palsy can be included comfortably within the regular classroom or how the diabetic teenager can juggle sports, eating out, and slumber parties.

In most areas where the community nurse works, the focus is on wellness. The children are basically well but may be going through growth and developmental crises. The nurse intervenes with children and family members to ease the transition from one stage to another. The nurse provides anticipatory guidance to family caregivers and emphasizes preventive health practices. Teaching health-promotion practices to children is another activity of primary importance.

Issues Facing Children and Families

Nurses who work in the community begin to see and interact with the other issues facing children and their families. Care giving activities in the community combine the uniqueness of the community setting with the knowledge the nurse gains from seeing the child in his or her own environment.

Poverty is a major issue that affects all aspects of recovery and response to care. For many families, a lack of resources takes its toll on children's health and hinders compliance. Services and resources may be inaccessible because of cost, location, lack of public or private transportation or the cost of transportation, or neighborhood safety; the family may see such services as unnecessary. Poverty, lack of information, questionable decisions about priorities, and deficient coping skills affect the health of children in significant ways; the results are often seen in the emergency department or the acute care beds of children's units.

The community nurse must explore these issues with the family caregivers. When a family does not follow up with an orthopedic appointment for a new cast application on the legs of a 6-month-old infant, what factors influenced their decision? When a family caregiver saves half of the antibiotic suspension for another child in the family with similar symptoms, what motivates this decision? When a single parent keeps a physically disabled and developmentally delayed 9-year-old son at home in one room of the apartment, what types of care giving services and information might be of benefit?

Rewards of Community-Based Nursing

Individual clients do not change as much in community-based settings. The clinic nurse may see the same family for different problems over many years. The camp or school nurse watches children grow and gets to know siblings and families over many years. A group home nurse works intensely with a group of developmentally disabled children who learn to know each one and rejoice in their small triumphs.

For the community nurse, rewards come slowly and in different ways. For 4 months, a school nurse may diligently work with a child and family and a community service organization to obtain a pair of glasses for the child. This nurse may feel rewarded when the child no longer comes into the nurse's office at school with headaches and is doing better in class work. The camp nurse may help a homesick new camper design a way to stay in touch with his or her parents and may encourage the camper to participate in camp activities. This nurse may also find reward when the camper returns each season. The nurse in a group home for teenage foster children with behavioral problems may help the teens develop a theater group that presents plays about safe sex and responsible teen dating to other group homes, high school classes, or community service organizations. This nurse may find reward after a year of work with the teens when they write the scripts, build the sets independently, and declare that they enjoy the theater group more than any other activity in the residence. This nurse may also find a deeper reward when he or she realizes that as a result of the theater group, there are fewer behavioral problems and the teens' self-esteem is high.

Community nurses work in many ways to prevent unnecessary hospitalization. Health problems that could have been prevented leave the nurse wondering why they were not prevented—like an auto accident involving a child not appropriately secured in a car seat, a toddler with a scalded face from grabbing a tablecloth and spilling a cup of coffee, a child who almost drowned in a backyard pool, an infant who fails to thrive because the parents do not know that infants need specific amounts of formula, or a pregnant teen who did not have safe sex. The community nurse helps families develop the skills and knowledge they need to make decisions that affect their lives and those of other family members. In this way, families can learn and practice preventive health care. With a focus on wellness, the community nurse provides a service that eventually improves the health of the entire community.

KEY POINTS

◗ Community-based health care focuses on wellness and prevention and is directed toward helping persons and families meet their health care needs.

◗ Community nurses focus on primary prevention followed by secondary prevention.

◗ The community offers many settings where children are cared for. Some focus on wellness care, others on specialized care for children with specific diagnoses.

◗ Shortened acute care stays have increased the number of children and families cared for by home nurses.

◗ School nurses provide classroom health teaching, perform health screenings, offer first aid to injured children, care for children who become ill in school, administer medications, care for mainstreamed children with chronic conditions, serve on professional panels, assist with sports physicals, and keep health records.

◗ In any community health care setting, the family and the child are the most important members of the health care team.

◗ Communication is one of the most important aspects of community health care.

◗ To establish rapport, the community nurse must understand and respond appropriately to cultural practices of community members.

◗ Community nurses spend much of their time teaching on a one-to-one basis or with a family, a small group, or a large group. The nurse must assess each audience and gear the teaching appropriately.

BIBLIOGRAPHY

Allender JA, Spradley BW (2000) *Community health nursing* (5th ed). Philadelphia: Lippincott Williams & Wilkins.

Anonymous. (2001) Boost for children's healthcare. *Nursing Standard*, 15(24), 7.

Children's Defense Fund. (2000) *The state of America's children.* Washington DC.

Hunt R. (2001) *Introduction to community-based nursing* (2nd ed). Philadelphia: Lippincott Williams & Wilkins.

Limerick M, Baldwin L (2000) Nursing in outpatient child and adolescent mental health. *Nursing Standard*, 15(24), 9.

McPherson G, Thorne S. (2000) Children's voices, can we hear them? *Journal of Pediatric Nursing*, 15(1), 22–9.

National Safety Council. (2000) *Report on injuries in America 2000.* Illinois. Available at: *http://www.nsc.org/library/rept2000.htn.*

Vessey JA (2000) Primary care approaches: Coordinated school health. *Pediatric Nursing*, 26(3), 303–4, 307.

Wong DL. (1998) *Whaley and Wong's nursing care of infants and children* (6th ed). St. Louis: Mosby.

Websites
www.health.discovery.com
www.kidshealth.org/kid
www.kinderstart.com

Workbook

NCLEX-STYLE REVIEW QUESTIONS

1. One role of the nurse in a community-based setting focuses on *primary* prevention. An example of *primary* prevention would be

   a. Screening children for vision in a preschool

   b. Teaching bicycle safety in an after-school program

   c. Identifying head lice in a child in elementary school

   d. Exploring financial help for a client in a home setting

2. One role of the nurse in a community-based setting focuses on *secondary* prevention. An example of *secondary* prevention would be

   a. Screening children for vision in a preschool

   b. Teaching about nutrition in an after-school program

   c. Recommending a group home setting for an adolescent

   d. Administering immunizations to infants in a clinic

3. One role of the nurse in a community-based setting focuses on *tertiary* prevention. An example of *tertiary* prevention would be

   a. Testing children for hearing loss in a preschool

   b. Teaching bicycle safety in an after-school program

   c. Administering immunizations to infants in a clinic

   d. Exploring financial help for a client in a home setting

4. A mother of a child being cared for in a home setting makes the following statements. Which statement BEST illustrates one of the positive aspects of home health care?

   a. "My family gets to visit once a week when my child is in the hospital."

   b. "I can do my child's care since you taught the procedure to me."

   c. "Our insurance pays for us to go to the well-child clinic."

   d. "The neighbor's child likes being in the group home."

5. When a nurse is doing teaching in a community-based setting, it is MOST important for the nurse to

   a. Ask questions about the histories of those present.

   b. Use posters that everyone in the group can read.

   c. Tell the participants about the nurse's background.

   d. Know the needs of the audience.

STUDY ACTIVITIES

1. Survey your community to discover the community-based health care providers available. Use the information you found to complete the following table.

Community-Based Health Care Providers	How Are They Funded?	What Types of Health Care for Children Do They Provide?

2. Using the information you obtained above, evaluate your community's health care services by answering the following:

   a. Does your community have adequate health care services for children?

   b. Are funding concerns an issue for your community? In what ways?

   c. What other services do you think are needed to care for the children in your community?

3. Select a community-based setting and outline the services that a nurse in that setting should ideally provide. Include the resources needed to provide the services.

CRITICAL THINKING

1. Identify the strengths you believe that a community nurse needs. Compare your nursing skills with these strengths, being as realistic as possible. Determine if your strengths meet those needed.
2. You are making a home visit to the Smith family because their newborn infant needs home phototherapy treatment for 3 to 5 days. You find 6-year-old Samantha ill with bronchitis. Both parents smoke. Outline a teaching plan for these caregivers regarding the health of their family.
3. Mrs. Perez, a second-grade teacher, asks you to teach a unit on personal hygiene to her class. Identify the information you will need from Mrs. Perez. Describe how you will present the lesson to these children.

Care of the Hospitalized Child

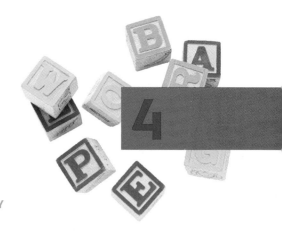

4

STUDENT OBJECTIVES

On completion of this chapter, the student will be able to

1. List nine possible influences on the family's response to a child's illness.
2. Explain the family caregivers' role in preparing a child for hospitalization.
3. Describe the benefits of rooming-in.
4. State the role that handwashing plays in infection control.
5. Identify four ways that pathogens are transmitted, and give an example of each.
6. Describe how the nurse can help ease the feelings of isolation a child may have when segregated by transmission-based precautions.
7. Identify and differentiate the three stages of response to separation seen in the young child.
8. Describe how a preadmission visit differs from an open house program.
9. State how the caregiver may be involved in the child's admission process.
10. Discuss the need for written discharge instructions for the caregiver.
11. State how family members should react to the post discharge child during this period of adjustment.
12. Describe how health professionals can help the adjustment of the child scheduled for surgery.
13. Discuss variations in preoperative preparation for children including skin, gastrointestinal, urinary, and medication preparation.
14. Identify behavioral characteristics that may indicate an infant or a young child is having pain.
15. Discuss the purpose of a hospital play program.
16. Describe therapeutic use for puppets.
17. State how stress affects the frequency of accidents and how this relates to a child's hospitalization.

KEY TERMS

anuria
child-life program
patient-controlled analgesia
play therapy
rooming-in
therapeutic play

ospitalization may cause anxiety and stress at any age. Fear of the unknown is always threatening. The child who faces hospitalization is no exception. Children are often too young to understand what is happening or are afraid to ask questions. Short hospital stays occur more frequently than extended hospitalization, but even during a short stay the child is often apprehensive. In addition, the child may pick up on the fears of family caregivers, and these negative emotions may hinder the child's progress.

The child's family suffers stress for a number of reasons. The cause of the illness, its treatment, guilt about the illness, past experiences of illness and hospitalization, disruption in family life, the threat to the child's long-term health, cultural or religious influences, coping methods within the family, and financial impact of the hospitalization all may affect how the family responds to the child's illness. Although these are concerns of the family and not specifically the child, they nevertheless influence how the child feels. Children are tuned in to the feelings and emotions of their caregivers.

The child's developmental level also plays an important role in determining how he or she handles the stress of illness and hospitalization. The nurse who understands the child's developmental needs may significantly improve the child's hospital stay and overall recovery. Many hospitals have a **child-life program** to make hospitalization less threatening for children and their parents. These programs are usually under the direction of a child-life specialist whose background is in psychology and early childhood development. This person works with nurses, physicians, and other health team members to help them meet the developmental, emotional, and intellectual needs of hospitalized children. The child-life specialist also works with students interested in child health care to help further their education. Sometimes, however, the best way to ease the stress of hospitalization is to ensure that the child has been well prepared for the hospital experience.

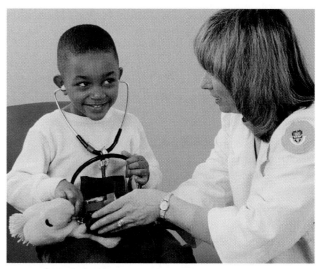

● **Figure 4.1** A nurse helps children learn what to expect from hospitalization during a prehospital program. (© B. Proud.)

regular open house programs for healthy children. Children may attend with parents or caregivers or in an organized community or school group. A room is set aside where children can handle equipment, try out call bells, try on masks and gowns, have their blood pressure taken to feel the squeeze of the blood-pressure cuff, and see a hospital pediatric bed and compare it with their bed at home. Hospital staff members explain simple procedures and answer children's questions (Fig. 4–1). A tour of the pediatric department including the playroom may be offered. Some hospitals have puppet shows or show slides or videos about admission and care. Child-life specialists, nurses, and volunteers help with these orientation programs.

Families are encouraged to help children at an early age develop a positive attitude about hospitals. The family should avoid negative attitudes about hospitals. Young children need to know that the hospital is more than a place where "mommies go to get babies"; it is also important to avoid fostering the view of the hospital as a place where people go to die. This is a particular concern if the child knows someone who died in the hospital. A careful explanation of the person's illness and simple, honest answers to questions about the death are necessary.

The Pediatric Unit Atmosphere

An effort by pediatric units and hospitals to create friendly, warm surroundings for children has produced many attractive, colorful pediatric settings. Walls are colorful, often decorated with murals, wallpaper, photos, and paintings specifically designed for children. Furniture is attractive, appropriate in size, and designed with safety in mind.

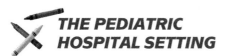

THE PEDIATRIC HOSPITAL SETTING

Early Childhood Education About Hospitals

Hospitals are part of the child's community, just as police and fire departments are. When the child is capable of understanding the basic functions of community resources and the people who staff them, it is time for an explanation. Some hospitals have

Curtains and drapes in appealing colors and designs are often coordinated with wall coverings.

The staff members of the pediatric unit often wear colored smocks, colorful sweatshirts, or printed scrub suits. Research has shown that children react with greatest anxiety toward the traditional white uniform. Children often are encouraged to wear their own clothing during the day. Colorful printed pajamas are provided for children who need to wear hospital clothing.

Treatments are performed in a treatment room, not in the child's room. Using a separate room to perform procedures promotes the concept that the child's bed is a "safe" place. All treatments, with no exceptions, should be performed in the treatment room to reassure the child.

A playroom or play area is a vital part of all pediatric units. The playroom should be a place that is safe from any kind of procedures. Some hospitals provide a person trained in therapeutic play to coordinate and direct the play activities.

Most pediatric settings provide **rooming-in** facilities and encourage parents or family caregivers to visit as frequently as possible (Fig. 4–2). This approach helps minimize the separation anxiety of the young child in particular. Caregivers are involved in much of the young child's care; they provide comfort and reassurance to the child. Many pediatric units use primary nursing assignments so that the same nurse is with a child as much as possible. This approach gives the nurse the opportunity to establish a trusting relationship with the child.

Planning meals that include the child's favorite foods, within the limitations of any special dietary restrictions, may perk up a poor appetite. In addition when space permits, several children may eat together at a small table. Younger children should be seated in high chairs or other suitable seats. Meals should be served out of bed, if possible, and in a

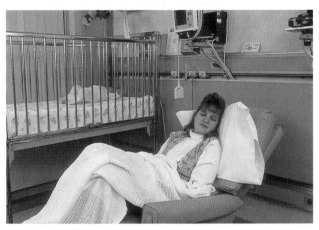

● **Figure 4.2** Rooming-in helps alleviate separation anxiety for both the child and the caregiver. (© B. Proud.)

A PERSONAL GLIMPSE

Hi my name is Jenni. I am 15 years old and would like to tell you about my experience in the hospital.

I am an asthmatic. I have been since my early childhood because of allergies (sic) to many things. Whenever I get a cold, it sometimes agrivates (sic) my asthma. I recently had an episode where I needed to be hospitalized because of an asthma attack.

I don't like hospitals. I could not wait until I was released. The IV hurt and needed to be put back in. The nurse had dry, scaly hands. It looked like she worked on a farm and then came to work at the hospital. The food was not too great either, not like Pizza Hut or McDonalds.

The person that made the hold (sic) ordeal tolerable was the respiratory therapist. I needed regular nebulizer treatments and it was a dream when he came into the room. Yes, he was good looking but what made the difference was his personality and sense of humor. It makes a big difference when it seems as if the staff person wants to be there and really cares rather than being cared by someone who is there just because it's a job and can't wait until the shift ends.

Jenni, age 15 years

> **LEARNING OPPORTUNITY:** What do you think are three important behaviors by the nurse or health care professional that indicate to a patient that he or she is cared about as a person?

pleasant atmosphere. Some pediatric units use the playroom to serve meals to ambulatory children.

Pediatric Intensive Care Units

A child's admission to a pediatric intensive care unit (PICU) may be overwhelming for both the child and the family, especially if the admission is unexpected. Highly technical equipment, bright lights, and the crisis atmosphere may be frightening. Visiting may be restricted. The many stressors present increase the effects on the child and the family. PICU nurses should take great care to prepare the family for how the child will look when they first visit. The family should be given a schedule of visiting hours so that they may plan permitted visits. Visiting hours should be flexible enough to accommodate the child's best interests. The family should be encouraged to bring in a special doll or child's toy to provide comfort and security. The child's developmental level must be assessed so that the nursing staff can provide appropriate explanations and reassurances before and during procedures. Positive reinforcements, such as stickers and small badges, may provide symbols of courage. The nurse also needs to interpret technical information for family members. The nurse should promote the relationship between the family caregiver and the child as much as possible. The caregiver should be encouraged to touch and talk to the child. If possible the caregiver may hold and rock the child ; if not, he or she can comfort the child by caressing and stroking.

Infection Control in the Pediatric Setting

Infection control is important in the pediatric setting. The ill child may be especially vulnerable to pathogenic (disease-carrying) microorganisms. Precautions must be taken to protect the children, families, and personnel. Microorganisms are spread by contact (direct, indirect, or droplet), vehicle (food, water, blood, or contaminated products), airborne (dust particles in the air), or vector (mosquitoes, vermin) means of transmission. Each type of microorganism is transmitted in a specific way, so precautions are tailored to prevent the spread of specific microorganisms.

In 1996, the U.S. Centers for Disease Control and Prevention and the Hospital Infection Control Practices Advisory Committee published new guidelines for isolation practices in hospitals. The guidelines were revised to include two levels of precautions: standard precautions and transmission-based precautions. Health care facilities continue to follow these guidelines.

Standard precautions blend the primary characteristics of universal precautions and body substance isolation. Standard precautions apply to blood, all body fluids, secretions, and excretions except sweat, nonintact skin, and mucous membranes. Standard precautions are geared toward reducing the risk of transmission of microorganisms from recognized or unrecognized sources of infection in hospitals. Standard precautions are used in the care of all patients.

Transmission-based precautions pertain to patients documented or suspected to have highly transmissible or other pathogens that require additional precautions beyond those covered under standard precautions. Transmission-based precautions include three types: airborne precautions, droplet precautions, and contact precautions. They may need to be combined to cover certain diseases. The infection control guidelines are presented in the Guidelines for Standard and Transmission-Based Precautions in Appendix E. See the Nursing Care Plan for the child placed on transmission-based precaution.

Handwashing is the cornerstone of all infection control. The nurse *must* wash his or her hands conscientiously between seeing each patient, even when gloves are worn for a procedure.

The child who is segregated by transmission-based precautions is subject to social isolation. Feelings of loneliness and depression are common. Every effort must be made to help reduce these feelings. The child must not think that being in a room alone is a punishment. The nurse can arrange to spend extra time in the room when performing treatments and procedures. While in the room, the nurse might read a story, play a game, or just talk with the child rather than going quickly in and out of the room.

Family caregivers should be encouraged to spend time with the child. The nurse might help them with gowning and other necessary precaution procedures so that they become more comfortable in the situation. Caregivers may need to have the precaution measures reviewed including handwashing, gowning, and masking as necessary. The nurse may encourage the family to bring the child's favorite dolls, stuffed animals, or toys. Most of these items can be sterilized after use. For the older child, electronic toys may help provide stimulation to ease the loneliness. The child should be encouraged to make phone calls to friends or family members to keep up social contacts. For the school-age child, family caregivers might be encouraged to contact the child's teacher so that classmates can send cards and other school items to keep the child involved. If the child's room has a window, move the bed so the child can see outside.

If masks or gloves are part of the necessary precautions, the child may experience even greater feelings of isolation. Before putting on the mask, the nurse should allow the child to see his or her face; that process will help the child easily identify the nurse. Gloves prevent the child from experiencing skin-to-skin contact; the nurse should talk to the child to draw out any of the youngster's feelings about this. Explaining at the child's level of understanding why gloves are necessary may help the child accept them. Gowns on the staff are generally not upsetting to the child, but the child may be bothered by the fact that caregivers must wear gowns. If this is the case, a careful explanation should help the child accept this. No matter what precautions are necessary, the nurse should always be alert to the child's loneliness and sadness and should be prepared to meet these needs.

Importance of Caregiver Participation

Research has shown that separating young children from their family caregivers, especially during times

NURSING CARE PLAN

for the Child Placed on Transmission-Based Precautions

TS is a 5-year-old girl who has a highly infectious illness resulting from an airborne microorganism. The child is placed on Airborne Transmission-Based Precautions.

NURSING DIAGNOSIS
Risk for Loneliness related to transmission-based precautions

GOAL: *The child will have adequate social contact.*

OUTCOME CRITERIA
• The child interacts with nursing staff and family.
• The child visits with friends and family via telephone.

NURSING INTERVENTIONS	*RATIONALE*
Identify ways in which the child can communicate with staff, family, and friends.	Frequent contact with family and staff helps to decrease the child's feeling of isolation.
Facilitate the use of telephone for the child to talk with friends.	Use of the telephone helps child feel connected with her friends.
Suggest family caregivers ask the child's preschool friends to send notes and drawings.	Notes, photos, and drawings are concrete signs to the child that her friends are thinking of her. It helps her stay in touch with her preschool.

NURSING DIAGNOSIS
Deficient Diversional Activity related to monotony of restrictions

GOAL: *The child will be engaged in age-appropriate activities.*

OUTCOME CRITERIA
• The child participates in age-appropriate activities.
• The child approaches planned activities with enthusiasm.

NURSING INTERVENTIONS	*RATIONALE*
Gather a collection of age-appropriate books, puzzles, and games. Consult with play therapist if available.	A variety of appropriate activities provide diversion and entertainment without boredom.
Encourage family caregivers to engage the child in activities she enjoys. Audiotapes can be made for (or by) playmates.	Family caregivers can use visiting time to help alleviate the monotony of isolation. Audiotapes make friends seem closer.
Plan nursing care to include time for reading or playing a game with the child.	Activities with a variety of persons (besides family caregivers) are welcome to the child.
Encourage physical exercise within the restrictions of the child's condition.	Physical activity helps to improve circulation and feelings of well-being.

NURSING DIAGNOSIS
Powerlessness related to separation resulting from required precautions

GOAL: *The child will have control over some aspects of the situation.*

OUTCOME CRITERIA
• The child will make choices about some of her daily routine.
• The child's family caregivers and the staff keep their promises about planned activities.

NURSING INTERVENTIONS	*RATIONALE*
Include the child in planning for daily activities such as bath routine, food choices, timing of meals and snacks, and other flexible activities.	The child will feel some control over her life if she is included in ways where she can have a choice.
Maintain the schedule after making the plan.	Keeping the schedule reinforces for the child that she really does have some control.
Plan a special activity with the child each day and keep your promise.	When the child can depend on the word of those in control, she is reassured about her own value.

of stress, may have damaging effects. Young children have no concept of time, so separation from their primary caregivers is especially difficult for them to understand. Three characteristic stages of response to the separation have been identified: protest, despair, and denial. During the first stage (protest), the young child cries, often refuses to be comforted by others, and constantly seeks the primary caregiver at every sight and sound. When the caregiver does not appear, the child enters the second stage—despair—and becomes apathetic and listless. Health care personnel often interpret this as a sign that the child is accepting the situation, but this is not the case; the child has given up.

In the third stage—denial—the child begins taking interest in the surroundings and appears to accept the situation. However, the damage is revealed when the caregivers do visit: the child often turns away from them, showing distrust and rejection. It may take a long time before the child accepts them again, and even then remnants of the damage linger. The child may always have a memory of being abandoned at the hospital. Regardless of how mistaken they may be, childhood impressions have a deep effect.

Rooming-in helps remove the young hospitalized child's hurt and depression. Although separation from primary caregivers is thought to cause the greatest upset in children younger than 5 years of age, children of all ages should be considered when setting up a rooming-in system.

One advantage of rooming-in is the measure of security the child feels as a result of the caregiver's care and attention. The primary caregiver may participate in bathing, dressing, and feeding, preparing the child for bed, and providing recreational activities. However, this system should not be used to relieve staff shortage. If treatments are to be continued at home, rooming-in creates an excellent opportunity for the caregiver to observe and practice before leaving the hospital.

Rules should be clearly understood before admission, and facilities for caregivers should be clearly explained. The hospital may provide a folding cot or reclining chair in the child's room. Provision for meals should be explained to the caregiver.

The nursing staff should be careful to avoid creating a situation in which they appear to be expecting the primary caregivers to perform as health care technicians. The primary caregiver's basic role is to provide security and stability for the child.

Many pediatric units also have recognized the importance of allowing siblings to visit the ill child. This policy benefits both the ill child and the sibling. The sibling at home may be imagining a much more serious illness than is actually the case. Visiting policies usually require that a family adult accompany and be responsible for the child and that the visiting period is not too long. There also should be a policy requiring that the visiting sibling does not have a cold or other contagious illness and is up to date in immunizations.

The nursing staff also should be aware of the caregiver's needs. The caregiver needs to be encouraged to leave for meals or a break or to go home, if possible, for a shower and rest. The child may be given a possession of the caregiver's to help reassure him or her that the caregiver will return. Some hospitals have established a program in which family caregivers receive pagers so that they can leave the immediate area of the child's room or waiting area but can be quickly paged to return if needed. This gives the family freedom with the reassurance of easy contact. This is particularly useful during periods when the caregivers must wait for procedures, surgery, or other activities.

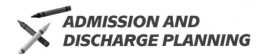

ADMISSION AND DISCHARGE PLANNING

Although admission may be a frightening experience, the child feels in much better control of the situation if the person taking the child to the hospital has explained where they are going and why and has answered questions truthfully. When the caregiver and the child arrive on the nursing unit, they should be greeted in a warm, friendly manner and taken to the child's room or to a room set aside specifically for the admission procedure. The caregiver and the child need to be oriented to the child's room, the nursing unit, and regulations (Box 4–1).

Planned Admissions

Preadmission preparation may make the experience less threatening and the adjustment to admission as smooth as possible. Children who are candidates for hospital admission may attend open house programs or other special programs that are more detailed and specifically related to their upcoming experience. It is important for family caregivers and siblings to attend the preadmission tour with the future patient to reduce anxiety in all family members.

During the preadmission visit, children may be given surgical masks, caps, shoe covers, and the opportunity to "operate" on a doll or other stuffed toy specifically designed for teaching purposes (Fig. 4–3). Many hospitals have developed special coloring

BOX 4.1	Guidelines to Orient Child to Pediatric Unit

1. Introduce the primary nurse.
2. Orient to the child's room:
    a. Demonstrate bed, bed controls, side rails.
    b. Demonstrate call light.
    c. Demonstrate television; include cost, if any.
    d. Show bathroom facilities.
    e. Explain telephone and rules that apply.
3. Introduce to roommate(s); include families.
4. Give directions to or show "special" rooms:
    a. Playroom—rules that apply, hours available, toys or equipment that may be taken to child's room
    b. Treatment room—explain purpose
    c. Unit kitchen—rules that apply
    d. Other special rooms
5. Explain pediatric rules; give written rules if available:
    a. Visiting hours, who may visit
    b. Mealtimes, rules about bringing in food
    c. Bedtimes, naptimes, or quiet time
    d. Rooming in arrangements
6. Explain daily routines:
    a. Vital signs routine
    b. Bath routine
    c. Other routines
7. Provide guidelines for involvement of family caregiver.

books to help prepare children for tonsillectomy or other specific surgical procedures. These books are given to children during the preadmission visit or sent to children at home before admission. Questions may be answered and anxieties explored during the visit. Children and their families often are hesitant to

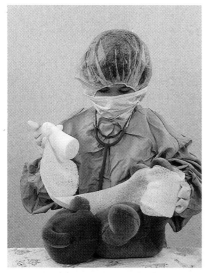

● **Figure 4.3** The child who is going to have surgery may act out the procedure on a doll, thereby reducing some of her fear. (© B. Proud.)

ask questions or express feelings; the staff must be sensitive to this problem and discuss common questions and feelings. Children are told that some things will hurt but that doctors and nurses will do everything they can to make the hurt go away. Honesty must be a keynote to any program of this kind. The preadmission orientation staff also must be sensitive to cultural and language differences and make adjustments whenever appropriate.

Emergency Admissions

Emergencies leave little time for explanation. The emergency itself is frightening to the child and the family, and the need for treatment is urgent. Even though a caregiver tries to act calm and composed, the child often may sense the anxiety. If the hospital is still a great unknown, it will only add to the child's fear and panic. If the child has even a basic understanding about hospitals and what happens there, the emergency may seem a little less frightening.

In an emergency, physical needs assume priority over emotional needs. When possible, the presence of a family caregiver who can conceal his or her own fear often is comforting to the child; however, the child may be angry that the caregiver does not prevent invasive procedures from being performed. Sometimes, however, it is impossible for the caregiver to stay with the child. A staff member may use this time to collect information about the child from the family member. This helps the family member to feel involved in the child's care.

Emergency department nurses must be sensitive to the needs of the child and the family. Recognizing the child's cognitive level and how it affects the child's reactions is important. In addition, the staff must explain procedures and conduct themselves in a caring, calm manner to reassure both the child and the family.

The Admission Interview

An admission interview is conducted as soon as possible after the child has been admitted. See Chapter 5, Assessment of the Child (Data Collection), for specific information related to the client interview and history. During the interview, an identification bracelet is placed on the child's wrist. If the child has allergies, an allergy bracelet must be placed on the wrist as well. The child must be prepared for even this simple procedure with an explanation of why it is necessary.

The nurse who receives the child on the pediatric unit should be friendly and casual, remembering that even a well-informed child may be shy and suspicious of excessive friendliness. The child who reacts with fear to well-meaning advances and who clings to the caregiver is telling the nurse to go more slowly with the acquaintance process. Children who know that the caregiver may stay with them are more quickly put at ease.

Through careful questioning, the interviewer tries to determine what the family's previous experience has been with hospitals and health care providers. It is also important to ascertain how much the caregiver and the child understand about the child's condition and their expectations of this hospitalization, what support systems are available when the child returns home, and any disturbing or threatening concerns on the part of the caregiver or the child. These findings, in addition to the client history and physical exam (see Chapter 5), form the basis for the patient's total plan of care while hospitalized.

The Admission Physical Examination

After the child has been oriented to the new surroundings by perhaps clinging to the family caregiver's hand or carrying a favorite toy or blanket, the caregiver may undress the child for the physical examination. This procedure may be familiar from previous health care visits. If comfortable with helping, the caregiver may stay with the child while the physical exam is being completed. See Chapter 5 for specific information related to the physical exam.

Discharge Planning

Planning for the child's discharge and care at home begins early in the hospital experience. Nurses and other health team members must assess the levels of understanding of the child and family and their abilities to learn about the child's condition and the care necessary after the child goes home. Giving medications, using special equipment, and enforcing necessary restrictions must be discussed with the person who will be the primary caregiver and with one other person, if possible. It is necessary to provide specific, written instructions for reference at home; the anxiety and strangeness of hospitalization often limit the amount of information retained from teaching sessions. The nurse must be certain the caregiver can understand the written materials too. If the treatment necessary at home appears too complex for the caregiver to manage, it may be helpful to arrange for a visiting nurse to assist for a period after the child is sent home.

Shortly before the child is discharged from the hospital, a conference may be arranged to review information and procedures with which the family caregivers must become familiar. This conference may or may not include the child, depending on his or her age and cognitive level. Questions and concerns must be dealt with honestly, and a resource such as a telephone number the caregiver can call should be offered for questions that arise after discharge.

The return home may be a difficult period of adjustment for the entire family. The preschool child may be aloof at first, followed by a period of clinging, demanding behavior. Other behaviors such as regression, temper tantrums, excessive attachment to a toy or blanket, night waking, and nightmares may demonstrate fear of another separation. The older child may demonstrate anger or jealousy of siblings. The family may be advised to encourage positive behavior and avoid making the child the center of attention because of the illness. Discipline should be firm, loving, and consistent. The child may express feelings verbally or in play activities. The family may be reassured that this is not unusual.

THE CHILD UNDERGOING SURGERY

Surgery frightens most adults, even though they understand why it is necessary and how it helps correct their health problem. Young children do not have this understanding and may become frightened of even a minor surgical procedure. If they are properly prepared, older children and adolescents are capable of understanding the need for surgery and what it will accomplish.

Many health care facilities have outpatient surgery facilities that are used for minor procedures and permit the patient to return home the day of the operation. These facilities reduce or eliminate the separation of parents and children, one of the most stressful factors in surgery for infants and young children. Whether admitted for less than 1 day or for several weeks, the child who has surgery needs sympathetic and thorough preoperative and postoperative care. When the child is too young to benefit from preoperative teaching, explanations should be directed to family caregivers to help relieve their anxiety and to prepare them to participate in the child's care after surgery.

Preoperative Care

Specific physical and psychological preparation of the child and the family varies according to the type of surgery planned. General aspects of care include patient teaching, skin preparation, preparation of the gastrointestinal and urinary systems, and preoperative medication.

Patient Teaching

The child admitted for planned surgery probably has had some preadmission preparation by the physician and family caregivers. Many families, however, have an unclear understanding of the surgery and what it involves, or they may be too anxious to be helpful. The health professionals involved in the child's care must determine how much the child knows and is capable of learning, help correct any misunderstandings, explain the preparation for surgery and what the surgery will "fix," as well as how the child will feel after surgery. This preparation must be based on the child's age, developmental level, previous experiences, and caregiver support. All explanations should be clear and honest and expressed in terms the child and the family caregivers can understand. Questions should be encouraged to ensure that the child and the family caregivers correctly understand all the information. If possible, preoperative teaching should be conducted in short sessions rather than trying to discuss everything at once.

Therapeutic play, discussed later in this chapter, is useful in preparing the child for surgery. Using drawings to identify the area of the body to be operated on helps the child have a better understanding of what is going to happen.

Children need to be prepared for standard preoperative tests and procedures such as radiographs and blood and urine tests. Nurses may explain the reason for withholding food and fluids before surgery so children do not feel they are being neglected or punished when others receive meal trays.

Children sometimes interpret surgery as punishment and should be reassured that they did not cause the condition. They also fear mutilation or death and must be able to explore those feelings, while recognizing them as acceptable fears. Children deserve careful explanation that the physician is going to repair only the affected body part.

It is important to emphasize that the child will not feel anything during surgery because of the special sleep that anesthesia causes. Describing the postanesthesia care unit (PACU or wake-up room) and any tubes, bandages, or appliances that will be in place after surgery lets the child know what to expect. If possible, the child should be able to see and handle the anesthesia mask (if this is the method to be used) and equipment that will be part of the postoperative experience.

Role playing, adjusted to the child's age and understanding, is helpful. This approach may include a trip on a stretcher and pretending to go to surgery. If the child requests, the nurse or play leader can pretend to be the patient.

The older child or adolescent may have a greater interest in the surgery itself, what is wrong and why, how the repair is done, and the expected postoperative results. Models of a child's internal organs or individual organs such as a heart are useful for demonstration, or the patient may be involved in making the drawing.

A child needs to understand that several people will be involved in preoperative, surgical, and postoperative care. If possible, staff members from the anesthesia department and the operating room, recovery room, or the ICU should visit the child preoperatively. Explaining what the people will be wearing (caps, masks, and gloves) and what equipment will be used (including bright lights) helps make the operating room experience less frightening. A preoperative tour of the ICU or PACU is also helpful.

Most patients experience postoperative pain, and children should be prepared for this experience. They also need to know when they may expect to be allowed to have fluids and food after surgery.

Children should be taught to practice coughing and deep-breathing exercises. Deep-breathing practice may be done with games that encourage blowing. Teaching children to splint the operative site with a pillow helps reassure them that the sutures will not break and allow the wound to open.

Children should be told where their family will be during and after surgery, and every effort should be made to minimize separation. Family caregivers should be encouraged to be present when the child leaves for the operating room.

Skin Preparation

Depending on the type of surgery, skin preparation may include a tub bath or shower and certainly includes special cleaning and inspection of the operative site. Shaving needed as part of the preparation usually is performed in the operating room. If fingers or toes are involved, the nails are carefully trimmed. The operative site may be painted with a special antiseptic solution as an extra precaution against infection, depending on the physician's orders and the procedures of the hospital.

Gastrointestinal and Urinary System Preparation

The surgeon may order a cleansing enema the night before surgery (see Chapter 6). An enema is an intrusive procedure and must be explained to the child before it is given. If old enough, the child should understand the reason for the enema.

Children usually receive nothing by mouth (NPO) 4 to 12 hours before surgery because food or fluids in the stomach may cause vomiting and aspiration particularly during general anesthesia. The child should be told that food and drink are being withheld to prevent an upset stomach. The NPO period varies according to the child's age; infants become dehydrated more rapidly than older children and thus require a shorter NPO period before surgery. Pediatric NPO orders should be accompanied by an intravenous (IV) fluid initiation order. Loose teeth are also a potential hazard and should be counted and recorded according to hospital policy.

In some instances, urinary catheterization may be performed preoperatively, but usually it is done while the child is in the operating room. The catheter is often removed immediately after surgery but can be left in place for several hours or days. Children who are not catheterized before surgery should be encouraged to void before the administration of preoperative medication.

Preoperative Medication

Depending on the physician's order, preoperative medications usually are given in two stages: a sedative is administered about 1.5 to 2 hours before surgery, and an analgesic-atropine mixture may be administered immediately before the patient leaves for the operating room. When the sedative has been given, the lights should be dimmed and noise minimized to help the child relax and rest. Family caregivers and the child should be aware that atropine could cause a blotchy rash and a flushed face.

Preoperative medication should be brought to the child's room when it is time for administration. At that time, the child is told that it is time for medication and that another nurse has come along to help the child hold still. Medication should be administered carefully and quickly because delays only increase the child's anxiety.

If hospital regulations permit, family caregivers should accompany the child to the operating room and wait until the child is anesthetized. If this is impossible, the nurse who has been caring for the child can go along to the operating room and introduce the child to personnel there.

Postoperative Care

During the immediate postoperative period, the child is cared for in the PACU or the surgical ICU. Meanwhile the room in the pediatric unit should be prepared with appropriate equipment for the child's return. Depending on the type of surgery performed, it may be necessary to have suctioning, resuscitation, or other equipment at the bedside.

When the child has been returned to the room, nursing care focuses on careful observation for any signs or symptoms of complications: shock, hemorrhage, or respiratory distress. Vital signs are monitored according to postoperative orders and recorded. The child is kept warm with blankets as needed. Dressings, IV apparatus, urinary catheters, and any other appliances are noted and observed. An IV flow sheet is begun that documents the type of fluid, the amount of fluid to be absorbed, the rate of flow, any additive medications, the site, and the site's appearance and condition. The IV flow sheet may be separate or incorporated into a general flow sheet for the pediatric patient. The first voiding is an important milestone in the child's postoperative progress because it indicates the adequacy of blood flow; it should be noted, recorded, and reported. Any irritation or burning also should be noted, and the physician should be notified if **anuria** (absence of urine) persists longer than 6 hours.

Postoperative orders may provide for ice chips or clear liquids to prevent dehydration; these may be administered with a spoon or in a small medicine cup. Frequent repositioning is necessary to prevent skin breakdown, orthostatic pneumonia, and decreased circulation. Coughing, deep breathing, and position changes are performed at least every 2 hours.

Pain Management

Pain is a concern of postoperative patients in any age group. Most adult patients can verbally express the pain they feel, so they request relief. However, infants and young children cannot adequately express themselves and need help to tell where or how great the pain is. Long-standing beliefs that children do not have the same amount of pain that adults have or that they tolerate pain better than adults have contributed to undermedicating infants and children in pain. Research has shown that children experience pain as keenly as adults do.

The nurse must be alert to indications of pain, especially in young patients. Careful assessment is necessary, for example noting changes in behavior such as rigidity, thrashing, facial expressions, loud crying or screaming, flexion of knees (indicating abdominal pain), restlessness, and irritability. Physiologic changes, such as increased pulse rate and blood pressure, sweating palms, dilated pupils, flushed or moist skin, and loss of appetite, also may indicate pain. Some children may try to hide pain because they fear an injection or because they are afraid that admitting to pain will increase the time they have to stay in the hospital.

Various tools have been devised to help children express the amount of pain they feel and allow nurses to measure the effectiveness of pain management efforts. These tools include the faces scale, the numeric scale, and the color scale. The first two scales are useful primarily with children 7 years of age and older (Fig. 4–4). To use the color scale, the young child is given crayons ranging from yellow to red or black. Yellow represents no pain, and the darkest color (or red) represents the most pain. The child selects the color that represents the amount of pain felt.

Pain medication may be administered orally, by routine intramuscular or IV routes, or by **patient-controlled analgesia,** a programmed IV infusion of narcotic analgesia that the child may control within set limits. A low-level dose of analgesia may be administered with the child able to administer a bolus as needed. Patient-controlled analgesia may be used for children 7 years of age or older who have no cognitive impairment and undergo a careful evaluation. Intramuscular injections are avoided if possible. Vital signs must be monitored, and the child's level of consciousness must be documented frequently following the standards of the facility.

Comfort measures should be used along with the administration of analgesics. The child is encouraged to become involved in activities that may provide distraction (Fig. 4–5). Such activities must be appropriate for the child's age, level of development, and interests. No child should be allowed to suffer pain

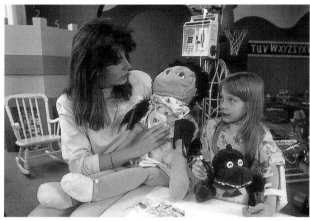

● *Figure 4.5* Distraction supplements pain control while a child is using PCA.

unnecessarily. Appropriate nonpharmacologic comfort measures may include position changes, massage, distraction, play, soothing touch, talk, coddling, and affection.

Surgical Dressings

Postoperative care includes close observation of any dressings for signs of drainage or hemorrhage and reinforcing or changing dressings as ordered. Wet dressings can increase the possibility of contamination; clean, dry dressings increase the child's comfort. If there is no physician's order to change the dressing, the nurse is expected to reinforce the moist original dressing by covering it with a dry dressing and taping the second dressing in place. If bloody drainage is present, the nurse should draw around the outline of the drainage with a marker and record the time and date. In this way the amount of additional drainage can be assessed when the dressings are inspected later.

Supplies needed for changing dressings vary according to the wound site and the physician's orders that specify the sterile or antiseptic technique to be used. Detailed procedures for these techniques

Numeric Scale

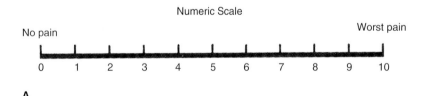

A

Faces Rating Scale

● *Figure 4.4* Pain scales: (*A*) numeric scale, (*B*) faces rating scale.

B

and the supplies to be used can be found in the facility's procedures manual.

As with all procedures, the nurse must explain to the child what will be done and why before beginning the dressing change. Some dressing changes are painful; if so, the child should be told that it will hurt and should be praised for behavior that shows courage and cooperation.

Patient Teaching

Postoperative patient teaching is as important as preoperative teaching. Some explanations and instructions given earlier must be repeated during postoperative care because the child's earlier anxiety may have prevented thorough understanding. Now that tubes, restraints, and dressings are part of the child's reality, they need to be discussed again: why they are important and how they affect the child's activities.

Family caregivers want to know how they can help care for the child and what limitations are placed on the child's activity. If caregivers know what to expect and how to aid in their child's recovery, they will be cooperative during the postoperative period.

As the child recuperates, the caregivers and child should be encouraged to share their feelings about the surgery, any changes in body image, and their expectations for recovery and rehabilitation.

When the sutures are removed, the nurse should reassure the child that the opening has healed and the child's insides will not "fall out," which is a common fear.

Before the child is discharged from the hospital, teaching focuses on home care, use of any special equipment or appliances, medications, diet, restrictions on activities, and therapeutic exercise (Fig. 4–6). Caregivers should demonstrate the procedures or repeat information so the nurse can determine if learning has occurred. The nursing process is used to assess the needs of the child and the family to plan appropriate postoperative care and teaching.

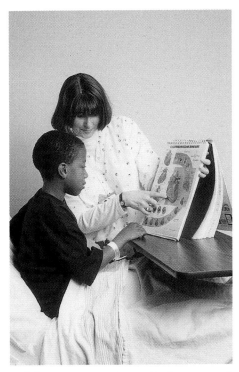

● **Figure 4.6** The nurse uses charts with pictures to perform patient teaching before the child goes home.

without the fear of being scolded by the nursing staff. Children who keep these negative emotions bottled up suffer much greater damage than those who are allowed to express them where they may be handled constructively. Children must feel secure enough in the situation to express negative emotions without fear of disapproval.

Children, however, must not be allowed to harm themselves or others. Although it is important to express acceptable or unacceptable feelings, unlimited permissiveness is as harmful as excessive strictness. Children rely on adults to guide them and set limits for behavior because this means the adults care about them. When behavior correction is necessary, it is important to make it clear that the child's action, not the child, is being disapproved.

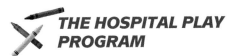

THE HOSPITAL PLAY PROGRAM

Play is the business of children and a principal way in which they learn, grow, develop, and act out feelings and problems. Playing is a normal activity; the more it can be part of hospital care, the more normal and more comfortable this environment becomes.

Play helps children come to terms with the hurts, anxieties, and separation that accompany hospitalization. In the hospital playroom, children may express frustrations, hostilities, and aggressions through play

The Hospital Play Environment

An organized and well-planned play area is of considerable importance in the overall care of the hospitalized child (Fig. 4–7). The play area should be large enough to accommodate cribs, wheelchairs, IV poles, and children in casts. It should provide a variety of play materials suitable for the ages and needs of all children. The child chooses the toy and the kind of play needed or desired; thus the selection and kind of play may usually be left unstructured. However, all children should participate, and the play leaders should ignore no one.

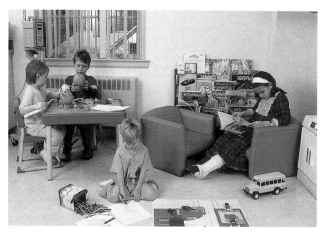

● *Figure 4.7* Children occupied in a hospital playroom. (© B. Proud.)

If possible, adolescents should have a separate recreation room or area. Ideally this is an area where adolescents may gather to talk, play pool or table tennis, drink soft drinks (if permitted), and eat snacks. Tables and chairs should be provided to encourage interaction among the adolescents. Television with a videocassette tape player, computer games, and shuffleboard are also desirable. These activities should be in an area away from young children. Rules may be clearly spelled out and posted. If adolescents must share the same recreation area with younger children, the area should be referred to as the "activity center" rather than the "playroom."

Although a well-equipped playroom is of major importance in any pediatric department, some children cannot be brought to the playroom, or some play programs may be cut due to cost-containment efforts. In these situations, nurses must be creative in providing play opportunities for children. Children may act out their fantasies and emotions in their own cribs or beds if materials are brought to them and someone (a nurse, student or volunteer) is available to give them needed support and attention. Children in isolation may be given play material, providing infection control precautions are strictly followed.

Therapeutic Play

The nurse should understand the difference between play therapy and therapeutic play. **Play therapy** is a technique of psychoanalysis that psychiatrists or psychiatric nurse clinicians use to uncover a disturbed child's underlying thoughts, feelings, and motivations to help understand them better. **Therapeutic play** is a play technique that play therapists, nurses, child-life specialists, or trained volunteers may use to help the child express feelings, fears, and concerns.

The play leader should be alert to the needs of the child who is afraid to act independently as a result of strict home discipline. Even normally sociable children may carry their fears of the hospital environment into the playroom. It could be some time before timid, fearful, or nonassertive children feel free enough to take advantage of the play opportunities. Too much enthusiasm on the part of the play leader in trying to get the child to participate may defeat the purpose and make the child withdraw. The leader must decide carefully whether to initiate an activity for a child or let the child advance at a self-set pace.

Often other children provide the best incentive by doing something interesting, so that the timid child forgets his or her apprehensions and tries it, or another child says, "Come and help me with this," and soon the other child becomes involved. A fearful child trusts a peer before trusting an adult, who represents authority. Naturally this fact does not mean that the adult ignores the child's presence. The leader shows the child around the playroom, indicating that the children are free to play with whatever they wish and that the leader is there to answer questions and to help when a child wishes help.

When group play is initiated, the leader may invite but not insist that the timid child participate. The leader must give the child time to adjust and gain confidence.

Play Material

Play material should be chosen with safety in mind; there should be no sharp edges and no small parts that can be swallowed or aspirated. Toys and equipment should be inspected regularly for broken parts or sharp edges. Constant supervision of children while they are playing is necessary for safety.

One important playroom function is that it gives the child opportunities to dramatize hospital experiences. One section of the playroom containing hospital equipment, miniature or real, gives the child an opportunity to act out feelings about the hospital environment and treatments. Stethoscopes, simulated thermometers, stretchers, wheelchairs, examining tables, instruments, bandages, and other medical and hospital equipment are useful for this purpose.

Dolls or puppets dressed to represent the people with whom the child comes in contact daily—a boy, girl, infant, adult family members, nurses, physicians, therapists, and other personnel—should be available. Hospital scrub suits, scrub caps, isolation-type gowns, masks, or other types of uniforms may be provided for children to use in acting out their hospital experiences. These simulated hospitals also serve an educational purpose: they may help a child who is to have surgery, tests, or special treatments to understand the procedures and why they are done.

Other useful materials include clay, paints, markers, crayons, stamps, stickers, sand art, cut-out books, construction paper, puzzles, building sets, and board games. Tricycles, small sliding boards, and seesaws may be fun for children who can be more physically active. Books for all age groups are also important.

Sometimes only a little imagination is needed to initiate an interesting playtime. Table 4–1 suggests activities for various age levels, most of which may be played in the child's room. These are especially useful for the child who cannot go to the playroom.

Puppets play an important part in the children's department. The use of hand puppets does much to orient or reassure a hospitalized child. The doctor or nurse puppet on the play leader's hand answers questions (and discusses feelings) that the puppet on the child's hand has asked. A child often finds it easier to express feelings, fears, and questions through a puppet than to verbalize them directly. A ready sense of magic can let the child make believe

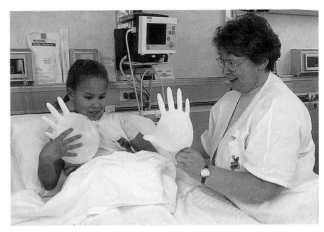

● **Figure 4.8** A puppet playgroup led by a pediatric nurse oncologist allows children to talk about what it's like to be in the hospital. Group sessions inform children that others have similar feelings. (© B. Proud.)

that the puppet is really expressing things that he or she hesitates to ask (Fig. 4–8).

TABLE 4.1	Games and Activities Using Materials Available on a Nursing Unit
Age	**Activity**
Infant	Make a mobile from roller gauze and tongue blades to hang over a crib.
	Ask the pharmacy or central supply for different size boxes to use for put-in, take-out toys. (Do not use round vials from pharmacy; if accidentally aspirated, these can completely occlude the airway.)
	Blow up a glove as a balloon; draw a smiling face on it with a marker. Hang it out of infant's reach.
	Play "patty cake," "So Big," "Peek-a-boo."
Toddler	Ask central supply for boxes to use as blocks for stacking.
	Tie roller gauze to a glove box for a pull toy.
	Sing or recite familiar nursery rhymes such as "Peter, Peter, Pumpkin Eater."
Preschool	Play "Simon Says" or "Mother, May I?"
	Draw a picture of a dog; ask child to close eyes; add an additional feature to the dog; ask child to guess the added part, repeat until a full picture is drawn.
	Make a puppet from a lunch bag or draw a face on your hand with a marker.
	Cut out a picture from a newspaper or a magazine (or draw a picture); cut it into large puzzle pieces.
	Pour breakfast cereal into a basin; furnish boxes to pour and spoons to dig.
	Furnish chart paper and a magic marker for coloring.
	Make modeling clay from 1 cup salt, ½ cup flour, ½ cup water from diet kitchen.
	Play "Ring-Around-the-Rosey" or "London Bridge."
School-age	Play "I Spy" or charades.
	Make a deck of cards to play "Go Fish" or "Old Maid"; invent cards such as Nicholas Nurse, Doctor Dolittle, Irene Intern, Polly Patient.
	Play "Hangman."
	Furnish scale or table paper and a magic marker for a hug drawing or sign.
	Hide an object in the child's room and have the child look for it (have the child name places for you to look if the child cannot be out of bed).
Adolescent	Color squares on a chart form to make a checker board.
	Have adolescent make a deck of cards to use for "Hearts" or "Rummy."
	Compete to see how many words the adolescent can make from the letters in his or her name.
	Compete to guess whether the next person to enter the room will be a man or woman, next car to go by window will be red or black, and so forth.
	Compete to see who can name the most episodes of the television show "Star Trek" or reruns of "The Brady Bunch."

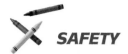

SAFETY

Safety is an essential aspect of pediatric nursing care. Accidents occur more often when people are in stressful situations; infants, children, and their caregivers experience additional stress when a child is hospitalized. They are removed from a familiar home environment, faced with anxieties and fear, and must adjust to an unfamiliar schedule. Consciously

assessing every situation for accident potential, the pediatric nurse must have safety in mind at all times.

The environment should meet all the safety standards appropriate for other areas of the facility including good lighting, dry floors with no obstacles that may cause falls, electrical equipment checked for hazards, safe bath and shower facilities, and beds in low position for ambulatory patients.

The child's age and developmental level must be considered. Toddlers are explorers whose developmental task is to develop autonomy. Toddlers love to put small objects into equally small openings, whether the opening is in their bodies, the oxygen tent, or elsewhere in the pediatric unit. Careful observation to eliminate dangers may prevent the toddler from having access to small objects. Toddlers are also often climbers and must be protected from climbing and falling. Toddlers and preschoolers must be watched to protect them from danger. Nurses also must encourage family members to keep the crib sides up when not directly caring for the infant in the crib. One unguarded moment may mean that the infant falls out of a crib. Box 4–2 presents a summary of pediatric safety precautions.

BOX 4.2	Safety Precautions for Pediatric Units

1. Cover electrical outlets.
2. Keep floor dry and free of clutter.
3. Use tape or Velcro closures when possible.
4. Always close safety pins when not in use.
5. Inspect toys (child's or hospital's) for loose or small parts, sharp edges, dangerous cords, or other hazards.
6. Do not permit friction toys where oxygen is in use.
7. Do not leave child unattended in high chair.
8. Keep crib sides up all the way except when caring for child.
9. If the crib side is down, keep hand firmly on infant at all times.
10. Use crib with top if child stands or climbs.
11. Always check temperature of bath water to prevent burns.
12. Never leave infant or child unattended in bath water.
13. Keep beds of ambulatory children locked in low position.
14. Turn off motor of electric bed if young children might have access to controls.
15. Always use safety belts or straps for children in infant seats, feeding chairs, strollers, wheelchairs, or stretchers.
16. Use restraints only when necessary.
17. When restraints are used, remove and check for skin integrity, circulation, and correct application at least every hour or two.
18. Never tie a restraint to the crib side; tie to bed frame only.
19. Keep medications securely locked in designated area; children should never be permitted in this area.
20. Set limits and enforce them consistently; do not let children get out of control.
21. Place needles and syringes in sharps containers; make sure children have no access to these containers.
22. Always pick up any equipment after a procedure.
23. Never leave scissors or other sharp instruments within child's reach.
24. Do not allow sleepy family caregivers to hold a sleeping child as they may fall asleep and drop the child.

KEY POINTS

▶ Many factors affect the way the family reacts to hospitalization of the child. These factors may place great stress on the child and the family.

▶ Preadmission education helps prepare the child for the event. Nevertheless, many anxieties persist. An child's emergency admission may be especially traumatic for both the child and the family.

▶ Liberal visiting policies, encouraging family caregivers to stay with young children, and sibling visits help decrease the stress of hospitalization.

▶ Conscientious handwashing is the cornerstone of infection control. Standard precautions are applied to all patients of every age and diagnosis.

▶ The family caregiver is an vital participant in the care of an ill child and should be included in planning of nursing care.

▶ The admission interview sets the stage for the hospitalization and provides information that helps the health care team give the best possible care to the child and help him or her adjust to the hospitalization.

▶ Discharge planning includes teaching the child and the family about care needed after discharge from the hospital. Discharge teaching should include written and verbal instructions; the nurse must be certain that instructions are fully understood.

Assessment of the Child (Data Collection)

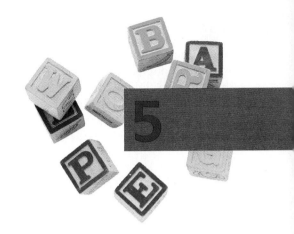

5

COLLECTING SUBJECTIVE DATA
  Conducting the Client Interview
  Obtaining a Client History
COLLECTING OBJECTIVE DATA
  General Status

Measuring Head Circumference
Vital Signs
Providing a Physical Examination
Assisting with Common Diagnostic
Tests

STUDENT OBJECTIVES

On completion of this chapter, the student will be able to

1. Describe the process for collecting subjective data from caregivers, children and adolescents.
2. Define chief complaint.
3. Explain the purpose of doing a review of systems when gathering data.
4. State how the caregiver may be involved in collecting objective data about the child.
5. Compare observations indicating health or illness of an infant or young child.
6. Describe three additional useful observations of the older child.
7. Discuss the reasons that height and weight are assessed on an ongoing basis.
8. List the types of patients on whom a rectal temperature should not be taken.
9. Identify the five types of respiratory retractions and the location of each.
10. State the purpose of pulse oximetry.
11. Name three methods of obtaining blood pressure.
12. Discuss the process of conducting a physical examination.
13. Explain the reason a physical exam is performed.
14. Identify the purpose of using the Glasgow coma scale for neurologic assessment.
15. Discuss the role of the nurse in assisting in common diagnostic tests and procedures.

KEY TERMS

fontanels
nutrition history
personal history
pinna
point of maximum impulse (PMI)
school history
social history
symmetry

Whether the setting is a hospital or other health care facility, it is important to gather information regarding the child's history and current status. Although data collection is continuous throughout a child's care, most data is collected during the interview, the physical examination, and from the results of diagnostic tests and studies.

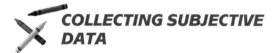

COLLECTING SUBJECTIVE DATA

Information spoken by the child or family is called subjective data. Interviewing the family caregiver and child allows the nurse to collect information that can be used to develop a plan of care for the child. The interview process is goal-directed.

Conducting the Client Interview

Most subjective data is collected through interviewing the family caregiver and the child. The interview helps establish a relationship between the nurse, the child, and the family. Listening and using appropriate communication techniques helps promote a good interview (see Chapter 1). Using focused questions and allowing time for answering will help the child and family feel comfortable. A private, quiet setting decreases distractions during the interview. The nurse should be introduced to the child and caregiver and the purpose of the interview stated. A calm, reassuring manner is important to establish trust and comfort. Past experiences with health care may influence the interview. The caregiver and the nurse should be comfortably seated, and the child should be included in the interview process (Fig. 5–1). The child may sit on the caregiver's lap or, if a crib is available, the child can be placed in the crib with the side-rails up. This will help to insure the safety of the infant or child during the interview. Age-appropriate toys and activities to keep young children occupied will allow the caregiver to focus on the questions asked. Being aware of the primary language spoken and using an interpreter when needed will help in gaining accurate information. Various cultural patterns, such as avoiding eye contact, should be noted and respected.

Interviewing Family Caregivers

The family caregiver provides most of the information needed in caring for the child, especially the infant or toddler. Rather than simply asking the caregiver to fill out a form, the nurse may ask the questions and write down the answers; this process gives the opportunity to observe the reactions of the child and the caregiver as they interact with each

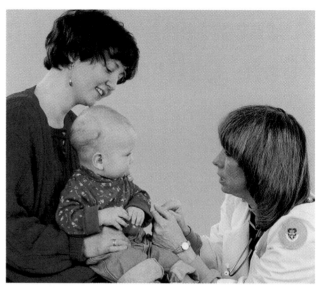

● **Figure 5.1** The child sits on the caregiver's lap during the interview process.

other and answer the questions. In addition, this eases the problem of the caregiver who cannot read or write. The nurse must be nonjudgmental, being careful not to indicate disapproval by verbal or nonverbal responses. While gathering information about the child's physical condition, the nurse also must allow the caregiver to express concerns and anxieties. If a certain topic seems uncomfortable for the caregiver to discuss in front of the child, that topic should be discussed later when the child cannot hear what is being said.

Interviewing the Child

It is important that the preschool child and the older child be included in the interview. Use age-appropriate questions when talking with the child. Showing interest in the child and what she or he says helps both the child and caregiver to feel comfortable. Using a doll or stuffed animal that the child is familiar with can help involve the child in the interview process. By being honest when answering the child's questions, the nurse establishes trust with the child. Using stories or books written at a child's level helps with understanding what the child is thinking or feeling. The child's comments should be listened to attentively, and the child should be made to feel important in the interview.

INTERNET EXERCISE 5.1

http://www.meddean.luc.edu/lumen/DeptWebs/emschild/stndrd-teaching.htm

Download Initial Pediatric Assessment Teaching Tool. Scroll down to section III General Approach to the Stable Pediatric Patient.

1. List five suggestions for the nurse to use in approaching the pediatric patient.

Scroll down to section V Initial inspection.

2. List five observations that the nurse would make when first approaching the child.

Interviewing the Adolescent

Adolescents can provide information about themselves; interviewing them in private often encourages them to share information that they might not contribute in front of their caregivers. This is especially true when asking questions of a sensitive nature such as information regarding drug use or the adolescent's sexual practices.

Obtaining a Client History

When a child is brought to any healthcare setting, it is important to gather information regarding the child's current condition as well as past medical history. This information is used to develop a plan of care for the child. In obtaining information from the child and caregiver, the nurse is developing a relationship as well as noting what the child and family know and understand about the child's health. Observations of the caregiver-child relationship can also provide important information.

Biographical Data

To begin obtaining a client history, the nurse collects and records identifying information about the child including the child's name, address, and phone number as well as information regarding the caregiver. This information is part of the legal record and should be treated as confidential. A questionnaire often is used to gather information such as the child's nickname, feeding habits, food likes and dislikes, allergies, sleeping schedule, and toilet-training status. Any special words the child uses or understands to indicate needs or desires, such as words used for urinating and bowel movements, would be included on the questionnaire. Figure 5–2 provides an example of an assessment form that may be used to collect information.

Chief Complaint

The reason for the child's visit to the health care setting is called the chief complaint. In a well-child setting, this reason might be a routine check or immunizations, whereas an illness or other condition might be the reason in another setting. The caregiver's primary concern is his or her reason for seeking health care for the child. To best care for the child, it is important to get the most complete explanation of what brought the child to the health care setting.

Repeating the caregiver's statement regarding the child's chief complaint will help to clarify that the nurse has correctly heard what the caregiver has said.

History of Present Health Concern

To help the nurse discover the child's needs, the nurse elicits information about the current situation, including the child's symptoms, when they began, how long the symptoms have been present, a description of the symptoms, their intensity and frequency, and treatments up to this time. The nurse should ask the questions in a way that encourages the caregiver to be specific. This is also the time for the nurse to ask the caregiver about any other concerns regarding the child.

Past Health History

Information regarding the mother's pregnancy and prenatal history are included in obtaining a past health history for the child. Any occurrences during the delivery can contribute to the child's health concerns. The child's mother is usually the best source of this information. Other areas the nurse asks questions about include common childhood, serious, or chronic illnesses; immunizations and health maintenance; feeding and nutrition; as well as hospitalizations and injuries.

Family Health History

Some diseases and conditions are seen in families and are important in prevention as well as detection for the child. The caregiver can usually provide information regarding family health history. The nurse uses this information to do preventative teaching with the child and family. Certain risk factors in families contribute to the development of health care concerns; risk factors addressed early in a child's life can often be monitored or changed to decrease the child's risk of getting these diseases or conditions.

Review of Systems for Current Health Problem

While the nurse is collecting subjective data, the caregiver or child is asked questions about each body system. Using a head-to-toe approach, information is gathered that helps to focus the physical exam as well as to get an overall picture of the child's current status. The body system involved in the chief complaint is reviewed in detail. As other body systems are discussed, it is important to reassure the caregiver that the chief complaint has not been forgotten or ignored. In doing a review of the body systems, the nurse needs to include the areas listed in Table 5–1.

Allergies, Medications, Substance Abuse

Allergic reactions to any foods, medications, or any other known allergies should be discussed to

PEDIATRIC NURSING ASSESSMENT FORM

1. Name _____ Date/Time of Admission _____ Via _____

2. Birth Date _____ Information obtained from:_____ Relationship to child _____

3. Child's legal guardian: _____ Child's Nickname: _____

VITAL SIGNS	Temp	Apical Pulse	Radial Pulse	Respirations	BP	Height	Weight	Head Circum

CURRENT CHIEF COMPLAINT/DIAGNOSIS:
Symptoms and Duration

Child's/Caregivers' Understanding of Condition:

PREVIOUS ILLNESS/INJURIES/DIAGNOSIS:
Illness, Symptoms, and Duration

Injuries or Surgery:

Anesthesia Complications?

Allergies and Reactions:	Immunizations	Dates:	Exposure to Infectious Disease	Date
	DPT (DT)		(chicken pox, measles, etc.)	
	Oral Polio			
	Hepatitis B			
	Hib (type)			
	MMR (measles, mumps, rubella)			
	TB skin test Result			

Medications: Name:	Dose	Frequency	Time of Last Dose

Child's reaction to previous hospitalizations: _____

Special fears of child about hospitalization? _____

Family History: (Check all that apply—indicate relationship to child)

_____ Cancer _____   _____ Seizures _____   _____ TB _____

_____ Heart disease _____   _____ Asthma _____   _____ Anesthesia complications_____

_____ Allergy _____   _____ Smoking _____   _____ Other (specify) _____

_____ Diabetes _____   _____ Hypertension _____

● *Figure 5.2* A sample pediatric nursing assessment form.

Living Facilities (check)

_____ House _____ Apartment _____ Trailer _____ Steps to travel? _____

Who does child live with? _____

Names, ages, of siblings in home _____

Names, ages of other children in home _____

Other persons in home _____

Special interests, toys, games, hobbies: _____

_____

Security object: _____ Was it brought to hospital? _____

Bowel/Bladder Habits:

Toilet Training (if applicable)

    Started _____ Yes _____ No

    Completed _____ Yes _____ No

Diapers:

    Day _____ Yes _____ No

    Night _____ Yes _____ No

Potty Chair: _____ Yes _____ No

Toilet: _____ Yes _____ No

Bedwetter: _____ Yes _____ No

Terms Used for:

Bowel Movement _____ Urination _____

Frequency of BM _____ Color _____ Consistency _____

Does child have problems with diarrhea or constipation? _____

_____

Does child have urinary frequency, burning, discomfort: _____ Yes _____ No

If yes, please explain: _____

_____

_____

Patterns of:

Sleep/rest:

Bedtime _____ Wakeup _____

Nap ____ Yes ____ No — When? _____

Activity:

Does infant roll over? _____

Does child stand/walk? _____

Does child climb? _____

Does child dress self? _____

Does child go up and down stairs? _____

Does child talk in formed sentences? _____

Eating Habits:

Does child: Feed self _____ Yes _____ No

Does child need help to eat? _____

Food and beverage:

    Likes: _____

_____

    Dislikes: _____

_____

Usual appetite? _____

Appetite now? _____

Last time child had food or beverage: _____

Items brought to hospital:

Glasses _____ Yes _____ No

Contacts _____ Yes _____ No

Hearing Aid _____ Yes _____ No

Dentures _____ Yes _____ No

Braces _____ Yes _____ No

Retainer _____ Yes _____ No

Special bottle _____ Yes _____ No

Own pacifier _____ Yes _____ No

Does child smoke or drink alcoholic beverages? _____ Yes _____ No

    If yes, please give details _____

_____

Does child use street drugs? _____ Yes _____ No

    If yes, please give details _____

_____

Other behavior habits of the child (Please check)

    Thumbsucking _____ ; Nailbiting _____ ; Headbanging _____

    Rituals (Explain) _____

_____

    Disposition (Describe) _____

_____

Skin Assessment:

_____ Jaundice _____ Cyanosis _____ Pallor _____ Redness

_____ Cool _____ Warm _____ Clammy _____ Dry

_____ Normal appearance

Describe: (Location and character)

    Rash _____

    Abrasions _____

    Lacerations _____

    Contusions _____

Respiratory Assessment:

_____ Clear _____ Stridor _____ Rales (___ moist, ___ dry) _____ Wheezing

_____ Rhonchi _____ Retractions (type) _____

_____ Coughing, Sneezing _____ Nasal Discharge (describe) _____

Child/Caregiver oriented to unit? _____ Yes _____ No; understanding verbalized by child _____, caregiver _____

Reviewed safety measures with child _____, caregiver _____; understanding verbalized by child _____, caregiver _____

Additional information nursing staff should know:

● **_Figure 5.2_** Continued

TABLE 5.1	Review of Systems
Areas to Be Reviewed	
General	Weight gain or loss, fatigue, colds, illnesses, behavior changes, edema
Skin	Itching, dryness, rash, color change
Head and neck	Headache, dizziness, injury, stiff neck, swollen neck glands
Eyes	Drainage, trouble focusing or seeing, rubbing, redness
Ears	Pulling, pain, drainage, difficulty hearing
Nose, mouth, throat	Nosebleeds, drainage, trouble breathing, toothache, sore throat, trouble swallowing
Chest and lungs—respiratory	Coughing, wheezing, shortness of breath, sputum, breast development, pain
Heart—cardiovascular	Cyanosis, fatigue, anemia, heart murmurs
Abdomen—gastrointestinal	Nausea, vomiting, pain
Genitalia and rectum	Pain or burning when voiding, blood in urine or stool, constipation, diarrhea
Back and extremities Musculoskeletal	Extremities—pain, difficult movement, swollen joints, broken bones, muscle sprains
Neurologic	Seizures, loss of consciousness

prevent the child being given any medications or substances that might cause an allergic reaction. Medications the child is taking or has taken in the past, whether prescribed by a care provider or over the counter, are recorded. This information will help avoid the possibility of overmedicating or causing drug interactions. It is important, especially in the adolescent, to assess the use of substances such as tobacco, alcohol or illegal drugs (substance abuse is covered in Chapter 19).

Lifestyle

School history includes information regarding the adolescent's current grade level and academic performance as well as behavior seen at school. Interactions between teachers and peers often give insight into areas of concern for the child that might affect the child's health.

Social history offers information about the environment that the child lives in including the home setting, parent's occupations, siblings, family pets, religious affiliations and economic factors. The persons who live in the home and those who care for the child are important data, especially in cases of separation or divorce.

Personal history relates to data collected about such things as the child's hygiene and sleeping and elimination patterns. Activities, exercise, special interests, and the child's favorite toys or objects are included. Questions about relationships and how the child emotionally handles certain situations can help in understanding the child. Any behaviors such as thumb sucking, nail biting, or temper tantrums are discussed.

Nutrition history of the child offers information regarding eating habits and preferences as well as nutrition concerns that might indicate illness.

Developmental Level

Gathering information about the child's developmental level is done by asking questions directly related to growth and development milestones. These milestones will be discussed in detail in the growth and development chapters of this text. Knowing normal development patterns will help the nurse determine if there are concerns that should be further assessed regarding the child's development.

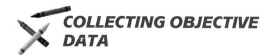

COLLECTING OBJECTIVE DATA

The collection of objective data includes the nurse doing a baseline measurement of the child's height, weight, blood pressure, temperature, pulse, and respiration. Data is also collected by examination of the body systems. Often the exam for a child is not done in a head-to-toe manner as in adults but rather in an order that takes the child's age and developmental needs into consideration. Aspects of the exam that might be more traumatic or uncomfortable for the child, such as examining the nose or mouth, are saved to be done last. The procedure of the physical exam may be familiar from previous health care visits. If comfortable with helping, the caregiver may be involved in helping with the data collection. For example the caregiver might help take a young child's temperature and obtain a urine specimen. Arrangements should be made so that the caregiver also may be present, if possible, for tests or examinations that need to be performed. Included in this initial exam is an inspection of the child's body. All observations are recorded. The nurse carefully documents any finding that is not within normal limits and describes in detail any unusual findings.

The nurse conducts or assists in conducting a complete physical exam with special attention to any symptoms that the caregiver has identified. The nurse's primary role in the complete assessment may be to support the child. All the information gathered is used to plan the child's care.

General Status

The nurse uses knowledge of normal growth and development to note if the child appears to fit the characteristics of the stated age. Interactions the child has with caregivers and siblings provide the nurse information about these relationships. The child's overall general appearance, facial expressions, speech, and behavior are noted as the nurse begins collecting information about the child.

Observing General Appearance

Observing physical appearance and condition can give clues to the child's overall health. The infant or child's face and body should be symmetrical (i.e., well balanced). Observe for nutritional status, hygiene, mental alertness and body posture and movements. Examine the skin for color, lesions, bruises, scars, and birthmarks. Observe hair texture, thickness and distribution.

Noting Psychological Status and Behavior

Carefully observing the child's behavior and recording those observations provide vital clues to a child's condition. Observation of behavior should include factors that influenced the behavior and how often the behavior is repeated. Physical behavior as well as emotional and intellectual responses should be noted. Also consider the child's age and developmental level, the abnormal environment of the health care facility, and if the child has been hospitalized previously or otherwise separated from family caregivers. It is important to note if the behavior is consistent or unpredictable and any apparent reasons for changed behavior.

Characteristic behaviors of the healthy infant or older child compared with behaviors that may indicate signs of illness are shown in Table 5–2. The nurse must be cautious when using the type of information shown in such a table because occasional evidence of one or more of the behaviors may not be significant. Any instance of behavior indicating illness needs to be documented and further evaluated in light of the behavior frequency as well as the infant's usual behavior. If the caregiver has indicated in the interview or on further questioning that this behavior is not out of the ordinary for the infant, it may not be indicative of a problem.

Measuring Height and Weight

The child's height and weight are helpful indicators of growth and development. Height and weight should be measured and recorded each time the child has a routine physical examination as well as at other health care visits. These measurements must be charted and compared with norms for the child's age (see Appendix A). Plotting the child's growth on a growth charts gives a good indication of the child's health status. This process gives a picture of how the child is progressing and often indicates wellness. Although the charts are indicators, the size of other family members, the child's illnesses, general nutritional status, and developmental milestones also must be considered.

In a hospital setting, the infant or child should be weighed at the same time each day on the same scales while wearing the same amount of clothing. An infant is weighed naked with no shirt or diaper. The nurse must keep a hand within 1 inch of the infant at all times to be ready to protect the infant from injury. The scale is covered with a fresh paper towel or clean sheet of paper as a means of infection control (Box 5–1). An older infant may sit up on the scale, but the nurse must still keep a hand ready to protect the infant from injury (Fig. 5–3A). A child who can stand alone steadily is weighed on platform-type scales. The child should be weighed without shoes. Bed scales may be used if the child cannot get out of bed. Weights are recorded in grams and kilograms or pounds and ounces.

The child who can stand usually is measured for height at the same time. The standing scales have a useful, adjustable measuring device (Fig. 5–3B). An infant is measured while lying on a flat surface. Usually examining tables have a measuring device mounted along the side of the table. The infant is measured flat with knees held flat to the table. Height is recorded in centimeters or inches according to the practice of the health care facility; the nurse must know which measuring system is used.

Measuring Head Circumference

The head circumference is measured routinely in children up to the age of 2 or 3 or in any child with a neurologic concern. A paper or metal tape measure is placed around the largest part of the head just above the eyebrows and around the most prominent part of the back of the head (Fig. 5–4). This measurement is recorded and plotted on a growth chart kept to monitor the growth of the child's head.

TABLE 5.2	Comparison of Observations of an Infant's Physical and Emotional Behavior	
Observation	Healthy Activity	Behavior Indicating Illness*
Activity	Constantly active; some infants are more intense and curious than others.	Lies quietly; little or no interest in surroundings; may stay in the same position
State of muscular tension	Muscular state is tense; grasp is tight; head is raised when prone; kicks are vigorous. When supine, there is a space between the mattress and the infant's back.	Lies relaxed with arms and legs straight and lax; makes no attempt to turn or raise head if placed in prone position; does not move about in crib
Constancy of reaction	Shows a constancy in reaction; does not regress in development; peppy and vigorous; interested in food; responds to caregiver's presence or voice	Not as peppy as usual; responds to discomfort and pain in apathetic manner; turns away from food that had once interested; turns head and cries instead of usual response
Behavior indicating pain	Appreciates being picked up Activity is not restlessness. Shows activity in every part of body	Cries or protests when handled; seems to want to be left alone. May cry when picked up, but settles down after being held for a time, indicating something hurts when moved Turns head fretfully from side to side; pulls ear or rubs head; turns and rolls constantly; seemingly to try to get away from pain
Cry	Strong, vigorous cry	Weak, feeble cry or whimper High-pitched cry; shrill cry may indicate increased intracranial pressure
Skin color	Healthy tint to skin; nail beds, oral mucosa, conjunctivae, and tongue are reddish-pink	Light-skinned babies may show unusual pallor or blueness around the eyes and nose. All babies may have dark or cyanotic nail beds; pale oral mucosa, conjuctivae, and tongue.
Appetite or feeding pattern	Exhibits an eagerness and impatience to satisfy hunger	May show indifference toward formula; sucks half-heartedly; vomits feeding; habitually regurgitates. May exhibit discomfort after feeding
Bizarre behavior		Any behavior that differs from expected for level of development; unusually good, or passive when in strange surroundings; responds with rejection to every overture, friendly or otherwise; extremely clinging, never satisfied with amount of attention received

*Any *one* manifestation in itself may not be significant. The important thing is whether this behavior is consistent with this particular child or is a change from previous behavior. The significance depends greatly on the constancy of the behavior.

BOX 5.1	Weighing the Infant

1. Prepare the scale by covering it with paper, cloth diaper, or sheet and by balancing it.
2. Place the naked infant on the scale and weigh the infant. *Always* hold your hand within an inch or so of the infant to be ready to take hold if necessary.
3. Pick up the infant and discard the scale cover.
4. Read the weight and record it on the worksheet or scrap paper.
5. Clean the scale according to the facility's policy. If the baby's weight varies significantly from the previous weight, have another person check it with you. Document and report the weight as appropriate. The ill infant often needs to be weighed daily to assess growth or fluid balance. Weights should be taken every day at the same time with the same scale.

Vital Signs

Vital signs including temperature, pulse, respirations, and blood pressure are taken at each visit and compared to the normal values for children of the same age as well as to that child's previous recordings. In a hospital setting, the vital signs are closely monitored and recorded; any changes are reported. Keeping in mind the child's developmental needs will increase the nurse's ability to take accurate vital sign measurements. It will usually be less traumatic for the infant if the nurse counts the respirations before the child is disturbed, then takes the pulse and the temperature.

Temperature

The method of measuring a child's temperature commonly is set by the policy of the health care

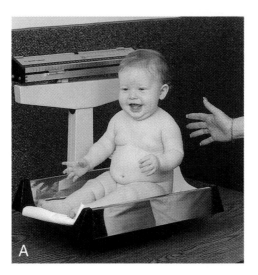
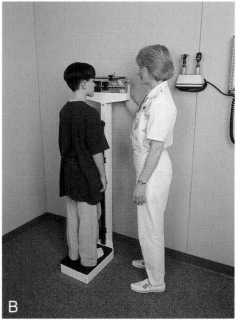

● **Figure 5.3 (A)** The nurse keeps a hand close to the infant while weighing. **(B)** The older child can be measured for weight and height on a standing scale.

setting. The temperature can be measured by oral, rectal, axillary, or tympanic method. Temperatures are recorded in Celsius or Fahrenheit according to the policy of the health care facility. A normal oral temperature range is 36.4°C to 37.4°C (97.6°F to 99.3°F). A rectal temperature is usually 0.5° to 1.0° higher than the oral measurement. An axillary temperature usually measures 0.5° to 1.0° lower than the oral measurement. The temperature measurement taken by the tympanic method is in the same range as the oral method. Any deviation from the normal range of

A PERSONAL GLIMPSE

I am 11 years old and I have already been in the hospital for four surgeries. I think I could be a nurse. One time a student nurse and her teacher came to do my vital signs. The teacher left and the student named Joan told me I was her first patient ever. She tried three of those electronic thermometers to take my temperature, but she said they were all broken. Then she tried to take my blood pressure with the blood pressure machine and she said it was broken. Then she used another blood pressure cuff and this time she put it on backwards. I knew it was wrong, but I just let her pump it up and up until it exploded off my arm. I laughed, but she almost cried. I showed her how to do it right and she seemed pretty glad that she finally got it to work. I was kind of happy when she left because I didn't know if I could teach her everything. A little while later she came back with her teacher and the teacher said, "Joan is going to give you your shot." "Uh Oh!" I thought, "here comes trouble." I just held my breath and hoped she won't do that wrong too. It wasn't too bad. Later, before she went home she brought me a pear, I am pretty sure she was relieved the day was over and I was too.

Abigail, age 11

▶ **LEARNING OPPORTUNITY:** What could this student nurse have done to be better prepared to take care of this patient? What feelings do you think this child might have had when the nurse came in with the medication?

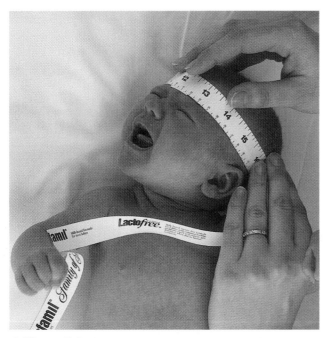

● **Figure 5.4** Measuring the head circumference.

temperature should be reported. Temperatures vary according to the method by which they are taken so it is important to record the method of temperature measurement as well as the measured temperature.

Mercury or electronic thermometers may be used to measure temperature by the oral, rectal, and axillary routes. Electronic thermometers have oral and rectal probes. The nurse should be careful to select the correct probe when using the thermometer. In pediatrics, oral temperatures usually are taken only on children older than 4 to 6 years of age who are conscious and cooperative. Oral thermometers should be placed in the side of the child's mouth. The child should not be left unattended while any temperature is being taken.

Tympanic thermometers are now used in many healthcare settings to measure temperature (Fig. 5–5A). The tympanic thermometer records the temperature rapidly (registering in about 2 seconds), is noninvasive, and causes little disturbance to the child. A tympanic measurement often can be obtained without awakening a sleeping infant or child. Tympanic thermometers are used according to the manufacturer's directions and the facility's policy. A disposable speculum is used for each child.

Rectal temperatures are measured in infants and children younger than 4 to 6 years of age. They are not desirable in the newborn because of the danger of irritation to the rectal mucosa. When a rectal temperature is taken, the bulb end should be lubricated with a water-soluble lubricant. The infant is placed in a prone position, the buttocks are gently separated with one hand, and the thermometer is inserted gently about ¼ to ½ inch into the rectum. If the nurse feels any resistance, he or she should remove the thermometer immediately, take the temperature by some other method, and notify the physician about the resistance. The nurse must keep one hand on the child's buttocks and the other on the thermometer during the entire time the rectal thermometer is in place. A mercury thermometer is left in place for 3 or 4 minutes. An electronic thermometer is removed as soon as it signals a recorded temperature.

Axillary temperatures are taken on newborns and on infants and children with diarrhea or when a rectal temperature is contraindicated. When taking an axillary temperature on an infant or child, the nurse must be certain to place the thermometer bulb well into the armpit and bring the child's arm down close to the body (Fig. 5–5B). The nurse must check to see that there is skin-to-skin contact with no clothing in the way. The thermometer is left in place for 10 minutes or until the electronic thermometer signals.

Pulse

Counting an apical rate is the preferred method to determine the pulse in an infant or young child. The nurse should try to accomplish this while the child is quiet. Approaching the child in a soothing, calm, quiet manner is helpful. The apical pulse should be counted before the child is disturbed for other procedures. A child can be held on the caregiver's lap for security for the full minute that the pulse is counted. The stethoscope is placed between the child's left nipple and sternum. A radial pulse may be taken on an older child. This pulse may be counted for 30 seconds and multiplied by two. A pulse that is unusual in quality, rate, or rhythm, should be counted for a full minute. Any rate that deviates from the normal rate should be reported. Pulse rates vary with age: from 100 to 180 beats per minute for a neonate (birth to 30 days old) to 50 to 95 beats per minute for the 14- to 18-year-old adolescent (Table 5–3).

Cardiac monitors are used to detect changes in cardiac function. Many of these monitors have a visual display of the cardiac actions. Electrodes must

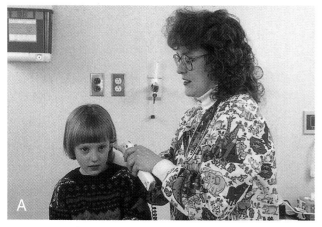
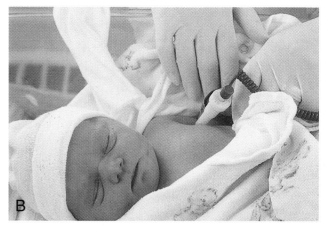

● **Figure 5.5** **(A)** Many facilities use a tympanic thermometer sensor to take the child's temperature. **(B)** Taking an axillary temperature on a newborn. (© B. Proud.)

TABLE 5.3	Normal Pulse Ranges in Children (bpm)	
Age	Normal Range	Average
0–24 hr	70–170 bpm	120 bpm
1–7 d	100–180 bpm	140 bpm
1 mo	110–188 bpm	160 bpm
1 mo–1 y	80–180 bpm	120–130 bpm
2 y	80–140 bpm	110 bpm
4 y	80–120 bpm	100 bpm
6 y	70–115 bpm	100 bpm
10 y	70–110 bpm	90 bpm
12–14 y	60–110 bpm	85–90 bpm
14–18 y	50–95 bpm	70–75 bpm

bpm = beats per minute

be placed properly to obtain accurate readings of the cardiac system. The skin is cleansed with alcohol to remove oil, dirt, lotions, and powder. Alarms are set to maximum and minimum settings above and below the child's resting heart rate. The electrode sites must be checked every 2 hours to detect any skin redness or irritation and to determine that the electrodes are secure. The child's cardiac status must be checked immediately when the alarm sounds (Fig. 5–6). Sometimes the monitor used will monitor both cardiac and respiratory function. Apnea monitors, which monitor respiratory function, will be discussed later in this chapter.

Respirations

Respirations of an infant or young child also must be counted during a quiet time. The child can be observed while lying or sitting quietly. Infants are abdominal breathers; therefore, the movement of the

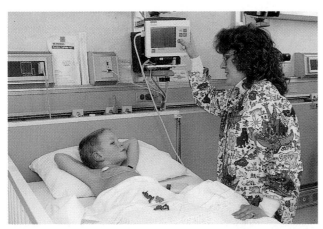

● *Figure 5.6* It is important for the nurse to frequently check the cardiopulmonary monitor, settings, and electrode sites. (© B. Proud.)

infant's abdomen is observed to count respirations. The older child's chest can be observed much as an adult's would be. The infant's respirations must be counted for a full minute because of normal irregularity. The chest of the infant or young child must be observed for retractions that indicate respiratory distress. Retractions are noted as substernal (below the sternum), subcostal (below the ribs), intercostal (between the ribs), suprasternal (above the sternum), or supraclavicular (above the clavicle) (Fig. 5–7).

Pulse Oximetry. Pulse oximetry measures the oxygen saturation of arterial hemoglobin. The probe of the oximetry unit can be taped to the toe or finger or clipped on the earlobe (Fig. 5–8). The pulse oximetry is taken and recorded with the other vital signs. In certain situations the probe is left in place to continually monitor the oxygen saturation. The site is changed at least every 4 hours to prevent skin irritation. In an infant, the foot may be used. The site should be checked every 2 hours to ensure that the probe is secure and tissue perfusion is adequate. Alarms can be set to sound when oxygen saturation registers lower than a predetermined limit. At the beginning of each shift and after transport of the patient, the nurse must check that alarms are accurately set and have not been inadvertently changed. This is true for all types of monitors.

Apnea Monitor. An apnea monitor detects the infant's respiratory movement. Electrodes or a belt are placed on the infant's chest where the greatest amount

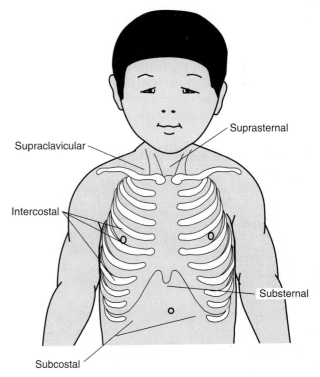

● *Figure 5.7* Sites of respiratory retraction.

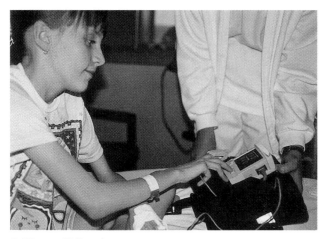

● *Figure 5.8* The pulse oximetry sensor measuring the oxygen saturation in the older child.

of respiratory movement is detected; the electrodes are attached to the monitor by a cable. An alarm is set to sound when the infant does not breathe for a predetermined number of seconds. These monitors can be used in a hospital setting and often are used in the home for an infant who is at risk for apnea or who has a tracheostomy (Fig. 5–9). Family caregivers are taught to stimulate the infant when the monitor sounds and to perform cardiopulmonary resuscitation if the infant does not begin breathing.

Blood Pressure

For children 3 years of age and older, blood-pressure monitoring is part of routine and ongoing data collection. Children of any age who come to a health care facility should have a baseline blood pressure taken. It is important for the nurse to offer the child an explanation of the procedure in terms the young child can understand. Referring to the blood pressure cuff as "giving your arm a hug" will help in the explanation. First taking a blood pressure on a stuffed animal or doll will further show the child the procedure is

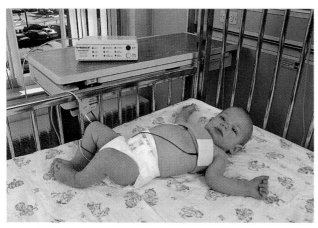

● *Figure 5.9* Apnea monitor being used in a hospital setting. (© B. Proud.)

not one to be feared. Obtaining a blood-pressure measurement in an infant or small child is difficult, but equipment of the proper size helps ease the problem. The cuff should be wide enough to cover about two thirds of the upper arm and long enough to encircle the upper arm without overlapping. The blood pressure is taken by the auscultation, palpation, or Doppler method (Box 5–2). The Doppler method is used with increasing frequency to monitor pediatric blood pressure, but the cuff still must be the correct size. Electronic blood pressure recording devices are used frequently in health care settings and provide accurate measurement. Normal blood-pressure values gradually increase from infancy through adolescence (Table 5–4).

Providing a Physical Examination

Data is also collected by examining the body systems of the child. The nurse provides the physical exam or assists the health care provider in doing the physical exam.

BOX 5.2 | Methods for Measuring Pediatric Blood Pressures

For any method of measuring blood pressure, allow the child to handle the equipment. Use terminology appropriate to the child's age. A preschool or young school-age child may want to use equipment to take the blood pressure of a doll or stuffed animal.

Auscultation
1. Place the correct size of cuff on the infant's or child's bare arm.
2. Locate the artery by palpating the antecubital fossa.
3. Inflate the cuff until radial pulse disappears or about 30 mmHg above expected systolic reading.
4. Place stethoscope lightly over the artery and slowly release air until pulse is heard.
5. Record readings as in adults.

Palpation
1. Follow steps 1 and 2 above.
2. Keep the palpating finger over the artery and inflate the cuff as above.
3. The point at which the pulse is felt is recorded as the systolic pressure.

Doppler
1. Obtain the monitor, dual air hose, and proper cuff size.
2. If monitor is not on a mobile stand, be certain that it is placed on a firm surface.
3. Plug in monitor (unless battery-operated) and attach dual hose if necessary.
4. Attach appropriate-size blood-pressure cuff and wrap around child's limb.
5. Turn on power switch. Record the reading.

TABLE 5.4	Normal Blood-Pressure Ranges (mmHg)	
Age	Systolic	Diastolic
Newborn—12 hr (< 1,000 g)	39–59	16–36
Newborn—12 hr (3,000 g)	50–70	24–45
Newborn—96 hr (3,000 g)	60–90	20–60
Infant	74–100	50–70
Toddler	80–112	50–80
Preschooler	82–110	50–78
School-age	84–120	54–80
Adolescent	94–140	62–88

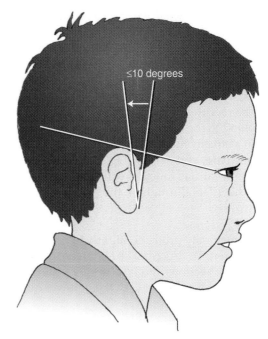

● *Figure 5.10* Normal alignment of the ear in the child.

Head and Neck

The head's general shape and movement should be observed. **Symmetry** or a balance is noted in the features of the face and in the head. Observe the child's ability to control the head and the range of motion. To see full range of motion, ask the older child to move her or his head in all directions. In the infant the nurse gently moves the head to observe for any stiffness in the neck. The nurse feels the skull to determine if the **fontanels** are open or closed and to check for any swelling.

Eyes. Observe the eyes for symmetry and location in relationship to the nose. Note any redness, evidence of rubbing, or drainage. Ask the older child to follow a light to observe her or his ability to focus. An infant will also follow a light with his or her eyes. Observe pupils for equality, roundness, and reaction to light. Neurologic considerations will be discussed later in this chapter. Routine vision screening is done in school settings. Screening helps identify vision concerns in children; with early detection, appropriate visual aids can be provided.

Ears. The alignment of the ears is noted by drawing an imaginary line from the outside corner of the eye to the prominent part of the child's skull; the top of the ear, known as the **pinna,** should cross this line (Fig. 5–10). Ears that are set low often indicate mental retardation (see Chapter 15). Note the child's ability to hear during normal conversation. A child who speaks loudly or responds inappropriately may have hearing difficulties that should be explored. Note any drainage or swelling.

Nose, Mouth, Throat. The nose is in the middle of the face. If an imaginary line were drawn down the middle, both sides of the nose should be symmetrical. Flaring of the nostrils might indicate respiratory distress and should be reported immediately. Observe for swelling, drainage, or bleeding. To observe the mouth and throat, have the older child hold her or his mouth wide open and move the tongue from side to side. With the infant or toddler, use a tongue blade to see the mouth and throat. Gently place the tongue blade on the side of the tongue to hold it down. Observe the mucous membranes for color, moisture, and any patchy areas that might indicate infection (see Chapter 11). Observe the number and condition of the child's teeth. The lips should be moist and pink. Note any difficulty in swallowing.

Chest and Lungs

Chest measurements are done on infants and children to determine normal growth rate. Take the measurement at the nipple level with a tape measure. Observe the chest for size, shape, movement of the chest with breathing, and any retractions (see respirations in this chapter). In the older school-age child or adolescent, note evidence of breast development. Evaluate respiratory rate, rhythm, and depth. Report any noisy or grunting respirations. Using a stethoscope, the nurse listens to breath sounds in each lobe of the lung, anterior and posterior, while the child inhales and exhales. Describe, document, and report absent or diminished breath sounds as well as unusual sounds such as crackling or wheezing. If the child is coughing or bringing up sputum, record the frequency, color and consistency of sputum.

Heart

In some infants and children, a pulsation can be seen in the chest that indicates the heartbeat. This point is called the **point of maximum impulse (PMI).** This point is where the heartbeat can be heard the best with a stethoscope. The nurse listens for the rhythm of the heart sounds and counts the rate for one full minute. Abnormal or unusual heart sounds or irregular rhythms might indicate the child has a heart murmur, heart condition, or other abnormality that should be reported. The heart is responsible for circulating blood to the body. To determine the heart function's effectiveness, the nurses assesses the pulses in various parts of the body (Fig. 5–11). Other indicators of good cardiac function will be discussed in specific disorders throughout the textbook.

Abdomen

The abdomen may protrude slightly in infants and small children. To describe the abdomen, divide the area into four sections and label sections with the terms left upper quadrant (LUQ), left lower quadrant

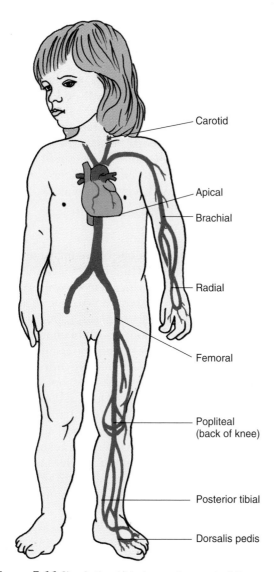

● **Figure 5.11** Sites in the child where pulses can be felt.

Labels on figure:
- Carotid
- Apical
- Brachial
- Radial
- Femoral
- Popliteal (back of knee)
- Posterior tibial
- Dorsalis pedis

(LLQ), right upper quadrant (RUQ), and right lower quadrant (RLQ). Using a stethoscope, the nurse listens for bowel sounds or evidence of peristalsis in each section of the abdomen and records what is heard. The umbilicus is observed for cleanliness and any abnormalities. Infants and young children sometimes have protrusions in the umbilicus or inguinal canal that are called hernias. Hernias will be discussed in Chapter 19. Report a tense or firm abdomen or unusual tenderness.

Genitalia and Rectum

When inspecting the genitalia and rectum, it is important to respect the child's privacy and take into account the child's age and the stage of growth and development. Keeping the child covered as much as possible is important. While wearing gloves, the nurse inspects the genitalia and rectum. Observe the area for any sores or lesions, swelling, or discharge. In male children the testes descend at varying times during childhood; if the testes cannot be palpated, this information should be reported. The nurse needs to be aware that unusual findings might indicate child abuse and should be further investigated (see Chapter 20).

Back and Extremities

The back should be observed for symmetry and for the curvature of the spine. In infants the spine is rounded and flexible. As the child grows and develops motor skills, the spine further develops. Screening is done in school age children to detect abnormal curvatures of the spine such as **scoliosis** (see Chapter 17). Note gait and posture when the child enters or is walking in the room. The extremities should be warm, have good color, and be symmetrical. By observing the child's movements during the exam, the nurse notes range of motion, movement of the joints and muscle strength. In infants, examine the hips and report any dislocation or asymmetry of gluteal skin folds. These could indicate a congenital hip dislocation (see Chapter 19).

Neurologic

Assessing the neurologic status of the infant and child is the most complex aspect of the physical exam. All the body systems function in relationship to the nervous system. The practitioner in the health care setting assesses the neurologic status of the child by doing a complete neurological exam. This exam includes detailed examination of the reflex responses as well as the functioning of each of the cranial nerves. The practitioner will perform a neurologic exam on children following a head injury, seizure, or on children who have metabolic conditions such as diabetes mellitus, drug ingestion, severe hemorrhage, or dehydration, where the child's neurologic status might be affected. A neurologic assessment is done to determine the level of the child's neurologic functioning. The nurse often is responsible for using neurologic assessment tools to monitor a child's neurologic status following the initial neurologic exam. The nurse uses a neurologic assessment tool such as the Glasgow coma scale for this. The use of a standard scale for monitoring permits the comparison of results from one time to another and from one examiner to another. Using this tool, the nurse monitors various aspects of the child's neurologic functioning (Fig. 5–12). If a child is hospitalized with a neurologic concern, the neurologic status is monitored closely and a neurologic assessment tool is used every 1 or 2 hours to observe for significant changes.

Assisting with Common Diagnostic Tests

Diagnostic tests and studies often are done to further evaluate the subjective and objective data collected. These diagnostic tests help the practitioner to determine more clearly the nature of the child's concern. The needs of the infant or child during these studies vary greatly from child to child. The role of the nurse in assisting with common diagnostic tests will be covered in Chapter 6.

KEY POINTS

- ‣ Interviewing the caregiver and the child is important in order to collect subjective data regarding the child.
- ‣ The chief complaint is the reason the child was brought to the healthcare setting and should be fully explored with the child and caregiver.
- ‣ When doing a review of systems, the nurse asks questions about each of the body systems using a head-to-toe approach.
- ‣ Although obtaining vital signs may seem like a routine procedure, the nurse must use good

judgment in selecting the means to measure each vital sign. The nurse also must document the vital signs promptly and accurately.

- ‣ To collect further objective data, the nurse does a physical exam on the child using the knowledge of normal growth and development as a basis for the exam.
- ‣ The nurse must become skilled in using a neurologic assessment tool, which is instrumental in monitoring the child's neurologic functioning.

BIBLIOGRAPHY

Barone MA, Rowe PC. (1999) Pediatric procedures.. In *Oski's pediatrics: Principles and practice* (3rd ed). Philadelphia: Lippincott Williams & Wilkins.

Craven RF, Hirnle CJ. (1999) *Fundamentals of nursing* (3rd ed.). Philadelphia: Lippincott Williams & Wilkins.

Gaynor, S. (2000) Pandora's box: Educational materials resources assessment. *Journal of Child and Family Nursing*, 3(2).

Heery K. (2000) Straight talk about the patient interview. *Nursing*. Retrieved from *http://www.findarticles.com*.

Houlder LC. (2000) Evidence-based practice: The accuracy and reliability of tympanic thermometry compared to rectal and axillary sites in young children. *Pediatric Nursing*, 26(3), 31–4.

Knies RC. (2001) Temperature measurement in acute care: The who, what, where, when, how, why and wherefore. Retrieved from *www.allnurses.com*.

Multon AH, Blactop J, Hall CM. (2001) Temperature taking in children. *Journal of Child Health Care*, 5(1), 5–10.

Pillitteri A. (1999) *Maternal and child health nursing* (3rd ed). Philadelphia: Lippincott Williams & Wilkins.

Wetzel GV. (1999) Red flags in common pediatric symptoms. *The American Journal of Maternal/Child Nursing*, 24(1).

Wong DL. (1998) *Whaley and Wong's nursing care of infants and children* (6th ed). St. Louis: Mosby.

Wong DL, Perry S, Hockenberry, M. (2002) *Maternal child nursing care* (2nd ed). St. Louis: Mosby.

Websites
http://health.discovery.com
Pediatric Assessment: *www.solutions-etc.com/PAO*
www.nurseone.com

GLASGOW COMA SCALES			MODIFIED COMA SCALE FOR INFANTS			
ACTIVITY	**BEST RESPONSE**		**ACTIVITY**	**BEST RESPONSE**		
Eye Opening	Spontaneous	4	Eye Opening	Spontaneous	4	
	To speech	3		To speech	3	
	To pain	2		To pain	2	
	None	1		None	1	
Verbal	Oriented	5	Verbal	Coos, babbles	5	
	Confused	4		Irritable	4	
	Inappropriate words	3		Cries to pain	3	
	Nonspecific sounds	2		Moans to pain	2	
	None	1		None	1	
Motor	Follows commands	6	Motor	Normal spontaneous movements	6	**PUPIL SIZE:**
	Localizes pain	5		Withdraws to touch	5	6mm ● 5mm ● 4mm ●
	Withdraws to pain	4		Withdraws to pain	4	
	Abnormal flexion	3		Abnormal flexion	3	3mm ● 2mm ● 1mm ●
	Extend	2		Abnormal extension	2	
	None	1		None	1	**REACTION: N**–normal, **S**–sluggish, **F**–fixed

		PUPIL SIZE		PUPIL REACTION		EXTREMITY MOVEMENT/ RESPONSE				GLASGOW COMA SCALE			VITAL SIGNS		
DATE	TIME	R	L	R	L	RA	LA	RL	LL	VERBAL RESP.	MOTOR RESP.	EYE OPENING	BP	PULSE	RESP.

GUIDE TO NEUROLOGIC EVALUATION

Pupils

Pupils should be examined in dim light

1. Compare each pupil with the size chart and record pupil size.
2. Use a bright flashlight to check the reaction of each pupil. Hold the flashlight to the outer aspect of the eye. While watching the pupil, turn the flashlight on and bring it directly over the pupil. Record the reaction. Repeat for the other eye. Report if either pupil is fixed or dilated.

Extremities

1. Observe the child for quality and strength of muscle tone in each upper extremity. Have child squeeze nurse's hand. Have child raise arms. Ask child to turn palms up, then palms down. Infant is observed for movement and position of arms when stroked or lightly pinched.
2. The child should be able to move each leg on command, and push against nurse's hands with each foot. Infant is observed for movement of legs and feet when stroked or lightly pinched.
3. Score the extremities using the motor scale appropriate for age (below).

Glasgow Coma Scale

Assess each response according to age

Eye opening

4 Opens eyes spontaneously when approached
3 Opens eyes to spoken or shouted speech
2 Opens eyes only to painful stimuli (nail bed pressure)
1 Does not open eyes in response to pain

Verbal

5 Oriented to time, place, person; infant responds by cooing and babbling, recognizes parent
4 Talks, not oriented to time, place, person; infant irritable, doesn't recognize parent
3 Words senseless, unintelligible; infant cries in response to pain
2 Responds with moaning and groaning, no intelligible words; infant moans to pain
1 No response

Motor

6 Responds to commands; infant smiles, responds
5 Tries to remove painful stimuli with hands; infant withdraws from touch
4 Attempts to withdraw from painful stimuli; infant withdraws from pain source
3 Flexes arms at elbows and wrists in response to pain (decorticate rigidity)
2 Extends arms at elbows in response to pain (cerebrate rigidity)
1 No motor response to pain

Check infant's fontanelle for bulging and record results

● *Figure 5.12* Neurologic flow sheet and neurologic evaluation guide.

Workbook

NCLEX-STYLE REVIEW QUESTIONS

1. The nurse is doing an admission interview with a toddler and the child's caregiver. Which of the following statements that the nurse makes to the caregiver indicates the nurse has an understanding of this child's growth and development needs?

   a. "You can sit in one chair and your child can sit in the other chair."

   b. "It would be best if you let the child play in the playroom while we are talking."

   c. "If you would like to hold your child on your lap, that would be fine."

   d. "I can find someone to take your child for a walk for a while."

2. When interviewing an adolescent, which of the following is the MOST important for the nurse to keep in mind. The adolescent

   a. will be able to give accurate details regarding her or his history.

   b. may feel more comfortable discussing some issues in private.

   c. may have a better understanding if books and pamphlets are provided.

   d. will be more cooperative if age-appropriate questions are asked.

3. In measuring an 18-month-old child's height and weight, which of the following actions by the nurse would be the HIGHEST priority. The nurse

   a. plots the measurements on a growth chart.

   b. keeps a hand within 1 inch of the child.

   c. has the child wear the same amount of clothing each time the procedure is done.

   d. covers the scale with a clean sheet of paper before placing the child on the scale.

4. In taking vital signs on a 6-month-old infant, the nurse obtains the following vital sign measurements. Which set of vital signs would the nurse be MOST concerned about?

   a. Pulse 90, temperature 36.9°C, blood pressure 80/50

   b. Pulse 114, temperature 37.6°C, blood pressure 88/60

   c. Pulse 148, temperature 38.0°C, blood pressure 92/62

   d. Pulse 162, temperature 38.5°C , blood pressure 96/56

5. When doing a physical exam on an infant, an understanding of this child's developmental needs are recognized when the exam is done by examining the

   a. heart before the abdomen

   b. chest before the nose

   c. extremities before the eyes

   d. neurologic status before the back

STUDY ACTIVITIES

1. Explain the step-by-step procedure you would follow to take vital signs on a 3-month-old infant. List the order in which you would take the vital signs and explain why you would do them in that order.

2. For each of the following body parts or systems, write a question that would be appropriate to ask a patient or caregiver when doing a review of systems as part of an interview.

Body Part or System	Question to Be Asked
General Skin Head and neck Eyes Ears Nose, mouth, throat Chest and lungs—respiratory Heart—cardiovascular Abdomen—gastrointestinal Genitalia and rectum Back and extremities Musculoskeletal Neurologic	

3. List four methods of taking a temperature and describe each method. Give an example of a reason that each method might be used to take a child's temperature.

CRITICAL THINKING

1. You are conducting an interview with the caregiver of a preschool-age child. Discuss the things you would say and do with the caregiver to get the important information you need to care for the child.
2. Explain the purpose of measuring the height and weight of a child at each healthcare visit. Discuss the purpose and significance of plotting height and weight on a pediatric growth chart.
3. Discuss the process of doing a physical exam on a child. How does the exam on a child differ from that of an adult? What are the most important considerations to keep in mind when doing a physical exam on a child?

Procedures and Treatments

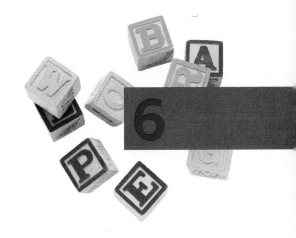

6

STUDENT OBJECTIVES

On completion of this chapter, the student will be able to:

1. Discuss the importance of preparing a child for a procedure or treatment.
2. List the responsibilities of the nurse when preparing a child for a procedure or treatment.
3. Describe the responsibilities of the nurse following a procedure or treatment.
4. List safety measures to consider when using restraints.
5. Describe methods of holding a child.
6. List four methods of reducing an elevated body temperature.
7. Explain the reason that accurate intake and output are monitored.
8. State how a nasogastric tube is measured to determine how far it is inserted.
9. Explain the reason that stomach contents are aspirated before a gastric tube feeding is done.
10. Discuss what is done with contents aspirated from the stomach.
11. Describe the reasons that gastrostomy tubes might be used in children.
12. List the methods used to administer oxygen to children.
13. Discuss the use of hot or cold therapy in relationship to circulation.
14. Describe three ostomies that are created that relate to elimination.
15. Describe four methods of collecting a urine specimen.
16. Discuss the role of the nurse in assisting with procedures related to diagnostic tests and studies.

KEY TERMS

clove hitch restraint
colostomy
elbow restraint
gastrostomy tube
gavage feedings
ileostomy
mummy restraint
papoose board
tracheostomy
urostomy

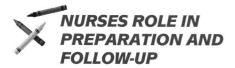

NURSES ROLE IN PREPARATION AND FOLLOW-UP

The role of the nurse in performing or assisting with procedures and treatments includes following guidelines set by the health care institution. These guidelines include the preparation before the procedure as well as the follow up needed when the procedure is completed. The nurse is responsible for following facility policies and ensuring patient safety before, during, and after all procedures and treatments.

Preparation for Procedures

The emotional support and information that the nurse offers often help to decrease anxiety for the child and family. Following the facility's policies regarding legal and safety factors is part of the nurse's responsibility, especially when working with children.

Psychological or Emotional Support

Many procedures in highly technological health care facilities may be frightening and painful to children. The nurse can be an important source of comfort to children who must undergo these procedures, even though it is difficult to assist with or perform procedures that cause discomfort or pain. It is also important for the nurse to explain the procedure and purpose of the procedure or treatment to the caregiver. When the caregiver's anxiety and concerns decrease, the child in turn often will have less anxiety. The child who is old enough to understand the purpose of the procedure and the expected benefit must have the procedure explained; he or she should be encouraged to ask questions and should be given complete answers. Infants can be soothed and comforted before and after the procedure.

The nurse caring for toddlers has a greater opportunity to explain procedures than when caring for infants, but at best the nurse will be only imperfectly understood. Even when toddlers grasp the words, they aren't likely to understand the meaning. The reality is the pain that occurs.

Sometimes children's interest can be diverted so that they may forget their fear. They must be allowed to cry if necessary, and they should always be listened to and have their questions answered. It takes maturity and experience on the nurse's part to know exactly which questions are stalling techniques and which call for firmness and action. Children need someone to take charge in a kind, firm manner that tells them the decision is not in their hands. They are too young to take this responsibility for themselves.

Nurses have conflicting feelings about the merit of giving some reward after a treatment. Careful thought is necessary. Children given a lollipop or a small toy after an uncomfortable procedure tend to remember the experience as not totally bad. This has nothing to do with their behavior. It is not a reward for being brave or good or big; it is simply a part of the entire treatment. The unpleasant part is mitigated by the pleasant. An older person's reward is contemplating the improved health that the procedure may provide, but the child does not have sufficient reasoning ability to understand future benefits.

Legal and Safety Factors

When the nurse is preparing to perform or assist with any procedures or treatments he or she follows certain steps no matter what the healthcare setting is. Most procedures require a written order before they are done. Orders should be clarified when needed. The child must always be identified prior to any treatment or procedure. The nurse identifies the child by checking the child's ID band and verifies that information by having the child or caregiver state the child's name. If consent is needed, the form is completed, signed, and witnessed. As stated earlier, the procedure is discussed with the child and family caregiver, and questions are answered. Washing hands before and after any procedure helps prevent or control the spread of microorganisms. The nurse gathers the needed supplies and equipment and reviews the steps for beginning the procedure. Safety for the child (see Chapter 4) is a priority. Standard precautions are followed for all procedures (see Appendix E).

Follow-Up for Procedures

When the procedure is completed, the child is left in a safe position with siderails raised and bed lowered. For the older child, the call light is put within her or his reach. Comforting and reassuring the child is important, particularly if the procedure has been uncomfortable or traumatic. The caregiver might have concerns or questions that need to be discussed. Equipment and supplies are removed and disposed of properly. Contaminated linens are handled according to facility policy. If a specimen is to be taken to another department, the specimen is labeled with the patient's name, identifying information, and the type of specimen in the container. The appropriate facility policies are followed. Often paperwork must go with the specimen, and certain precautions are taken to prevent any exposure from the specimen. Documentation includes the procedure, the child's response, and the description and characteristics of any specimen obtained. If specimens were sent to another department in the facility, this information is also recorded.

PERFORMING PROCEDURES RELATED TO POSITION

Safety is the nurse's most important responsibility when performing procedures related to positioning a child. The child's safety and comfort must be a priority when using restraints or transporting children. Safety is also an important factor when holding or positioning children for sleep.

Restraints

Restraints often are needed to protect a child from injury during a procedure or an examination or to ensure the infant's or child's safety and comfort. Restraints should never be used as a form of punishment. When possible, restraining by hand is the best method. However, mechanical restraints must be used to secure a child during IV infusions, to protect a surgical site from injury such as cleft lip and cleft palate, or when restraint by hand is impractical.

Various types of restraints may be used. Whatever the type of restraint, however, caution is essential. Close and conscientious observation is a necessary part of nursing care. The nurse also must be alert to family concerns when the child is in restraints. Explanations about the need for restraints will help the family understand and be cooperative. The caregiver may wish to restrain the child physically to prevent use of restraints, and this action is often possible. Each situation must be judged individually.

Mummy Restraints and Papoose Boards

Mummy restraints are used for an infant or small child during a procedure (Fig. 6–1). This device is a snug wrap that is effective when performing a scalp venipuncture, inserting a nasogastric tube, or performing other procedures that involve only the head or neck. **Papoose boards** are used with toddlers or preschoolers.

Clove Hitch Restraints

Clove hitch restraints are used to secure an arm or leg, most often when a child is receiving an IV infusion. The restraint is made of soft cloth formed in a figure eight. Padding under the restraint is desirable if the child puts any pull on it. The site should be checked and loosened at least every 2 hours. Commercial restraints also are available for this purpose. This restraint should be secured to the lower part of the crib or bed, not to the side rail, to avoid possibly causing injury when the siderail is raised or lowered.

Elbow Restraints

Elbow restraints often are made of muslin in two layers. Pockets wide enough to hold tongue depressors are placed vertically in the width of the fabric. The top flap folds over to close the pockets. The restraint is wrapped around the child's arm and tied securely to prevent the child from bending the elbow. Care must be taken that the elbow restraints fit the child properly. They should not be too high under the axillae. They may be pinned to the child's shirt to keep them from slipping. Commercially made elbow restraints may also be used.

Jacket Restraints

Jacket restraints are used to secure the child from climbing out of bed or a chair or to keep the child in a horizontal position. The restraint must be the correct size for the child. A child in a jacket restraint should be checked frequently to prevent him or her from slipping and choking on the neck of the jacket. Ties must be secure to the bed frame, not the sides, so that the jacket is not pulled when the sides are moved up and down.

Transporting

When moving infants and small children in a health-care setting, the safety of the child is the biggest concern. It is best to carry the infant or place him or her in a crib or bassinet. Often in pediatric settings wagons are used to transport children; the wagon ride is functional as well as enjoyable for the child. The toddler may be transported in a crib with high siderails or a high-topped crib. Strollers or wheelchairs are used when the child is able to sit. Older children are placed on stretchers or may be moved in their beds. Often a hospitalized child who is in traction, which cannot be removed, can go to the playroom or other areas in the hospital in this manner.

Holding

When a child is held, it is most important to be sure the child is safe and feels secure. The three most common methods of holding a child are the horizontal position, upright position, or the football hold (Fig. 6–2). When holding an infant, always support the head and back. During and after feedings, the infant to be burped is sometimes held in a sitting position on the lap. The infant is held leaning forward against the nurse's hand while the nurse's thumb and finger support the infant's head. This

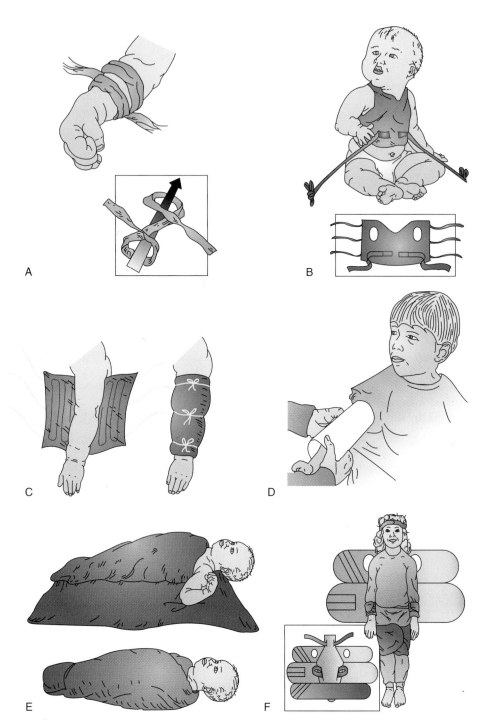

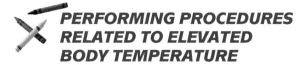

● *Figure 6.1 (A)* Clove hitch restraint. *(B)* Jacket restraint. *(C)* Elbow restraint. *(D)* Commercial elbow restraint. *(E)* Mummy restraint. *(F)* Papoose board.

leaves the other hand free to gently pat the infant's back (Fig. 6–3).

Sleeping

Infants should be positioned on their backs or supported on their sides for sleeping. The nurse working with family caregivers teaches and reinforces this information. These positions seem to have decreased the incidence of crib death or SIDS (see Chapter 11) in infants.

PERFORMING PROCEDURES RELATED TO ELEVATED BODY TEMPERATURE

Significant alterations in body temperature can have severe consequences for children. "Normal" body temperature varies from 97.6°F (36.4°C) orally to 100.3°F (37.9°C) rectally. The body temperature generally should be maintained below 101°F (38.3°C) orally or 102°F (38.9°C) rectally, although the health

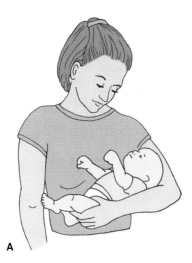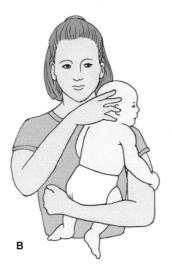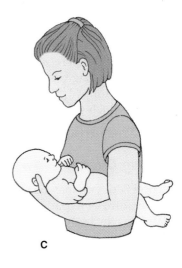

A   B   C

● *Figure 6.2* Positions to hold an infant or child: *(A)* horizontal position, *(B)* upright position, *(C)* football hold.

care facility or practitioner may set lower limits. Methods used to reduce fever include maintaining hydration by encouraging fluids and administering acetaminophen. Because of their ineffectiveness in reducing fever and the discomfort they cause, tepid sponge baths are no longer recommended for reducing fever. Because many children have a fever but do not need hospitalization, family caregivers need instructions on fever reduction (see Family Teaching Tips: Reducing Fever).

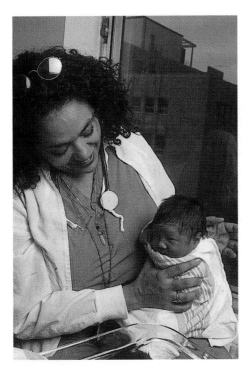

● *Figure 6.3* The nurse holds the infant in a sitting position to burp the baby.

INTERNET EXERCISE 6.1

www.vh.org/Providers/Simulations/VirtualPedsPatients/PedsVPHome.html

"The Virtual Pediatric Patient"
Scroll down to and click on Case 7—A child with a fever.
Read the sections discussing the patient and the problem.
Read the section entitled "Approach to the Child with Fever."

1. List six "common" causes of fever in children.

2. At what body temperature is it considered that a child has an elevation?

Control of Environmental Factors

Excess coverings should be removed from the child with fever to permit additional cooling through

FAMILY TEACHING TIPS

Reducing Fever

1. Do not overdress or heavily cover child. Diaper, light sheet, or light pajamas are sufficient.
2. Encourage child to drink fluids.
3. Keep room environment cool.
4. Use acetaminophen or other antipyretics according to physician's directions. Do not give aspirin.
5. Wait for 30 minutes and take temperature again.
6. Call physician at once if child's temperature is 105°F (40.6°C) or higher.
7. Call physician if child has history of febrile seizures.

evaporation. Changing to lightweight clothes, removing clothes, lowering the room temperature, or applying cool compresses to the forehead may help to lower the temperature. If a child begins to shiver, whatever is being used to lower the temperature should be stopped. Shivering indicates the child is chilling, which will cause the body temperature to increase.

Cooling Devices

A cooling device may be used to lower an elevated temperature. A hypothermia pad or blanket lowers or maintains the body temperature. The child's temperature is monitored closely and checked frequently with a regular thermometer. The blanket is always covered before being placed next to the child's skin so moisture can be absorbed from the skin. The baseline and temperature measurements are documented as well as information regarding the child's response to the treatment.

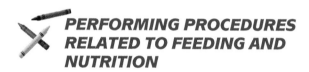

PERFORMING PROCEDURES RELATED TO FEEDING AND NUTRITION

Monitoring the intake of fluids and nutrients is important in both maintaining and promoting appropriate growth in children. The nurse is responsible for accurately documenting both a child's intake and output. If a child is unable to consume adequate amounts of fluid or foods, gavage or gastrostomy feedings are given to meet the child's nutrient needs and promote normal growth.

Intake and Output

Accurately measuring and recording intake and output are especially important in working with the ill or hospitalized child. In a well child setting, the caregiver can provide information about the child's usual patterns of intake and output. With the ill or hospitalized child, more exact measurements of fluid intake and output are required. In many settings these measurements are recorded as often as every hour, and a running total is kept to closely monitor the child.

Oral fluids, feeding tube intake, IV fluids, and foods that become liquid at room temperature are all measured and recorded (Fig. 6–4). Urine, vomitus, diarrhea, gastric suctioning, and any other liquid drainage are measured and considered output. The color and characteristics of the output are described and recorded.

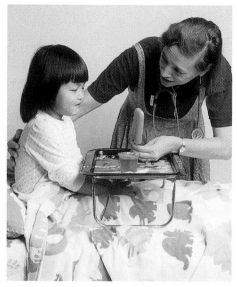

● **Figure 6.4** The nurse offers the child foods that are liquid at room temperature and will be recorded as intake.

To measure the output of an infant wearing a diaper, the wet diaper is weighed and the weight of the dry diaper is subtracted before the amount is recorded.

Gavage Feeding

Sometimes infants or children who have had surgery or have a chronic or serious condition are unable to take adequate food and fluid by mouth and must receive nourishment by means of gavage feedings. **Gavage feedings** provide nourishment directly through a tube passed into the stomach. This procedure is particularly appropriate in infants. If gavage feedings are not well tolerated, the nurse should report it and await alternate orders from the provider.

Whether the tube is inserted nasally or orally, the measurement is the same: from the tip of the child's nose to the earlobe and down to the tip of the sternum (Fig. 6–5). This length may be marked on the tube with tape or a marking pen. The end of the tube to be inserted should be lubricated with sterile water or water-soluble lubricating jelly, never an oily substance because of the danger of oil aspiration into the lungs.

To prepare the child for gavage feeding, elevate the head and place a rolled-up diaper behind the neck. Turn the head and align the body to the right.

After inserting the tube, verify its position by aspirating stomach contents or by inserting 1 to 5 mL of air (using an Asepto syringe) and listening with a stethoscope. If the tube is properly placed, gurgling or growling sounds will be heard as air enters the stomach. If stomach contents are aspirated, these

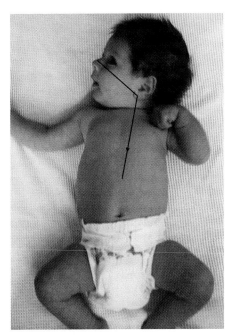

● *Figure 6.5* Measurement of tubing for nasogastric tube insertion.

should be measured and replaced and, in a very small infant, subtracted from the amount ordered for that particular feeding.

The nurse may hold the tube in place if it is going to be removed immediately after the feeding. If the tube is left in position for further use, it should be secured to the infant's nose using adhesive tape (Fig. 6–6). The correct position must be verified before each feeding.

The feeding syringe is inserted into the tube, and the feeding, which has been warmed to room temperature, is allowed to flow by gravity. The entire feeding should take 15 to 20 minutes after which the infant must be burped and positioned on the right side for at least 1 hour to prevent regurgitation and aspiration.

The type and amount of contents aspirated by the nurse, the amount of formula fed, the infant's tolerance for the procedure, and the positioning of the infant after completion should be recorded on the chart. The feeding tube and any leftover formula should be discarded at the completion of the procedure.

Gastrostomy Feeding

Children who must receive tube feedings over a long period may have a **gastrostomy tube** surgically inserted through the abdominal wall into the stomach (Fig. 6–7). This procedure is performed under general anesthesia. It also is used in children who have obstructions or surgical repairs in the mouth, pharynx, esophagus, or cardiac sphincter of the stomach or who are respirator-dependent.

The surgeon inserts a catheter, usually a Foley or mushroom, that is left unclamped and connected to gravity drainage for 24 hours. Meticulous care of the wound site is necessary to prevent infection and irritation. Until healing is complete, the area must be covered with a sterile dressing. Ointment, Stomadhesive, or other skin preparations may be ordered for application to the site. The child may need to be restrained to prevent pulling on the catheter, which may cause leakage of caustic gastric juices.

Procedures for positioning and feeding the child with a gastrostomy tube are similar to those for gavage feedings. The residual stomach contents are aspirated, measured, and replaced at the beginning of the procedure. The child's head and shoulders are elevated during the feeding. After each feeding, the child is placed on the right side or in Fowler's position.

When regular oral feedings are resumed, the tube is surgically removed, and the opening usually closes spontaneously.

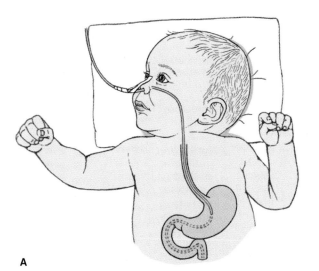

A

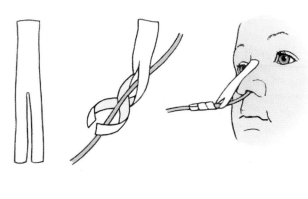

B

● *Figure 6.6* **(A)** Nasogastric tube placement. **(B)** Adhesive tape used to secure nasogastric tube.

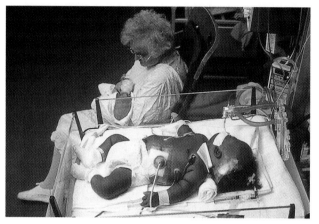

● **Figure 6.7** A gastrostomy tube is placed when long-term feedings will be needed.

For long-term gastrostomy feedings, a gastrostomy button may be inserted. Some advantages of buttons are that they are more desirable cosmetically, are simple to care for, and cause less skin irritation.

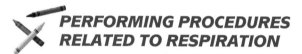

PERFORMING PROCEDURES RELATED TO RESPIRATION

Oxygen administration, nasal and oral suctionings, and caring for the child with a tracheostomy are procedures the nurse might be called on to perform for the child with a respiratory condition. The nurse is responsible for monitoring and maintaining adequate oxygenation.

Oxygen Administration

Oxygen is administered to treat symptoms of respiratory distress or when the oxygen saturation level in the blood is below normal (see Chapter 5 for measurement of O_2 saturation). Depending on the child's age and oxygen needs, many different methods are used to deliver oxygen. The infant is often given oxygen while in an isolette or incubator. Infants as well as older children might have oxygen administered by nasal cannula or prongs, mask, or via an oxygen hood (Table 6–1). Oxygen tents may also be used to deliver oxygen. An advantage of using an oxygen tent for the toddler and school-age child is that no device has to be put over the child's nose or face. The oxygen concentration is more difficult to maintain in the tent because it is opened many times throughout the day. The tent is frightening to children so they must be reassured frequently (Fig. 6–8). Whatever equipment is used to administer oxygen, the procedure and equipment must be explained to the child and the caregiver. Letting the child hold and feel the equipment and flow of oxygen through the device helps decrease the child's fear and anxiety about the procedure. The device warms and humidifies oxygen to prevent the recipient's nasal passages from becoming dry. The nurse closely monitors children receiving oxygen therapy; when oxygen is to be discontinued, it is done so gradually. Equipment is checked frequently to ensure proper functioning, cleanliness, and correct oxygen content. Exposure to high concentrations of oxygen can be dangerous to small infants and children with other respiratory diseases. Many times children

TABLE 6.1	Methods of Oxygen Administration	
Method	**Age or Reason to Use**	**Nursing Concerns When Using**
Isolette/Incubator	Newborn or infant	
Nasal prongs/cannula	Many sizes available	Not humidified; causes dryness
	Nasal prongs fit into child's nose	Keep nasal prongs clean and clear of secretions
	Toddlers may pull out of nose, other method better	Monitor nostrils for irritation
Mask	Various sizes available	Not used in comatose children
	Covers mouth and nose, not eyes	
	Humidified, decreases dryness	
Hood	Fits over head and neck of child	May be frightening for child
	Clear so child can be seen	
Oxygen Tent/croupette	Equipment does not come in contact with face	Difficult to see child in tent
	Allows for movement inside tent	Difficult for child to see out
		Child feels isolated
		Change clothing and linen often
		Keep siderails up
Tracheostomy	Used in emergencies or when long-term oxygen is needed	Must be kept clean with airway patent
		Suction when needed

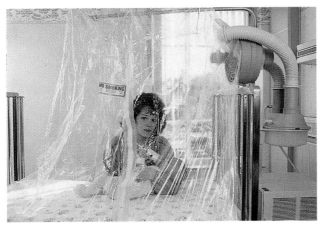

● *Figure 6.8* The child in the oxygen tent must be reassured often.

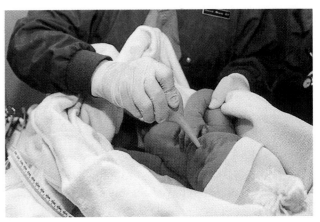

● *Figure 6.9* A bulb syringe is used to remove secretions from the nose and mouth.

are cared for in a home setting while on oxygen. The nurse teaches the family caregiver regarding oxygen administration, equipment, and safety measures (see Family Teaching Tips: Oxygen Safety).

Nasal/Oral Suctioning

Excess secretions in the nose or mouth can obstruct the infant or child's airway and decrease respiratory function. Coughing often clears the airway, but when the infant or child is unable to remove secretions, the nurse must remove secretions by suctioning. A bulb syringe is used to remove secretions from the nose and mouth (Fig. 6–9). Sterile normal saline drops may be used to loosen dried nasal secretions. Nasotracheal suctioning with a sterile suction catheter may be needed if secretions cannot be removed by other methods.

Tracheostomy

A **tracheostomy** is a surgical procedure in which an opening is made into the trachea so that a child with a

respiratory obstruction can breathe. A tracheostomy is performed in emergency situations or in conditions where infants or children have a blocked airway. Children with a tracheostomy are cared for initially in a hospital setting; children with a long-term condition often are cared for at home. The tracheostomy tube is suctioned to remove mucous and secretions and to keep the airway patent. The plastic or metal trach tube must be cleaned often to decreases the possibility of infection. Care of the skin around the site will prevent breakdown. A tracheostomy collar or mist tent provides moisture and humidity. The tracheostomy prevents the child from being able to cry or speak, so the nurse must closely monitor and find alternative methods of communicating with the child.

PERFORMING PROCEDURES RELATED TO CIRCULATION

After a provider has written an order for heat or cold therapy, the nurse is responsible for applying the treatment, closely monitoring the effects of the treatment, and documenting those observations.

Heat Therapy

The local application of heat increases circulation by vasodilatation and promotes muscle relaxation, thereby relieving pain and congestion. It also speeds the formation and drainage of superficial abscesses.

Artificial heat should never be applied to the child's skin without a specific order. Tissue damage can occur particularly in fair-skinned people or those who have suffered sensory loss or impaired circulation. Children should be closely monitored, and none should receive heat treatments longer than 20

FAMILY TEACHING TIPS

Oxygen Safety

1. Keep equipment clean. Dirty equipment can be a source of bacteria.
2. Use signs noting that oxygen is in use.
3. Give good mouth care. Use swabs and mouthwash.
4. Offer fluids frequently.
5. Keep nose clean.
6. Don't use electric or battery-powered toys.
7. Don't allow smoking, matches, or lighters nearby.
8. Don't keep flammable solutions in room.
9. Don't use wool or synthetic blankets.

minutes at a time unless specifically ordered by the provider.

Moist heat produces faster results than does dry heat and is usually applied in the form of a warm compress or soak. Towels should not be warmed in the microwave because the microwave may unevenly heat the towels, which in turn may burn the child.

Dry heat may be applied by means of an electric heating pad, a K-pad (a unit that circulates warm water through plastic-enclosed tubing), or a hot water bottle. Many children have been burned because of improper use of hot water bottles; therefore, these devices are not recommended. Electric heating pads and K-pads should be covered with a pillowcase, towel, or stockinette. Documentation includes the application type, start time, therapy duration, and the skin's condition before and after the application.

Cold Therapy

As with heat, a provider must order the use of cold applications. In addition to reducing body temperature (see Cooling Devices, page 82), the local application of cold also may help prevent swelling, control hemorrhage, and provide an anesthetic effect. Intervals of about 20 minutes are recommended for both dry cold (ice bag and commercial instant-cold preparation) and moist cold (compress, soak, and bath) treatments. Dry cold applications should be covered lightly to protect the child's skin from direct contact. Because cold decreases circulation, prolonged chilling may result in frostbite and gangrene.

The child's skin must be inspected before and after the cold application to detect skin redness or irritation. Documentation includes the application type, start time, therapy duration, and the skin's condition before and after the application.

Detailed instructions for the therapeutic application of cold and heat may be obtained in the procedures manual of each facility and from manufacturers of commercial devices.

PERFORMING PROCEDURES RELATED TO ELIMINATION

The nurse in the pediatric setting might be responsible for performing procedures related to elimination. The nurse might administer an enema to a child as a treatment or as a preop procedure. When a child has a colostomy, ileostomy, or urostomy, the nurse cares for the ostomy site and documents the output from the ostomy.

Enema

The pediatric nurse may administer an enema to an infant or child as treatment for some disorders or before a diagnostic or surgical procedure. The procedure can be uncomfortable and threatening, so it is important for the nurse to discuss the procedure with the child before giving the enema. The type and amount of fluid, as well as the distance the tube is inserted, vary according to age. The tube is well lubricated with a water-soluble jelly before insertion. Because the infant or child cannot retain the solution, the nurse holds the buttock for a short time to prevent the fluid from being expelled. A diaper or bedpan is used and the child's back and head supported by a pillow. With an explanation before the procedure, the older child can usually hold the solution. A bedpan or bathroom should be available before the enema is started.

Ostomies

Infants and children may have an ostomy created for various disorders and conditions. A **colostomy** is made by bringing a part of the colon through the abdominal wall to create an outlet for fecal material elimination. Colostomies can be temporary or permanent. A new colostomy may be left to open air or a bag, pouch, or appliance used to collect the stool. An **ileostomy** is a similar opening in the small intestine. The drainage from the ileostomy contains digestive enzymes so the stoma must be fitted with a collection device to prevent skin irritation and breakdown. It is important to teach the child or caregiver how to care for the stoma and skin with any ostomy. Preventing skin breakdown is a priority. A **urostomy** may be created to help in the elimination of urine. Ostomies bags should be checked for leakage, emptied frequently, and changed when needed. A variety of collection bags and devices are available to be used with ostomies. The products used and the procedure for changing the bags or appliances should be reviewed and institution procedures followed. The output from any ostomy is recorded accurately.

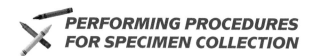

PERFORMING PROCEDURES FOR SPECIMEN COLLECTION

The nurse is often responsible for collecting or assisting in the collection of specimens. Standard precautions (see Appendix E) are followed in collecting and transporting specimens, no matter what the source of the specimen.

Nose and Throat Specimen

Specimens from the nose and throat are used to help diagnosis infection. To collect a specimen, the nose or the back of the throat and tonsils are swabbed with a special collection swab. The swab is placed directly into a culture tube and taken to the lab for analysis. If epiglottitis (Chapter 13) is suspected, a throat culture should not be done because of possible trauma and airway occlusion. To diagnose RSV (Chapter 11), a nasal washing may be done. A small amount of saline is instilled into the nose then the fluid is aspirated and placed into a sterile specimen container.

Urine Specimens

Urine is collected for a variety of reasons including urinalysis, urine cultures, specific gravity, and dip-sticking urine for glucose, protein, and pH. Several methods can be used to obtain specimens. To monitor the intake and output, all urine is collected and measured whether voided into a diaper, urinal, bedpan, or toilet collection device (see intake and output). If urine specimens are needed for diagnostic purposes, other methods of collection may be used. Cotton balls can be placed in the diaper of an infant; the urine squeezed from the cotton ball can be collected and used for many urine tests. Because toddlers and young children cannot usually void on command, they should be offered fluids 15 to 20 minutes before the urine specimen is needed. When requesting a specimen, the nurse uses the word the child knows to identify urination, such as "pee-pee" or "potty," so the child will understand. Offering privacy to the older child and adolescent is important when obtaining a urine specimen.

In preparation for collecting a urine specimen, the infant or child is positioned so that the genitalia are exposed and the area can be cleansed. On the male patient, the tip of the penis is wiped with a soapy cotton ball, followed by a rinse with a cotton ball saturated with sterile water. In the female patient, the labia majora are cleansed front to back using one cotton ball for each wipe. The labia minora are then exposed and cleansed in the same fashion. The area is rinsed with a cotton ball saturated with sterile water. The male or female genitalia are permitted to air-dry before collection methods are followed (see below).

Following the collection, the specimen may be sent to the laboratory in the plastic collection container or in a specimen container preferred by the laboratory. Appropriate documentation includes the time of specimen collection, the amount and color of the urine, the test to be performed, and the condition of the perineal area.

Collection Bag

To collect a urine specimen from infants and toddlers who are not potty trained, a pediatric urine collection bag is used (Fig. 6–10). For the collection bag to stay in place, the skin must be clean, dry, and free of lotions, oils, and powder. The device is a small, plastic bag with a self-adhesive material to apply it to the child's skin. The paper backing is removed from the urine collection container, and the adhesive surface is applied over the penis in the male and the vulva in the female. The child's diaper is replaced. Usually within a short period of time, the child will void and the specimen can be obtained. The collection device should be removed as soon as the child voids.

Clean Catch

If a urine specimen is needed for a culture, the older child may be able to cooperate in the collection of a midstream specimen. Instruct the child as to the procedure so she or he understands what to do. The genital area is cleaned (as above), the child urinates a small amount, stops the flow, then continues to void into a specimen container.

Catheterization

Occasionally children must be catheterized to obtain a specimen, particularly if a sterile specimen is required. If the catheter is only needed to get a specimen, often a small sterile feeding tube is used. If an indwelling or Foley catheter is needed after catheterization, the catheter is left in place, the balloon inflated, and a collection bag attached.

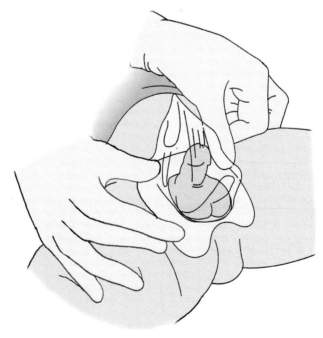

● **Figure 6.10** The skin must be clean and dry in order for the urine collection bag to adhere to the child's skin.

24-Hour Urine Collection

Timed urine collections are sometimes done for a period of as long as 24 hours. The caregiver can often assist the nurse and should be instructed in the procedure. The urine is kept on ice in a special bag or container during the collection time period. At the end of the timed collection, the entire specimen is sent to the lab.

Stool Specimens

Stool specimens are tested for various reasons including the presence of occult blood, ova and parasites, bacteria, glucose, or excess fat. Using a tongue blade, the nurse puts on gloves, collects these specimens from a diaper or bedpan, and places them in clean specimen containers. Stool specimens must not be contaminated with urine, and they must be labeled and delivered to the laboratory promptly. Documentation includes the time of specimen collection; stool color, amount, consistency, and odor; the test to be performed; and the skin condition.

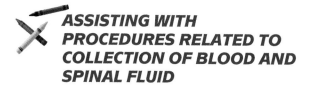

ASSISTING WITH PROCEDURES RELATED TO COLLECTION OF BLOOD AND SPINAL FLUID

One role of the pediatric nurse is to assist with procedures performed on children. The nurse might assist with the collection of blood samples or in holding and supporting a child during a lumbar puncture.

Blood Collection

Blood tests are part of almost every hospitalization experience and many times must be done in other settings to help with diagnosis. Although laboratory personnel or a physician usually obtains the specimens, the nurse must be familiar with the general procedure to explain it to the child. The nurse may be asked to help hold or restrain the child during the procedure. Blood specimens are obtained either by pricking the heel, great toe, earlobe, or finger or by venipuncture. In infants, the jugular or scalp veins are most commonly used; sometimes the femoral vein is used (Fig. 6–11). In older children, the veins in the arm are used.

Lumbar Puncture

When analysis of cerebrospinal fluid is necessary, a lumbar puncture is performed. During this procedure, the nurse must restrain the child in the position shown in Figure 6–12 until the procedure is completed. The nurse grasps the child's hands with the hand that has passed under the child's lower extremities and holds the child snugly against his or her chest. This position enlarges the intervertebral spaces for easier access with the aspiration needle. Children undergoing this procedure may be too young to understand the nurse's explanation. The nurse should tell the child, however, that it is important to hold still and the child will have help to do this. The lumbar puncture is performed with strict asepsis. A sterile dressing is applied when the procedure is complete. The child must remain quiet for 1 hour after the procedure. Vital signs, level of consciousness, and motor activity should be monitored frequently for several hours after the procedure.

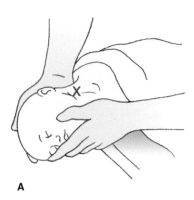

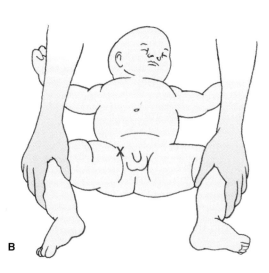

● *Figure 6.11* **(A)** Position of infant for jugular venipuncture. **(B)** Position of infant for femoral venipuncture.

A PERSONAL GLIMPSE

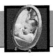

I have been sick so many times that I don't know which one to write about. When I had hapetitis, I was very sick for a very long time. I missed a lot of school. I had to get blood tests, urine tests, and medications all the time, and I slept a lot, because I felt tired all the time. Every time I had to get a blood test I would cry because I didn't want to go. After a very long time, I got well enough to go back to school, but I couldn't play any gym games or activities because I couldn't get hit in my belly.

Justin, age 9 years

▶ **LEARNING OPPORTUNITY:** What approach would be appropriate for the nurse to take with this patient if he were to become ill again and need medical care? What would you say to him before any treatment or procedure was done?

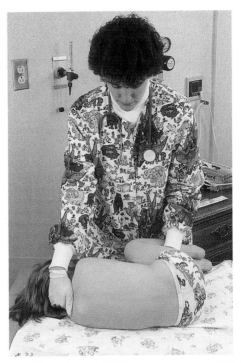

● **Figure 6.12** Position of child for lumbar puncture. (© B. Proud.)

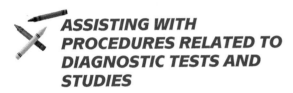

ASSISTING WITH PROCEDURES RELATED TO DIAGNOSTIC TESTS AND STUDIES

A variety of healthcare personnel in the radiology, nuclear imaging, and other departments of the healthcare setting perform many diagnostic tests and procedures. These diagnostic studies include X-rays, arteriograms, computed tomography (CT) scans, intravenous pyelograms, bone or brain scans, EKGs, EEGs, MRIs, and cardiac catheterizations. The nurse's role often is to teach and prepare the child and the caregiver for the procedures to be done. After orders have been written, the nurse requests and schedules the tests or studies to be done. The required paperwork is completed and consents are signed. If the child must be NPO prior to the study, the nurse ensures that the NPO status is maintained. Any allergies are clarified and documented on the consent and requisition forms. During the procedure the nurse might be called on to support and comfort or restrain the child. Following the procedure, the nurse performs and documents the care needed.

- Following guidelines and policies is important in preparation and in follow-up of procedures and treatments.
- When administering physical care, doing procedures, and assisting with treatments for a child, the nurse calls on a wide variety of skills that must be modified to meet the child's growth and developmental level.
- When restraints are necessary, care including regular, careful observation must be taken to protect the child from injury.
- In teaching a family caregiver about methods to relieve an elevated temperature in a child, the nurse must be certain to include safety measures.
- Accurately measuring and documenting intake and output are important tasks for the pediatric nurse.
- Oxygen is administered in a variety of ways to children. Careful monitoring of the child and equipment is necessary.
- When collecting specimens of any type of body secretion, it is important to follow standard precautions in handling and transporting specimens.
- The nurse's role in assisting with procedures and treatments is often one of supporting the child as well as the caregiver.

KEY POINTS

- Preparation of the child for procedures and treatments includes preparing the child emotionally.

BIBLIOGRAPHY

(2000) *Nursing procedures* (3rd ed). Springhouse, PA: Springhouse Corporation.

Barone MA, Rowe PC. (1999) Pediatric procedures, *Oski's pediatrics: Principles and practice* (3rd ed). Philadelphia: Lippincott Williams & Wilkins.

Champi C, Gaffney-Yocum P. (2001) Managing febrile seizures in children. *Dimensions of Critical Care Nursing,* 20(5).

Chandler, T. (2000) Oxygen saturation monitoring. *Pediatric Nursing,* 12(8). 37–42

Craven RF, Hirnle CJ. (1999) *Fundamentals of nursing* (3rd ed). Philadelphia: Lippincott Williams & Wilkins.

Pillitteri A.(1999) *Maternal and child health nursing* (3rd ed). Philadelphia: Lippincott Williams & Wilkins.

Wilson L. (2000) Nurse-assisted PEG in pediatric patients. *Gastroenterology Nursing,* 23(3), 121.

Wong DL, Hess C. (2000) *Wong and Whaley's clinical manual of pediatric nursing* (5th ed). St. Louis: Mosby.

Wong DL, Perry S, Hockenberry M. (2002) *Maternal child nursing care* (2nd ed). St. Louis: Mosby.

Woodring BC. (2001) Humane treatment of children. *Journal of Child and Family Nursing,* 4(3).

Websites

www.wwnurse.com

www.nursetonurse.com

http://nursing.about.com/library/blhowto.htm

Workbook

NCLEX-STYLE REVIEW QUESTIONS

1. When the nurse is performing or assisting the care provider in doing a treatment, which of the following actions by the nurse would be the HIGHEST priority? The nurse

   a. explains the procedure to the child

   b. gathers the needed supplies

   c. identifies the child prior to beginning the procedure

   d. documents the procedure immediately after completion

2. The nurse is inserting a nasogastric tube on a toddler. Which of the following restraints would be the MOST appropriate for the nurse to use with this child during this procedure?

   a. mummy restraint

   b. clove hitch restraint

   c. elbow restraint

   d. jacket restraint

3. After giving instructions to the child's caregiver regarding methods used to reduce an elevated temperature, the caregiver makes the following statements. Which statement would require follow-up by the nurse?

   a. "The last time my child had shots I gave her Tylenol."

   b. "When my older child had a fever, I always gave him a cold bath."

   c. "I never have had trouble getting my child to drink juice."

   d. "My child does not like lots of blankets over her."

4. When caring for a 3½-year-old child who is receiving oxygen in an oxygen tent, which of the following toys or activities would be best to offer this child?

   a. A radio playing soothing music

   b. Age appropriate books to look at

   c. A favorite blanket belonging to the child

   d. Board games the child can play alone

5. The practical nurse is participating in the development of a plan of care for a child who has a new ileostomy. Of the following nursing diagnosis, which would be the HIGHEST priority for this child?

   a. 'Risk for altered development"

   b. "Ineffective family coping'

   c. "Bowel incontinence"

   d. "Risk for impaired skin integrity"

STUDY ACTIVITIES

1. Using the table below, list the types of restraints, describe each restraint, and explain the purpose of using this type of restraint in the pediatric patient.

Type of Restraint	Description	Purpose

2. Develop a teaching plan to be used in teaching a group of caregivers about caring for a child who has a fever. Include in your plan when and how to take a temperature, what to do to reduce the fever, and when it would be important for the caregiver to call the health care provider.

3. Make a list of games and activities that a child who is in an oxygen tent could play or do. Develop a game or activity that would be appropriate to use with a child who is in an oxygen tent.

CRITICAL THINKING

1. Three-year-old Denise has an elevated temperature of 104.4 °F (40.2°C). Describe the steps you would take to care for her. Include the explanations you would give the child and the caregiver for what you are doing.

2. The caregiver of a 2-year-old child seems upset when you enter the patient's room. The child has a feeding tube in place as well as an intravenous line. The caregiver says, "My child does not like to have her hands tied down. Why don't you just untie her?" What explanation would you give to the caregiver? What could you do to help reassure this caregiver and support this child?

3. What factors must be considered when providing activities for a child who must be in an oxygen tent? Explain why these factors must be considered.

Medication Administration and IV Therapy

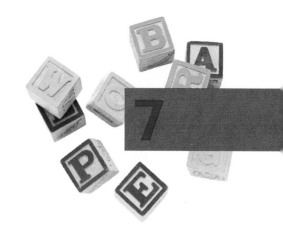

MEDICATION ADMINISTRATION
  Computing Dosages
  Oral Medication
  Intramuscular Medication
  Other Routes of Medication
  Administration

INTRAVENOUS THERAPY
  Fundamentals of Fluid Balance
  Intravenous Fluid Administration
  Intravenous Medication
  Intravenous Sites
  Infusion Control

STUDENT OBJECTIVES

On completion of this chapter, the student will be able to

1. Identify the six "rights" of medication administration.
2. Convert pounds to kilograms of body weight to use in pediatric dosage calculation.
3. Calculate low and high dosages of medications using body weight.
4. Identify a variety of medication administration routes.
5. Identify the muscle preferred for intramuscular injections in the infant.
6. Discuss fluid balance in pediatric patients.
7. State the reason that a pediatric intravenous set-up has a burette chamber in the line.

KEY TERMS

acid-base balance
acidosis
alkalosis
azotemia
body surface area method
electrolytes
extracellular fluid
extravasation
homeostasis
induration
intermittent infusion device
interstitial fluid
intracellular fluid
intravascular fluid
total parenteral nutrition
West nomogram

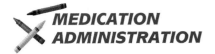

MEDICATION ADMINISTRATION

Caring for children who are ill challenges every nurse to function at the highest level of professional competence. Giving medications is one of the most important nursing responsibilities; medication administration calls for accuracy, precision, and considerable psychological skill. Basic to administering medications to a person of any age are the following six "rights" of medication administration:

- The right medication. Check the drug label to confirm that it is the correct drug. Do not use a drug that is not clearly labeled. Check the expiration date of the drug.
- The right patient. Check the identification bracelet *each* time that a medication is given to confirm identification of the patient. In settings where an ID bracelet is not worn, always verify the child's name with the caregiver.
- The right dose. Always double-check the dose by calculating the dosage according to the child's weight. Question the order if it is unclear. Have another qualified person double-check any time that a divided dosage is to be given or for insulin, digoxin, and other agents governed by the facility's policy. Use drug references or check with a physician or pharmacist for the appropriateness of the dose. Orders must be questioned *before* the drug is given.
- The right route. Give the drug only by the route ordered. Question the order if it is unclear or confusing. If a child is vomiting or a drug needs to be given by an alternate route, always get an order from the provider before administration.
- The right time. Administering a drug at the correct time helps to maintain the desired blood level of the drug. When giving a prn medication, always check the last time it was given and clarify how much has been given over the past 24 hours.
- The right documentation. Recording the administration of the medication, especially prn medications, is critical to avoid potential errors in medication administration.

Administering medications to children is much more complex than these guidelines indicate. Accurate administration of medications to children is especially critical because of the variable responses to drugs that children have as a result of immature body systems. The nurse must understand the factors that influence or alter how the child absorbs, metabolizes and excretes the medication, and any allergies that the child has. The nurse is responsible for the admin-

istration of medications and, therefore, is legally liable for errors of medication. It is also important to teach the patient and the family caregivers about the effects and possible side effects of medications given.

Nine rules to guide the nurse in administering medications are presented in Box 7–1. The nurse should evaluate each child from a developmental point of view to administer medications successfully. Understanding, planning, and implementing nursing care that considers the child's developmental level and coping mechanisms contribute to administering medications with minimal trauma to the child (Table 7–1).

Medication errors can occur because nurses are human and not perfect. To admit an error is often difficult, especially if there has been carelessness concerning the rules. A person may be strongly tempted to adopt a "wait and see" attitude, which is the gravest error of all. Nurses must accept responsibility for their own actions. Serious consequences for the child may be avoided if a mistake is disclosed promptly.

BOX 7.1	**Nine Rules of Medication Administration in Children**

1. Never give a child a choice of whether or not to receive medicine. The medication is ordered and is necessary for recovery, therefore, there is no choice to be made.
2. Do give choices that allow the child some control over the situation such as the kind of juice or the number of bandages.
3. Never lie. Do not tell a child that an injection will not hurt.
4. Keep explanations simple and brief. Use words that the child will understand.
5. Assure the child that it is all right to be afraid and that it is okay to cry.
6. Do not talk in front of the child as though he or she were not there. Include the child in the conversation when talking to family caregivers.
7. Be positive in approaching the child. Be firm and assertive when explaining to the child what will happen.
8. Keep the time between explanation and execution to a minimum. The younger the child, the shorter the time should be.
   Keep the explanation simple.
   Preparations such as setting up an injection, solutions, or instrument trays should be done out of the child's sight.
9. Obtain cooperation from family caregivers. They may be able to calm a frightened child, persuade the child to take the medication, and achieve cooperation for care.

TABLE 7.1	Developmental Considerations in Medication Administration

Age	Behaviors	Nursing Actions
Birth–3 mo	Reaches randomly toward mouth and has a strong reflex to grasp objects	The infant's hands must be held to prevent spilling of medications.
	Poor head control	The infant's head must be supported while medications are given.
	Tongue movement may force medication out of mouth	A syringe or dropper should be placed along the side of the mouth.
	Sucks as a reflex with stimulation	Use this natural sucking desire by placing oral medications into a nipple and administering in that manner.
	Stops sucking when full	Administer medications before feeding when infant is hungry. Be aware that some medications' absorption is affected by food.
	Responds to tactile stimulations	The likelihood that the medication is taken will increase if the infant is held in a feeding position.
3–12 mo	Begins to develop fine muscle control and advances from sitting to crawling	Medication must be kept out of reach to avoid accidental ingestion.
	Tongue may protrude when swallowing	Administer medication with a syringe.
	Responds to tactile stimuli	Physical comfort (holding) given after a medication is helpful.
12–30 mo	Advances from independent walking to running without falling	Allow the toddler to choose position for taking medication.
	Advances from messy self-feeding to proficient feeding with minimal spilling	Allow the toddler to take medicine from a cup or spoon.
	Has voluntary tongue control; begins to drink from a cup	Disguise medication in a small amount of food to decrease incidence of spitting out medication.
	Develops second molars	Chewable tablets may be an alternative.
	Exhibits independence and self-assertiveness	Allow as much freedom as possible. Use games to gain confidence. Use a consistent, firm approach. Give immediate praise for cooperation.
	Responds to sense of time and simple direction	Give direction to "Drink this now" and "Open your mouth."
	Responds to and participates in routines of daily living	Involve the family caregivers and include the toddler in medicine routines.
	Expresses feelings easily	Allow for expression through play.
30 mo–6 y	Knows full name	Ask the child his or her name before giving medicine.
	Is easily influenced by others when responding to new foods or tastes	Approach the child in a calm, positive manner when giving medications.
	Has a good sense of time and a tolerance of frustration	Use correct immediate rewards for the young child and delayed gratification for the older child.
	Enjoys making decision	Give choices when possible.
	Has many fantasies; has fear of mutilation	Give simple explanations. Stress that the medication is not being given because the child is bad.
	Is more coordinated	Child can hold cup and may be able to master pill-taking.
	Begins to lose teeth	Chewable tablets may be inappropriate because of loose teeth.
6–12 y	Strives for independence	Give acceptable choices. Respect the need for regression during hospitalization.
	Has concern for bodily mutilation	Give reassurance that medication, especially injectables, will not cause harm. Reinforce that medications should be taken only when given by nurse or family caregiver.
	Can tell time	Include the child in daily schedule of medication. Make the child a poster of medications and time due so he or she can be involved in care.
	Is concerned with body image and privacy	Provide private area for administration of medication, especially injections.
	Peer support and interaction are important.	Allow child to share experiences with others.
12+ years	Strives for independence	Write a contract with the adolescent, spelling out expectations for self-medication.
	Can understand abstract theories	Explain why medications are given and how they work.

TABLE 7.1 (continued)	Developmental Considerations in Medication Administration	
Age	**Behaviors**	**Nursing Actions**
12+ years	Decisions are influenced by peers	Encourage teens to talk with their peers in a support group. Work with teens to plan medication schedule around their activities. Differentiate pill-taking from drug-taking.
	Questions authority figures	Be honest and provide medication information in writing.
	Is concerned with sex and sexuality	Explain relationships between illness, medications, and sexuality. For example, emphasize, "This medication will not react with your birth-control pills."

INTERNET EXERCISE 7.1

www.findarticles.com

Go to the space next to *for* and type in *Medication Errors DOSING ERROR.*
Scroll down to Medication Errors DOSING ERROR.

1. What does the author say should always be written before a decimal for doses that are less than 1?

Scroll down to RESPONDING TO ERRORS.

2. List four disciplinary actions that can occur following a medication error.

Computing Dosages

Commercial unit-dose packaging sometimes does not include dosages for children, so the nurse must calculate the correct dosage. Two methods of computing dosages are used to determine accurate pediatric medication dosages. Nurses use these methods to clarify that dosages ordered are appropriate and accurate. The first method uses the child's weight to determine dosage. To use this method, the child's weight in kilograms must be calculated if the weight has been recorded in pounds. The second method uses the child's body surface area.

Conversion of Pounds to Kilograms

To use the body weight method of dosage calculation, a child's weight recorded in pounds has to be converted into kilograms. To do this, set up a proportion using the number of pounds in a kilogram in one fraction and the known weight in pounds and the unknown weight in kilograms in the other fraction. For a child weighing 42 pounds, the conversion is set up as follows:

$$\frac{2.2 \text{ lbs}}{1 \text{ kg}} = \frac{42 \text{ lbs}}{X \text{ kg}}$$

The fractions are then cross-multiplied:

$$2.2 \text{ lb} \times X \text{ kg} = 1 \text{ kg} \times 42 \text{ lb}$$

The problem is solved for X. Divide each side by 2.2 and cancel the units that are in both the numerator and the denominator

$$\frac{2.2 \text{ lb} \times X \text{ kg}}{2.2 \text{ lb}} = \frac{1 \text{ kg} \times 42 \text{ lb}}{2.2 \text{ lb}}$$

$$X = \frac{42}{2.2}$$

$$x = 19 \text{ kg}$$

(adapted from [2000] *Springhouse Nurse's Drug Guide*)

The child who weighs 42 pounds weighs 19 kilograms.

Body Weight Method

The first method of computing dosages uses the child's weight. Often drug companies provide a dosage range of milligrams of a medication to number of kilograms the child weighs. To calculate an accurate dose for a child, the nurse uses the dosage range provided by the drug manufacturer. The child's weight in kilograms is used to calculate a safe dose range for that child. For example if a dosage range of 10 to 30 mg/kg of body weight is a safe dosage range and a child weighs 20 kgs, calculate the low safe dose using the following:

$$\frac{10 \text{ mg}}{1 \text{ kg}} = \frac{X \text{ mg}}{20 \text{ kg}}$$

Cross multiply the fractions:

$$10 \text{ mg} \times 20 \text{ kg} = 1 \text{ kg} \times X \text{ mg}$$

Solve for X by dividing each side of the equation by 1 (canceling the units that are in both the numerator and the denominator):

$$\frac{10 \text{ mg} \times 20 \text{ kg}}{1 \text{ kg}} = \frac{1 \text{ kg} \times X \text{ mg}}{1 \text{ kg}}$$

$$200 \times 1 = 1X$$

$$200 = X$$

The low safe dose range of this medication for the child who weighs 20 kilograms is 200 milligrams.

To calculate the high safe dose for this child, use the following:

$$\frac{30 \text{ mg}}{1 \text{ kg}} = \frac{X \text{ mg}}{20 \text{ kg}}$$

Cross multiply the fractions:

$$30 \text{ mg} \times 20 \text{ kg} = 1 \text{ kg} \times X \text{ mg}$$

Solve for X by dividing each side of the equation by 1 (canceling the units that are in both the numerator and the denominator):

$$\frac{30 \text{ mg} \times 20 \text{ kg}}{} = \frac{1 \text{ kg} \times X \text{ mg}}{1 \text{ kg}}$$

$$600 \times 1 = 1X$$

$$600 = X$$

The high safe dose range of this medication for the child who weighs 20 kilograms is 600 milligrams.

The safe dosage range for this medication for the child who weighs 20 kg is 200 mg to 600 mg. (Adapted from [2000] *Springhouse Nurse's Drug Guide*.)

Body Surface Area Method

The second formula used to calculate dosages is the **body surface area (BSA) method.** The **West nomogram,** commonly used to calculate BSA, is a graph with several scales arranged so that when two values are known, the third can be plotted by drawing a line with a straight edge (Fig. 7–1). The child's weight is marked on the right scale, the height on the left scale. Use a straight edge to draw a line between the two marks. The point where the lines cross the column labeled *SA* (surface area) is the BSA expressed in square meters (m²). The average adult BSA is 1.7 m²; thus, the formula to calculate the appropriate dosage for a child is

$$\text{Estimated child's dose} = \frac{\text{child's BSA (m}^2)}{1.7 \text{ (adult BSA)}}$$

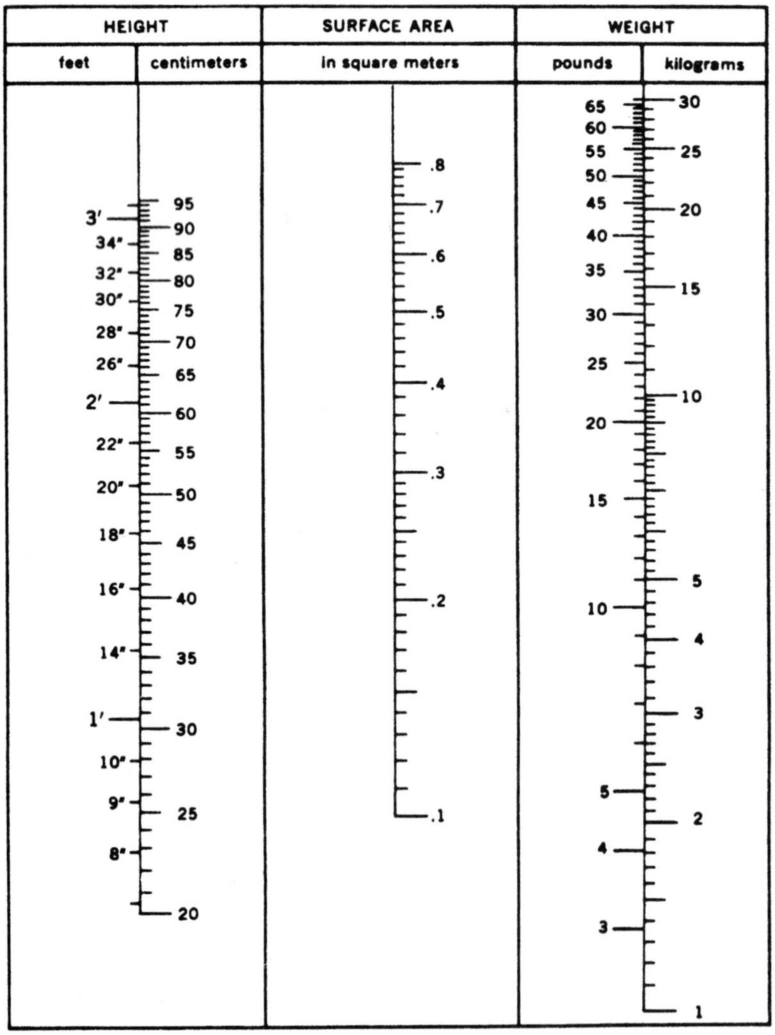

● *Figure 7.1* West nomogram for estimating surface area of infants and young children. To determine the body surface area, draw a straight line between the point representing the child's height on the left scale to the child's weight on the right scale. The point at which this line intersects the middle scale is the child's body surface area in square meters.

For example, a child is 37 inches (95 cm) tall and weighs 34 lb (15.5 kg). The usual adult dose of the medication is 500 mg. Place and hold one end of a straight edge on the first column at 37 inches and move it so that it lines up with 34 lb in the far right column. On the SA column, the straight edge falls across 0.64 (m²). You are ready to do the calculation.

$$\frac{0.64}{1.7} = 0.38$$

You now know that the child's BSA is 0.38 that of the average adult. You are ready to calculate the child's dose by multiplying 0.38 times 500 mg.

$$0.38 \times 500 = 190$$

The child's dose is 190 mg.

After computing any dosage, the nurse should *always* have the computation checked by another staff person qualified to give medication or someone in the department who is delegated for this purpose. Errors are easy to make and easy to overlook. A second person should do the computation separately, then both results should be compared.

Oral Medication

Small babies who are hungry are not too particular about the taste of food. Almost anything liquid may be sucked through a nipple including liquid medicines unless they are bitter. Medications that are available in syrup or fruit-flavored suspensions are easily administered this way. Another method of administering oral medications is to drop them slowly into the baby's mouth with a plastic medicine dropper or oral syringe. When using a syringe, place it on the side of the tongue and slowly drip the medication into the infant's mouth (Fig. 7–2).

Elixirs contain alcohol and are apt to cause choking unless they are diluted. Syrups and suspensions are thick and may need dilution to ensure that the child gets the full dose. Always check with the pharmacist before diluting any medication.

When a child is old enough to swallow a pill, make sure that the pill is actually swallowed. When asked to open their mouths, children usually cooperate so well and open so wide that their tonsils can be inspected. While the mouth is open, the nurse can look under the tongue to be sure the medication is not hidden. Chewable tablets work well for the preschool child.

It usually is best to give medicine in solution form to a small child. Tablets, if used, must be dissolved in water. Do not use orange juice for a solvent unless specifically ordered to do so; the child may always associate the taste of orange juice with the unpleasant medicine. If the medicine is bitter,

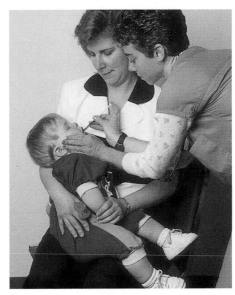

● **Figure 7.2** A syringe may be used to administer an oral medication by placing the syringe at the side of the tongue.

corn syrup may disguise the taste. The child may develop a dislike for corn syrup, but that is not as important as a lifelong dislike of orange juice.

There is little excuse for restraining a small child and forcing a medication down the child's throat. The child can always have the last word and bring it up again. The danger of aspiration is real. Of even greater importance are the antagonism and helplessness that build up in the child subject to such a procedure. A child's sense of dignity must be respected as much as that of an adult. Refer to Table 7–1 to review the developmental characteristics to be considered at each age.

Intramuscular Medication

Children have the same fear of needles as do adults. Inexperienced nurses are reluctant to hurt children and often cause the pain they are trying to prevent by inserting the needle slowly. A swift, sure thrust with insertion is the best way to minimize pain, but the nurse must stay calm and sure and be prepared for the child's squirming. It is best to have a second nurse help hold the child if he or she is younger than school age or if this is his or her first injection.

Injections should be given to a child in the treatment room rather than in bed or in the playroom. The bed and playroom should be "safe" places for the child. The nurse may have a ready Band-Aid to cover the injection site. This technique prevents young children from worrying that they might "leak out" of the hole, and the bandage serves as a badge of courage or bravery for the older child.

Figures 7–3 through 7–6 illustrate each intramuscular injection site and how to locate them.

COMMUNICATIONS BOX 7.1

Three-year-old Nickie must have an intramuscular injection. He is crying and protesting loudly.

LESS EFFECTIVE COMMUNICATION	*MORE EFFECTIVE COMMUNICATION*

LESS EFFECTIVE COMMUNICATION

Nurse: Nickie, I have to give you an injection to help make you better.

Nickie: No! Get away from me!

Nurse: Oh, come on, Nickie! Show me what a big boy you can be.

Nickie: (Protesting even louder) No! I hate you! I don't want a shot!

Nurse: You have to have it, Nickie. Turn over so we can get it over with.

Nickie: No!! (Kicking)

Nurse: I'll have to have Miss Jones hold you down so I can give it to you. It's only going to feel like a little sting.

Nickie: Shots hurt a lot. I want my Mommy.

Nurse: No, I'll just have Miss Jones help hold you still. Your mother can wait out in the hall.

Nickie: I want my Mommy!

Nurse: Just wait till we finish here and she can come back in.

> *(The injection is accomplished with two nurses holding Nickie while he loudly protests). In this scenario, the nurse charges Nickie to be a big boy. The nurse does not acknowledge his fears or offer him any sense of control. The nurse even refuses to let Nickie have his mother for consolation.*

MORE EFFECTIVE COMMUNICATION

Nurse: Nickie, I have to give you an injection to help make you better.

Nickie: No! Get away from me!

Nurse: Getting an injection is scary for you. You are afraid it's going to hurt.

Nickie: Yes! Get away!

Nurse: It will hurt a little when it goes in, but I'll be very quick about it, and we can put a bandage on it when we are finished.

Nickie: But I don't want it. (Beginning to quiet a little)

Nurse: I know. You can choose which hip to use. How would it be if you hold the bandage for me till we're finished?

Nickie: Well, OK, but I want Mommy to hold my hand.

Nurse: Sure, and I'll need you to help me by lying very still while Miss Jones helps you keep your legs still. Can you count to ten for me while I give it to you?

Nickie: OK.

> *In this scenario, the nurse acknowledges Nickie's feelings of fear and pain. The nurse lets him know that she will listen to him and offers him some control by allowing him to choose the site and hold the bandage. The nurse also agrees to his request for his mother. The nurse admits the injection may be painful, but suggests ways to reduce the pain.*

Vastus Lateralis

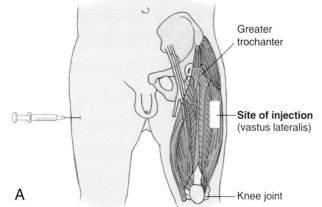

Greater trochanter

Site of injection
(vastus lateralis)

Knee joint

A

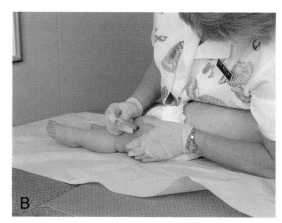

B

● *Figure 7.3* **(A)** Vastus lateralis muscle. **(B)** Intramuscular injection into the vastus lateralis.

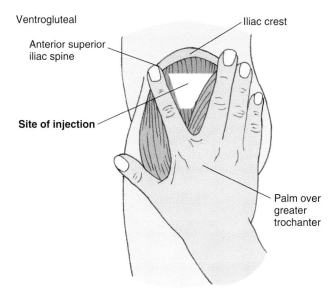

● *Figure 7.4* Locating the ventrogluteal intramuscular injection site.

Table 7–2 describes each of these sites, how to locate them, the suggested needle size, and the amount of medication.

Other Routes of Medication Administration

With few variations, the principles of administering medications by other routes are much the same as those for adults. Eye, ear, and nose drops should be warmed to room temperature before being administered. The infant or young child may need to be restrained for safe administration. This restraint may

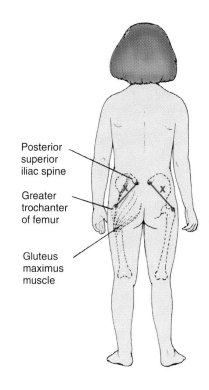

A

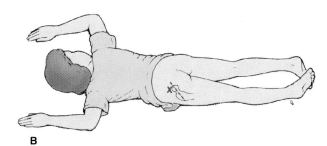

B

● *Figure 7.6* **(A)** Locating the dorsogluteal intramuscular injection site. **(B)** Child in position for dorsogluteal intramuscular injection. The site is marked by an X.

be accomplished with a mummy restraint or the assistance of a second person. The nurse must realize that these are invasive procedures and that the young child may be resistant. Approaching the child with patience, explanations, and praise for cooperation helps gain the child's cooperation. Documentation must be completed after the administration of any medication.

Eye Drops or Ointment

The child is placed in a supine position. To instill the drops, the lower lid is pulled down to form a pocket, and the solution is dropped into the pocket (Fig. 7–7). The eye is held shut briefly, if possible, to help distribute the medication to the conjunctiva. Ointment is applied from the inner to the outer canthus with care not to touch the eye with the tip of the dropper or tube.

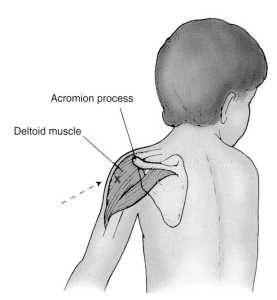

● *Figure 7.5* Location of the deltoid intramuscular injection site. The site is marked by an X.

TABLE 7.2 | Intramuscular Injection Sites

Muscle Site	Needle Size	Maximum Amount	Procedures
Vastus lateralis (Fig. 7–3)	Infant: 25 gauge, ⅝ inch or 23 gauge, 1 inch	1 mL	This main thigh muscle is used almost exclusively in infants for intramuscular injections but is used frequently in children for all ages. Locate the trochanter (hip joint) and knee as landmarks. Divide the area between landmarks into thirds. Inject into the middle third section, using the lateral aspect. Inject at a 90-degree angle.
	Older: 22 gauge, 1 inch to 1.5 inches	2 mL	
Ventrogluteal (Fig. 7–4)	Assess child's muscle mass. 22–25 gauge, ⅝ inch to 1 inch		With thumb facing the front of child, place forefinger on the anterior superior iliac spine with middle finger on the iliac crest and the palm centered over the greater trochanter. Inject at a 90-degree angle below the iliac crest within the triangle defined. No important nerves are in this area.
	Infant:	½–¾ mL	
	Toddler:	1 mL	
	School-age and older:	1½–2 mL	
Deltoid (Fig. 7–5)	Not recommended for infants		Expose entire arm. Locate the acromion process at the top of the arm. Give the injection in the densest part of the muscle below the acromion process and above the armpit. Not recommended for repeated injections. Can be used for one-time immunizations. Angle needle slightly toward the shoulder.
	Older: 22–25 gauge, 0.5 inch to 1 inch	Small muscle limits amount to ½–1 mL	
Dorsogluteal (Fig. 7–6)	This site is not recommended in children who have not been walking for at least 1 to 2 yrs. Not recommended for infant or toddler.		Because of the location of the sciatic nerve, use of this site is discouraged in younger children. Place child on abdomen with toes pointing in; this relaxes the gluteus. Locate the posterior superior iliac crest and the greater trochanter of the femur. Draw an imaginary line between the two. Give the injection above and to the outside of this line. The needle should be inserted at a 90-degree angle.
	School-age and older: 20–25 gauge, 0.5 inch to 1.5 inches	1½–2 mL	

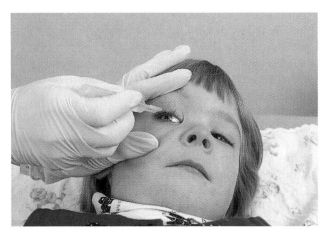

● **Figure 7.7** Administering eye drops. (© B. Proud.)

Nose Drops

Before nose drops are instilled, the nostrils should be wiped free of mucus. For instillation, an infant may be held in the nurse's arms with the head tilted over the arm. For a toddler or older child, the head may be placed over a pillow while the child is lying flat. The infant or child should maintain the position for at least 1 minute to ensure distribution of the medication.

Ear Drops

The infant or young child is placed in a side-lying position with the affected ear up. In an infant or toddler, the pinna (the outer part of the ear) is pulled *down* and back to straighten the ear canal. In a child older than 3 years of age, the pinna is pulled *up* and back, as with adults, to straighten the canal (Fig. 7–8).

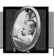

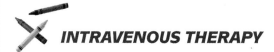

When I was 5 years old I went to the doctors office. I had to get shots my Mom said for school. I don't know what they were for. I felt scared before I went. My Mom told me ideas to think about when I got the shots so I wouldn't think about it hurting. She told me to think about my puppy dog and flowers and sailing ships. The nurse told me it would hurt a little. It hurt when the nurse stuck a needle in my leg. It didn't hurt as much as I thought it would. The nurse was nice and told me I was a brave girl. I am glad I thought about my dog Cheeto. I was happy to go to kindergarten.

Adriel, age 6

▶ **LEARNING OPPORTUNITY:** Why is it important to prepare children for medication administration? What would you include when teaching a child prior to giving IM injections?

After instilling the drops, gently massage the area in front of the ear. The child should be kept in a position with the affected ear up for 5 to 10 minutes. A cotton pledget may be loosely inserted into the ear to prevent leakage of medication, but care should be taken to avoid blocking drainage from the ear.

Rectal Medications

For the administration of rectal medications, the child is placed in a side-lying position, and the nurse must wear gloves or a finger cot. The suppository is lubricated, then inserted into the rectum, followed by a finger, up to the first knuckle joint. The little finger

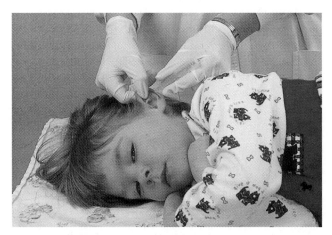

● *Figure 7.8* Positioning for ear drops. The pinna is pulled up and back. (© B. Proud.)

should be used for insertion in infants. After the insertion of the suppository, the buttocks must be held tightly together for 1 or 2 minutes until the child's urge to expel the suppository passes.

INTRAVENOUS THERAPY

Fluids and medications are often administered intravenously (IV) to infants and children. Planning nursing care for the child receiving IV therapy requires knowledge of the physiology of fluids and electrolytes as well as the child's developmental level and an understanding of the emotional aspects of IV therapy for children. Intravenous therapy is commonly administered in the pediatric patient for the following reasons:

- To maintain fluid and electrolyte balance
- To administer antibiotic therapy
- To provide nutritional support
- To administer chemotherapy or anticancer drugs
- To administer pain medication

Candidates for IV therapy include children who have poor gastrointestinal absorption caused by diarrhea, vomiting, and dehydration; those who need a high serum concentration of a drug; those who have resistant infections that require IV medications; those with emergency problems; and those who need continuous pain relief.

Fundamentals of Fluid Balance

Maintenance of fluid balance in the body tissues is essential to health. Uncorrected, severe imbalance causes death, as in patients with serious dehydration resulting from severe diarrhea, vomiting, or loss of fluids in extensive burns. The fundamental concepts of fluid and electrolyte balance in body tissue are reviewed briefly to help the student understand the importance of adequate fluid therapy for the sick child.

Water

A continuous supply of water is necessary for life. At birth, water accounts for about 77% of body weight. Between ages 1 and 2 years , this proportion decreases to the adult level of about 60%.

In health, the body's water requirement is met through the normal intake of fluids and foods. Intake is regulated by the person's thirst and hunger. Normal body losses of fluid occur through the lungs (breathing) and the skin (sweating) and in the urine and feces. In the normal state of health, intake and output amounts balance each other, and the body is said to be in a state of **homeostasis** (a uniform state). Homeostasis signifies biologically the dynamic equilibrium of the healthy organism. This balance is achieved by appropriate shifts in fluid and electrolytes across the cellular membrane and by elimination of the end products of metabolism and excess electrolytes.

Body water, which contains electrolytes, is situated within the cells, in the spaces between the cells, and in the plasma and blood. Imbalance (failure to maintain homeostasis) may be the result of some pathologic process in the body. Some of the disorders associated with imbalance are pyloric stenosis, high fever, persistent or severe diarrhea and vomiting, and extensive burns. Retention of fluid may occur through impaired kidney action or altered metabolism.

Intracellular Fluid. Intracellular fluid is contained within the body cells. Nearly half the volume of body water in the infant is intracellular. Intracellular fluid accounts for about 40% of body weight in both infants and adults. Each cell must be supplied with oxygen and nutrients to keep the body healthy. In addition, the body's water and salt levels must be kept constant within narrow parameters.

A semipermeable membrane that retains protein and other large constituents within the cell surrounds cells. Water, certain salts and minerals, nutrients, and oxygen enter the cell through this membrane. Waste products and useful substances produced within the cell are excreted or secreted into the surrounding spaces.

Extracellular Fluid. Extracellular fluid is situated outside the cells. It may be **interstitial fluid** (situated within the spaces or gaps of body tissue) or **intravascular fluid** (situated within the blood vessels or blood plasma). Blood plasma contains protein within the walls of the blood vessels and water and mineral salts that flow freely from the vascular system into the surrounding tissues.

Interstitial fluid (also called intercellular or tissue fluid) has a composition similar to plasma except that it contains almost no protein. This reservoir of fluid outside the body cells decreases or increases easily in response to disease. An increase in interstitial fluid results in edema. Dehydration depletes this fluid before the intracellular and plasma supplies are affected.

In the infant, about 25% to 35% of body weight is due to interstitial fluid. In the adult, interstitial fluid accounts for only about 15% of body weight (Fig. 7–9). Infants and children become dehydrated much more quickly than do adults. In part, this dehydration occurs because of a greater fluid exchange caused by the rapid metabolic activity associated with infants' growth and because of the relatively larger ratio of

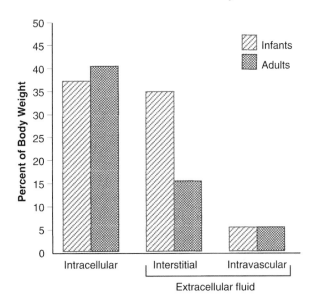

Fluid Distribution in Body

● *Figure 7.9* Graph indicating distribution of fluid in body compartments. Comparison between the infant and adult fluid distribution in body compartments shows that the adult total is about 60% of body weight, whereas the infant total is more than 70% of body weight.

skin surface area to body fluid volume, which is two or three times that of adults.

Because of these factors, the infant who is taking in no fluid loses an amount of body fluid equal to the extracellular volume in about 5 days or twice as rapidly as does an adult. The infant's relatively larger volume of extracellular fluid may be designed to compensate partially for this greater loss.

Electrolytes

Electrolytes are chemical compounds (minerals) that break down into ions when placed in water. An ion is an atom having a positive or a negative electrical charge. Important electrolytes in body fluids are sodium (Na^+), potassium (K^+), magnesium (Mg^{++}), calcium (Ca^{++}), chloride (Cl), phosphate (PO_4), and bicarbonate (HCO_3). Electrolytes have the important function of maintaining acid-base balance. Each water compartment of the body has its own normal electrolyte composition.

Acid-Base Balance

Acid-base balance is a state of equilibrium between the acidity and the alkalinity of body fluids. The acidity of a solution is determined by the concentration of hydrogen (H^+) ions. Acidity is expressed by the symbol pH. Neutral fluids have a pH of 7.0, acid fluids lower than 7.0, and alkaline fluids higher than 7.0. Normally body fluids are slightly alkaline. Internal body fluids have a pH of 7.35 to 7.45. Body excretions, however, are products of metabolism and become acid; the normal pH of urine, for example, is 5.5 to 6.5.

Defects in the acid-base balance result either in **acidosis** (excessive acidity of body fluids) or **alkalosis** (excessive alkalinity of body fluids). Acidosis may occur in conditions such as diabetes, kidney failure, and diarrhea. Hypochloremic alkalosis may occur in pyloric stenosis because of the decrease in chloride concentration and increase in carbon dioxide.

In normal health, the fluid and electrolyte balance is maintained through the intake of a well-balanced diet. The kidneys play an important part in regulating concentrations of electrolytes in the various fluid compartments. In illness, the balance may be disturbed because of excessive losses of certain electrolytes. Replacement of these minerals is necessary to restore health and maintain life. When the infant or child can take sufficient fluids orally, that is the preferred route; often though it is necessary to administer fluids IV.

Intravenous Fluid Administration

Intravenous fluids are administered to provide water, electrolytes, and nutrients that the child needs. **Total parenteral nutrition** (TPN), chemotherapy, and blood products also are administered IV. Total parenteral nutrition (TPN) is the administration of dextrose, lipids, amino acids, electrolytes, vitamins, minerals, and trace elements into the circulatory system to meet the nutritional needs of a child whose needs cannot be met through the gastrointestinal tract.

These solutions often are given through a central venous line. Medications are not given by the central venous line but must be given through a peripheral site. A central venous line passes directly into the subclavian vein through the jugular or subclavian vein. The line is inserted by surgical technique. Caring for a child with a central venous line calls for skilled nursing care because of the danger of complications such as contamination, thrombosis, dislodgement of the catheter, and **extravasation** (fluid escaping into surrounding tissue). The infant or child must be closely monitored for hyperglycemia, dehydration, or **azotemia** (nitrogen-containing compounds in the blood).

Peripheral vein total parenteral nutrition may occasionally be used on a short-term basis. Extra care must be taken to avoid infiltration because tissue sloughing may be severe.

For long-term administration of TPN, a venous access device such as a Hickman or Broviac catheter may be inserted into the jugular or subclavian vein in a surgical procedure under anesthesia. These catheters may exit through a tunnel in the subcutaneous tissue on the right chest. Children can be discharged from the hospital on TPN therapy after family caregivers have been instructed in the care of the device, thus reducing hospitalization time and expense.

Dressing changes are routinely performed on the external site of a central venous device. The institution's policies must always be clarified and followed; often the practical nurse assists with this dressing change. This is a sterile procedure so sterile gloves and forceps are used. Following the dressing change, the procedure is documented as well as the skin condition including any redness, swelling, drainage, or irritation.

Intravenous Medication

Intravenous medications often are administered to pediatric patients. Some drugs must be administered IV to be effective; in some patients the quick response gained from IV administration is important. Delivering medications IV is actually less traumatic than administering multiple intramuscular injections. Extra caution is necessary to observe for irritation of small pediatric veins from irritating medications. The nurse must double-check the medication label before hanging the IV fluid bottle to ensure that the medication is correct for the correct patient, that it is being administered at the correct time, and that it is not outdated.

Intravenous Sites

Site selection in the pediatric patient varies with the child's age. The best choice of sites is the one that least restricts the child's movements. Sites used include the hand, the wrist, forearm, the foot, and the ankle. The antecubital fossa, which restricts movement, is sometimes used only if other sites aren't available. The scalp vein may be used if no other site can be accessed. This site has an abundant supply of superficial veins in infants and toddlers. When a scalp vein is used, the infant's hair is shaved over a small area; family caregivers can be reassured that the infant's hair will grow back quickly. An inverted medicine cup or a paper cup with the bottom cut out is often taped over the site to protect it. The needle is stabilized with U-shaped taping, and a loop of the tubing is taped so that if the child pulls on the tubing, the loop will absorb the pull and the site will remain intact (Fig. 7–10A, B). The older infant's hands may need to be restrained.

If a site in the hand, foot, or arm is used, the limb should be stabilized on an armboard before insertion is attempted (Fig. 7–10C, D). These sites restrict the child's movement much more than the scalp site.

The use of a plastic cannula or winged, small-vein needle has reduced the need for surgical

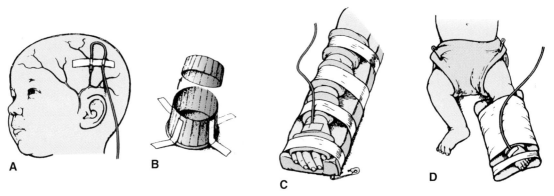

● **Figure 7.10 (A)** Scalp vein IV site. **(B)** Paper cup taped over IV site for protection. **(C)** Armboard restraint used when IV site is in the hand. **(D)** Infant's leg taped to a sandbag to secure IV site in the leg.

cutdowns. In a surgical cutdown, a small incision is made usually in the foot or hand to provide access to a vein. A physician performs the cutdown procedure under sterile conditions.

Older children may be permitted some choice of site, if possible. The child should be involved in all aspects of the procedure within age-appropriate capabilities. The preschool child often can cooperate if given adequate explanation. Play therapy in preparation for IV therapy may be helpful. Honesty is essential with children of any age. The older school-age child and adolescent may have many questions that should be answered at their level of understanding. Family caregivers also need explanations and should be included in the preparation for the procedure. By their presence and reassurance, family caregivers may provide the emotional support the child needs and may help the child remain calm throughout the procedure.

In preparation for starting an IV line, the nurse must collect all the equipment that may be needed including the IV tubing, any necessary extension tubing, the container of solution, the equipment to stabilize the site, a tourniquet, cleansing supplies used by the institution such as povidone-iodine or alcohol swabs, sterile gauze, adhesive tape, cling roll gauze, an IV pole, an infusion pump or controller, and a plastic cannula or winged small-vein needle usually between 21-gauge and 25-gauge (depending on the child's size).

Only nurses skilled in the procedure should start an IV infusion in children. An unskilled nurse should not attempt the procedure unless under the direct supervision of a person skilled in pediatric IV administration. It is sometimes difficult to gain access to children's small veins, and they may easily be "blown." Venipuncture requires practice and expertise. The staff nurse may serve as the child's advocate when the physician or IV nurse comes to start an infusion. The staff nurse who has cared for the child has the child's confidence and knows the child's preferences.

Infusion Control

A variety of IV infusion pumps are suitable for pediatric use. The rate of infusion for infants and children must be carefully monitored. To avoid overloading the circulation and inducing cardiac failure, the IV drip rate must be slow for the small child. Various adapting devices are available that decrease the size of the drop to a "mini" or "micro" drop of 1/50 or 1/60 mL, thus delivering 50 or 60 minidrops or microdrops per milliliter rather than the 15 drops per milliliter of a regular set. Many IV sets also contain a control chamber (or burette) that holds 100 to 150 mL of fluid and is designed to deliver controlled volumes of fluid, avoiding the accidental entrance of too great a fluid volume into the child's system (Fig. 7–11).

Regardless of the control systems and safeguards, the child and the IV infusion should be monitored as frequently as every hour. The IV site must be checked to see that it is intact and observed for redness, pain, **induration** (hardness), flow rate, moisture at the site, and swelling. Documentation is sometimes done on an IV flow sheet that lists the flow rate, the amount in the bottle, the amount in the burette, the amount infused, and the condition of the site. It is important to accurately document IV fluid intake on any child undergoing IV therapy.

For the administration of an IV medication, a heparin lock or **intermittent infusion device** may be used (Fig. 7–12). This method allows the child more freedom and frees him or her from IV tubing between medication administrations. The veins on the back of the hand are often used for heparin lock insertion. Medication is administered through the lock; when the administration is completed, the needle and tubing are removed and the heparin lock is flushed. A

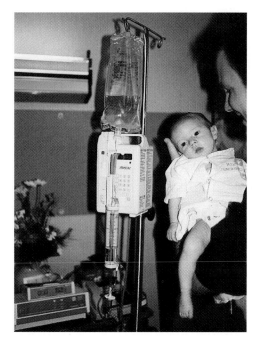

● *Figure 7.11* An infant with an infusion pump and an infusion chamber. The infusion chamber has a "mini" dropper to reduce the size of the drops.

self-healing rubber stopper closes the heparin lock so that it does not leak between administrations. This method also may be used for a child who must have frequent blood samples drawn. The heparin lock is

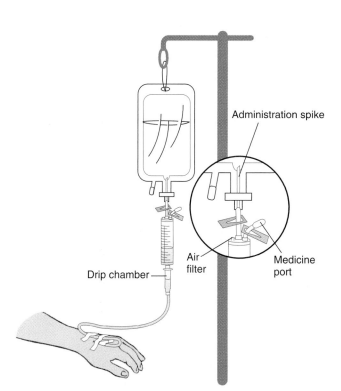

● *Figure 7.12* Secondary administration through a volume control set into a heparin lock.

flushed every 4 to 8 hours with saline or heparin, according to the facility's procedure.

KEY POINTS

▶ The six "rights" of medication administration are basic to administering medications to anyone, but administering medications to children is much more complex because of their immature body systems and varying sizes.

▶ The nurse should always have another person check his or her computations of drug dosage before administering it to a child.

▶ Administration of IV fluids requires careful observation of the child's appearance, vital signs, intake and output, and the fluid's flow rate, because the child's fluid balance can fluctuate very rapidly.

▶ Intravenous infusion sites must be monitored to avoid infiltration and tissue damage.

BIBLIOGRAPHY

Craven RF, Hirnle CJ. (1999) *Fundamentals of nursing* (3rd ed). Philadelphia: Lippincott Williams & Wilkins.

Johnson C, Horton S. (2001) Owning up to errors: Put an end to the blame game. *Nursing,* 31(6), 54.

Pillitteri A.(1999) *Maternal and child health nursing* (3rd ed). Philadelphia: Lippincott Williams & Wilkins.

Roach S, Scherer J. (2000) *Introductory clinical pharmacology* (6th ed). Philadelphia: Lippincott Williams & Wilkins.

(2000) *Springhouse nurse's drug guide* (3rd ed). Springhouse, PA: Springhouse Corporation.

Steward D. (2001) Taking the "ouch" out of injection for children: Using distraction to decrease pain. *The American Journal of Maternal/Child Nursing,* 26(2).

Teplitsky B. (2001) Avoiding the hazards of look-alike drug names. *Nursing,* 31(9), 56.

VanHulle VC. (2001) Nurses' analgesic practices with hospitalized children. *Journal of Child and Family Nursing,* 4(2), 79.

Wong DL, Hess C. (2000) *Wong and Whaley's clinical manual of pediatric nursing* (5th ed). St. Louis: Mosby.

Wong DL, Perry S, Hockenberry M. (2002) *Maternal child nursing care* (2nd ed). St. Louis: Mosby.

Websites
Drug Calculations
  www.geocites.com/HotSprings/8517/Quiz/quiz.htm
Nursing Library, Doing Two Step Dosage Calculations,
  www.findarticles.com

Workbook

NCLEX-STYLE REVIEW QUESTIONS

1. The pediatric nurse is administering medications to a 4-year-old. Which of the following statements by the nurse indicates an understanding of the child's developmental level?

   a. "Your Mom will help me hold your hands."

   b. "Would you like orange or apple juice to drink after you take your medicine?"

   c. "You can make a poster of the schedule for all your medications."

   d. "This booklet tells all about how this medicine works."

2. The nurse is doing a dosage calculation for an infant who weights 16 pounds. How many kilograms does the child weigh?

   e. 0.72 kg

   f. 1.7 kg

   g. 7.3 kg

   h. 9.0 kg

2. The dosage range of Demerol for a school-age child is 1.1 mg/kg to 1.8 mg/kg. Of the following, which dosage would be appropriate to give a school-age child who weighs 76 pounds?

   a. 24.4 mg

   b. 30.0 mg

   c. 60 mg

   d. 110 mg

3. When administering an IM injection to a 4-month-old infant, the BEST injection site to use would be the

   a. vastus lateralis

   b. ventrogluteal

   c. deltoid

   d. dorsogluteal

4. Infusion pumps and volume control devices are used when children are given IV fluids. The MOST important reason these devices are used is to

   a. regulate the rate of the infusion

   b. decrease the size of the drops delivered

   c. reduce the chance of infiltration

   d. administer medications

STUDY ACTIVITIES

1. Catlin weighs 28.5 lb (13 kg) and measures 35.5 inches (90 cm). Find her BSA using the West nomogram. Calculate the dose of a medication for her if the adult dosage is 750 mg.

2. Describe how you would approach each of the following children when giving oral medications and intramuscular medications.

	Oral Medications	Intramuscular Medications
6-month-old Kristi 18-month-old Jared 3-year-old Sarah 4½-year-old Miguel 8-year-old Nicole 16-year-old Jon		

3. Identify each of the intramuscular injection sites, state how to locate each of the sites, and name the landmarks used.

CRITICAL THINKING

1. Discuss the importance of the six "rights" of medication administration

2. What do you think are the most important responsibilities of the nurse when medicating children?

3. Describe the steps you would take if you discovered that you had made a medication error. Discuss with your peers legal responsibilities related to medication errors.

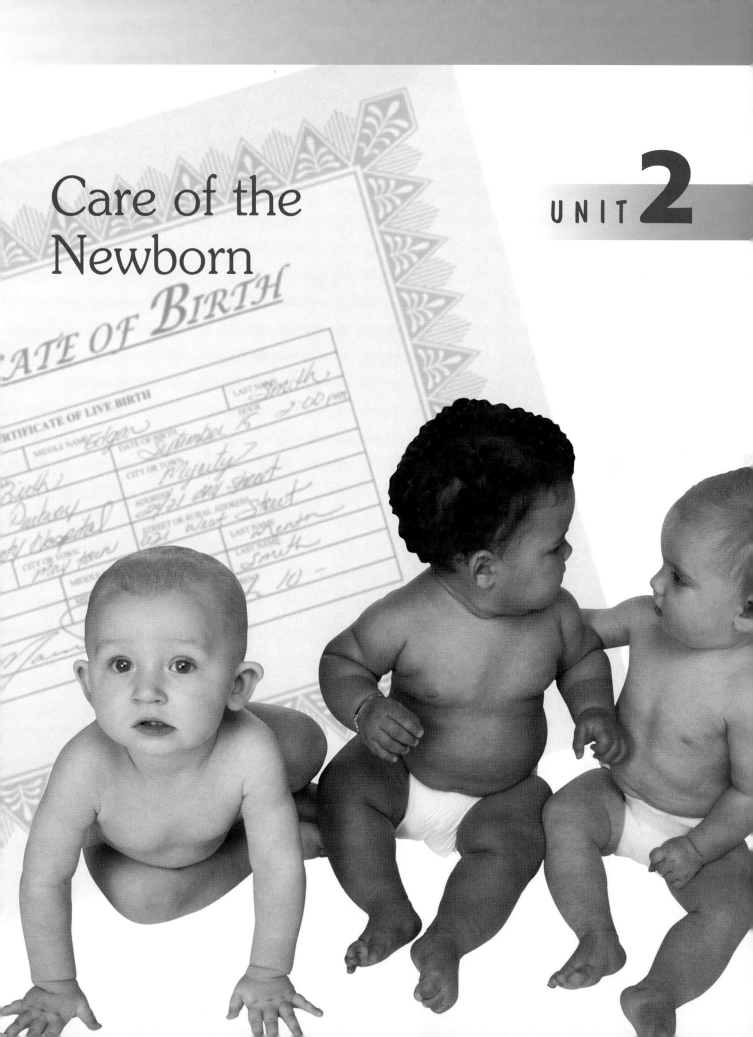

Care of the Newborn

The Normal Newborn

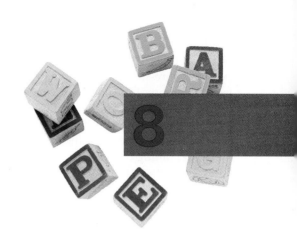

8

PHYSIOLOGIC CHARACTERISTICS OF THE NEWBORN
Head and Skull
Chest
Bony Structure
Body Temperature
Respiratory System
Circulatory System
Gastrointestinal Tract
Genitourinary Tract
Nervous System: Reflexes
Special Senses
Skin

NEWBORN-PARENT BEHAVIOR
Newborn Activity
Mother-Infant Interaction
Father-Infant Interaction
NEWBORN FEEDING
Breast-Feeding
Formula Feeding
TEACHING THE NEW PARENT
FAMILY ADJUSTMENT
The Parents' Adjustment
The Infant's Adjustment
The Sibling's Adjustment

STUDENT OBJECTIVES

On completion of this chapter, the student will be able to

1. State the average weight and length of a newborn.
2. List three advantages and three disadvantages of circumcision.
3. Describe the general appearance of the newborn's (a) head, (b) genitalia, and (c) skin.
4. Describe six normal neonatal reflexes.
5. Explain physiologic jaundice (icterus neonatorum).
6. Discuss the importance of parent-infant interaction.
7. State seven advantages of breast-feeding.
8. List the points that should be covered when teaching about (a) skin rashes, (b) infections, and (c) stools.
9. Describe the procedure for giving a sponge bath.

KEY TERMS

acrocyanosis
areola
Babinski reflex
bonding
caput succedaneum
cavernous hemangioma
cephalhematoma
circumcision
colostrum
cradle cap
en face position
erythema toxicum
fontanelle
forceps marks
gag reflex
lanugo
meconium
milia
mongolian spots
Moro reflex
mutual gazing
palmar grasp reflex
petechiae
phimosis
physiologic jaundice
plantar grasp reflex
pseudomenses
pseudostrabismus
regurgitation
rooting reflex
smegma
startle reflex
step reflex
sucking reflex
suture
tonic neck reflex
vascular nevus
vernix caseosa

From the moment of conception until full maturity, human life proceeds in an orderly pattern of growth and development. This pattern and the person that results from it are shaped by various factors that precede and follow conception. Genetic influences help determine a child's physical and intellectual characteristics, as do environmental influences.

Birth is hard work for the mother and the baby; therefore, calling the birth process labor is accurate. After 9 months in the warm, dark security of the uterus, the newborn suddenly enters a strange, bright, cooler world. Is it any wonder that a cry is forthcoming? This cry fulfills a biologic need: by drawing air into the lungs with the first breath, the breathing process is initiated, which is one big step the infant takes toward maintaining life. Although totally helpless in comparison with other baby mammals, the human infant is physically equipped to survive outside the uterus—to regulate temperature, eat, sleep, and respond to certain stimuli—provided that someone else is ready to meet all his or her needs. The newborn is also ready to develop social relationships, usually beginning with the parents.

The health care personnel in both the delivery room and in the newborn nursery play an important role in the transition period from intrauterine to extrauterine life. Nurses who care for the laboring and postpartum mother have specialized training, and some nurses specialize in caring for the newborn following delivery. The first few minutes of life are a critical period in which the immediate needs of the newborn are a priority. The newborn is closely assessed and given care. In this text, the characteristics of the normal newborn will be discussed as well as the child's patterns of normal growth and development. Refer to a maternal-child textbook for detailed information regarding pregnancy, birth, care of the newborn, and the role of the nurse.

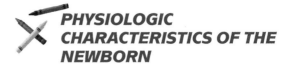

PHYSIOLOGIC CHARACTERISTICS OF THE NEWBORN

Approximately 95% of newborns born at term weigh 5.5 to 10 lb (2.5 to 4.6 kg) and measure 18 inches to 23 inches (45 to 55 cm) long. Normal head circumference is about 12 inches to 14 inches (33 to 35 cm). The crown-to-rump measurement is about equal to the head circumference.

Head and Skull

The six bones of the newborn's skull are not united but can mold and overlap to permit the large head to pass through the birth canal. Narrow bands of connective tissue called **sutures** divide these bones. At the juncture of these bones are small spaces called **fontanelles.** At birth, the two palpable fontanelles, or soft spots, are the anterior fontanelle at the juncture of the frontal and parietal bones and the posterior fontanelle at the juncture of the parietal and occipital bones (Fig. 8–1).

During delivery, the head is molded along the suture lines and may appear asymmetric or elongated (Fig. 8–2). Usually normal shape is assumed after a few days. The sections of the bony skull calcify and join during the first months of life. The posterior triangle-shaped fontanelle closes in about 1.5 to 3 months of life; the anterior diamond-shaped fontanelle closes between 12 and 18 months.

The brain is covered with a tough membrane, making it difficult to injure the child's head through the fontanelles by ordinary handling. Mothers need to be reassured that the baby's scalp may be washed with soap and water (*not* baby oil) over these areas without harm. Ordinary cleansing may be helpful to

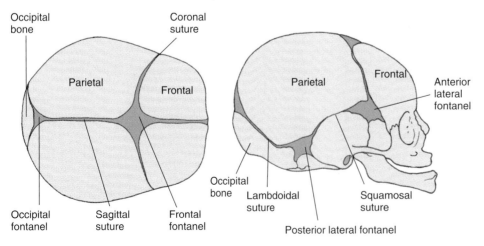

● **Figure 8.1** Infant skull showing fontanelles and cranial sutures.

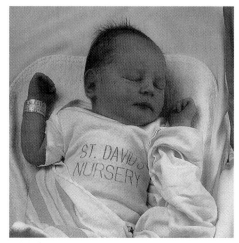

● *Figure 8.2* Molding: the head of this newborn is elongated due to the pressure of passage through the birth canal.

prevent **cradle cap** (seborrheic dermatitis), an accumulation of oil, serum, and dirt that often forms on an infant's scalp.

Chest

The chest of the newborn has a smaller circumference than the head. The breasts of both male and female newborns may be engorged as a result of maternal estrogens in the bloodstream, and a pale, milky fluid (witches' milk) may be secreted. This condition disappears within 4 to 6 weeks, but until it does the breasts should be handled gently and should not be manipulated in any way.

Bony Structure

The arms and legs of the newborn are short in comparison with the trunk. Prenatal development proceeds in a cephalocaudal (head-to-toe) progression and in a proximal (nearest to center) to distal (remote) sequence (Fig. 8–3). This means that the head and trunk are well developed at birth, but the distal areas (arms, hands, legs, and feet) develop later. Development always proceeds from the general to the specific: gross muscle control, for instance, comes before fine muscle control.

Body Temperature

At delivery, the infant's body temperature is generally the same as the mother's, but it drops rapidly after the infant enters a cooler environment. As mentioned earlier, a warm, stable environment is necessary until the neonate has adjusted to independent living. In the delivery room, the infant is usually wrapped in a warm blanket or placed in a heated

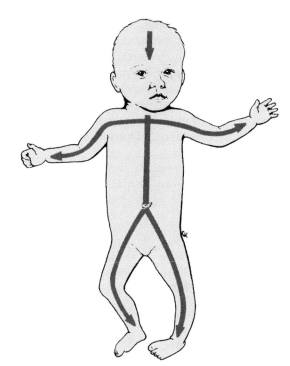

● *Figure 8.3* *Arrows* indicate the cephalocaudal and proximodistal progress of infant development.

crib. Because of an immature nervous system, body temperature varies with the environment, with a range from 97.5° to 98.6°F (36.4° to 37°C). It usually stabilizes in a few days. Normal newborn axillary temperature, after stabilization, varies from 96.8° to 99° F (36° to 37.2° C).

The newborn's temperature may be taken by rectum, axilla, or tympanic. In most newborn nurseries, the first temperature is taken rectally to determine the patency of the anal opening. There may be a shallow opening in the anus, however, with the rectum ending in a blind pouch. In this instance, the ability to insert a thermometer into the rectum does not signify a patent rectum. When a temperature is measured rectally, care must be taken to insert the thermometer only just beyond the bulb of the thermometer. Axillary and tympanic temperatures are obtained using the procedure outlined in Chapter 5.

Respiratory System

The first and most important task of the neonate is to oxygenate the red blood cells; this occurs with the first cry. Although respiratory movements appear in fetal life, there is no *functional* respiration before birth. Breathing in the healthy newborn is quiet and shallow, and variations in rate and rhythm are normal. In normal infants, the rate may vary from 20 to 100 breaths per minute, according to whether the infant is sleeping or awake, crying, lying passively, or vigorously moving the arms and legs. Because the rate fluctuates rapidly, respirations should be counted for a full minute. Persistent rates greater than 60 or less than 30 breaths per minute should be called to the care provider's attention because this may indicate cardiac or pulmonary difficulty. Sternal retractions are considered abnormal and should also be reported.

The newborn's breathing is diaphragmatic (abdominal), so respirations may be counted most easily by watching the rise and fall of the abdomen rather than the chest. Parents should be informed of this characteristic to prevent any alarm about what may seem to them to be abnormal breathing.

Circulatory System

The changes that occur in the circulatory system at birth are primarily due to oxygenating the blood through the pulmonary system and to discarding the placenta, umbilical vein, and arteries. Shortly after birth, blood flows through the infant's circulatory system in the same manner as that of an adult. **Acrocyanosis** (cyanosis of the hands and feet) is common and occurs because of the immature peripheral circulatory system. When the infant cries, however, the skin becomes rosy red.

At birth, an infant's heart rate may reach 180 beats per minute, then decrease to 100 to 120. Usually by the second day of life, the pulse is 90 to 160, depending on whether the infant is asleep or awake and active. Blood pressure is difficult to measure in the newborn unless it is taken with specialized equipment using ultrasonography such as a Doppler and an oscillometer. An initial blood-pressure measurement should be taken, however, to provide a baseline and to alert the staff to any cardiac problems.

Gastrointestinal Tract

The gastrointestinal tract is functional at birth, and within 8 to 24 hours the infant usually passes **meconium** (a sticky, greenish-black substance composed of bile, mucus, cellular waste, intestinal secretions, fat, hair, and other materials swallowed during fetal life combined with amniotic fluid). The time of the first stool should be recorded to confirm anal patency. If no stool is passed during the first 24 hours after birth, the provider should be notified because some obstruction may exist in the intestinal tract.

The neonate can digest the fat, protein, and carbohydrates in breast milk or in a modified formula. **Regurgitation,** spitting up of small quantities of milk, occurs rather easily in the young infant and is different from vomiting. An air bubble in the infant's stomach, too-rapid nursing, or overfeeding may cause regurgitation.

Vomiting differs from regurgitation in that a larger amount of fluid is expelled. Although this also may result from rapid feeding or inadequate burping, frequent or persistent vomiting may signal an abnormal condition and should be reported to the physician.

The neonate hiccups easily, most likely from feeding too rapidly. Hiccupping does, however, also occur in fetal life. Burping the infant to bring up swallowed air or nursing for another minute usually controls the hiccups, but they eventually stop without treatment.

Genitourinary Tract

The kidneys secrete urine before birth, and some urine collects in the bladder after birth. A record of the first urination is important to confirm adequate kidney function and the absence of severe constrictions somewhere in the urinary system.

The male testes are usually descended into the scrotum at birth, but occasionally one or both are in the process of descending or remain in the abdomen. These testes usually descend spontaneously during the first year of life.

In the newborn, the foreskin of the penis is normally tight. **Phimosis,** adherence of the foreskin to the glans penis, is normal in early infancy, and forceful retraction should not be attempted. The foreskin usually becomes retractable by 3 years of age. If minor irritations develop, cleansing with soap and water is all that is needed. One danger of forceful retraction of the foreskin during early infancy is that the elastic fibers at the tip of the foreskin may tear and bleed. The result will be that the foreskin heals by scarring, perhaps making circumcision necessary later.

In 1975, the American Academy of Pediatrics opposed the routine **circumcision** (surgical removal of all or part of the prepuce, or foreskin, of the penis) of the newborn, stating that there is no sound medical reason for the procedure, that good personal hygiene is adequate, and that nonremoval prevents the infant from the possible risks related to having a surgical procedure. The Academy changed its position in 1989, stating that circumcision for the newborn has potential medical advantages and benefits as well as disadvantages and risks. Today the discussion over circumcision continues. Parents should be thoroughly informed by the physician about both the risks and benefits of the procedure

TABLE 8.1	Advantages and Disadvantages of Neonatal Circumcision
Advantages	**Disadvantages**
Prevention of Penile cancer Inflammation of glans and prepuce Complications of later circumcision Possible decrease of Urinary tract infections in males Sexually transmitted disease Preserves male body image (to be same as circumcised father or peers when older)	Complications of Hemorrhage Infection Dehiscence Meatitis from loss of protective foreskin Adhesions Concealed penis Urethral fistula Meatal stenosis Pain at time of procedure

(Table 8–1). Most notably, those of the Jewish faith perform circumcision of the newborn frequently for religious reasons. Circumcision prevents the accumulation of the secretions collectively called **smegma.** If the foreskin of the newborn is so tight that it obstructs the urinary system, circumcision is performed at once.

In the female neonate, the labia are prominent due to the effect of the mother's estrogens during intrauterine life. The infant may have a slight red-tinged vaginal discharge called **pseudomenses,** which results from a decline in the hormonal level compared with the higher concentration in the maternal hormone environment. Unless the mother understands why this happens, she may become alarmed. She should be told that although it does not appear in all newborn females, the discharge is a natural manifestation resulting from hormonal transfer and will disappear in a few days. It should be emphasized that this discharge is not due to any trauma or infection.

Nervous System: Reflexes

The neonate normally exhibits several reflexes that are triggered by an immature nervous system. For example, all newborns smile even if they are blind and all infants tightly grasp objects placed in their palms. Infants should be tested for the most common reflexes because absence of reflex may indicate a disturbance in the nervous system. Most of the reflexes disappear during the first year of life.

The **rooting reflex,** which is present at birth, is seen when the cheek is stroked and the infant responds by turning the head toward that side and opening the mouth (Fig. 8–4). When the mother or nurse places a hand on the infant's cheek to turn the head toward the breast, the infant turns instead toward the person's hand.

The **sucking reflex** is so well developed at birth that personnel in the delivery room are often startled by the loud sucking noises coming from the newborn's crib.

The **gag reflex** is present at birth and continues throughout life. Any stimulation of the posterior pharynx by food, suction, or passage of a tube causes gagging.

The **palmar** (palm of the hand) **grasp reflex** causes the infant's fingers to curl around the examiner's finger when it is placed in the palm of the infant's hand. The palmar grasp reflex (Fig. 8–5) is so

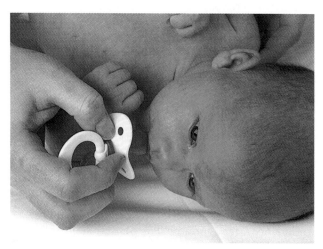

● **Figure 8.4** The rooting reflex is elicited when the newborn's lip or cheek is touched; the newborn turns the head and opens the mouth.

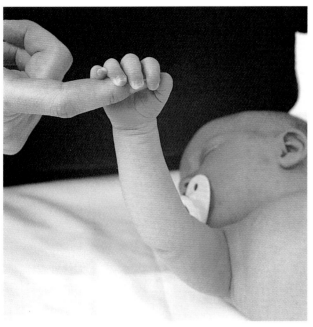

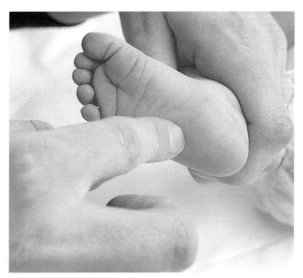

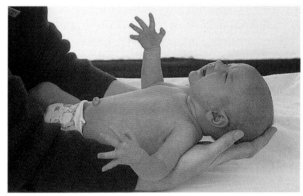

● **Figure 8.6** Babinski reflex occurs when the lateral plantar surface is stroked; the toes flare open.

● **Figure 8.5** Palmar grasp reflex is present in all normal newborns and is sufficiently strong enough to lift them from the examining table.

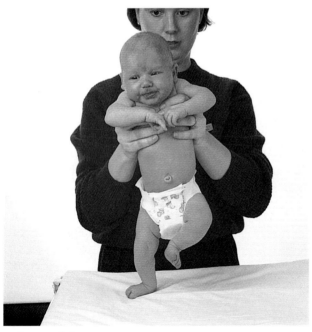

● **Figure 8.8** Moro reflex is elicited by sudden jarring or change in equilibrium. Arms abduct at the shoulder and extend at the elbow. All digits extend except the index finger and the thumb, which curve into a C-shape.

● **Figure 8.7** Step, or dance, reflex simulates walking when the infant is held so that the sole of the foot touches the examining table.

strong in a healthy infant that the infant can be lifted off the examining table. The palmar grasp reflex diminishes after 3 months. The **plantar** (sole of the foot) **grasp reflex** occurs when pressure is placed on the sole of the foot at the base of the toes, causing the toes to curl downward. The plantar grasp reflex persists until 9 to 12 months of age.

The **Babinski reflex** (Fig. 8–6) occurs when the side of the sole of the foot is stroked beginning at the heel and toward the toes in an inverted "J" curve; the toes flare open. This is called a positive Babinski's sign. If this sign is absent, a neurologic problem may be present. This reflex usually disappears by the age of 6 to 12 months.

Until 6 weeks of age, most normal infants held in an upright position make stepping movements (Fig. 8–7). This movement is called the **step** (or dance) **reflex.**

Any sudden jarring or abrupt change in equilibrium elicits the **Moro reflex** in the normal newborn. Moro reflex consists primarily of abduction and extension of the arms. All digits extend except the index finger and the thumb, which are flexed to form a C shape (Fig. 8–8). If the response is not immediate, bilateral, and symmetric, injury to the brachial plexus,

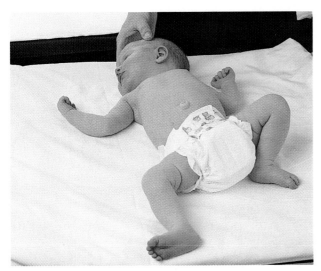

● **Figure 8.9** Tonic neck reflex is present when the infant lies on his or her back with the head turned to one side, with the arm and leg on the same side extended and the arm on the opposite side flexed.

the humerus, or the clavicle may be present. Persistence of this reflex after 6 months of age may indicate brain damage.

Similar to the Moro reflex, the **startle reflex** follows any loud noise and consists of abduction of the arms and flexion of the elbows. Unlike the Moro reflex, the hands remain clenched. Absence of this reflex may indicate hearing impairment.

Not always apparent during the first weeks of life, the **tonic neck reflex,** also called the fencing reflex, may be observed when the infant lies on the back. With the head turned to one side, the infant's arm and leg extend on the same side and the opposite arm flexes as if in a fencing position (Fig. 8–9). Usually this reflex disappears between 3 and 4 months of age.

Special Senses

The senses of sight, hearing, smell, taste, and touch are developed to a great extent in the newborn.

Sight

Research has shown that the unborn baby can distinguish light from dark; at birth, the infant can see. The rod cells in the retina of the eyes, which are responsible for light perception, are functional at birth; however, the retina, the newborn's organ of visual perception, is not fully developed until about 16 weeks of age. The neonate's head turns toward light, and the neonate blinks and closes his or her eyes at bright light. The infant follows a bright moving object momentarily, but fixation and coordination come much later. The nerves and muscles that control focusing and coordination are not completely

developed until the sixth month and account for the cross-eyed look (**pseudostrabismus**) that babies sporadically show. Parents have no cause for alarm if their infant's eyes occasionally don't coordinate with their movements, but if lack of focusing remains at 4 months, the pediatrician should be alerted.

Most dark-skinned infants have brown eyes at birth, whereas most light-skinned newborn's eyes are slate gray or dark blue. Tears are produced constantly at birth but are completely disposed of through the nasolacrimal duct until about 2 or 3 months of age, when tear production increases. Newborns have about 20/500 vision, compared with a normal-seeing adult's vision of 20/20. This means that most distant objects appear very fuzzy. Close vision is much better, and the infant can see most of the features of a human face clearly at a distance of 7 inches to 15 inches (17–38 cm). This is one reason why the **en face position** (in which the caregiver and the infant establish eye contact in the same vertical plane) is so important to parent-infant attachment immediately after birth.

Hearing

A newborn stops crying momentarily at the sound of a soothing voice and is startled and cries at a loud noise. By the age of 3 days, the infant can distinguish the mother's voice from that of other females. The sense of hearing certainly contributes to the infant's emotional reactions to fear and to comforting. It is not known exactly how early the infant hears soft voices and other faint sounds, but infants 2 or 3 days old stop crying momentarily when talked to soothingly.

Smell

The sense of smell is not highly developed at birth, but research has shown that the newborn infant does turn toward the mother's breast because of the breast milk's smell. A neonate can differentiate the smell of his or her mother's breast milk from that of other females. Strong smells also bring about reaction, and a newborn turns away from smells such as vinegar and alcohol.

Taste

Because much of taste depends on the sense of smell, the infant's sense of taste is probably not highly developed at birth. Some studies have shown, however, that breathing, sucking, and swallowing patterns are different when infants are fed formula than when they are fed breast milk. In addition, neonates have produced the expected reaction of distaste for sour or bitter solutions and pleasure at a sweet solution. They definitely prefer glucose and water to unflavored (sterile) water.

Touch

Sensitivity to touch is present from birth particularly in the lips and tongue. The sense of pain is also present at birth, but infants, like adults, vary in their sensitivity to pain. Newborns react to painful pinpricks. Sensitivity appears to increase during the first few days of life as part of individual development. The infant cries loudly when suffering gastrointestinal discomfort.

Skin

The newborn's skin has specific characteristics noted in its normal appearance. Skin blemishes in the newborn are frequently seen but are often only temporary.

Normal Appearance

Sluggish peripheral circulation and vasomotor instability are manifested in the deep-red color the infant acquires when crying as well as in the pale hands and feet of many newborns. The skin is usually red to dark pink in white newborns. African American newborns have reddish-brown skin, and Hispanic infants have an olive or yellowish tint to the skin. The skin should feel elastic when picked up between the examiner's fingers.

Fine, downy hair called **lanugo** covers the skin of the fetus. It is usually not present in a full-term infant but may be seen on a premature infant.

A greasy, cheese-like substance called **vernix caseosa** protects the skin during fetal life. Vernix caseosa is a mixture of oil and water containing cells flaked from the skin and fatty substances secreted by the sebaceous glands. At birth, vernix may cover the skin or remain only in the folds of the skin. In most hospitals, not all of the vernix is removed with the first bath, but it is left on as a protective agent. It eventually is absorbed or rubs off.

Skin Blemishes

Newborns may have various temporary skin blemishes. One of the most common is a **vascular nevus** ("strawberry mark"). A nevus is a circumscribed new growth of the skin of congenital origin; it may be either vascular or nonvascular. The strawberry mark is a slightly raised, bright-red collection of blood vessels that does not blanch completely on pressure. It may be present at birth or may appear during the first 6 months of life. This blemish may enlarge during the first 6 months of life but after it stops growing, fibrosis replaces the capillaries and the lesion shrinks. Treatment usually is not indicated because most of these marks regress and disappear by 10 years of age. If the lesion is so large as to cause emotional trauma in the child, the physician may suggest removal.

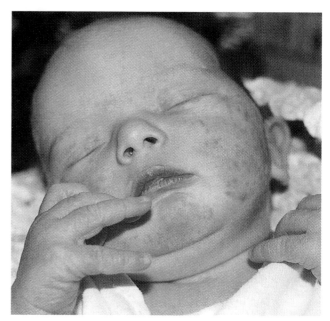

● *Figure 8.10* Erythema toxicum is a fine rash seen in most newborns.

Erythema toxicum (fine rash of the newborn) (Fig. 8–10) may appear over the trunk, back, abdomen, and buttocks. It appears in about 24 hours and disappears in several days. It is not infectious and needs no treatment.

Vascular nevi are sometimes present in **cavernous hemangiomas,** subcutaneous collections of blood vessels with bluish overlying skin. Although these lesions are benign tumors, they may become so large and extensive as to interfere with the functions of the body part where they appear. Small hemangiomas ("stork bites") are often seen on the eyelids or the back of the neck (Fig. 8–11). They disappear within 6 to 12 months without treatment. In infants of African, Mediterranean, Native American, or Asian descent, **mongolian spots** (areas of bluish-black pigmentation resembling bruises) may be seen most often over the sacral or gluteal region. They usually fade within a year or two.

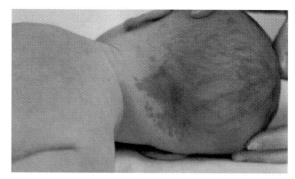

● *Figure 8.11* Small hemangiomas ("stork bites") are often seen on the eyelids or the back of the neck.

Milia are pearly white cysts appearing on the face in about 40% of newborns. They are usually retention cysts of sebaceous glands or hair follicles and disappear in a few weeks without treatment.

Petechiae are small bluish-purple spots caused by tiny broken capillaries. They may be seen on the face as a result of excess pressure on the head during a rapid or difficult delivery. They disappear in a day or so.

Forceps marks may be noticeable on the infant's face if forceps were used during delivery (Fig. 8–12). These marks ordinarily disappear in a day or two. After a difficult delivery, bruises and edema may be present on the head or scalp or on the buttocks and the genitalia after a breech delivery. Although these gradually clear up without treatment, such bruises may be distressing to the parents, who may not understand the relative insignificance of these marks. The nurse may carefully and simply explain that they are minor bruises and will fade quickly.

Occasionally the infant's head is misshapen by its passage through the birth canal. The mother is naturally distressed and needs to know that this is temporary and is caused by the head's inability to accommodate to the narrow passage. The head acquires a normal rounded shape in a few days.

Caput succedaneum is an edematous swelling of the soft tissues of the scalp caused by prolonged pressure of the occiput against the cervix during labor and delivery. The edema disappears in a few days. **Cephalhematoma** is a collection of blood between the periosteum and the skull. The swelling of the overlying scalp usually is not visible until several hours after birth. This swelling also may frighten the caregivers, who may think some injury has occurred. The edema of caput succedaneum may spread across the scalp, but the swelling of cephalhematoma is contained by the periosteum and cannot cross suture lines. Most cephalhematomas are reabsorbed within 2

weeks to 3 months depending on their size. Aspiration, incision, or any other treatment is contraindicated because the only serious complication may be the introduction of infection.

Physiologic jaundice (icterus neonatorum) occurs in many newborns and has no medical significance. It is believed to result from the breakdown of fetal red blood cells. It must, however, be observed carefully and reported in an effort to distinguish it from a serious jaundice condition. The nursing staff may do a simple heel stick to perform a microbilirubin examination that may confirm or rule out an elevated bilirubin level. Physiologic jaundice with yellowing of the skin does not appear until after the second day of life, which may be after the newborn goes home. Caregivers should be advised to report to the physician any jaundice appearing during the first 3 days.

A PERSONAL GLIMPSE

When my daughter was born, she was jaundiced, but her bilirubin level was not high enough to put her under the "lights." The doctors wanted to monitor her with heel prick blood tests twice a day. In between the tests at the hospital, I was to go home and put her in the sunlight (unfortunately, it was overcast all that week) and nurse her as much as possible. They said that would help. Each time she was tested, we waited at the hospital an hour for the test results, only to find that the level went up a little, but not enough to put her under the lights. We did this twice a day for 5 days, back and forth to the hospital. I was stressed out from listening to my infant wail at the heel pricks, having my sleep interrupted every 2 hours to nurse her, and crashing postpartum hormones. Add to that the trips back and forth and I was a mess. On the fourth day, after they jabbed my baby's heel once again and once again she wailed in pain, I burst into tears and said that maybe she wasn't fighting off the jaundice because of me, because my breasts were not making enough milk. The nurse got very firm and said, "Lift up your blouse." I did and we both looked down on my more-than-ample breasts. She said, "You have more than enough milk for that baby." We both laughed.

Nancy

> **LEARNING OPPORTUNITY:** Explain the factors that you think were affecting this mother. In giving this new mother an opportunity to laugh, the nurse helped to decrease her anxiety. What else could the nurse do to support this mother?

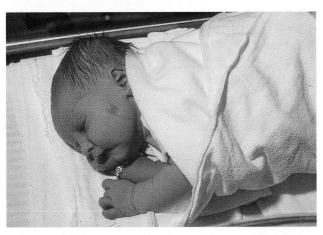

● *Figure 8.12* Forceps marks may be noticeable on the infant's face if forceps were used during delivery.

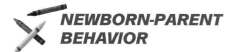

NEWBORN-PARENT BEHAVIOR

The newborn's activity and behaviors often initiate the mother-infant interaction as well as the father-infant interaction. These interactions help establish the parent-infant attachment known as **bonding.**

Newborn Activity

The healthy newborn, if placed face down, lifts or turns the head to one side to clear the airway. The infant exercises in uncoordinated, random movements involving the entire body in the activity. The muscles are taut, and the infant finds it difficult to extend the extremities manually. The infant momentarily ceases activity at the sound of a nearby voice.

The newborn may yawn, hiccup, stretch, blink, cough, and sneeze to clear the nasal passages. The fetus learned to suck and swallow during intrauterine life.

The infant's only way of expressing tension from hunger, cold, pain, or other discomfort is by crying. Prompt comforting and attention to the infant's needs usually restores composure and alleviates the discomfort. It is often in these first moments of comforting and soothing that the parent-child attachment process begins.

INTERNET EXERCISE 8.1

http://www.babycenter.com/infant

Caring for your Newborn
Click on Survival Tactics.
Click on seven reasons infants cry.
Read the section on seven reasons infants cry and how to soothe them.

1. List seven things that you could share with new parents about why infants cry.

2. Describe ideas and suggestions that you could offer to parents about ways to soothe their infants.

Mother-Infant Interaction

Even though infant and mother have been physically inseparable for 9 months, their emotional togetherness and the beginning of mutual love and attachment start after delivery, ideally in the first few hours. This attachment or bonding is vital to the infant's psychological development. Many babies are alert for a short time after delivery, offering a good opportunity for sensory contact with the mother.

Research indicates that early attachment activities have a significant effect on the long-term parent-child relationship. This does not mean that early attachment guarantees a satisfactory lifetime relationship or that lack of opportunity for early attachment seriously threatens the family's chances for a strong relationship. It simply means that the family relationship is given the best possible start if the mother, the father, and the infant are together during this early period in their new life as a family (Fig. 8–13).

Touch is a highly significant part of the attachment process. Shortly after delivery, the nude infant may be placed on the mother's abdomen and chest and held to the mother's breast if the mother plans to breast-feed. Touching provides warmth, comfort, and a sense of security; all are vital for the vulnerable newborn.

Studies have shown that the mother is likely to follow a predictable pattern of touching her new baby—first using only the fingertips to touch the extremities, then gradually moving her fingers over the infant's entire body, and finally using her entire hand to massage the trunk of the body. Next she tries to reposition herself and the baby in the en face position. This is also referred to as **mutual gazing.** The attachment process is affected by many factors such as the mother's physical and emotional condition and the infant's condition and behavior following the birth. The attachment or bonding

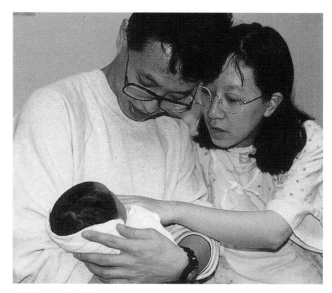

● **Figure 8.13** Bonding between the mother, partner or father, and infant should be encouraged whenever possible.

process continues through infancy and childhood as the infant and parent get to know each other.

During her pregnancy every woman imagines what her baby will look like, how he or she will act, what the child will eventually accomplish, and how she and others in the family will be affected by this new person. This imaginary baby is likely to be different from the real infant she meets soon after delivery. At first sight, the infant seldom resembles the chubby, well-formed baby pictured by the world in general. The newborn may appear completely self-centered and displeased over this abrupt introduction to the world. Such a first impression may summon feelings of guilt in the mother that she does not feel the expected gush of love and tenderness. If the baby is quiet and passive and the mother had imagined an awake, alert, active child, she may be disappointed; she may give less attention and stimulation than she would to an infant who more closely resembled the imagined child.

Both parents must understand that each infant is unique with individual characteristics and potential. Studies have shown that pointing out to parents their child's unique characteristics may help develop a more positive attitude, reduce feeding and sleeping problems, and bring about greater activity and alertness in the infant.

One widely used guide for assessing neonatal activity is the Brazelton Neonatal Behavioral Assessment Scale (Fig. 8–14). Special training is necessary to use the test. The Brazelton criteria also help the parents tune in to their baby and learn more about this budding personality and how their responses affect their adjustment to each other.

Father-Infant Interaction

Fathers who are involved during pregnancy, delivery, and the postpartum period also develop a strong attachment to the infant. The father's attachment behavior is similar to the mother's: touching, holding the infant in the en face position, observing the beauty of the child (particularly any features that resemble the father), and expressing feelings of elation and satisfaction (Fig. 8–15). Many fathers indicate that they want to share the responsibility of raising the baby.

Some cultures dictate that men not show emotion, so some fathers may need encouragement to express their feelings about their infant. Nurses should reinforce any positive attachment behavior displayed by either parent and should show, whenever necessary, the soothing effect of cuddling, stroking, rocking, and talking to the baby.

BRAZELTON SCALE CRITERIA

1. Response decrement to light
2. Response decrement to rattle
3. Response decrement to bell
4. Response decrement to pinprick
5. Orientation response—inanimate visual
6. Orientation response—inanimate auditory
7. Orientation—animate visual
8. Orientation—animate auditory
9. Orientation—animate-visual and auditory
10. Alertness
11. General tonus
12. Motor maturity
13. Pull-to-sit
14. Cuddliness
15. Defensive movements
16. Consolability with intervention
17. Peak of excitement
18. Rapidity of buildup
19. Irritability (to aversive stimuli: uncover, undress, pull-to sit, prone, pinprick, TNR, Moro, defensive reaction)
20. Activity
21. Tremulousness
22. Amount of startle during exam
23. Lability of skin color
24. Lability of states
25. Self-quieting activity
26. Hand to mouth facility
27. Smiles

● *Figure 8.14* Brazelton Neonatal Behavioral Assessment Scale.

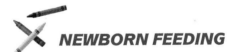

NEWBORN FEEDING

Feeding time is an occasion that provides stimulation and builds confidence for both the infant and caregiver. The infant touches and makes eye-to-eye

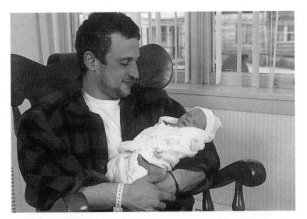

● *Figure 8.15* This father gets to know his child by holding the infant in the en face position, observing the beauty of the child.

contact with the caregiver, while the caregiver looks, touches, explores, and talks to the infant. The infant learns to trust through repeated touch, fondling, and warm physical comfort. The infant's response to parental comforting care gives the mother and father a sense of satisfaction and confidence. Eventually, when the infant learns that signals of need are answered promptly, he or she can wait after crying for the response. The infant should not be made to wait too long, however, because the newly developed sense of trust is fragile if not reinforced soon.

At one time, mothers were told to put the baby on a feeding schedule and never to deviate from it. When the baby cried, they were told to check and see if anything was disturbing him or her, then to put the infant down and let the baby cry. Unfortunately the infant did not know about being trained to conform to a schedule. The baby knew only that hunger demanded satisfaction. The infant's discomfort and sense of aloneness needed comfort and reassurance. Routine did nothing to satisfy needs, but it did potentially shake the infant's trust and belief that the world was a safe and caring place. Attitudes have changed; infants are now fed primarily on a demand schedule, and a routine is eventually established.

Both breast-fed and formula-fed infants need to suck, and sometimes feeding does not satisfy this need. Pacifiers may be given to the infant to help satisfy this need. This decision depends on the parents' attitudes, but often the use of pacifiers is considered more desirable than having the infant suck on the fingers or a thumb. Only commercial pacifiers, however, should be used. Makeshift pacifiers constructed from nipples and plastic collars from infant formula bottles are dangerous. Deaths of infants have occurred from the aspiration, or drawing into the lungs, of such nipples.

Family caregivers should be informed that the infant normally loses 5% to 10% of his or her body weight during the first few days of life. This loss is expected, and the weight should be regained within about 2 weeks.

Breast-Feeding

Breast-feeding is the ideal form of infant nutrition. Whether to breast-feed or to use formula, however, is the decision of the mother or the couple unless there is a contraindication to either method. During pregnancy the mother often decides which method to use and frequently consults her mate, family members, or other persons with whom she can review the advantages and possible disadvantages of breast-feeding (Table 8–2).

When breast-feeding is chosen, the infant is usually put to the breast shortly after birth in the delivery or birthing room. The infant's sucking promotes early secretion of milk, is a source of security and comfort to the infant and satisfaction to the mother, and stimulates uterine contractions. During this time, the infant is often placed skin to skin with the mother, enhancing the bonding process.

Nursing on demand seems to work best for most infants. The mother should be instructed to expect to nurse every 2 to 3 hours for the first few days. The time may be increased gradually until the infant nurses 10 to 15 minutes on the first breast (to empty it) and as the infant desires on the second breast.

The mother must wash her hands before each feeding. If this is the mother's first child, she will

TABLE 8.2	Advantages and Disadvantages of Breast-Feeding
Advantages	**Disadvantages**
1. Nutritionally best for baby 2. Provides protection against allergies 3. Provides antibodies against illness 4. Helps to develop a special bond between mother and infant 5. Promotes involution of uterus (return of uterus to its prepregnant state) 6. Easily digested 7. Convenient, always ready, inexpensive, sterile 7. Breast-feeding makes demands on mother's time. 8. Correct temperature 9. Provides times for mother to rest while nursing 10. Mother gains a sense of accomplishment and satisfaction 11. Obesity is infrequent in breast-fed children	1. Mother may be sensitive to nursing when others are around. 2. Neonatal jaundice may occur from inadequate fluid intake. 3. Mother must watch what medications she takes. 4. Mother must be careful about diet, limiting caffeine and other foods that may upset the infant. 5. Mother cannot take oral contraceptives. 6. Mother's nipples may become sore and cracked.

need help and support when she first attempts to nurse. At first, it is usually easier for the mother to nurse while lying flat with a pillow under her head and cradling the infant's head. The nurse may instruct the mother to turn to one side, place her nipple between her index and third finger, and bring the nipple toward the infant's mouth. As the nipple brushes near the newborn's lips, the baby will actively seek it.

A considerable portion of the **areola** (the darkened area around the nipple) should be drawn into the infant's mouth because this stimulates the mammary glands and helps prevent sore nipples. If the mother's breasts are large and soft, pressing against the breast while trying to nurse may obstruct the infant's nose. The mother may be shown how to press her breast away from the infant's nose with her finger so that breathing is comfortable (Fig. 8–16).

The mother may find that she prefers sitting in bed with a pillow support for her arm or in a chair with arms at a comfortable level. The infant is held in a position lying entirely on the side facing the mother, with the mother's nipple directly in front of the infant's mouth.

For the first 2 or 3 days, the mother's breasts secrete **colostrum,** a yellowish, watery fluid with a higher protein, vitamin A, and mineral content and a lower fat and carbohydrate content than breast milk. It also contains antibodies that may play a part in the newborn's immune mechanism. Its laxative effect helps promote evacuation of meconium from the infant's bowel.

Until lactation begins, both breasts should be used at each feeding to stimulate the secretion of milk. Later when the breasts are full, one breast is generally sufficient at a feeding. That breast should be emptied at each feeding to stimulate refilling. Many physicians do not want infants to have any supplemental formula feedings during this initial period, so that they will be hungry and will nurse vigorously to stimulate milk production.

Whether breast milk or formula is used, some air is swallowed during nursing, and the infant needs burping to help expel it. After feeding, the infant may be held up on the mother's shoulder, may sit upright on her lap with the head supported, or may lie face down across her lap. With the baby in any of these positions, the mother gently rubs the infant's back. Some infants who nurse eagerly may need more than one burping during a feeding.

The mother who wishes to have support for breast-feeding after leaving the facility may appreciate a referral to the LaLeche League, a national organization dedicated to helping breast-feeding mothers have a successful experience. Most healthcare facilities have the names of local members who are happy to consult with new mothers.

Formula Feeding

If the mother does not breast-feed for whatever reason, caregivers may still provide all the necessary nutrients through a formula. As they hold and bottle-feed the infant, caregivers may also furnish the same comfort and security the infant experiences when breast-fed (Fig. 8–17). The caregivers should be warned of the problems created by "propping" the bottle and should be taught to always hold the infant when feeding. The practice of propping the bottle deprives the infant of the comfort and security of being held and may cause aspiration if the infant is left unattended. Infants who nurse from propped bottles are more prone to develop middle ear infections; formula pooling in the infant's mouth and pharynx provides a medium for bacterial growth.

Formula may be purchased already prepared in individual bottles, but this can be quite expensive. More economical formulas are prepared from dry powder or cans of formula that may be mixed with water. Water used to mix the formula should be boiled. The person preparing the formula must wash his or her hands before starting the preparation. All equipment to be used must be washed and rinsed thoroughly. Disposable bottles are available but add

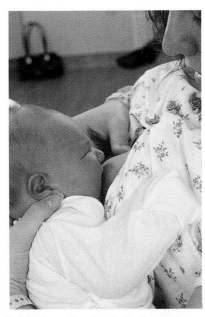

● *Figure 8.16* When offered a nipple, the newborn responds immediately and vigorously owing to the rooting and sucking reflexes. The mother presses her breast away from the infant's nose to enable more comfortable breathing while feeding.

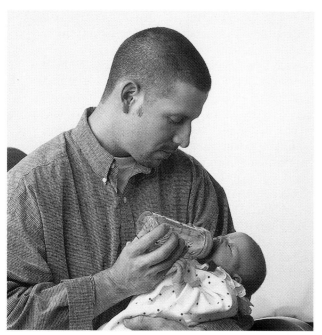

● *Figure 8.17* Bottle-fed babies can feel warmth and closeness from a caregiver.

to the cost of infant feeding. The best plan is to prepare one bottle at a time and use it immediately.

Formula may be given to the infant at room temperature or warmed, if desired. Bottles should never be warmed in a microwave oven, however, because they may explode or the formula may become too hot. Formula remaining in the bottle should not be saved from one feeding to the next because of the risk of bacterial growth. Open cans of formula may be covered and refrigerated until the next feeding.

Bottle-fed infants should be burped after every ½ to 1 oz they consume. The newborn takes about 2 oz at each feeding, and the feeding should take about 15 to 20 minutes. After the feeding, the infant should be positioned on the right side to minimize regurgitation and to allow swallowed air to rise above the level of fluid and escape. If the bottle is tilted so that formula fills the nipple, the amount of air swallowed is reduced.

The new caregiver should be encouraged to find a comfortable position with arm support when preparing to feed the infant. The caregiver's comfort transfers to the infant and makes feeding time more pleasant for both of them. The father or other support person may need encouragement to help with feeding.

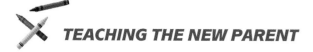

TEACHING THE NEW PARENT

Nurses have a major responsibility for patient teaching, so it is of the utmost importance that the

nurse is well informed. Most new parents are eager to learn all they can about their new roles. Many realize suddenly that they have taken on a tremendous task in raising a healthy, well-adjusted child. Although many may have attended parenting classes, caregivers bluntly face the reality of their responsibilities when their child is born. Some parents who have older children feel comfortable in their ability to care for a new infant. Others may want an update on infant care. Some parents have definite ideas about how they want to care for their infants, so nurses should be objective in the way they present information. Information and instruction should be made available to all the infant's prospective caretakers, if possible.

The most effective teaching often occurs on an individual basis when the nurse, mother, and father or support person are all together with the infant. In addition to determining how much the parent already knows, the nurse needs to know if the family has any anxieties or any misunderstandings and misinformation that need to be corrected.

Short stays have created additional problems finding time to teach infant care, so teaching often is done in community settings. Audiovisual materials such as slide-and-tape programs and videocassettes are used in many healthcare settings. The nurse must take care to follow up after these programs, encouraging questions and clarifying any misunderstandings. The nurse must be familiar with the information these materials contain in order to handle questions effectively.

Written materials are also widely used, but the nurse must not assume that all patients can read and understand these materials. With the goal of making the information clear to all, the nurse must be sensitive to possible reading problems and language differences. See the Family Teaching Tips displays on skin rashes, infections, stools, and bathing.

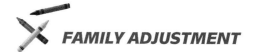

FAMILY ADJUSTMENT

The family is reshaped each time an infant is born, because every member of that family is affected by the presence of this new person. The family also shapes the child. First-time parents probably have the greatest anxieties because they have totally new roles to learn. Early research on parent-infant attachment studied the "mothering" aspect of the relationship; more recent studies of neonatal behavior indicate that the infant also has a definite role in the attachment process. Fathers have also been the subject of increasing research, all of which has aided the understanding of how relationships are formed, what factors help or hinder the process, and how to avoid potential problems.

FAMILY TEACHING TIPS

Skin Rashes—Points to Cover

1. The infant may break out with heat rash when dressed too warmly. Dress infant with light covering or diapers only, especially in warm weather.
2. The plastic in disposable diapers may cause some infants to develop a rash. Observe infant for rash if using disposable diapers. Switching brands may help but if the rash persists, cloth diapers may be necessary.
3. Cloth diapers may also cause a rash. Keep infant as dry as possible. If cloth diapers are used, close the safety pins when removing them and insert pins into the diaper with points outward.
4. Good laundry practices are important.
   a. Wash baby's clothing separate from the rest of the laundry. Use a mild soap and rinse well (twice if possible).
   b. Avoid using softeners or strong detergents on baby's clothes.
   c. White vinegar (⅔ cup) may be added to the final wash rinse as a fabric softener. It softens the clothes without leaving an odor.
5. If the infant develops diaper rash, keep the area dry and expose it to air if possible. Urine irritates diaper rash. A soothing ointment (such as A&D or lanolin) may be used to protect the skin. If the rash persists, notify the physician, who may order a special ointment.
6. Dry skin may be soothed with an over-the-counter ointment.

FAMILY TEACHING TIPS

Infections—Points to Cover

1. One way that infants get infectious diseases is through handling by other people. Be careful who handles the baby. No one with any type of infection should visit. Avoid taking the baby into crowded places for the first month or so. Newborns may have low resistance to some diseases.
2. If you think your infant is getting sick, note the symptoms. Take the infant's temperature and call the baby's pediatrician.
3. Check with the baby's care provider before giving any medications to be certain of the type and amount of medicine to use.
4. Handwashing carried out by anyone who is going to handle the infant is one of the most important ways to avoid infections.
5. Anything that is going into the infant's mouth should be washed before being given to the child.

ity—she is likely to feel resentful, then guilty for resenting the new baby. Although the new mother loves the baby, no one has prepared her for the normal resentment that the responsibility of total care for a helpless, demanding infant often brings.

Rather than deny her resentment and what she considers to be unworthy feelings, the mother needs help to admit feelings and, furthermore, to understand that resentment is a normal reaction. She needs to understand that as she grows into her task and as she and her child begin to adjust to each other, resent-

FAMILY TEACHING TIPS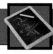

Stools—Points to Cover

1. Breast-fed infants average two to four stools a day, with a range of one to seven for the first few months. Occasionally an infant may have one movement every few days and still be comfortable and normal. After breast-feeding is established, the stool will be yellow to golden with a consistency of liquid paste and an odor of sour milk.
2. Bottle-fed infants average one to four stools per day. An infant may have more or less and still be normal. The stool may range from pale yellow to light brown, and the consistency may be firmer and more solid than stools from a breast-fed baby.
3. When solid food is added, stools tend to become darker, firmer, and stronger in odor.
4. Constipation is rare. A change in the stool's consistency (hard or dry and difficult to pass) rather than the stools frequency, is the sign of constipation. Notify the care provider for treatment.

Although early contact has been carefully studied, no definite conclusions have been reached; parents and families should not be made to feel that all is lost if early bonding does not take place for some reason.

The Parents' Adjustment

Regardless of how much preparation the mother has had for her new role, it is still a totally new experience. She is prepared to love her child, but having a new child who needs total care 24 hours a day is a terrific responsibility.

The new mother may expect a surge of motherly love to enable her instinctively to love and care for her baby without any doubt or trouble. This does not happen on the first day, however, or even after a week; it does develop over time. If she has had a previous child, she may find that this child does not "measure up" in the same way that the previous child did, and this reaction may contribute to feelings of guilt and self-doubt. When she feels inadequate, exhausted, and discouraged—as many people do when confronted with a new and seemingly overwhelming responsibil-

FAMILY TEACHING TIPS

Sponge Bath

PURPOSES OF THE BATH
1. The bath removes waste products from the infant's skin and removes odors.
2. The bath is a time when the bath giver can inspect the infant's body carefully and note any changes such as rashes, discolorations, and abnormal movements of the extremities.
3. The infant has the opportunity to kick and exercise.
4. The bath is a time to be alone with the infant and become acquainted. It is also a time for the baby to begin to feel more secure. Talking, cooing, cuddling, and stroking are important parts of the bath procedure. The more the bath giver can relax and enjoy the infant, the happier the time will be for both of them.
5. Until the cord stump falls off and the navel is healed, the baby should only have sponge baths because the cord stump should be kept as dry as possible.

Assemble the necessary articles on the bathing table. Any sturdy table covered with a clean cloth can be used. Articles needed are the following:
- Basin of warm water, warm to the elbow, 100 to 105°F (37.5°B40.6°C). The basin should be used for this purpose only.
- Mild, unscented soap to be used only if needed
- Soft washcloth; towel for drying baby; large soft towel or cotton blanket on table on which to lay baby
- Alcohol—70% (rubbing)
- Cotton balls
- Comb and/or brush
- Ointment such as A&D for dry skin
- Clean clothes for baby

PROCEDURE
1. Before handling and touching the infant, wash hands and arms well. Anyone with any type of infection should be discouraged from handling the baby.
2. Have everything ready before picking up the baby. *Never* leave the baby on the table unattended. Small infants can easily roll off the table; keep one hand on the infant at all times.
3. Place the baby on the blanket or towel and wash the face with clear water. If eyes have been draining, sponge them with a clean piece of cotton, wiping from the inner canthus outward. Use clean cotton for each eye. Wash the outer folds of the ears and behind them, but do not poke in the infant's ear because that can cause serious harm. Remember, "Nothing smaller than your elbow in the ear."
4. If the infant has a nasal discharge, wash the edge of nostrils with cotton but do not poke in the nose. To dislodge dried mucus just inside the nostril, cleanse with a small piece of cotton dipped in water. This will usually make the infant sneeze and dislodge any mucus lodged further up in the nose.
5. Pick up baby and slide an arm under the baby up toward the head; with hand under head, lift the infant up. One comfortable method of holding a baby is the *football hold*, in which the infant's head rests in the palm of the holder's hand and the body lies along the inside of the holder's arm with the infant resting on the holder's hip.

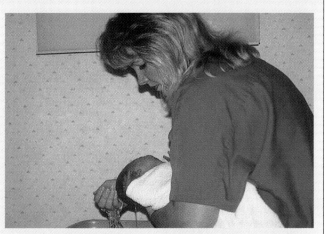

The football hold supports the infant's head and back and leaves the caregiver's other hand free.

6. Wet the head, lather with soap, rinse well, and dry. Combing the hair gently with a fine-toothed comb helps loosen and rid the scalp of debris that could cause cradle cap. *Do not* use shampoo until the infant is 1 month old.
7. Undress the baby. Cleanse the diaper area with a clean wet cloth if the diaper is soiled. Always clean from front to back to avoid contamination of the urinary system with fecal material. Before continuing the bath, wash hands. (It is a good idea to have another small basin of water nearby for handwashing.)
8. Wash the baby's arms, trunk, and legs. Lather the body with soap if needed, getting into skin folds such as in the neck and underarms. Rinse soap from the skin and dry thoroughly, making certain to dry well in the skin folds and in the groin.
9. Wash the genital area, cleansing in the creases. Gently cleanse around the labia of girls, but do not try to retract the foreskin in an uncircumcised boy unless under the pediatrician's specific direction. Circumcision care should be performed on circumcised boys.
10. Dry the infant, then turn him or her on the abdomen and wash the back of the neck, the trunk, and lastly the buttocks including cleansing around the rectum.
11. Wet a cotton ball with alcohol, and wipe the cord stump and the skin immediately around it. This should be done until the cord falls off. The cord may take 3 to 4 weeks to dry and fall off. If a few drops of blood appear when the cord falls off, simply wipe the area with alcohol. There should not be any drainage the next day.
12. Use of baby powders and lotions is discouraged because they can irritate the infant's skin. They should be used only after consultation with the infant's provider.
13. Remove the wet towel on which the baby had been lying, and dress the baby according to the season. Fold the undershirt up and the diaper down so that the cord is exposed to the air to promote drying.

ment and feelings of inadequacy will fade away. When a woman is able to acknowledge her feelings as normal following the birth of her child, she has started the process of accepting those feelings and finding a balance in her life.

Another way to help is to find some way in which the mother may be relieved of some of the burden until she is stronger. The father or another support person may help give some relief from care responsibilities each day. The new mother will need to spend time with older children, perhaps while the newborn is sleeping, but she still needs time completely for herself.

Even a father who loves his new baby very much may feel left out and neglected when the mother and the baby come home and all the mother's time and attention seem to be devoted to the baby. The father may resent the fact that the mother seems exhausted unless he understands just how much effort caring for a helpless infant requires. This is especially true of the first-time father. Like the mother, he needs to be encouraged to admit his feelings and understand that they are normal reactions to the situation. He also needs to be encouraged to give the mother a break or to arrange for someone to come in to give her a break. If a family member or other person will relieve them for short periods regularly, the couple should take advantage of this and do something together, even if it is only taking a walk. These small breaks can do much to refresh the spirit.

The Infant's Adjustment

Each infant affects and reacts to the family environment uniquely. The infant's primary developmental task, according to Erikson, is to develop a sense of trust. After 9 months of security, the infant has been thrust into a world in which needs must be made known, with no assurance that they will be met. At birth, the infant entered a strange country where the language, customs, and rules are unknown. The infant is sensitive to attitudes that alter the caretakers' touch or the tone of voice. Likewise, the caretakers are affected by the infant's reactions and characteristics. The infant needs reassurance that this is a friendly world.

The Sibling's Adjustment

Sibling attachment and adjustment are as important as those of other family members. Sibling rivalry and the detrimental effects of separation anxiety make it important to include the other children in the events surrounding the birth of a new family member. The practice of allowing siblings to witness the actual birth is controversial, but policies generally allow siblings to visit after the birth (Fig. 8–18). Many

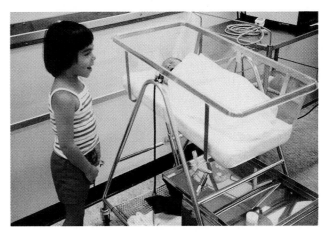

● **Figure 8.18** Shortly after birth, big sister meets her baby brother.

hospitals provide prenatal sibling classes in which the prenatal instructor talks about the feelings of new babies, how they look, how they behave, how to handle them, the amount of care they take, and feelings of rivalry. The classes often include a tour of the obstetric department to see where the mother will be. Studies indicate that newborns that have direct contact with their siblings have no higher incidence of infection than do those who have contact with adults.

Siblings are often more concerned about the reunion with their mother than about meeting the newborn. After reassurances from the mother, the child usually accepts the new infant. Children who had established prenatal relationships with the fetus demonstrate a higher frequency of attachment behavior with the newborn than do siblings who had not established such a relationship. Depending on the sibling's age, these prenatal relationships can be established by encouraging the sibling to be part of the preparation process for the baby's birth. Siblings often help to prepare the baby's room, call the sibling by name if a name has been chosen, listen to the heartbeat of the unborn child, and express their feelings about the arrival of a new brother or sister.

KEY POINTS

▸ The neonate is an intriguing, exciting being. Although helpless and vulnerable, the neonate is complex and capable of responding to and eliciting many responses from caregivers.

▸ One goal of family-centered care is to create a positive atmosphere in which the family is helped to learn about, care for, appreciate, and enjoy their infant. The new family has much to learn, and the nurse has a great responsibility to aid in that process. Shortened hospital stays make this learning process intense, but it must be thorough.

♦ All members of the family have adjustments to make to include the newest family member. Family members will find that as they make adjustments in their lives, they can learn to live in harmony with each other.

BIBLIOGRAPHY

Berger KS. (2001) *The developing person through the life span* (5th ed). New York: Worth Publishers.

Brazelton TB, Greenspan S. (2001) *The irreducible needs of children: What every child must have to grow, learn, and flourish.* Cambridge, MA: Perseus Publishing.

Craven RF, Hirnle CJ. (1999) *Fundamentals of nursing* (3rd ed). Philadelphia: Lippincott Williams & Wilkins.

Dudek SG. (2000) *Nutrition essentials for nursing practice* (4th ed). Philadelphia: Lippincott Williams & Wilkins.

Dworkin P. (2000) *Pediatrics* (4th ed). Philadelphia: Lippincott Williams & Wilkins.

Ivey JB. (2001) Somebody's grandma and grandpa: Children's response to contacts with elders. *The American Journal of Maternal/Child Nursing*,26(1), 23.

Pillitteri A. (1999). *Maternal and child health nursing* (3rd ed). Philadelphia: Lippincott Williams & Wilkins.

Spock B, et al. (1998) *Dr. Spock's baby and child care.* New York: Pocket Books.

Wong DL. (1998) *Whaley and Wong's nursing care of infants and children* (6th ed). St. Louis: Mosby.

Wong DL, Perry S, Hockenberry, M. (2002) *Maternal child nursing care* (2nd ed). St. Louis: Mosby.

Websites
www.babycenter.com
www.lamaze.com
www.oxygen.com/family/babies

Workbook Chapter 8

NCLEX-STYLE REVIEW QUESTIONS

1. Examining the head and body of the normal newborn, the nurse would expect to find which of the following?

   a. An open posterior fontanel

   b. Head circumference equal to chest measurement

   c. 2 to 4 deciduous (baby) teeth erupted

   d. Abdominal circumference of approximately 20 inches

2. The rooting reflex is usually present at birth in the normal newborn. Of the following behaviors, which one is an example of the rooting reflex? The infant

   a. turns head to side when the cheek is stroked

   b. makes sucking noises when lying in crib

   c. gags when food stimulates the pharynx

   d. abducts arms following a loud noise

3. When assisting with a neurologic exam on a newborn, the nurse notes that the infant can be lifted off the examining table when pressure is put on the palms of the newborn's hands. This is an example of which reflex?

   a. palmar grasp reflex

   b. Babinski reflex

   c. Moro reflex

   d. tonic neck reflex

4. A nurse is teaching a group of parents of newborns about common skin blemishes. Which of the following statements by the caregiver would indicate an understanding of what happens with most skin blemishes seen in newborns?

   a. "We will just have to get used to our baby having that mark that looks like a strawberry."

   b. "If they wouldn't have had to use forceps, my baby would not have to always live with that spot on her face."

   c. "It is reassuring to hear that those little purple spots on his face will go away in a few days."

   d. "I am concerned that the yellow color of his skin is a serious disease."

5. When teaching about the control of infection to a group of caregivers of newborns, which of the following should the nurse reinforce? The caregiver should

   a. encourage family members to hold the newborn to increase the newborn's resistance to disease.

   b. check the newborn's temperature two or three times a day.

   c. wash her or his hands frequently especially before handling the newborn.

   d. sterilize any toy the newborn puts into his or her mouth at least once a week.

STUDY ACTIVITIES

1. List and compare the eight neurologic reflexes seen in the newborn infant. Include the description and characteristic signs of the reflex and if and when the reflex disappears.

Reflex	Description and Characteristic Signs of Reflex	Age Reflex Disappears

2. You are working with a new mother who needs guidance with breast-feeding. List the points you will talk about with this mother. Describe in detail the steps you will follow to help her with breast-feeding her infant.

3. You are teaching Rosa about infant care. She is upset by her baby's caput succedaneum. Describe the teaching you will offer Rosa and her family about this condition.

CRITICAL THINKING

1. You walk by Mary Greene's room and notice that her baby is crying loudly while Mary apparently is watching a television soap opera. Discuss some of the possible feelings and emotions this mother might be going through. Write out a therapeutic conversation you might have with this mother.

2. The parent of a dark-skinned infant questions you about a large area on the infant's right buttock that appears to be a bruise. What response will you give to this parent to provide reassurance?

3. The parents of a newborn boy are discussing whether they should or should not circumcise their child. They ask you what you think about circumcision. What will you say in response to these parents? Discuss your thoughts and opinions regarding circumcision with your peers.

Health Problems of the Newborn

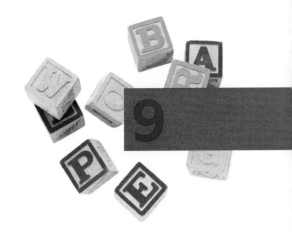

9

CONGENITAL ANOMALIES
Facial Deformities
Nursing Process for the Infant with
    Cleft Lip and Cleft Palate
Digestive Tract Defects
Central Nervous System Defects
Nursing Process for the Infant With
    Myelomeningocele
Nursing Process for the Postoperative
    Infant With Hydrocephalus

Cardiovascular System Defects
Nursing Process for the Infant With
    Congestive Heart Failure
Skeletal System Defects
Nursing Process for the Infant in an
    Orthopedic Device or Cast
Genitourinary Tract Defects
CONGENITAL DISORDERS
Infections
Inborn Errors of Metabolism

STUDENT OBJECTIVES

On completion of this chapter, the student will be able to

1. Differentiate between cleft lip and cleft palate.
2. Identify the early signs that indicate the presence of an esophageal fistula.
3. Name the greatest preoperative danger for infants with tracheoesophageal atresia.
4. List and describe the five types of hernias that infants may have.
5. Differentiate the three types of spina bifida that may occur.
6. Name the type of spina bifida that is most difficult to treat, and state why this is so.
7. Describe the two types of hydrocephalus that may occur.
8. State the most obvious symptoms of hydrocephalus.
9. Describe two types of shunting performed for hydrocephalus.
10. State the signs and symptoms of congestive heart failure in the child with congenital heart disease.
11. List five common types of congenital heart defects and trace the blood flow of each defect, indicating whether blood is oxygen-poor or oxygen-rich.
12. State the two most common skeletal deformities in the newborn.
13. Discuss the importance of early treatment for clubfoot.
14. List three signs and symptoms of congenital dislocation of the hip.
15. Describe the treatment for congenital dislocation of the hip.
16. List the infections included in the acronym TORCH.
17. State the cause of gonorrheal ophthalmia neonatorum.
18. Describe the best treatment for syphilis.
19. Discuss the ways in which hepatitis B and HIV are transmitted to the newborn.
20. Describe congenital rubella, and discuss its prevention.
21. State the effect of herpes simplex virus on the newborn.
22. Identify the test to detect phenylketonuria in the newborn.
23. Describe the treatment for phenylketonuria.
24. Name the tests performed on newborns to detect congenital hypothyroidism.
25. State the one serious outcome that is common to untreated phenylketonuria, congenital hypothyroidism, and galactosemia.

KEY TERMS

atresia
bilateral
chordee
congestive heart failure (CHF)
cyanotic heart disease
ductus arteriosus
ductus venosus
foramen ovale
galactosemia
hernia
hip dysplasia
hypothermia
imperforate anus
interstitial keratitis
overriding aorta
phenylketonuria
pulmonary stenosis
right ventricular hypertrophy
spina bifida
supernumerary
talipes equinovarus
unilateral
ventricular septal defect
ventriculoatrial shunting
ventriculoperitoneal shunting

A high-risk neonate is defined as any neonate who is in danger of serious illness or death as a result of prenatal, perinatal, or neonatal conditions regardless of birth weight or gestational age. Only technologically advanced, expert care by skilled health professionals and a controlled environment can offer such an infant hope of realizing a normal life potential. These infants are cared for in intensive care settings and the nurses and healthcare professionals are highly skilled and specially trained. The largest numbers of high-risk newborns, who are usually preterm or premature, are those who have a low birth weight. Other high-risk conditions in the neonate are caused by conditions present in the mother during pregnancy and at the time of delivery. Because of the seriousness of the conditions in these infants, many of them do not survive. The special needs of the premature newborn, the newborn with high-risk conditions, and care of the high-risk newborn are covered in-depth in maternal child textbooks and references.

Those newborns who survive these high-risk conditions often have long-term disorders that affect them through life. These disorders will be discussed throughout this textbook in the disease and disorder chapters.

Malformations that occur during the prenatal period and are present at birth are termed congenital anomalies. Many times these can be corrected during the first months or years of life. A congenital disorder is a condition that is present at birth and is often caused by a maternal infection. Some congenital conditions are termed inborn errors of metabolism, which are hereditary disorders that affect metabolism.

The birth of an infant with a congenital defect (anomaly) or birth injury is a crisis for parents and caregivers. Depending on the defect, immediate or early surgery may be necessary. Early, continuous, skilled observation and highly skilled nursing care are required. Rehabilitation of the infant and education of the family caregivers in the infant's care are essential. The emotional needs of the infant and the family must be integrated into the plans for nursing care. Many of these infants have a brighter future today as a result of increased diagnostic and medical knowledge and advances in surgical techniques.

Family caregivers experience a grief response whether the infant's defect is a result of injury at birth or of abnormal intrauterine development. They mourn the loss of the perfect child of their dreams, question why it happened, and may wonder how they will show the infant to family and friends without shame or embarrassment. This grief may interfere with the process of parent-infant attachment.

Parents need to understand that their response is normal and that they are entitled to honest answers to their questions about the infant's condition. Other children in the family should be informed gently but honestly about the infant and should be allowed to visit the infant when accompanied by adult family members. Sufficient time and attention must be devoted to the older siblings to avoid jealousy toward the infant.

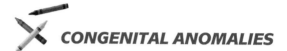

CONGENITAL ANOMALIES

Congenital anomalies may be caused by genetic or environmental factors. These anomalies include facial deformities, such as cleft lip and palate, and defects of the gastrointestinal, central nervous, cardiovascular, skeletal, and genitourinary systems. Defects such as facial deformities and severe neural tube defects are apparent at birth, but others may be discovered only after a complete physical examination. Congenital anomalies account for a large percentage of the health problems seen in infants and children.

Facial Deformities

The birth of an infant with a facial deformity may change the atmosphere of the delivery from one of joyous anticipation to one of awkward tension. The most common facial malformations, cleft lip and cleft palate, occur either alone or in combination. Cleft lip occurs in about one in 1,000 live births and is more common in males. Cleft palate occurs in one infant in 2,500, more often in females. Their cause is not entirely clear; they appear to be genetically influenced but sometimes occur in isolated instances with no genetic history.

Cleft Lip and Cleft Palate

Parents and family are naturally eager to see and hold their newborn infant and must be prepared for the shock of seeing the disfigurement of a cleft lip. Their emotional reaction to such an obvious malformation is usually much stronger than to a "hidden" defect such as congenital heart disease. They need encouragement and support as well as considerable instruction about the infant's feeding and care. The child born with a cleft palate but with an intact lip does not have the external disfigurement that may be so distressing to the new parent, but the problems are more serious.

Although a cleft lip and a cleft palate often appear together, either defect may appear alone. In embryonic development, the palate closes later than the lip, and the failure to close occurs for different reasons.

The cleft lip and palate defects result from failure of the maxillary and premaxillary processes to fuse during the fifth to eighth week of intrauterine life. The cleft may be a simple notch in the vermilion line, or it may extend up into the floor of the nose (Fig. 9–1). It may be either **unilateral** (one side of the lip) or **bilateral** (both sides). Cleft palate occurs with a cleft lip about 50% of the time, most often with bilateral cleft lip. Cleft palate, which develops sometime between the seventh and 12th weeks of gestation, is often accompanied by nasal deformity and dental disorders such as deformed, missing, or **supernumerary** (excessive in number) teeth.

In an 8-week-old embryo, there is still no roof to the mouth; the tissues that are to become the palate are two shelves running from the front to the back of the mouth and projecting vertically downward on either side of the tongue. The shelves move from a vertical position to a horizontal position; their free edges meet and fuse in midline. Later bone forms within this tissue to form the hard palate.

Normally the palate is intact by the 10th week of fetal life. Exactly what happens to prevent this closure is not known for sure. The incidence of cleft palates is higher in the close relatives of people with the defect than it is in the general population, and some evidence indicates that environmental and hereditary factors play a part in this defect.

Clinical Manifestations and Diagnosis. The physical appearance of the infant confirms the diagnosis of cleft lip. Diagnosis of cleft palate is made at birth with the close inspection of the newborn's palate. To be certain that a cleft palate is not missed, the examiner must insert a gloved finger into the newborn's mouth to feel the palate to determine that it is intact. If a cleft is found, consulta-

tion is set up with a clinic specializing in cleft palate repair.

Treatment. Surgery, usually performed by a plastic surgeon, is a major part of the treatment of a child with a cleft lip, palate, or both (Fig. 9–2). Total care involves many other specialists including pediatricians, nurses, orthodontists, prosthodontists, otolaryngologists, speech therapists, and occasionally psychiatrists. Long-term, intensive, multidisciplinary care is needed for infants with major defects.

Plastic surgeons' opinions differ as to the best time for repair of the cleft lip. Some surgeons favor early repair, before the infant is discharged from the hospital; they believe early repair can alleviate some of the family's feelings of rejection of the infant. Other surgeons prefer to wait until the infant is 1 or 2 months old, weighs about 10 lb, and is gaining weight steadily. Infants who are not born in large medical centers with specialists on the staff are discharged from the birth hospital and referred to a center or physician specializing in cleft lip and palate repair.

If early surgery is contemplated, the infant should be healthy and of average or above-average weight. The infant must be observed constantly, because a newborn has a higher likelihood of aspiration than does an older infant. These infants must be cared for by competent plastic surgeons and experienced nurses.

The goal in repairing the cleft palate is to give the child a union of the cleft parts to allow intelligible

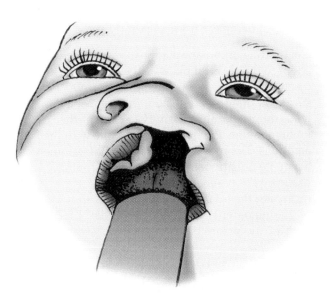

● *Figure 9.1* A cleft lip may extend up into the floor of the nose.

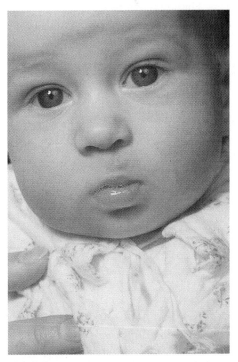

● *Figure 9.2* Infant with a surgical repair of a cleft lip.

and pleasant speech and to avoid injury to the maxillary development. The timing of cleft palate repair is individualized according to the size, placement, and degree of deformity. The surgery may need to be done in stages over several years to achieve the best results. The optimal time for surgical repair of the cleft palate is considered to be between 6 months and 5 years of age. Because the child cannot make certain sounds when starting to talk, undesirable speech habits are formed that are difficult to correct. If surgery must be delayed beyond the third year, a dental speech appliance may help the child develop intelligible speech.

● Nursing Process for the Infant With Cleft Lip and Cleft Palate

ASSESSMENT

One primary concern in the nursing care of the infant with a cleft lip with or without a cleft palate is the emotional care of the infant's family. In interviewing the family and collecting data, the nurse must include exploration of the family's acceptance of the infant. Practice active listening with reflective responses, accept the family's emotional responses, and demonstrate complete acceptance of the infant.

The family caregivers who return to the hospital with the young infant for the beginning repair of a cleft palate have already faced the challenges of feeding their infant. Conduct a thorough interview with the caregivers that includes a question about the methods they found to be most effective in feeding the infant.

Physical exam of the infant includes temperature, apical pulse, and respirations. Listen to breath sounds to detect any pulmonary congestion. Observe skin turgor and color, noting any deviations from normal. Also, observe the child's neurologic status, noting alertness and responsiveness. Document a complete description of the cleft.

NURSING DIAGNOSES

Formulation of nursing diagnoses depends partly on the timing of the initial cleft lip surgery. If the infant is to be discharged from the hospital before surgery, nursing diagnoses are directed to the feeding and nutrition of the infant and the emotional care of the family. If the newborn is to have lip repair surgery before discharge, nursing diagnoses would include

those related to preoperative care as well as those related to the operative plans.

Nursing diagnoses for the newborn infant preoperatively may include:
- Imbalanced Nutrition: Less than Body Requirements related to inability to suck secondary to cleft lip
- Compromised Family Coping related to visible physical defect
- Anxiety of family caregivers related to the child's condition and surgical outcome
- Deficient Knowledge of family caregivers related to care of child preoperatively and surgical procedure

Some postoperative nursing diagnoses applicable to the infant following the surgical repairs are:
- Risk for Aspiration related to a reduced level of consciousness postoperatively
- Ineffective Breathing Pattern related to anatomic changes
- Risk for Deficient Fluid Volume related to NPO status postoperatively
- Imbalanced Nutrition: Less than Body Requirements related to difficulty in feeding postoperatively
- Acute Pain related to surgical procedure
- Risk of Injury to the operative site related to infant's desire to suck thumb or fingers and anatomic changes
- Risk for Infection related to operative site
- Risk for Delayed Growth and Development related to hospitalizations and surgery
- Deficient Knowledge of family caregivers related to long-term aspects of cleft palate

OUTCOME IDENTIFICATION AND PLANNING: PREOPERATIVE CARE

Goal setting and planning must be modified to adapt to the surgical plans. If the infant is to be discharged from the birth hospital to have surgery a month or two later, the nurse may focus on preparing the family to care for the infant at home and helping them cope with their emotions. The major goals include maintaining adequate nutrition, increasing family coping, reducing the parents' anxiety and guilt regarding the infant's physical defect, and preparing parents for the future repair of the cleft lip and palate.

IMPLEMENTATION

Maintaining Adequate Nutrition. The infant's nutritional condition is important to the planning of surgery because the infant must be in good condition before surgery can be scheduled. Feeding the infant with a cleft lip before repair, however, is a challenge: the procedure may be time-consuming and tedious because the infant's ability to suck is inadequate. Breast-feeding may be successful because the breast tissue may mold to close the gap. If the infant cannot breast-feed, the mother's breast milk may be expressed and used instead of formula until after the surgical repair heals. Various nipples may be tried to find the method that works best. A soft nipple with a crosscut made to promote easy flow of milk or formula may work well. Lamb's nipples (extra-long nipples) as well as special cleft palate nipples molded to fit into the open palate area to close the gap have been used with success. One of the simplest and most effective methods may be the use of an eyedropper or an Asepto syringe with a short piece of rubber tubing on the tip (Breck feeder) (Fig. 9–3). The dropper or syringe is used carefully to drip formula into the infant's mouth at a rate slow enough to allow the infant to swallow. As the infant learns to eat, much coughing, sputtering, and choking may occur. The nurse or family caregiver feeding the infant must be alert for signs of aspiration.

Whatever feeding method is used, the experience may be frustrating for both the feeder and the infant. Have family caregivers practice the feeding techniques under supervision. During the teaching process, give them ample opportunity to ask questions so they feel able to care for the infant (see Family Teaching Tips: Cleft Lip/Cleft Palate).

Promoting Family Coping. Encourage family members to verbalize their feelings regarding the defect and their disappointment. Convey to the family that their feelings are acceptable and normal. While caring for the infant, demonstrate behavior that clearly displays acceptance of the infant. Serve as a model for the family caregivers' attitudes toward the child.

Reducing Family Anxiety. Give the family caregivers information about cleft repairs.

FAMILY TEACHING TIPS

Cleft Lip/Cleft Palate

1. Sucking is important to speech development.
2. Holding the baby upright while feeding helps avoid choking.
3. Burp the baby frequently because a large amount of air is swallowed during feeding.
4. Don't tire the baby. Limit feeding times to 20 to 30 minutes maximum. If necessary, feed the baby more often.
5. Feed strained foods slowly from the side of the spoon in small amounts.
6. Don't be alarmed if food seeps through the cleft and out the nose.
7. Have baby's ears checked any time he or she has a cold or upper respiratory infection.
8. Talk normally to baby (no "baby talk"). Talk often; repeat baby's babbling and cooing. This helps in speech development.
9. Try to understand early talking without trying to correct baby.
10. Good mouth care is very important.
11. Early dental care is essential to observe teething and prevent caries.

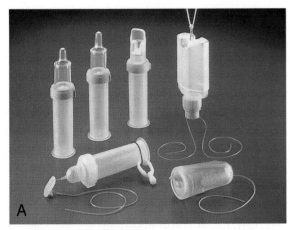

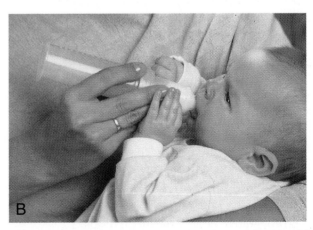

● **Figure 9.3** Specialty feeding devices used for the infant with a cleft lip or palate include **(A)** special nipples and devices and **(B)** a special feeder.

Pamphlets are available that present photographs of before-and-after corrections that will answer some of their questions. Encourage them to ask questions and reassure them that any question is valid.

Providing Family Teaching. By the time the infant is actually admitted for the repair, the family will have received a great amount of information, but all families need additional support throughout the procedure. Explain the usual routine of preoperative, intraoperative, and postoperative care. Written information is helpful, but be certain the parents understand the information. Simple things are important: show families where they may wait during surgery, inform them how long the surgery should last, tell them about the postanesthesia care unit procedure, and let them know where the surgeon will expect to find them to report on the surgery.

OUTCOME IDENTIFICATION AND PLANNING: POSTOPERATIVE CARE

Major goals for the postoperative care of the infant who is hospitalized for surgical repair of cleft lip or palate include preventing aspiration, improving respiration, maintaining adequate fluid volume and nutritional requirements, relieving pain, preventing injury and infection to the surgical site, promoting normal growth and development, and increasing the family caregivers' knowledge about the child's long-term care.

IMPLEMENTATION

Preventing Aspiration. To facilitate drainage of mucus and secretions, position the infant on the side, never on the abdomen, after a cleft lip repair. The infant may be placed on the side after a cleft palate repair. Watch the infant closely in the immediate postoperative period. Do not put anything in the infant's mouth to clear mucus because of the danger of damaging the surgical site, particularly with a palate repair.

Changing Breathing Pattern. Immediately after a palate repair, the infant must change from a mouth-breathing pattern to nasal breathing. This change may frustrate the infant, but the infant positioned to ease breathing and given encouragement should be able to adjust quickly.

Monitoring Fluid Volume. In the immediate postoperative period, the infant needs parenteral fluids. Follow all the usual precautions: check placement, discoloration of the site, swelling, and flow rate every 2 hours. Document intake and output accurately. Parenteral fluids are continued until the infant can take oral fluids without vomiting.

Maintaining Adequate Nutrition. As soon as the infant is no longer nauseated (vomiting should be avoided if possible), the surgeon usually permits clear liquids.

Sucking is important to the development of speech muscles, so it should be encouraged. If the infant does not have a cleft lip or if the lip has had an early repair, sucking may be learned more easily even though the suction generated is not as good as in the infant with an intact palate. A large nipple with holes that allow the milk to drip freely makes sucking easier. If the cleft is unilateral, the nipple should be aimed at the unaffected side.

For an infant who has had a palate repair, no nipples, spoons, or straws are permitted; only a drinking glass or a cup is recommended. A favorite cup from home may be reassuring to the infant. Offer clear liquids such as flavored gelatin water, apple juice, and synthetic fruit-flavored drinks. Red juices should not be given because they may conceal bleeding. Infants do not usually like broth. The diet is increased to full liquid, and the infant is usually discharged on a soft diet. When permitted, foods such as cooked infant cereals, ice cream, and flavored gelatin are often favorites. The surgeon determines the progression of the diet. Nothing hard or sharp should be placed in the infant's mouth.

Relieving Pain. Observe the infant for signs of pain or discomfort from the surgery. Administer ordered analgesics as needed. Relieving pain not only comforts the infant, but may also prevent crying, which is important because of the danger of disrupting the suture line. Make every effort to prevent the infant with a lip repair from crying to prevent excessive tension on the suture line.

Preventing Postoperative Injury. Continuous, skilled observation is essential. Swollen mouth tissues cause excessive secretion of mucus that is poorly handled by a small infant. For the first few postoperative hours, never leave the infant alone because aspiration of mucus occurs quickly and easily. Because nothing is permitted in the infant's mouth, particularly the thumb or finger, elbow restraints are necessary. The thumb, though comforting, may quickly undo the repair or cause undesirable scarring along the suture line. The infant's ultimate happiness and well-being must take precedence over immediate satisfaction. Accustoming the infant to elbow restraints gradually before admission is helpful.

Elbow restraints must be applied properly and checked frequently (see Fig. 6–1 in Chap. 6). The restraints should be placed firmly around the arm and pinned to the infant's shirt or gown to prevent them from sliding down below the elbow. The infant's arms can move freely but cannot bend at the elbows to reach the face. Apply the restraint snugly but do not allow the circulation to be hindered. The older infant may need to be placed in a jacket restraint. The use of restraints must be documented.

Remove restraints at least every 2 hours, but remove them only one at a time and control the released arm so that the thumb or fingers do not pop into the mouth. Comfort the infant and explore various means of comforting. Talk to the infant continuously while providing care. Playing "Peek-a-Boo" and other baby games may be helpful; however, "Patty Cake" does not work well with an infant in elbow restraints! Inspect and massage the skin, apply lotion, and perform range-of-motion exercises. Replace restraints when they become soiled.

Preventing Infection. Gentle mouth care with tepid water or clear liquid may be recommended to follow feeding. This care helps clean the suture area of any food or liquids to promote a cleaner incision for optimal healing.

Care of Lip Suture Line. The lip suture line is left uncovered after surgery and must be kept meticulously clean and dry to prevent infection and subsequent scarring. A wire bow called a Logan bar or a butterfly closure is applied across the upper lip and attached to the cheeks with adhesive tape to prevent tension on the sutures caused by crying or other facial movement (Fig. 9–4). Carefully clean the sutures after feeding and as often as necessary to prevent collection of dried formula or serum. Frequent cleaning is essential as long as the sutures are in place. Clean the sutures gently with sterile cotton swabs and saline or the solution of the surgeon's choice. Application of an ointment such as bacitracin may also be ordered. Care of the suture line is extremely important because it has a direct effect on the

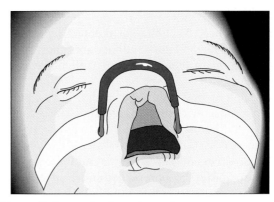

● *Figure 9.4* Logan bar for easing strain on sutures.

cosmetic appearance of the repair. Teach the family how to care for the suture line, because the infant will probably be discharged before the sutures are removed (7 to 10 days after surgery). The infant probably will be allowed to suck on a soft nipple at this time.

Aseptic technique is important while caring for the infant undergoing lip or palate repair. Good handwashing technique is essential. Instruct the family caregivers about the importance of preventing anyone with an upper respiratory infection from visiting the infant. Observe for signs of otitis media that may occur from drainage into the eustachian tube.

Promoting Sensory Stimulation. The infant needs stimulating, safe toys in the crib. The nurse and family caregivers must use every opportunity to provide sensory stimulation. Talking to the infant, cuddling and holding him or her, and responding to cries are important interventions. Provide freedom from restraints within the limitations of safety as much as possible. One caregiver should be assigned to provide stability and consistency of care. Family caregivers and health care personnel must encourage the older child to use speech and help enhance the child's self-esteem. A baby suffers emotional frustration because of restraints, so satisfaction must be provided in other ways. Rocking, cuddling, and other soothing techniques are an important part of nursing care. Family members and other caregivers are the best people to supply this loving care.

Providing Family Teaching. After effective surgery and skilled, careful nursing care, the appearance of the baby's face should be greatly improved. The scar fades in time. Family caregivers need to know that the baby will probably need a slight adjustment of the vermilion line in later childhood, but they can expect a repair that is barely, if at all, noticeable (see Fig. 9–2).

Cleft lip and cleft palate centers have teams of specialists who can provide the services that these children and their families need through infancy, preschool, and school years. Explain to the caregivers the services offered by the pediatrician, plastic surgeon, orthodontist, speech therapist, nutritionist, and public or home health nurse. These professionals can give explanations and counseling about the child's diet, speech training, immunizations, and general health. Encourage family caregivers to ask them any questions they may have. Be alert for any evidence that the caregivers need additional information, and arrange appropriate meetings.

Dental care for the deciduous teeth is even more important than usual. The incidence of dental caries is high in children with a cleft palate, but preservation of the deciduous teeth is important for the best results in speech and appearance.

EVALUATION: GOALS AND OUTCOME CRITERIA

Preoperative

- *Goal:* The infant will show appropriate weight gain.
  Criteria: The infant's weight increases at a predetermined goal of 1 oz or more per day.
- *Goal:* The family will demonstrate acceptance of the infant.
  Criteria: Family caregivers verbalize their feelings about the infant and cuddle and talk to the infant.
- *Goal:* The family caregiver anxiety will be reduced.
  Criteria: Family caregivers ask appropriate questions about surgery, openly discuss their concerns, and voice reasonable expectations.
- *Goal:* The family will learn how to care for the infant and will have an understanding of surgical procedures.
  Criteria: Family caregivers ask appropriate questions, demonstrate how to feed the infant preoperatively, and describe the surgical procedures.

Postoperative

- *Goal:* The infant's respiratory tract will remain clear, the infant will breathe easily, and the respiratory rate will be within normal limits.
  Criteria: The infant has clear lung sounds with no aspiration and the respiratory rate stays within normal range.
- *Goal:* The infant will adjust his or her breathing pattern.
  Criteria: The infant breathes nasally with little stress and maintains normal respirations.
- *Goal:* The infant will show signs of adequate hydration during NPO period.
  Criteria: The infant's skin turgor is good, mucous membranes are moist, and urine output is adequate; there is no evidence of parenteral fluid infiltration.
- *Goal:* The infant will have adequate caloric intake and retain and tolerate oral nutrition.
  Criteria: The infant gains 0.75 to 1 oz (22–30 g) per day if under 6 months of age or 0.5 to 0.75 oz (13–22 g) per day if over 6 months of age and does not experience nausea or vomiting
- *Goal:* The infant's pain and discomfort will be minimized.
  Criteria: The infant rests quietly, does not cry, and is not fretful.
- *Goal:* The surgical site will remain free of injury.
  Criteria: The surgical site is intact; the infant puts nothing into the mouth such as straws, sharp objects, thumb, or fingers.
- *Goal:* The infant will remain free from signs and symptoms of infection.
  Criteria: The incisional site is clean with no redness or drainage. The infant's temperature is within normal limits. The caregivers and family members practice good handwashing and aseptic technique.
- *Goal:* The infant will show evidence of normal growth and development.
  Criteria: The infant is content most of the time and responds appropriately to the caregiver and family. The infant engages in age- and development-appropriate activities within the limits of restraints.
- *Goal:* The family will learn how to care for the infant's long-term needs.
  Criteria: The family caregivers ask appropriate questions, respond appropriately to staff queries, and describe services available for the child's long-term care.

Digestive Tract Defects

Most digestive tract anomalies are apparent at birth or shortly thereafter. The anomalies are often the result of embryonic growth interrupted at a crucial stage. Many of these anomalies interfere with the normal nutrition and digestion essential to the infant's normal growth and development. Many anomalies require immediate surgical intervention.

Esophageal Atresia

Atresia is the absence of a normal body opening or the abnormal closure of a body passage. Esophageal atresia with or without fistula into the trachea is a serious congenital anomaly and is among the most common anomalies causing respiratory distress. This condition occurs in about one in 2,500 live births. Several types of esophageal atresia occur; in more than 90% of affected infants, the upper, or proximal, end of the esophagus ends in a blind pouch and the lower, or distal, segment from the stomach is connected to the trachea by a fistulous tract (Fig. 9–5).

Clinical Manifestations and Diagnosis. Any mucus or fluid that an infant swallows enters the blind pouch of the esophagus. This pouch soon fills and overflows, usually resulting in aspiration into the trachea. Few other conditions depend so greatly on careful nursing observation for early diagnosis and, therefore, improved chances of survival. The infant with this disorder has frothing and excessive drooling and periods of respiratory distress with choking and cyanosis. Many newborns have difficulty with mucus, but the nurse should be alert to the possibility of an anomaly and report such difficulties immediately. No feeding should be given until the infant has been examined.

If early signs are overlooked and feeding is attempted, the infant chokes, coughs, and regurgitates as the food enters the blind pouch. The newborn becomes deeply cyanotic and appears to be in severe respiratory distress. During this process, some of the formula may be aspirated, resulting in pneumonitis and increasing the risk of surgery. This infant's life may depend on the careful observations of the nurse. If there is a fistula of the distal portion of the esophagus into the trachea, the gastric contents may reflux into the lungs and cause a chemical pneumonitis.

Treatment. Surgical intervention is necessary to correct the defect. Timing of the surgery depends on the surgeon's preference, the anomaly, and the infant's condition. Aspiration of mucus must be prevented, and continuous, gentle suction may be used. The infant needs intravenous fluids to maintain optimal hydration. The first stage of surgery may involve a gastrostomy and a method of draining the proximal esophageal pouch. A chest tube is inserted to drain chest fluids. An end-to-end anastomosis is sometimes possible. If the repair is complex, surgery may need to be done in stages.

Often these defects occur in premature infants, so additional factors may complicate the surgical repair and prognosis (Fig. 9–6). If there are no other major problems, the long-term outcome should be good. Regular follow-up is necessary to observe for and dilate esophageal strictures that may be caused by scar tissue.

Imperforate Anus

Early in intrauterine life, the membrane between the rectum and the anus should be absorbed, and a clear passage from the rectum to the anus should exist. If the membrane remains and blocks the union between the rectum and the anus, an **imperforate anus** results. In an infant with imperforate anus, the rectal pouch ends blindly at a distance above the anus; there is no anal orifice. A fistula may exist between the rectum and the vagina in females or between the rectum and the urinary tract in males.

Diagnosis. In some newborns, only a dimple indicates the site of the anus (Fig. 9–7A). When the initial rectal temperature is attempted, it is apparent that there is no anal opening. A shallow opening may occur in the anus, however, with the rectum ending in a blind pouch some distance higher (Fig. 9–7B). Thus, being able to pass a thermometer into the rectum does not guarantee that the rectoanal canal is normal. More reliable presumptive evidence is obtained by watching carefully for the first meconium stool. If the infant does not pass a stool within the first 24 hours, the physician should be notified. Abdominal distention also occurs. Definitive diagnosis is made by radiographic studies.

Surgical Treatment. If the rectal pouch is separated from the anus by only a thin membrane, the surgeon may repair the defect from below. For a high defect, abdominoperineal resection is indicated. In these infants, a colostomy is performed, and extensive abdominoperineal resection is delayed until the age of 3 to 5 months or later.

Home Care. When the infant goes home with a colostomy, the family must learn how to give colostomy care. Teach caregivers to keep the area around the colostomy clean with soap and water and to diaper the baby in the usual way. A protective ointment is useful to protect the skin around the colostomy.

Hernias

A **hernia** is the abnormal protrusion of a part of an organ through a weak spot or other abnormal opening in a body wall. Complications occur depending on the amount of circulatory impairment involved and how much the herniated organ impairs the functioning of another organ. Most hernias can be repaired surgically.

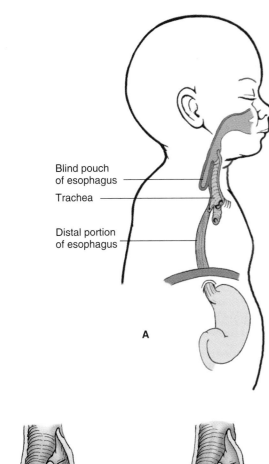

Blind pouch
of esophagus

Trachea

Distal portion
of esophagus

A

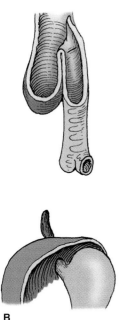

B

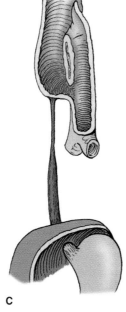

C

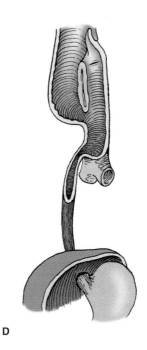

D

● **Figure 9.5 (A)** The most common form of esophageal atresia. **(B)** Both segments of the esophagus are blind pouches. **(C)** Esophagus is continuous but with narrowed segment. **(D)** Upper segment of esophagus opens into trachea.

Diaphragmatic Hernia. In a congenital hernia of the diaphragm, some of the abdominal organs are displaced into the left chest through an opening in the diaphragm. The heart is pushed toward the right, and the left lung is compressed. Rapid, labored respirations and cyanosis are present on the first day of life, and breathing becomes increasingly difficult. Surgery is essential and may be performed as an emergency procedure. During surgery, the abdominal viscera are withdrawn from the chest and the diaphragmatic defect is closed.

This defect may be minimal and easily repaired or so extensive that pulmonary tissue has failed to develop normally. The outcome of surgical repair depends on the degree of pulmonary development. The prognosis in severe cases is guarded.

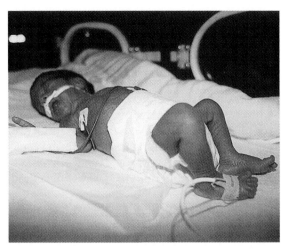

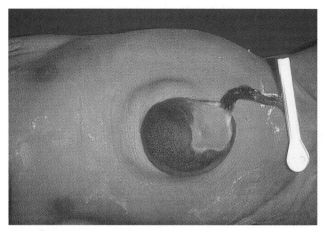

● *Figure 9.8* Large omphalocele with liver and intestine.

● *Figure 9.6* Repair of tracheal esophageal atresia in premature infants may be complicated by other factors.

Hiatal Hernia. More common in adults than in newborns, hiatal hernia is caused when the cardiac portion of the stomach slides through the normal esophageal hiatus into the area above the diaphragm. This action causes reflux of gastric contents into the esophagus and subsequent regurgitation. If upright posture and modified feeding techniques do not correct the problem, surgery is necessary to repair the defect.

Omphalocele. Omphalocele is a relatively rare congenital anomaly. Some of the abdominal contents protrude through into the root of the umbilical cord and form a sac lying on the abdomen. This sac may be small with only a loop of bowel or large and containing much of the intestine and the liver (Fig. 9–8). The sac is covered with peritoneal membrane instead of skin. These defects may be detected during prenatal ultrasonography so that prompt repair may be anticipated. At birth, the defect should be covered

immediately with gauze moistened in sterile saline then may be covered with plastic wrap to prevent heat loss. Surgical replacement of the organs into the abdomen may be difficult with a large omphalocele because there may not be enough space in the abdominal cavity. Other congenital defects are often present.

With large omphaloceles, surgery may be postponed and the surgeon will suture skin over the defect, creating a large hernia. As the child grows, the abdomen may enlarge enough to allow replacement.

Umbilical Hernia. Normally the ring that encircled the fetal end of the umbilical cord closes gradually and spontaneously after birth. When this closure is incomplete, portions of omentum and intestine protrude through the opening. More common in preterm and African-American infants, umbilical hernia is largely a cosmetic problem (Fig. 9–9). While upsetting to parents, umbilical hernia is associated with little or no morbidity. In rare

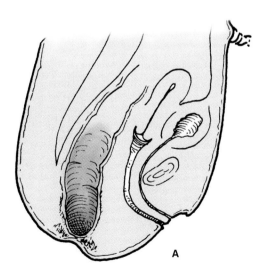

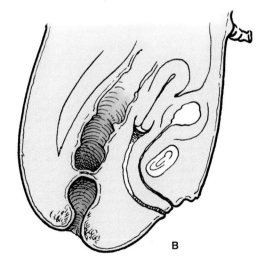

● *Figure 9.7* Imperforate anus (anal atresia). **(A)** Membrane between anus and rectum. **(B)** Rectum ending in a blind pouch at a distance above the perineum.

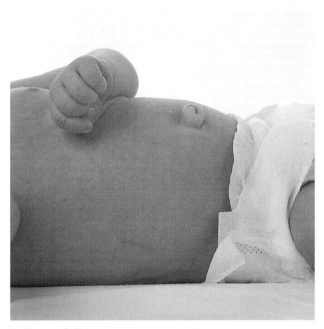

● **Figure 9.9** Small umbilical hernia in infant.

instances, the bowel may strangulate in the sac and require immediate surgery. Almost all these hernias close spontaneously by the age of 3 years; hernias that do not close should be surgically corrected before the child enters school.

Inguinal Hernia. Primarily common in males, inguinal hernias occur when the small sac of peritoneum surrounding the testes fails to close off after the testes descend from the abdominal sac into the scrotum. This failure allows the intestine to slip into the inguinal canal, with resultant swelling. If the intestine becomes trapped (incarcerated) and the circulation to the trapped intestine is impaired (strangulated), surgery is necessary to prevent intestinal obstruction and gangrene of the bowel. As a preven-

tive measure, inguinal hernias normally are repaired as soon as they are diagnosed.

Central Nervous System Defects

Central nervous system defects include disorders caused by an imbalance of cerebrospinal fluid (as in hydrocephalus) and a range of disorders (often called neural tube defects) resulting from malformations of the neural tube during embryonic development. These defects vary from mild to severely disabling.

Spina Bifida

Caused by a defect in the neural arch generally in the lumbosacral region, **spina bifida** is a failure of the posterior laminae of the vertebrae to close; this leaves an opening through which the spinal meninges and spinal cord may protrude (Fig. 9–10).

Clinical Manifestations. A bony defect that occurs without soft-tissue involvement is called *spina bifida occulta*. In most instances it is asymptomatic and presents no problems. A dimple in the skin or a tuft of hair over the site may cause one to suspect its presence or it may be entirely overlooked.

When part of the spinal meninges protrudes through the bony defect and forms a cystic sac, the condition is termed *spina bifida with meningocele*. No nerve roots are involved, so no paralysis or sensory loss below the lesion appears. The sac may, however, rupture or perforate, introducing infection into the spinal fluid and causing meningitis. For this reason as well as for cosmetic purposes, surgical removal of the sac with closure of the skin is indicated.

In *spina bifida with myelomeningocele*, there is a protrusion of the spinal cord and the meninges, with nerve roots embedded in the wall of the cyst (Fig. 9–11). The effects of this defect vary in severity from sensory loss or partial paralysis below the lesion to

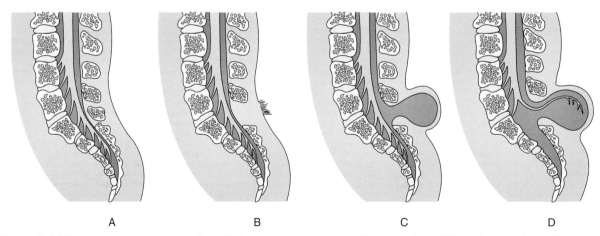

| A | B | C | D |

● **Figure 9.10** Degrees of spinal cord anomalies. **(A)** The normal spinal closure. **(B)** Occulta defect. **(C)** Meningocele defect. **(D)** Myelomeningocele defect clearly shows the spinal cord involvement.

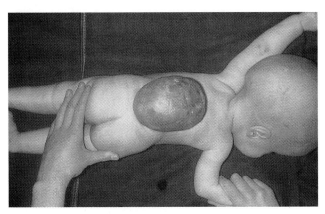

● *Figure 9.11* An infant with a myelomeningocele and hydro-cephalus.

complete flaccid paralysis of all muscles below the lesion. Complete paralysis involves the lower trunk and legs as well as bowel and bladder sphincters.

Making a clear-cut differentiation in diagnosis between a meningocele and a myelomeningocele on the basis of symptoms alone is not always possible. Myelomeningocele may also be termed *meningomyelocele;* the associated "spina bifida" is always implied but not necessarily named. *Spina bifida cystica* is the term used to designate either of these protrusions.

Diagnosis. Elevated maternal alphafetoprotein (AFP) levels followed by ultrasonographic examination of the fetus may show an incomplete neural tube. An elevated AFP level in the maternal serum or amniotic fluid indicates the probability of central nervous system abnormalities. Further examination may confirm this and allow the pregnant woman the opportunity to consider terminating the pregnancy. The best time to perform these tests is between 13 to 15 weeks' gestation when peak levels are reached. Most obstetricians perform AFP testing.

Diagnosis of the newborn with spina bifida is made from clinical observation and examination. Further evaluation of the defect may include magnetic resonance imaging (MRI), ultrasonography, computed tomography (CT) scanning, and myelography. The newborn needs to be examined carefully for other associated defects particularly hydrocephalus, genitourinary defects, and orthopedic anomalies.

Treatment. Many specialists are involved in the treatment of these infants, especially in the case of myelomeningocele. These specialists may include neurologists, neurosurgeons, orthopedic specialists, pediatricians, urologists, and physical therapists. After a thorough evaluation of the infant, a plan of surgical repair and treatment is developed.

Highly skilled nursing care is necessary in all aspects of the infant's care. The child requires years of ongoing follow-up and therapy. Surgery is required to close the open defect but may not be performed

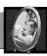

A PERSONAL GLIMPSE

A child with "special needs." I never thought I would have to understand just what that really means. Courtney was our second child. A perfect pregnancy. Absolutely no problems. I didn't drink, never smoked, so I planned on a perfectly healthy baby. Until the AFP test. I will never forget that test now. I was 4 months pregnant and went in for the routine test. A few days later the results were in. A neurotube defect. . . . what in the world was that?

I have been asked many times if I was glad I knew before I had Courtney that she would have problems. I've thought a lot about it and even though it made the last several months of the pregnancy a little (well, maybe more than a little) worrisome, yes, I'm very glad we knew. Courtney was born C-section at a regional medical center that is about 60 miles from home. She was in surgery just a few hours after she was born.

Words like spina bifida, hydrocephalus, v. p. shunt, catheterizations, glasses, walkers, braces, kidney infections, all became everyday words at our home. We have learned a lot in the last 5 years. Courtney has frequent doctor visits to all her specialists. She is the only 5-year-old concerned if her urine is cloudy and making sure her mom gives her medication on time.

A little over 5 years ago a "special" child was born and we feel very blessed she was given to us!!

Rhonda

▶ **LEARNING OPPORTUNITY:** What reactions do you think the nurse might anticipate in working with a pregnant woman who finds her child will be born with "special needs"? In what ways could the nurse encourage this mother to share with other parents in similar situations?

immediately, depending on the surgeon's decision. Waiting several days does not seem to cause additional problems, and this period gives the family an opportunity to adjust to the initial shock and become involved in making the necessary decisions.

● Nursing Process for the Infant With Myelomeningocele

ASSESSMENT

A routine newborn exam is conducted with emphasis on neurologic impairment. When collecting data during the exam, observe the movement and response to stimuli of the lower extremities. Carefully measure the head circumference and examine the fontanelles. Thoroughly document the observations made. When the infant is handled, take great care to prevent injury to the sac.

The family needs support and understanding during the infant's initial care as well as for the many years of care during the child's life. Determine the family's knowledge and understanding of the defect as well as their attitude concerning the birth of an infant with such serious problems.

NURSING DIAGNOSES

The nursing diagnoses suggested here are appropriate for the newborn infant. Because this child will be hospitalized periodically throughout his or her life, suitable diagnoses will vary and need to be made at each admission after careful examination. Possible nursing diagnoses include:

- Risk for Infection related to vulnerability of the myelomeningocele sac
- Risk for Impaired Skin Integrity related to exposure to urine and feces
- Risk for Injury related to neuromuscular impairment
- Compromised Family Coping related to the perceived loss of the perfect newborn
- Deficient Knowledge of the family caregivers related to the complexities of caring for an infant with serious neurologic and musculoskeletal defects

OUTCOME IDENTIFICATION AND PLANNING: PREOPERATIVE CARE

The preoperative goals for care of the infant with myelomeningocele include preventing infection, maintaining skin integrity, preventing trauma related to disuse, increasing family coping skills, education about the condition, and support.

IMPLEMENTATION

Preventing Infection. Monitor the infant's vital signs, neurologic signs, and behavior frequently to observe for any deviations from normal that may indicate an infection. Prophylactic antibiotics may be ordered. Carry out routine aseptic technique with conscientious handwashing, gloving, and gowning as

appropriate. Until surgery is performed, the sac must be covered with a sterile dressing moistened in a warm sterile solution (often sterile saline). Change this dressing every 2 hours; do not allow it to dry to avoid damage to the covering of the sac. The dressings may be covered with a plastic protective covering. Maintain the infant in a prone position so that no pressure is placed on the sac. After surgery, continue this positioning until the surgical site is well healed.

Diapering is not advisable with a low defect, but the sac must be protected from contamination with fecal material. Placing a protective barrier between the anus and the sac may prevent this contamination. If the anal sphincter muscles are involved, the infant may have continual loose stools, which adds to the challenge of keeping the sac free from infection.

Promoting Skin Integrity. The nursing interventions discussed in the previous section on infection also are necessary to promote skin integrity around the area of the defect as well as the diaper area. As mentioned earlier, leakage of stool as well as urine may be continual. This leakage causes skin irritation and breakdown if the infant is not kept clean and the diaper area is not free of stool and urine. Scrupulous perineal care is necessary.

Preventing Contractures of Lower Extremities. Infants with spina bifida often have talipes equinovarus (clubfoot) and congenital hip dysplasia (dislocation of the hips), both of which are discussed later in this chapter. If there is loss of motion in the lower limbs due to the defect, conduct range-of-motion exercises to prevent contractures. Position the infant so that the hips are abducted and the feet are in a neutral position. Massage the knees and other bony prominences with lotion regularly, then pad them, and protect them from irritation. When handling the infant, avoid putting pressure on the sac.

Promoting Family Coping. The family of an infant with such a major anomaly is in a state of shock on first learning of the problems. Be especially sensitive to their needs and emotions. Encourage family members to express their feelings and emotions as openly as possible. Recognize that some families express emotions much more freely than others do, and adjust your responses to the family with this in mind. Provide privacy as needed for the family to mourn together over their loss, but do not avoid the family because this only exaggerates their feelings of loss and depression. If possible, encourage the family members to cuddle or touch the infant using proper precautions for the safety of the defect. With the permission of the physician, the infant may be held chest to chest to provide closer contact.

Providing Family Teaching. Give family members information about the defect and encourage them to discuss their concerns and ask questions. Provide information about the infant's present state, the proposed surgery, and follow-up care. Remember that anxiety may block understanding and processing knowledge, so information may need to be repeated. Information should be provided in small segments to facilitate comprehension.

After surgery, the family needs to be prepared to care for the infant at home. Teach the family to hold the infant's head, neck, and chest slightly raised in one hand during feeding. Also teach them that stroking the infant's cheek helps stimulate sucking. Showing the family how to care for the infant, allowing them to participate in the care, and guiding them in performing return demonstrations are all methods to use in family teaching.

For long-term care and support, refer the family to the Spina Bifida Association of America (*http://www.sbaa.org*). Give them materials concerning spina bifida. These children need long-term care involving many aspects of medicine and surgery as well as education and vocational training. Although children with spina bifida have many long-term problems, their intelligence is not affected; many of these children grow into productive young adults who may live independently (Fig. 9–12).

EVALUATION: GOALS AND OUTCOME CRITERIA

- *Goal:* The infant will be free from signs and symptoms of infection.
  Criteria: The infant's vital signs and neurologic signs are within normal limits; the infant shows no signs of irritability or lethargy.
- *Goal:* The infant will have no evidence of skin breakdown.
  Criteria: The infant's skin will remain clean, dry, and intact and will have no areas of reddening or signs of irritation.

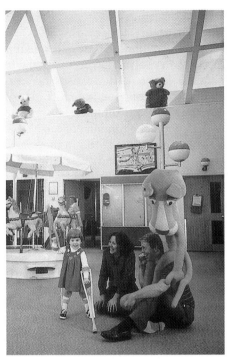

● *Figure 9.12* Learning to use new braces and a crutch, this girl underwent successful surgery for repair of a myelomeningocele during infancy.

- *Goal:* The infant remains free from injury.
  Criteria: The infant's lower limbs show no evidence of contractures.
- *Goal:* The family caregivers will show positive signs of beginning coping.
  Criteria: The family members verbalize their anxieties and needs and hold, cuddle, and soothe the infant as appropriate.
- *Goal:* The family caregivers will learn to care for the infant.
  Criteria: The family demonstrates competence in performing care for the infant, verbalizes understanding of the signs and symptoms that should be reported, and has information about support agencies.

Hydrocephalus

Hydrocephalus is a condition characterized by an excess of cerebrospinal fluid (CSF) within the ventricular and subarachnoid spaces of the cranial cavity. Normally a delicate balance exists between the rate of formation and absorption of CSF: the entire volume is absorbed and replaced every 12 to 24 hours. In hydrocephalus, this balance is disturbed.

Cerebrospinal fluid is formed mainly in the lateral ventricles by the choroid plexus and is absorbed into the venous system through the arachnoid villi. Cerebrospinal fluid circulates within the ventricles and the subarachnoid space. It is a colorless fluid consisting of water with traces of protein, glucose, and lymphocytes.

In the *noncommunicating* type of congenital hydrocephalus, an obstruction occurs in the free circulation of CSF. This blockage causes increased pressure on the brain or spinal cord. The site of obstruction may be at the foramen of Monro, the aqueduct of Sylvius, the foramen of Lushka, or the foramen of Magendie (Fig. 9–13). In the *communicating* type of hydrocephalus, no obstruction of the free flow of CSF exists between the ventricles and the spinal theca; rather the condition is caused by defective absorption of CSF, thus causing increased pressure on the brain or spinal cord. Congenital hydrocephalus is most often the obstructive or noncommunicating type.

Hydrocephalus may be recognized at birth, or it may not be evident until after a few weeks or months of life. The condition may not be congenital but instead may occur during later infancy or during childhood as the result of a neoplasm, a head injury, or an infection such as meningitis.

When hydrocephalus occurs early in life before the skull sutures close, the soft, pliable bones separate to allow head expansion. This condition is manifested by a rapid increase in head circumference. The fact that the soft bones can yield to pressure in this manner may partially explain why many of these infants fail to show the usual symptoms of brain pressure and may exhibit little or no damage in mental function until later in life. Other infants show severe brain damage, which often has occurred before birth.

Clinical Manifestations. An excessively large head at birth is suggestive of hydrocephalus. Rapid head growth with widening cranial sutures is also strongly suggestive and may be the first manifestation of this condition. An apparently large head in itself is not necessarily significant. Normally every infant's head is measured at birth, and the rate of growth is checked at subsequent examinations. If an infant's head appears to be abnormally large at birth or appears to be enlarging, it should be measured frequently.

As the head enlarges, the suture lines separate and the spaces may be felt through the scalp. The anterior fontanelle becomes tense and bulging, the skull enlarges in all diameters, and the scalp becomes shiny and its veins dilate (Fig. 9–14). If pressure continues to increase without intervention, the eyes appear to be pushed downward slightly with the sclera visible above the iris–the so-called "setting sun" sign.

If the condition progresses without adequate drainage of excessive fluid, the head becomes increasingly heavy, the neck muscles fail to develop sufficiently, and the infant has difficulty raising or turning the head. Unless hydrocephalus is arrested, the infant becomes increasingly helpless and symptoms of increased intracranial pressure (IICP) develop. These symptoms may include irritability, restlessness, personality change, high-pitched cry, ataxia, projectile vomiting, failure to thrive, seizures, severe headache, changes in level of consciousness, and papilledema.

Diagnosis. Clinical manifestations, particularly an excessive increase in the head circumference, are indications of hydrocephalus. Positive diagnosis is made with CT and MRI. Echoencephalography and

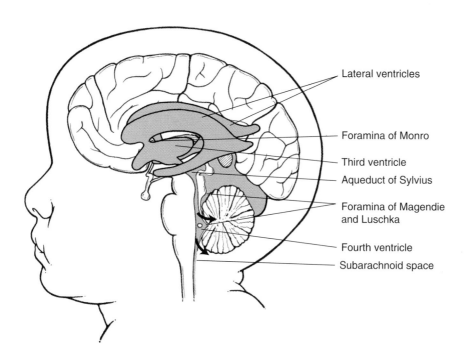

Lateral ventricles

Foramina of Monro

Third ventricle
Aqueduct of Sylvius

Foramina of Magendie
and Luschka

Fourth ventricle
Subarachnoid space

● *Figure 9.13* Ventricles of the brain and channels for the normal flow of cerebrospinal fluid.

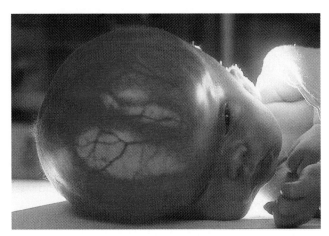

● *Figure 9.14* An infant with hydrocephalus. Note the pull on the eyes giving the "setting sun" appearance.

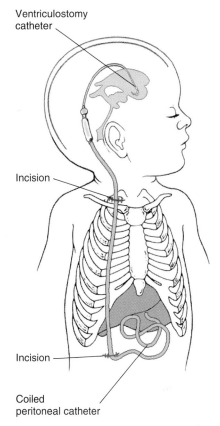

● *Figure 9.15* Ventriculoperitoneal shunt.

ventriculography also may be performed for further definition of the condition.

Treatment. Surgical intervention is the only effective means of relieving brain pressure and preventing further damage to the brain tissue. If minimal brain damage has occurred, the child may be able to function within a normal mental range. Motor function is usually retarded. In some instances, surgical intervention may remove the cause of the obstruction, such as a neoplasm, a cyst, or a hematoma, but most children require placement of a shunting device that bypasses the point of obstruction, draining the excess CSF into a body cavity. This procedure arrests excessive head growth and prevents further brain damage.

Shunting Procedures. Many shunt procedures use a silicone rubber catheter that is radiopaque so that its position may be checked by radiographic examination. The silicone rubber catheter reduces the problem of tissue reaction. A valve or regulator is an essential part of each catheter that prevents excessive build-up of fluid or too-rapid decompression of the ventricle.

The most common procedure, particularly for infants and small children, is **ventriculoperitoneal shunting** (VP shunt). In this procedure, the CSF is drained from a lateral ventricle in the brain; the CSF runs subcutaneously and empties into the peritoneal cavity. This procedure allows the insertion of some excess tubing to accommodate growth. As the child grows, the catheter needs to be revised and lengthened (Fig. 9–15).

In **ventriculoatrial shunting,** CSF drains into the right atrium of the heart. This procedure cannot be used in children with pathologic changes in the heart. The CSF drained from the ventricle is absorbed into the bloodstream.

Other pathways of drainage have been used with varying degrees of success. All types of shunts may have problems with kinking, blocking, moving, or shifting of tubing. The danger of infection in the tubing is a constant concern. Children with shunts must be constantly observed for signs of malfunction or infection.

The long-term outcome for a child with hydrocephalus depends on several factors. If untreated, the outcome is very poor, often leading to death. With shunting, the outcome depends on the initial cause of the increased fluid, the treatment of the cause, the brain damage sustained before shunting, complications with the shunting system, and continued long-term follow-up. Some of these children can lead relatively normal lives if they have follow-up and revisions as they grow.

● Nursing Process for the Postoperative Infant With Hydrocephalus

ASSESSMENT

Obtaining accurate vital and neurologic signs is necessary preoperatively and postoperatively.

Measurement of the infant's head is essential. If the fontanelles are not closed, carefully observe them for any signs of bulging. Observe, report, and document all signs of IICP. If the child has returned for revision of an existing shunt, obtain a complete history preoperatively from the family caregiver to provide a baseline of the child's behavior.

Determine the level of knowledge family members have about the condition. For the family of the newborn or young infant, the diagnosis will probably come as an emotional shock. Conduct the interview and exam of the infant with sensitivity and understanding.

NURSING DIAGNOSES

The nursing diagnoses vary with the results of the data collected, the child's age, and the procedure to be performed (first placement of a shunt or a revision). Possible nursing diagnoses may be:

- Risk for Injury related to increased ICP
- Risk for Impaired Skin Integrity related to pressure from physical immobility
- Risk for Infection related to the presence of a shunt
- Risk for Delayed Growth and Development related to impaired ability to achieve developmental tasks
- Anxiety related to the family caregivers fear of the surgical outcome
- Deficient Knowledge related to the family's understanding of the child's condition and home care

OUTCOME IDENTIFICATION AND PLANNING

The goals for the postoperative care of the infant with shunt placement for hydrocephalus include preventing injury, maintaining skin integrity, preventing infection, maintaining growth and development, and reducing family anxiety. Family goals include increasing knowledge about the condition and providing loving, supportive care to the infant.

IMPLEMENTATION

Preventing Injury. At least every 2 to 4 hours, the infant's level of consciousness is monitored. Check the pupils for equality and reaction, monitor the neurologic status, and observe for a shrill cry, lethargy, or irritability. Measure and record the head circumference daily. Carry out

appropriate procedures to care for the shunt as directed. To prevent a rapid decrease in ICP, keep the infant flat. Observe for signs of seizure, and initiate seizure precautions. Keep suction and oxygen equipment convenient at the bedside.

Promoting Skin Integrity. After a shunting procedure, keep the infant's head turned away from the operative site until the physician allows a change in position. If the infant's head is enlarged, prevent pressure sores from forming on the side where the child rests. Support the head when the child is moved or picked up. Egg-crate pads, lamb's wool, or a special mattress may be used, if necessary, to prevent pressure and breakdown of the scalp. Reposition the infant at least every 2 hours as permitted. Inspect the dressings over the shunt site immediately after the surgery, every hour for the first 3 to 4 hours, and then at least every 4 hours.

Preventing Infection. Infection is the primary threat after surgery. Closely observe for and promptly report any signs of infection: redness, heat, or swelling along the surgical site, fever, and signs of lethargy. Perform wound care meticulously as ordered. Administer antibiotics as prescribed.

Promoting Growth and Development. Every infant has the need to be picked up and held, cuddled, and comforted. An uncomfortable or painful experience increases the need for emotional support. An infant perceives such support principally through physical contact made in a soothing, loving manner.

The infant needs social interaction and needs to be talked to, played with, and given the opportunity for activity. Provide toys appropriate for his or her physical and mental capacity. If the child has difficulty moving about the crib, place toys within easy reach and vision: a cradle gym, for example, may be tied close enough for the infant to maneuver its parts.

Unless the infant's nervous system is so impaired that all activity increases irritability, the infant needs stimulation just as any child does. If repositioning from side to side means turning the infant away from the sight of activity, the crib may be turned around so that vision is not obstructed.

An infant who is given the contact and support that all infants require develops a pleasing personality because he or she is nourished by emotional stimulation. Use the time spent on physical care as a time for social interaction. Talking, laughing, and playing with the infant are important aspects of the infant's care. Make frequent contacts, and do not limit them to the times when physical care is being performed.

Reducing Family Anxiety. Explain to the family the condition and the anatomy of the surgical procedure in terms they can understand. Discuss the overall prognosis for the child. Encourage family members to express their anxieties and ask questions. Giving accurate, non-technical answers is extremely helpful. Give the family information about support groups such as the National Hydrocephalus Foundation, and encourage them to contact the groups.

Providing Family Teaching. Demonstrate care of the shunt to the family caregivers, and have them perform a return demonstration. Provide them with a list of signs and symptoms that should be reported. Review these with the family members and make sure they understand them. Discuss appropriate growth and developmental expectations for the child, and stress realistic goals.

EVALUATION: GOALS AND OUTCOME CRITERIA

- *Goal:* The infant will be free from injury related to complications of excessive cerebrospinal fluid.
  Criteria: The infant has no signs of IICP, such as lethargy, irritability, and seizure activity, and has a stable level of consciousness.
- *Goal:* The infant's skin will remain intact.
  Criteria: The infant's skin shows no evidence of pressure sores, redness, or other signs of skin breakdown.
- *Goal:* The infant will remain free of infection.
  Criteria: The infant shows no signs of infection; vital signs are stable; and there is no redness, drainage, or swelling at the surgical site.
- *Goal:* The infant will have age appropriate growth and development.
  Criteria: The infant's social and developmental needs are met. The infant interacts and plays appropriately with toys and surroundings.
- *Goal:* The family caregiver's anxiety will be reduced.

Criteria: The family expresses fears and concerns and interacts appropriately with the infant.
- *Goal:* The family will learn care of the child.
  Criteria: The family participates in the care of the infant, asks appropriate questions, and lists signs and symptoms to report.

Cardiovascular System Defects

Cardiovascular system defects range from mild to severe. They may be detected immediately at birth or may not be detected for several months.

Congenital Heart Disease

When a newborn is suspected of having a heart abnormality, the family is understandably upset. The heart is *the* vital organ; a person can live without a number of other organs and appendages, but life itself depends on the heart. The family caregivers will have many questions: some may be answered by the nurse; others must be answered by the physician. Many answers will not be available until after various evaluation procedures have been conducted.

Technological advances have progressed rapidly in this field, making earlier detection and successful repair much more likely. Heart defects are, however, still the leading cause of death from congenital anomalies in the first year of life.

A brief discussion of the development and function of the embryonic heart is useful to understanding the malformations that occur.

Pathophysiology. The heart begins beating early in the third to eighth week of intrauterine life. When first formed, the heart is a simple tube receiving blood from the placenta and pumping it out into its developing body. During this period, it rapidly develops into the normal, but complex, four-chambered heart.

Adjustments in circulation must be made at birth. During fetal life the lungs are inactive, requiring only a small amount of blood to nourish their tissues. Blood is circulated through the umbilical arteries to the placenta, where waste products and carbon dioxide are exchanged for oxygen and nutrients. The blood is then returned to the fetus through the umbilical vein.

At birth, the umbilical cord is cut, and the infant's own independent circulatory system is established. Certain circulatory bypasses, such as the **ductus arteriosus,** the **foramen ovale,** and the **ductus venosus,** are no longer necessary. They close and atrophy during the first several weeks after birth. In addition, the pressure in the heart, which has been higher on the right side during fetal life, now changes so that the left side of the heart has the higher pressure (Fig. 9–16).

During this period of complex development, any error in formation may cause serious circulatory difficulty. The incidence of cardiovascular malformations is about eight in 1,000 live births.

Etiology. Rubella in the expectant mother during the first trimester is a common cause of cardiac malformation. Maternal alcoholism, maternal irradiation, ingestion of certain drugs during pregnancy, maternal diabetes, and advanced maternal age (older than 40 years) also increase the incidence. Maternal malnutrition and heredity are also contributing factors. Recent studies have shown that the offspring of mothers who had congenital heart anomalies have a much higher risk of having congenital heart anomalies. If one child in the family has a congenital heart abnormality, later siblings have a very high risk for such a defect.

The newborn with a severe abnormality, such as a transposition of the great vessels, is cyanotic from birth and requires oxygen and special treatment. A less seriously affected child, whose heart can compensate to some degree for the impaired circulation, may not have symptoms severe enough to call attention to the difficulty until he or she is a few months older and more active. Others may live a fairly normal life and not be aware of any heart trouble until a murmur or an enlarged heart is discovered during physical examination in later childhood. Some abnormalities are slight and allow the person to lead a normal life without correction. Others cause little apparent difficulty but need correction to improve the chance for a longer life and for optimal health. Some severe anomalies are incompatible with life for more than a short time; others may be helped but not cured by surgery.

Clinical Manifestations. A cardiac murmur discovered early in life necessitates frequent physical examinations. This murmur may be a functional, "innocent" murmur that may disappear as the child grows older or it may be the chief manifestation of an abnormal heart or an abnormal circulatory system. The most common parental complaint is that of feeding difficulties. Infants with cardiac anomalies severe enough to cause circulatory difficulties have a history of being poor eaters, tiring easily from the effort to suck, and failing to grow or thrive normally.

Manifestations of **congestive heart failure** (CHF) may appear during the first year of life in infants with conditions such as large ventricular septal defects, coarctation of the aorta, and other defects that place an increased workload on the ventricles. One indication of CHF in infancy is easy fatigability, which is manifested by feeding problems. The infant tires, breathes hard, and refuses a bottle after 1 or 2 oz but soon becomes hungry again. Lying flat causes stress, and the infant appears to be more comfortable if held upright over an adult's shoulder.

Other signs are failure to gain weight; a pale, mottled, or cyanotic color; a hoarse or weak cry; and tachycardia. Rapid respiration (with an expiratory grunt), flaring of the nares, and the use of accessory respiratory muscles with retractions at the diaphragmatic and suprasternal levels are other clinical manifestations of CHF. Edema is a factor, and the heart generally shows enlargement. Anoxic attacks (fainting spells) are common.

Diagnosis. The clinical symptoms of CHF are the primary basis for diagnosis of most congenital heart diseases. Chest radiographs that reveal an enlarged heart and electrocardiography indicate ventricular hypertrophy.

Treatment. Treatment of CHF includes digitalization to improve the cardiac function, removing excess fluids with the use of diuretics, decreasing the workload on the heart by limiting physical activity and improving oxygenation. Digoxin (Lanoxin) is used to improve the cardiac efficiency. ACE inhibitors (angiotensin-converting enzyme inhibitors) such as captopril (Capoten) and enalapril (Vasotec) are given to increase vasodilatation. Diuretics, such as

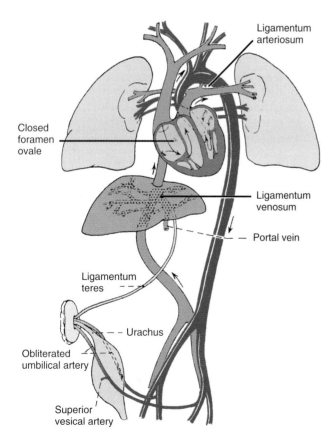

● *Figure 9.16* Normal blood circulation. Highlighted ligaments indicate pathways that should close at or soon after birth. *Arrows* indicate normal flow of blood.

furosemide (Lasix) or spironolactone (Aldactone), and fluid restriction in the acute stages of CHF help to eliminate excess fluids. The infant should be placed with the head elevated and energy requirements should be minimized to ease the workload of the heart. Often the infant is placed on bedrest. Small, frequent feedings improve nutrition with minimal energy output. Oxygen is administered to increase oxygenation of tissues.

Advances in medical technology have enabled heart repairs to be performed in infants as young as less than 1 day old. Miniaturization of instruments, earlier diagnosis through the use of improved diagnostic techniques, pediatric intensive care facilities staffed with highly skilled nurse specialists, and more sophisticated monitoring techniques have all contributed to these advances.

Most physicians now think it is important to operate as early as possible to repair defective hearts. Inadequate circulation may prevent adequate growth and development and cause permanent, irreparable physical, mental, and emotional damage. If the child is diagnosed early and correction or repair is possible, CHF may be avoided.

Care at Home Before Surgery. A child with congenital heart disease may show easy fatigability and retarded growth. If the child has a cyanotic type of heart disease with clubbing of the fingers or toes, periods of cyanosis and reduced exercise tolerance are evident. This young child may assume a squatting position, which reduces the return flow to the heart, thus temporarily reducing the workload of the heart.

Such a child should be allowed to lead as normal a life as possible. Families are naturally apprehensive and find it difficult not to overprotect the child. They often increase the child's anxiety and cause fear in the child about participating in normal activities. Children are rather sensible about finding their own limitations and usually limit their activities to their capacity if they are not made unduly apprehensive.

Some families can adjust well and provide guidance and security for the sick child. Others may become confused and frightened and show hostility, disinterest, or neglect; these families need guidance and counseling. The nurse has a great responsibility to support the family. The nurse's primary goal is to reduce anxiety in the child and family. This goal may be accomplished through open communication and ongoing contact.

Routine visits to a clinic or a physician's office become a way of life, and the child may come to feel different from other people. Physicians and nurses have a responsibility both to the family caregivers and the child to give clear explanations of the defect, using readily understandable terms and diagrams, pictures, or models. A child who knows what is happening can accept a great deal and can continue with the business of living.

Cardiac Catheterization. Cardiac catheterization may be performed before heart surgery to obtain more accurate information about the child's condition. The child or infant is sedated or anesthetized for this process, and a radiopaque catheter is inserted through a vein into the right atrium. In the infant or young child, the femoral vein often is used. Close observation of the child after the procedure is essential. Carefully monitor the site used and check the extremity for pulses, edema, skin temperature and color, and any other signs of poor circulation or infection. Vital signs are monitored closely.

Preoperative Preparation. When a child enters the hospital for cardiac surgery, that is seldom a first admission; generally, it has been preceded by cardiac catheterization or perhaps other hospitalizations. The child may be admitted a few days before surgery to allow time for adequate preparation. With the current emphasis on cost containment, however, many preoperative procedures are done on an outpatient basis. Preoperative teaching should be intensive for the family and the child at an age appropriate level. They should understand that blood might be obtained for typing and cross-matching and for other determinations as ordered. Additional x-ray studies may be done.

The equipment to be used after surgery should be described with drawings and pictures. If possible, the family caregivers and the child should be taken to a cardiac recovery room and shown chest tubes and an oxygen tent. They should meet the nursing personnel and see the general appearance of the unit. Of course, nurses should use good judgment about the timing and the extent of such preparation; nothing is gained by arousing additional anxiety with premature or excessively graphic descriptions. A young child may become familiar with the surgical clothing worn by personnel and with the oxygen tent and can perhaps listen to a heartbeat. The child should be taught how to cough and should practice coughing. He or she should understand that coughing is important after surgery and must be done regularly, even though it may hurt.

INTERNET EXERCISE 9.1

http://www.pediheart.org

Click on Parent's Place.
Click on Prepare for Surgery.
Read the section Preparing Your Child for Surgery.
Read the section Helpful Parent Tips.

1. List eight tips to share with parents whose child is having heart surgery.

2. List three books that parents could use with the child who is having heart surgery.

Cardiac Surgery. Open-heart surgery using the heart-lung machine has made extensive heart correction possible for many children who otherwise would have been disabled throughout their limited lives. Machines have been refined for use with infants and small children. Heart transplants may be performed when no other treatment is possible.

Hypothermia—reducing the body temperature to 68° to 78.8°F (20° to 26C)—is a useful technique that helps to make early surgery possible. A reduced body temperature increases the time that the circulation may be stopped without causing brain damage. The blood temperature is reduced by the use of cooling agents in the heart-lung machine. This also provides a dry, bloodless, motionless field for the surgeon.

Postoperative Care. At the end of surgery, the child is taken to the pediatric intensive care unit for skillful nursing by specially trained personnel for as long as necessary. Children who have had closed-chest surgery need the same careful nursing as those who have had open-heart surgery.

By the time the child returns to the regular pediatric unit, chest drainage tubes usually have been removed and the child has started taking oral fluids and is ready to sit up in bed or in a chair. The child probably feels weak and helpless after such an experience and needs encouragement and reassurance. With recovery, however, a child is usually ready for activity. Family caregivers usually need to reorient themselves and to accept their child's new status. This attitude is not easy to acquire after what seemed like a long period of anxious watching. The surgeon and the surgical staff evaluate the results of the surgery and make any necessary recommendations regarding resumption of the child's activities. Plans should be made for follow-up and supervision as well as counseling and guidance.

Common Types of Congenital Heart Defects

Traditionally congenital heart defects have been described as cyanotic or acyanotic conditions. **Cyanotic heart disease** implies an oxygen saturation of the peripheral arterial blood of 85% or less. This condition occurs when a heart defect allows any appreciable amount of oxygen-poor blood in the right side of the heart to mix with the oxygenated blood in the left side of the heart. Defects that permit right-to-left shunting may occur at the atrial, ventricular, or aortic level. However, because defects are often complex and occur in various combinations, this is an inadequate means of classification. A more clear-cut classification system is based on blood flow characteristics. These are (1) increased pulmonary blood flow (e.g., ventricular septal, atrial septal, and patent ductus arteriosus), (2) obstruction of blood flow out of the heart (e.g., coarctation of the aorta), (3) decreased pulmonary blood flow (e.g., tetralogy of Fallot), and (4) mixed blood flow, where saturated and desaturated blood mix in the heart, aorta, and pulmonary vessels (e.g., transposition of the great arteries).

Because defects often occur in combination, they give rise to complex situations. Most nurses may never see many of the complex defects and most of the rare, isolated defects. The conditions discussed here are common enough that the pediatric nurse needs to be familiar with their diagnosis and treatment.

Ventricular Septal Defect. Ventricular septal defect is the most common intracardiac defect. It consists of an abnormal opening in the septum between the two ventricles that allows blood to pass directly from the left to the right ventricle. No unoxygenated blood leaks into the left ventricle, so cyanosis does not occur (Fig. 9–17).

Small, isolated defects are usually asymptomatic and often are discovered during a routine physical examination. A characteristic loud, harsh murmur associated with a systolic thrill occasionally is heard on examination. A history of frequent respiratory infections may occur during infancy, but growth and

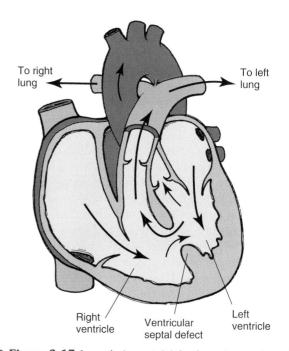

To right lung

To left lung

Right ventricle   **Ventricular septal defect**   **Left ventricle**

● *Figure 9.17* A ventricular septal defect is an abnormal opening between the right and left ventricle. Ventricular septal defects vary in size and may occur in the membranous or muscular portion of the ventricular septum. Owing to higher pressure in the left ventricle, a shunting of blood from the left to the right ventricle occurs during systole. If pulmonary vascular resistance produces pulmonary hypertension, the shunt of blood is then reversed from the right to the left ventricle, with cyanosis resulting.

development are unaffected. The child leads a normal life.

Corrective surgery may be postponed until the age of 18 months to 2 years, when the surgical risk is less than that for infants. Surgical techniques have improved, however, to the degree that the repair may be made in the first year of life with high rates of success. The child is observed closely and may be placed on prophylactic antibiotics to prevent frequent respiratory infections. If pulmonary involvement becomes a problem, the repair is done without further delay. Repairs in children who are at high risk are done by the use of cardiac catheterization procedures.

Atrial Septal Defects. In general, left-to-right shunting occurs in all true atrial septal defects. Many healthy people, however, have a patent **foramen ovale** that is situated in the atrial septum and normally causes no problems. This is because the valve of the foramen ovale is anatomically structured to withstand left chamber pressure, making the patent foramen ovale functionally closed (Fig. 9–18).

True atrial septal defects are common heart anomalies and may occur as isolated defects or in combination with other heart anomalies.

Atrial septal defects are amenable to surgery with a low surgical mortality risk. Since the advent of the heart-lung bypass machine, this repair may be performed in a dry field, replacing the older "blind"

technique. The opening is closed with sutures or a Dacron patch.

Patent Ductus Arteriosus. The **ductus arteriosus** is a vascular channel between the left main pulmonary artery and the descending aorta. In fetal life it allows blood to bypass the nonfunctioning lungs and go directly into the systemic circuit. After birth the duct normally closes, eventually becoming obliterated and forming the ligamentum arteriosum. If the ductus arteriosus remains patent, however, blood continues to be shunted from the aorta into the pulmonary artery. This situation results in a flooding of the lungs and an overloading of the left heart chambers (Fig. 9–19).

Normally the ductus arteriosus is nonpatent after the first or second week of life and should be obliterated by the fourth month. Why it fails to close is unknown. Patent ductus arteriosus is common in infants who exhibit the rubella syndrome, but most infants with this anomaly have no history of exposure to rubella during fetal life. It is also common in preterm infants weighing less than 1,200 g and in infants with Down syndrome.

Symptoms of patent ductus arteriosus are often absent during childhood. Growth and development may be retarded in some children with an easy fatigability and dyspnea on exertion. The diagnosis may be based on a characteristic machinery-like murmur over the pulmonary area, a wide pulse pressure, and

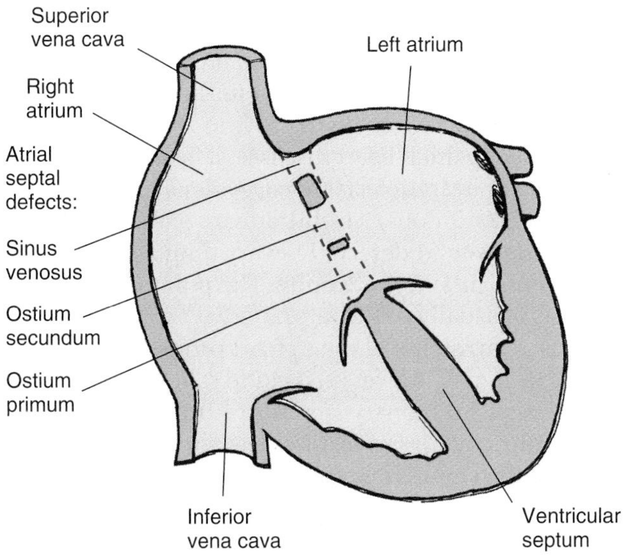

● **Figure 9.18** An atrial septal defect is an abnormal opening between the right and left atria. Basically, three types of abnormalities result from incorrect development of the atrial septum. An incompetent foramen ovale is the most common defect. The ostium secundum defect results from abnormal development of the septum secundum and causes an opening in the middle of the septum. Improper development of the septum primum produces an opening at the lower end of the septum known as an ostium primum defect, frequently involving the atrioventricular valves. In general, left-to-right shunting of blood occurs in all atrial septal defects.

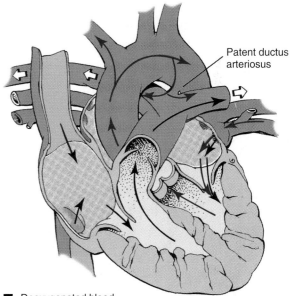

■ Deoxygenated blood
■ Oxygenated blood
☐ Mixed blood

● **Figure 9.19** The patent ductus arteriosus is a vascular connection that, during fetal life, short-circuits the pulmonary vascular bed and directs blood from the pulmonary artery to the aorta. Functional closure of the ductus normally occurs soon after birth. If the ductus remains patent after birth, the higher pressure in the aorta reverses the direction of blood flow in the ductus.

a bounding pulse. Cardiac catheterization is diagnostic but is not required in the presence of classic clinical features.

Surgery is indicated in all diagnosed cases, even if they are asymptomatic. Some persons live a normal life span without correction, but the risks involved far outweigh the surgical ones. Indomethacin (Indocin), a prostaglandin inhibitor, may be administered with some success to premature infants with respiratory distress syndrome to promote closure of the ductus arteriosus. If this fails to close the ductus, surgery is performed. Surgical correction consists of closure of the defect by ligation or by division of the ductus. Division is the method of choice if the child's condition permits because the ductus occasionally reopens after ligation. The optimal age for surgery is before the age of 2 years, with earlier surgery for severely affected infants. Prognosis is excellent after a successful repair.

Coarctation of the Aorta. This congenital cardiovascular anomaly consists of a constriction or narrowing of the aortic arch or the descending aorta usually adjacent to the ligamentum arteriosum (Fig. 9–20).

Most children with this condition are asymptomatic until later childhood or young adulthood. A few infants have severe symptoms in their first year of life; they show dyspnea, tachycardia, and cyanosis, which are all signs of developing CHF.

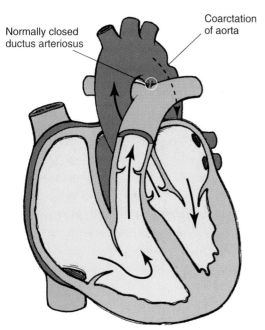

● **Figure 9.20** Coarctation of the aorta is characterized by a narrowed aortic lumen. It exists as a preductal or postductal obstruction, depending on the position of the obstruction in relation to the ductus arteriosus. Coarctations exist with great variation in anatomic features. The lesion produces an obstruction to the flow of blood through the aorta, causing an increased left ventricular pressure and workload.

In older children, the condition is easily diagnosed based on hypertension in the upper extremities and hypotension in the lower extremities. The radial pulse is readily palpable, but the femoral pulses are weak or even impalpable. Blood pressure is normal or elevated in the arms and is low or undetectable in the legs. A high-pitched systolic murmur is usually present and heard over the base of the heart and over the interscapular area of the back. The diagnosis may be confirmed by aortography.

Obstruction to blood flow caused by the constricted portion of the aorta does not cause early difficulty in an average child because the blood bypasses the obstruction by way of collateral circulation. The bypass is chiefly from the branches of the subclavian and carotid arteries that arise from the arch of the aorta. Eventually the enlarged collateral arteries erode the rib margins, and the rib notching may be visualized by radiographic examination.

Uncorrected coarctation may cause hypertension and cardiac failure later in life. The optimal age for elective surgery is before the age of 2 years. Early surgery may be necessary for a gravely ill infant who presents with severe CHF. In early infancy, the mortality rate depends on the presence of other congenital heart problems.

Surgery consists of resection of the coarcted area with an end-to-end anastomosis of the proximal and distal ends of the aorta. Occasionally a long defect may necessitate an end-to-end graft using tubes of Dacron or similar material. Prognosis is excellent for the restoration of normal function after surgery.

Tetralogy of Fallot. This is a fairly common congenital heart defect involving 50% to 70% of all cyanotic congenital heart diseases. It consists of a grouping of heart defects (*tetralogy* denotes four abnormal conditions): (1) **pulmonary stenosis,** (2) **ventricular septal defect,** (3) **overriding aorta,** and (4) **right ventricular hypertrophy.** The pulmonary stenosis is usually of the infundibular type in which there is a narrowing of the upper portion of the right ventricle; it may, however, include stenosis of the valve cusps. Pulmonary stenosis results, in turn, in right ventricular hypertrophy. The aorta appears to straddle the ventricular septum, overriding the ventricular septal defect. This defect allows a shunt of unsaturated blood from the right ventricle into the aorta or into the left ventricle (Fig. 9–21).

The child with tetralogy of Fallot may be precyanotic in early infancy with the cyanotic phase starting at 4 to 6 months of age. Some severely affected infants, however, may show cyanosis earlier. As long as the ductus arteriosus remains open, enough blood apparently passes through the lungs to prevent cyanosis.

Normally closed ductus arteriosus

Coarctation of aorta

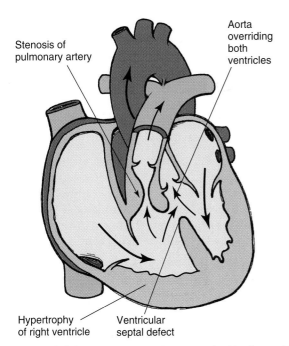

Stenosis of pulmonary artery

Aorta overriding both ventricles

Hypertrophy of right ventricle

Ventricular septal defect

● **Figure 9.21** Tetralogy of Fallot is characterized by the combination of four defects: (1) pulmonary stenosis, (2) ventricular septal defect, (3) overriding aorta, and (4) hypertrophy of the right ventricle. It is the most common defect causing cyanosis in patients surviving beyond 2 years of age. The severity of symptoms depends on the degree of pulmonary stenosis, the size of the ventricular septal defect, and the degree to which the aorta overrides the septal defect.

The infant presents with feeding difficulties and poor weight gain, resulting in retarded growth and development. Dyspnea and easy fatigability become evident. Exercise tolerance depends in part on the severity of the disease; some children become fatigued after little exertion. In the past, on experiencing fatigue, breathlessness, and increased cyanosis, the child was described as assuming a squatting posture for relief. Squatting apparently increased the systemic oxygen saturation. However, squatting rarely is seen today because these infants' defects usually are repaired by the time they are 2 years old.

Attacks of paroxysmal dyspnea are common during infancy and early childhood. An anoxic spell is heralded by sudden restlessness, gasping respiration, and increased cyanosis that lead to a loss of consciousness and, possibly, convulsions. These attacks, called "tet spells," last from a few minutes to several hours and appear to be unpredictable, although stress does seem to trigger some episodes.

The history and clinical manifestations are usually sufficient to make a diagnosis. However, cardiac catheterization, electrocardiography, chest radiography, and laboratory tests to determine polycythemia and arterial oxygen saturation may be performed for further definition.

The preferred repair of these defects is total surgical correction. This procedure may be carried out only in a dry field, requiring the use of a cardiopulmonary bypass machine. The heart is opened and extensive resection is done. The septal defect is closed by use of a patch, and the valvular stenosis and infundibular chamber are resected.

Successful total correction transforms a grossly abnormal heart into a functionally normal one. Most of these children, however, are left without a pulmonary valve.

In infants who cannot withstand the total surgical correction until they are older, the Blalock-Taussig procedure is performed. This procedure is an end-to-end anastomosis of a vessel arising from the aorta, usually the subclavian artery, to the corresponding right or left pulmonary artery. These shunts are now only seen occasionally because total surgical repair is meeting with much greater success and lower mortality rates.

Transposition of the Great Arteries. This severe defect is usually fatal. In transposition of the great arteries, the aorta arises from the right ventricle instead of the left, and the pulmonary artery arises from the left ventricle instead of the right. These infants are usually cyanotic from birth and, depending on the extent of the defects, have a low rate of survival.

● Nursing Process for the Infant With Congestive Heart Failure

ASSESSMENT

The interview of the family caregiver of an infant with CHF must include the gathering of information about the present illness and any previous episodes. Ask about any problems the infant may have during feeding, episodes of rapid or difficult respirations, episodes of turning blue, and difficulty with lying flat. Determine if the infant has been gaining weight. Avoid causing any feelings of guilt in the caregiver.

The physical exam of the infant includes a complete measurement of vital signs. Note the quality and rhythm of the apical pulse. Observe respiratory status including any use of accessory muscles, retractions, breath sounds, rate, and type of cry. Examine the skin and extremities for color, skin temperature, and evidence of edema. Observe the infant closely for signs of easy fatigability or an increase in symptoms on exertion.

NURSING DIAGNOSES

Some infants are so acutely ill on admission that they are admitted immediately to the pediatric intensive care unit, if one is available. The nursing diagnoses depend on the severity of the symptoms that determine the priority of care. Some diagnoses that may be useful include:

- Decreased Cardiac Output related to structural defects of the heart
- Ineffective Breathing Pattern related to pulmonary congestion and anxiety
- Risk for Imbalanced Nutrition: Less than Body Requirements related to fatigue and dyspnea
- Activity Intolerance related to insufficient oxygenation secondary to heart defects
- Deficient Knowledge of caregivers related to the infant's life-threatening illness

OUTCOME IDENTIFICATION AND PLANNING

The major goals include improving cardiac output and oxygenation, relieving inadequate respirations, maintaining adequate nutritional intake, and conserving energy. The family's goals include increasing understanding of the condition and its prognosis.

IMPLEMENTATION

Monitoring Vital Signs. Monitor vital signs regularly to detect symptoms of decreased cardiac output. If digoxin is ordered, count the apical pulse for a full minute before administering digoxin. Withhold digoxin and notify the physician if the apical rate is lower than the established norms for the child's age and baseline information (90 to 110 beats per minute for infants, 70 to 85 beats per minute for older children). Always check the dosage of digoxin with another nurse before administering it. Regularly observe the child for evidence of periorbital or peripheral edema. Before the first feeding of the day, weigh the undressed infant daily early in the morning using the same scale every time. Maintain careful intake and output measurements. If diuretics are administered, monitor serum electrolyte levels especially potassium levels.

Improving Respiratory Function. Elevate the head of the crib mattress so that it is at a 30-degree to 45-degree angle. Do not allow the infant to shift down in the crib and become "scrunched up," which causes decreased expansion room for the chest. Avoid constricting clothing. Administer oxygen as ordered. Monitor respirations at least every 4 hours, paying close attention to breath sounds, dyspnea, tachypnea, retractions and inspecting the nail beds for cyanosis. Monitor oxygen saturation levels with pulse oximetry.

Maintaining Adequate Nutrition. Give frequent feedings in small amounts to avoid overtiring the infant. Use a soft nipple with a large opening to ease the infant's workload. If adequate nutrition cannot be taken during feedings, gavage feedings may be necessary.

Promoting Energy Conservation. Nursing care is planned so that the infant has long periods of uninterrupted rest. While carrying out nursing procedures, talk to the infant softly and soothingly and handle him or her gently with loving care. Respond to the infant's cries quickly to avoid the infant's tiring.

Providing Family Teaching. The family of this infant has reason to be apprehensive and anxious. Be understanding, empathetic, and nonjudgmental when communicating with them. Give them information about CHF in a way that they can understand. Repeat information about signs and symptoms and offer explanations as many times as necessary. Include teaching about medication, feeding and care techniques, growth and development expectations, and future plans for correction of the defect, if known. Involve the family in the infant's care as much as possible within the limitations of the infant's condition.

EVALUATION: GOALS AND OUTCOME CRITERIA

- *Goal:* The infant's cardiac output will improve and be adequate to meet infant's needs.
  Criteria: The infant's heart rate is within the normal limits for age; no arrhythmia or evidence of edema exists. Peripheral perfusion is adequate.
- *Goal:* The infant's respiratory function will improve.
  Criteria: The infant's respirations are regular with no retractions; breath sounds are clear; oxygen saturation is within acceptable range for infant's status.
- *Goal:* The infant's caloric intake will be adequate to maintain nutritional needs for growth.

Criteria: The infant consumes most of the feeding each time and feeds with minimal tiring. The infant has appropriate weight gain for age.

- *Goal:* The infant will have increased levels of energy.
  Criteria: The infant rests quietly during uninterrupted periods of rest and does not become overly tired when awake.
- *Goal:* The family caregivers are prepared for the infant's home care.
  Criteria: The family verbalizes anxieties, asks appropriate questions, participates in the infant's care, and discusses infant's condition.

Skeletal System Defects

Infants or children with congenital skeletal defects usually receive primary treatment in the general pediatric unit; thus, nurses need to understand the nature and treatment of these anomalies. Children with these conditions and their parents often face long periods of exhausting, costly treatment; they, therefore, need continuing support, encouragement, and education.

The two most common and important skeletal defects are congenital **talipes equinovarus** (clubfoot) and congenital **hip dysplasia** (dislocation of the hip).

Congenital Talipes Equinovarus

Congenital clubfoot is a deformity in which the entire foot is inverted, the heel is drawn up, and the forefoot is adducted. The Latin *talus,* meaning ankle, and *pes,* meaning foot, make up the word *talipes,* which is used in connection with many foot deformities. Equinus, or plantar flexion, and varus, or inversion, denote the kind of foot deformity present in this condition. The equinovarus foot has a clublike appearance, hence the term clubfoot (Fig. 9–22*A*).

Congenital talipes equinovarus is the most common congenital foot deformity, occurring in about seven in 1,000 births. It appears as a single anomaly or in connection with other defects such as myelomeningocele. It may be bilateral (both feet) or unilateral (one foot). The cause is unclear, though a hereditary factor occasionally is observed. A hypothesis that has received some acceptance proposes an arrested embryonic growth of the foot during the first trimester of pregnancy.

Diagnosis. Talipes equinovarus is easily detected in a newborn infant but must be differentiated from a persisting "position of comfort" assumed in utero. The positional deformity may be easily corrected by the use of passive exercise, but the true clubfoot deformity is fixed. The positional deformity should be explained to the parents at once to prevent anxiety.

Nonsurgical Treatment. If treatment is started during the neonatal period, correction usually may be accomplished by manipulation and bandaging or by application of a cast. The cast often is applied while the infant is still in the neonatal nursery. While the cast is applied, the foot is first gently moved into as nearly normal a position as possible. Force should not be used. If the family caregiver can be present to help hold the infant while the cast is applied, the caregiver will have the opportunity to understand what is being done. The very young infant gets satisfaction from sucking, so a pacifier helps prevent squirming while the cast is applied.

The cast is applied over the foot and ankle (and usually to mid-thigh) to hold the knee in right-angle flexion (Fig. 9–22*B*). Casts are changed frequently to provide gradual, atraumatic correction—every few days for the first several weeks, then every week or

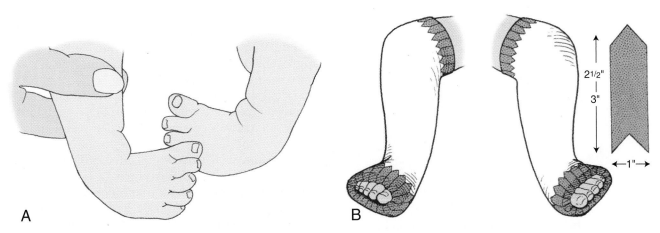

● *Figure 9.22* **(A)** Bilateral clubfoot. **(B)** Casting for clubfoot in typical overcorrected position showing petalling of cast.

two. Treatment is continued usually for a matter of months until radiograph and clinical observation confirm complete correction.

Any cast applied to a child's body should have some type of waterproof material protecting the skin from the cast's sharp plaster edges. One method is to apply strips of adhesive vertically around the edges of the cast in a manner called petaling. To pedal a cast, strips of adhesive are cut 2 inches or 3 inches long and 1 inch wide. One end is notched and the other end is cut pointed to aid in smooth application. Family caregivers must be taught cast care.

After correction with a cast, a Denis Browne splint with shoes attached may be used to maintain the correction for another 6 months or longer (Fig. 9–23). After over-correction has been attained, the child should wear a special clubfoot shoe, which is a laced shoe whose turning out makes it appear that the shoe is being worn on the wrong foot. The Denis Browne splint still may be worn at night, and the caregivers should carry out passive exercises of the foot. The older infant may resist wearing the splint, so family caregivers must be taught the importance of gentle, but firm, insistence that the splint be worn.

Surgical Treatment. Children who do not respond to nonsurgical measures, especially older children, need surgical correction. This approach involves several procedures depending on the age of the child and the degree of the deformity. It may involve lengthening the Achilles tendon, capsulotomy of the ankle joint, release of medial strictures, and operating on the bony structure for the child older than 10 years. Prolonged observation after correction by either means should be carried out at least until adolescence; any recurrence is treated promptly.

Congenital Hip Dysplasia

Congenital hip dysplasia results from defective development of the acetabulum with or without dislocation. The malformed acetabulum permits dislocation

with the head of the femur becoming displaced upward and backward. The condition is difficult to recognize during early infancy. When there is a family history of the defect, increased observation of the young infant is indicated. The condition is often bilateral and about seven times more common in girls than in boys.

Diagnosis. Early recognition and treatment before an infant starts to stand or walk are extremely important for successful correction. The first examination should be part of the newborn examination. Experienced examiners may detect an audible click when examining the newborn using the Bartow and Ortolani tests. These tests, used together on one hip at a time, involve dislocating and relocating the acetabulum in adduction and abduction and should be conducted only by an experienced practitioner. The tests are effective only for the first month, then the clicks disappear. Signs that are useful after this include:

1. Asymmetry of the gluteal skin folds (higher on the affected side) (Fig. 9–24*A*)
2. Limited abduction of the affected hip (Fig. 9–24*B*). This is tested by placing the infant in a dorsal recumbent position with the knees flexed then abducting both knees passively until they reach the examination table without resistance. If dislocation is present, the affected side cannot be abducted more than 45 degrees.
3. Apparent shortening of the femur (Fig. 9–24*C*)

After the child has started walking, later signs include lordosis, swayback, protruding abdomen, shortened extremity, duck-waddle gait, and a positive Trendelenburg sign. To elicit this sign, the child stands on the affected leg and raises the normal leg. The pelvis tilts down rather than up toward the unaffected side.

X-ray studies usually are made to confirm the diagnosis in the older infant. Uncorrected dislocation causes limping, easy fatigue, hip and low back discomfort, and postural deformities.

Treatment. When the dislocation is discovered during the first few months, treatment consists of manipulation of the femur into position and the application of a brace. The most common type of brace used is the Pavlik harness (Fig. 9–25). The physician assesses the infant weekly while the infant is in the harness and adjusts the harness to align the femur gradually. Sometimes no further treatment is needed.

If treatment is delayed until after the child has started to walk or if earlier treatment is ineffective, open reduction followed by application of a spica cast usually is needed. After the cast is removed, a metal or plastic brace is applied to keep the legs in wide abduction.

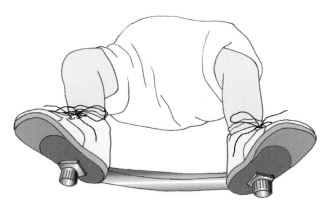

● *Figure 9.23* A Denis Browne splint with shoes attached is used to correct clubfoot.

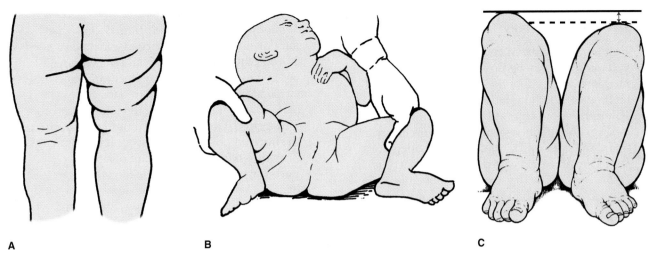

A   B   C

● **Figure 9.24** Congenital hip dislocation. **(A)** Asymmetry of the gluteal folds of the thighs. **(B)** Limited abduction of the affected hip. **(C)** Apparent shortening of the femur.

● Nursing Process for the Infant in an Orthopedic Device or Cast

ASSESSMENT

Although the actual hospitalization of the infant is relatively short (if no other abnormalities require hospitalization), the nurse must teach the family about cast care or care of the infant in an orthopedic device such as a Pavlik harness. Determine the family caregiver's ability to understand and cooperate in the infant's care. Emotional support of the family is important.

The observation of the infant varies depending on the orthopedic device or cast

used. Immediately after the application of a cast, observe for signs that the cast is drying evenly. Check the toes for circulation and movement. Check the skin at the edges of the cast for signs of pressure or irritation. If an open reduction has been performed, observe the child for signs of shock and bleeding in the immediate postoperative period.

NURSING DIAGNOSES

The nursing diagnoses depend on the defect and the type of treatment. Some diagnoses that may be used are:
● Acute Pain related to discomfort of orthopedic device or cast
● Risk for Impaired Skin Integrity related to pressure of the cast on the skin surface
● Risk for Delayed Growth and Development related to restricted mobility secondary to orthopedic device or cast
● Deficient Knowledge of family caregivers related to home care of the infant in the orthopedic device or cast

OUTCOME IDENTIFICATION AND PLANNING

Goals include relieving pain and discomfort, maintaining skin integrity, promoting growth and development, and increasing family knowledge about the infant's home care. Goals for the family focus on the desire for correction of the defect with minimal disruption to the infant's growth and development and care of the infant at home.

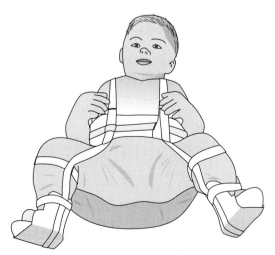

● **Figure 9.25** Proper positioning of an infant in a Pavlik harness. The harness is composed of shoulder straps, stirrups, and a chest strap. It is placed on both legs, even if only one hip is dislocated.

IMPLEMENTATION

Providing Comfort Measures. The infant may be irritable and fussy because of the restricted movement caused by the device or cast. Useful methods of soothing the infant include nonnutritive sucking, stroking, cuddling, and talking. If irritability seems excessive, check the infant for signs of irritation from the device or cast. The infant in a cast may be held after the cast is completely dry. Do not remove the harness unless specific permission for bathing is granted by the provider. Teach the family caregivers how to reapply the harness correctly. The infant in a Pavlik harness is not as difficult to handle as the infant in a cast.

Promoting Skin Integrity. For the first 24 to 48 hours after application of a cast, place the infant on a firm mattress and support position changes with firm pillows. When handling the cast, use the palms of the hands to avoid excessive pressure on the cast. Carefully inspect the skin around the cast edges for signs of irritation, redness, or edema. Petal the edges of the cast around the waist and toes and protect the cast with plastic covering around the perineal area. Take great care to protect the diaper area from becoming soiled and moist. If the covering becomes soiled, remove it, wash and dry thoroughly, then reapply or replace it. With the Pavlik harness, monitor the skin under the straps frequently and massage it gently to promote circulation. To relieve pressure under the shoulder straps, place extra padding in this area.

Avoid using powders and lotions because caking of the powder or lotion can cause areas of irritation. Daily sponge baths are important and must include close attention to the skin under the straps of the device or around the edge of the cast.

Observe the infant in a cast carefully for any restriction of breathing caused by tightness over the abdomen and lower chest area. Vomiting after a feeding may be an indication that the cast is too tight over the stomach. In either case, the cast may have to be removed and reapplied.

Prevent the older infant or child from pushing any small particles of food or toys down into the cast.

Diapering can be a challenge for the infant in a cast. Disposable diapers are usually the most effective way to provide good protection of the cast and prevent leakage.

Providing Sensory Stimulation. Because the infant will be in the device or cast for an extended period when much growth and development occur, provide him or her with stimulation of a tactile nature. Provide mobiles, musical toys, and stuffed toys. Do not permit the infant to cry for long periods. Keep feeding times relaxed. Hold the infant if possible and encourage interaction. Provide a pacifier if the infant desires it. Encourage activities that use the infant's free hands. The older infant may enjoy looking at picture books and interacting with siblings.

Diversionary activities should include transporting the infant to other areas in the home or in the car. Strollers and car seats may be adapted to allow safe transportation. For toddlers, a wagon or a large skateboard may provide a movable base to explore the environment and encourage independence.

Providing Family Teaching. Determine the family caregiver's knowledge and design a thorough teaching plan because the infant will be cared for at home for most of the time. Use complete explanations, written guidelines, demonstrations, and return demonstrations. Provide the family with a resource person who may be called when a question arises and encourage them to feel free to call that person. Make definite plans for return visits to have the device or cast checked. The caregiver needs to understand the importance of keeping these appointments. Provide a public or home health nurse referral when appropriate (see Nursing Care Plan).

EVALUATION: GOALS AND OUTCOME CRITERIA

- *Goal:* The infant will show signs of being comfortable.
  Criteria: The infant is alert and content with no long periods of fussiness. The infant interacts with caregivers with cooing, smiling, and eye contact.
- *Goal:* The infant's skin will remain intact.
  Criteria: The infant's skin around the edges of the cast shows no signs of redness or irritation. The diaper area is clean, dry and intact, and protected from soiling.
- *Goal:* The infant will attain appropriate developmental milestones.
  Criteria: The infant responds positively to audio, visual, and diversionary activities. The infant shows age-appropriate development.

NURSING CARE PLAN

for the Infant With an Orthopedic Cast

Six-month-old MD has right congenital hip dysplasia. After a trial with a Pavlik harness, she has been placed in a hip spica cast. The cast has just been applied. This is a new experience for her and her caregiver.

NURSING DIAGNOSIS
Acute Pain related to discomfort of hip spica cast

GOAL: *The infant will show signs of being comfortable.*

OUTCOME CRITERIA
- The infant is alert and contented.
- The infant has no long periods of fussiness.
- The infant interacts with caregivers by cooing, smiling, and eye contact.

NURSING INTERVENTION	*RATIONALE*
Check edges of cast for smoothness; pedal edges of cast.	Rough edges can cause irritation and discomfort.
Soothe by stroking, cuddling, and talking to infant.	These comfort measures help the infant feel safe, secure, and loved and provide distraction from discomfort and restriction of cast.
Provide infant with a pacifier.	Nonnutritive sucking is a means of self-comfort.

NURSING DIAGNOSIS
Risk for Impaired Skin Integrity related to pressure of the cast on the skin surface

GOAL: *The infant's skin will remain intact.*

OUTCOME CRITERIA
- The infant's skin around the cast shows no signs of redness or irritation.
- The infant's skin in the diaper area is clean, dry, and intact with no signs of perineal redness or irritation.

NURSING INTERVENTIONS	*RATIONALE*
Place infant on firm mattress for 24 to 48 hours until cast is dry.	The cast is still pliable until dry. Undue pressure on any point must be avoided.
Use palms when handling damp cast.	Using palms instead of fingers prevents excessive pressure in any one area.
Petal all edges of cast.	Petalling provides a smooth edge along cast to avoid irritation.
Inspect skin around the cast edges for redness and irritation during each shift.	Early signs of irritation indicate areas that may need added protection.
Protect perineal area of cast with waterproof covering.	Urine and feces can easily cause irritation, skin breakdown, or a softened and malodorous cast.
Remove, wash, and thoroughly dry perineal covering if wet or soiled.	A clean, dry perineal cast protective covering decreases the problem of breakdown.

NURSING DIAGNOSIS
Risk for Delayed Growth and Development related to restricted mobility secondary to hip spica cast

GOAL: *The infant will attain appropriate developmental milestones.*

OUTCOME CRITERIA
- The infant responds positively to audio, visual, and diversional activities.
- The infant smiles, coos, and squeals in response to family caregivers.
- The infant shows age appropriate development.

NURSING INTERVENTIONS	*RATIONALE*
Provide mobiles, musical toys, stuffed toys, and toys infant can manipulate.	Visual, tactile, and auditory stimulation are important for infant development.

nursing care plan continues on page 160

NURSING CARE PLAN continued

for the Infant With an Orthopedic Cast

Six-month-old MD has right congenital hip dysplasia. After a trial with a Pavlik harness, she has been placed in a hip spica cast. The cast has just been applied. This is a new experience for her and her caregiver.

NURSING INTERVENTIONS	RATIONALE
Encourage caregiver to interact with infant during feeding.	Interacting (babbling, cooing) with others in her or his environment encourages development.
Plan activities that include changes of environment such as moving to the playroom in the hospital or to a different room in the home.	Environmental variety provides increased visual, auditory, and tactile stimulation.

NURSING DIAGNOSIS
Deficient Knowledge of family caregivers related to the home care of the infant in a cast

GOAL: *The family caregivers will learn home care of the infant.*

OUTCOME CRITERIA
• The family caregivers demonstrate care of the infant in the hip spica cast.
• The family caregivers ask pertinent questions.
• The family caregiver identifies a resource person to call.

NURSING INTERVENTIONS	RATIONALE
Determine the family caregivers' knowledge level and design a teaching plan.	An effective teaching plan is tailored to begin with the knowledge base of the family.
Choose teaching methods most suited to family caregivers recognized needs and learning style.	The family's ability to read, understand, and follow directions and their cognitive abilities affect the results.
Before discharge, schedule follow-up appointment for return visit to have the cast checked.	Scheduling the follow-up appointment emphasizes to family caregivers the importance of close follow-up.

• *Goal:* The family caregivers will learn home care of the infant.
Criteria: The family demonstrates care of the infant in the orthopedic device or cast, asks pertinent questions, and identifies a resource person to call.

Genitourinary Tract Defects

Most congenital anomalies of the genitourinary tract are not life-threatening but may present social problems with lifelong implications for the child and family. Thus, early recognition and supportive, understanding care are essential.

Hypospadias and Epispadias

Hypospadias is a congenital condition in which the urethra terminates on the ventral (underside) surface of the penis instead of at the tip. A cordlike anomaly (a **chordee**) extends from the scrotum to the penis,

pulling the penis downward in an arc. Urination is not affected, but the boy cannot void while standing in the normal male fashion. Surgical repair is desirable between the ages of 6 and 18 months before body image and castration anxiety become problems. Microscopic surgery makes early repair possible.

Surgical repair is often accomplished in one stage and is often done as outpatient surgery. These infants should not be circumcised, because the foreskin is used in the repair. Severe hypospadias may require additional surgical procedures.

In epispadias, the opening is on the dorsal (top) surface of the penis. This condition often occurs with exstrophy of the bladder. Surgical repair is indicated.

Exstrophy of the Bladder

This urinary tract malformation occurs in one in 30,000 live births in the United States and is usually accompanied by other anomalies such as epispadias, cleft scrotum, cryptorchidism (undescended testes), a shortened penis, and cleft clitoris. It is also associated with malformed pelvic musculature, resulting in a prolapsed rectum and inguinal hernias. Children with this defect have a widely split symphysis pubis and posterolaterally rotated hip sockets, causing a waddling gait.

In this condition, the anterior surface of the urinary bladder lies open on the lower abdomen (Fig. 9–26). The exposed mucosa is red and sensitive to touch and allows direct passage of urine to the outside. This condition makes the area vulnerable to infection and trauma. Surgical closure of the bladder is preferred within the first 48 hours of life. Final surgical correction is completed before the child goes to school. If bladder repair is not done early in the child's life, the family caregivers must be taught how to care for this condition and how to deal with their feelings toward this less-than-perfect child. Their emotional reaction may be further complicated if the malformation is so severe that the sex of the child may be determined only by a chromosome test (see the following section on sexual ambiguity).

Nursing care of the infant with exstrophy of the bladder should be directed toward preventing infection, preventing skin irritation around the seeping mucosa, meeting the infant's need for touch and cuddling, and educating and supporting the family during this crisis.

Sexual Ambiguity

Although rare, the birth of an infant with ambiguous genitalia presents a highly charged emotional climate and has possible long-range social implications. Regardless of the cause, it is important to establish the genetic sex and the sex of rearing as early as possible, so that surgical correction of anomalies may occur before the child begins to function in a sex-related social role. Authorities believe that the infant's anatomic structure, rather than the genetic sex, should determine the sex of rearing. It is possible to construct a functional vagina surgically and to administer hormones to offer an anatomically incomplete female a somewhat normal life. Currently it is impossible to offer comparable surgical reconstruction to males with an inadequate penis. Parents may feel guilt, anxiety, and confusion about their child's condition and need empathic understanding and support to help them cope with this emergency.

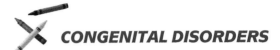

CONGENITAL DISORDERS

Disorders present at birth (congenital) include certain infections: many that the infant acquires from the mother during the prenatal period or at the time of delivery, others are inborn errors of metabolism caused by hereditary disorders that affect metabolism.

Infections

There are numerous maternally derived infections associated with congenital conditions. Many of these infections are represented by the acronym TORCH. These include toxoplasmosis, other (gonorrhea, syphilis, varicella, hepatitis B, HIV), rubella, cytomegalovirus, and herpes simplex virus. Nursing care for these infants focuses on prompt diagnosis, strict adherence to infection control guidelines, and routine care as for any newborn. Anxious caregivers often require support, education regarding treatment and prevention, and preparation for long-term care.

Toxoplasmosis

Toxoplasmosis infections in humans are caused by hand-to-mouth contact with contaminated feces usually from cat litter. The pregnant mother transmits the disease to the unborn baby. Many infants who are affected have mental retardation and other serious conditions following birth.

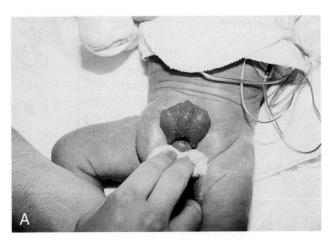

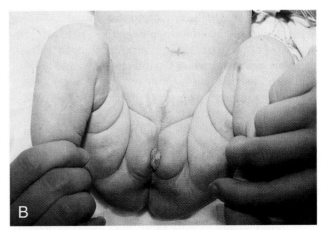

● *Figure 9.26* Exstrophy of the bladder. **(A)** Prior to surgery, note the bright-red color of the bladder. **(B)** Following surgical repair.

Gonorrheal Ophthalmia Neonatorum

Gonorrheal eye infection in the newborn is a serious condition usually resulting in blindness if prophylactic treatment at birth is omitted. The infectious agent is the gonococcus *Neisseria gonorrhoeae.* The infant becomes infected while passing through the birth canal of an infected mother.

Clinical Manifestations and Diagnosis. Symptoms are acute redness and swelling of the conjunctiva with a purulent discharge from the eyes occurring within 36 to 48 hours after birth. These symptoms usually indicate gonorrheal eye infection; however, inspection of the eye should be followed by a culture and smear to determine the causative organism. The condition is communicable for 24 hours after specific therapy is instituted or, when no therapy is used, until discharge from the eyes has ceased.

Prevention and Treatment. In the United States, all states have laws requiring the use of specific preparations instilled into the eyes at birth. Instillation of antibiotic drops or ophthalmic ointments, such as tetracycline and erythromycin, is used to prevent infection.

Congenital Syphilis

Syphilis, whether congenital or acquired, is caused by the spirochete *Treponema pallidum.* Fetal anomalies rarely occur because fetal infections usually are not present before the fourth month of fetal life, which is after the organs have been formed. The infection is contracted from the mother through placental transfer. About one fourth of infected infants are stillborn. Surviving infants may not show any clinical symptoms for months or years.

Clinical Manifestations. In early congenital syphilis, symptoms may appear before the sixth week of life. Rhinitis with a profuse, mucopurulent nasal discharge is usually the first symptom. A maculopapular skin rash appears next and is heaviest over the back, buttocks, and backs of the thighs. Bleeding ulcerations and mucous membrane lesions appear around the mouth, the anus, and the genital areas. Anemia is present; pseudoparalysis and pathologic fractures may occur. These symptoms usually subside without treatment while the infectious organism lies latent in the child's tissues.

Late symptoms appearing after infancy involve the skeletal framework, the eyes, and the central nervous system. The child may acquire a flat bridge of the nose known as "saddle nose." The permanent teeth are affected in that the incisors are peg-shaped (Hutchinson's teeth). A condition of the eyes called **interstitial keratitis,** inflammation of the cornea, often occurs later in the disease with lacrimation, photophobia, and opacity of the lens that may lead to blindness.

Diagnosis. A VDRL (Venereal Disease Research Laboratory) or Wassermann test on cord blood at delivery is done when congenital syphilis is suspected. Passively acquired antibodies may give false-positive results; therefore, other serologic tests are conducted subsequently. If results are doubtful, treatment usually is instituted to avoid a full-blown infection.

Treatment. Ideally treatment is preventive and consists of penicillin therapy for the affected mother early in pregnancy. The physician may order the test to be repeated later in pregnancy if infection is suspected; if the test is positive, penicillin therapy is instituted at this point. Treatment for the affected infant consists of a course of penicillin therapy. Strict isolation of the infant is required.

Early congenital syphilis usually responds to vigorous treatment, and growth and development are not affected. Late congenital syphilis responds well to treatment, but pathologic changes in the bones, eyes, and nervous system are permanent.

Hepatitis B

The hepatitis B virus can be transmitted to the newborn during delivery when the mother is positive for the virus. The infected vaginal blood carries the virus and thus infects the infant. These infants can then become carriers of the virus. The newborn is given immune serum globulin soon after birth to decrease the chances of infection. Infants are now being routinely given hepatitis B immunizations before they leave the hospital to help reduce the spread of hepatitis B.

Human Immunodeficiency Virus (HIV)

The newborn of a human immunodeficiency virus (HIV) positive mother may not show any signs of infection at birth and appears much the same as any other newborn. Human immunodeficiency virus may be transmitted to the fetus across the placenta, from the mother's body fluids during birth, or through breast milk. If the mother is known to be positive for HIV, she should not breast-feed her newborn. The infant's test results are positive for HIV antibodies for as long as 15 months because he or she has passively acquired antibodies from the mother. Only 25% to 30% of infants born to known HIV-infected mothers are infected themselves.[1] Signs of HIV infection usually are not seen in infants younger than 4 to 6 months of age. By 1 year of age, about half of those who are infected are symptomatic; by 2 years of age, most HIV-infected infants become symptomatic. The prognosis is poor for infants who have symptoms before 1 year of age and those who develop opportunistic infections such as *Pneumocystis carinii* pneumonia. Bacterial infections, such as pneumonia, meningitis, and bacteremia, are common in infected newborns. These infants also commonly have thrush, mouth sores, and severe diaper rash. Personnel must follow standard precautions when performing the first bath on every newborn and when they perform any procedure with possible exposure to blood or body fluids (see Chap. 19 for further discussion of HIV-infected children).

Congenital Rubella

The rubella virus infection acquired by the fetus in utero generally persists throughout fetal life and for as long as 18 months after delivery. Persons coming into close contact with these babies may develop the disease; therefore, all women of childbearing age who are not immune to rubella should avoid contact with an infected infant.

The congenital rubella syndrome comprises a large variety of malformations including cataracts and other eye defects such as glaucoma. Other complications include deafness, cardiac anomalies (especially patent ductus arteriosus), septal defects, intrauterine growth retardation, subnormal head circumference, and retarded functional development.

Symptoms of childhood rubella may be mild and many rashes resemble rubella, therefore, it is unreliable to assume that a person has an immunity because of a presumed attack of rubella during childhood. Children now receive rubella vaccine as part of their immunizations at 12 months of age. Testing for the presence of rubella serum antibody is routine in all pregnant women. A positive reaction shows the person to be immune either as a result of the disease itself or from immunization. As a result of these concentrated efforts, neonates are protected from this devastating disease.

Cytomegalovirus

The cytomegalovirus is the most common cause of congenital viral infections in humans. Most infected infants do not have symptoms at birth but later on in life can exhibit hearing problems and learning difficulties.

Herpes Simplex Virus

Herpes simplex virus, most frequently caused by herpesvirus type 2, is transmitted to the neonate during vaginal delivery by a mother who has an active genital lesion. Cesarean delivery before rupture of membranes is considered a preventive measure, although a small possibility remains that the fetus could have been infected before delivery. The infant usually has no apparent signs of the disease until 6 to 9 days after delivery. In the newborn nursery, infants who have had possible exposure should be segregated or cared for in the mother's private room.

The infection may be generalized, resembling sepsis. The infant may or may not have lesions, which are highly contagious. The mortality rate is high. Infants who survive have a high probability for ocular and neurologic damage.

Inborn Errors of Metabolism

Inborn errors of metabolism include phenylketonuria, galactosemia, congenital hypothyroidism, maple syrup urine disease, and homocystinuria. Nursing care for the infant involves prompt diagnosis and initiation of treatment. Family teaching might include dietary guidelines, information about the disorder, and genetic counseling. The family also needs support and information to prepare for the long-term care of a chronically ill child (see Chap. 21).

Phenylketonuria

Phenylketonuria (PKU) is a recessive hereditary defect of metabolism that, if untreated, causes severe mental retardation in most but not all affected children. It is uncommon, appearing in about one in 10,000 births. Children with this condition lack the enzyme that normally changes the essential amino acid phenylalanine into tyrosine.

As soon as the newborn with this defect begins to take milk (either breast or cow's milk), phenylalanine is absorbed in the normal manner. Because the affected infant cannot metabolize this amino acid, however, phenylalanine builds up in the blood serum to as much as 20 times the normal level. This build-up occurs so quickly that increased levels of phenylalanine appear in the blood after only 1 or 2 days of ingestion of milk. Phenylpyruvic acid appears in the urine of these infants between the second and the sixth week of life.

Most untreated children with this condition develop severe and progressive mental deficiency, apparently because of the high serum phenylalanine level. The infant appears normal at birth but begins to show signs of mental arrest within a few weeks. Therefore, this disorder must be diagnosed as early as possible and the child must be placed immediately on a low-phenylalanine formula.

Clinical Manifestations. Untreated infants may experience frequent vomiting and have aggressive and hyperactive traits. Severe, progressive retardation is characteristic. Convulsions may occur, and eczema is common particularly in the perineal area. There is a characteristic musty smell to the urine.

Diagnosis. Most states require newborns to undergo a blood test to detect the phenylalanine level. This screening procedure called the Guthrie inhibition assay test uses blood from a simple heel prick. The test is most reliable after the infant has ingested some form of protein. The accepted practice is to perform the test on the second or third day of life. If the infant leaves the hospital before this time, the infant is brought back to have the test performed. The test may be repeated in the third week of life if the first test was done before the infant was 24 hours old. Health practitioners caring for infants not born in a hospital are responsible for screening these infants. When screening indicates an increased level of phenylalanine, additional testing is done to make a firm diagnosis.

Treatment. Dietary treatment is required. A formula low in phenylalanine should be started as soon as the condition is detected; Lofenalac and Phenyl-free are low-phenylalanine formulas. Best results are obtained if the special formula is started before the infant is 3 weeks of age. A low-phenylalanine diet is a very restricted one: foods to be omitted are breads, meat, fish, dairy products, nuts, and legumes. The diet should be carefully supervised by a nutritionist and should be continued well into the school years. Routine blood testing is done to maintain the serum phenylalanine level at 2 to 8 mg/dL.

Maintaining the infant on the restricted diet is relatively simple compared with the problems that arise as the child grows and becomes more independent. As the child ventures into the world beyond home, more and more dietary temptations are available, and dietary compliance is difficult. The family and child need support and counseling throughout the child's developmental years. The length of time that the restrictions are necessary remains unclear. Although difficult, it seems best to follow the diet into adolescence.

Galactosemia

Galactosemia is a recessive hereditary metabolic disorder in which the enzyme necessary to convert galactose into glucose is missing. The infants generally appear normal at birth but experience difficulties after ingesting milk (breast, cow's, or goat's) because one of the component monosaccharides of milk lactose is galactose.

Clinical Manifestations and Diagnosis. Early feeding difficulties with vomiting and diarrhea severe enough to produce dehydration and weight loss and jaundice are primary manifestations. Unless milk is withheld early, other difficulties include cataracts, liver and spleen damage, and mental retardation with a high mortality rate early in life. A screening test (Beutler test) can be used to test for the disorder.

Treatment. Galactose must be omitted from the diet, which in the young infant means a substitution for milk. Nutramigen and Pregestimil are formulas that provide galactose-free nutrition for the infant. The diet must continue to be free of lactose when the child moves on to table foods, but the diet allows more variety than the phenylalanine-free diet.

Congenital Hypothyroidism

At one time referred to by the now unacceptable term cretinism, congenital hypothyroidism is associated with either the congenital absence of a thyroid gland or the inability of the thyroid gland to secrete thyroid hormone. The incidence is about one in 5,000 births or about twice as common as PKU.

Diagnosis. Most states require a routine test for triiodothyronine (T_3) and thyroxine (T_4) levels to determine thyroid function in all newborns before discharge for early diagnosis of congenital hypothyroidism. This test is done as part of the heel stick screening, which includes the Guthrie screening test for PKU.

Clinical Manifestations. The infant appears normal at birth, but clinical signs and symptoms begin to be noticeable at about 6 weeks of life. The facial features are typical: depressed nasal bridge, large tongue, and puffy eyes. The neck is short and thick (Fig. 9–27). The voice (cry) is hoarse, the skin is dry and cold, and the infant has slow bone development. Two common features are chronic constipation and abdomen enlargement due to poor muscle tone. The infant is a poor feeder and often characterized as a "good" baby by the parent or caretaker because he or she cries very little and sleeps for long periods.

Treatment. The thyroid hormone must be replaced as soon as the diagnosis is made. Levothyroxine sodium, a synthetic thyroid replacement, is the drug most commonly used. Blood levels of T_3 and T_4 are monitored to prevent overdosage. Unless therapy is started in early infancy, mental retardation and slow growth occur. The later that therapy is started, the more severe the mental retardation. Therapy must be continued for life.

Maple Syrup Urine Disease

Maple syrup urine disease (MSUD) is an inborn error of metabolism of the branched chain amino acids. It is

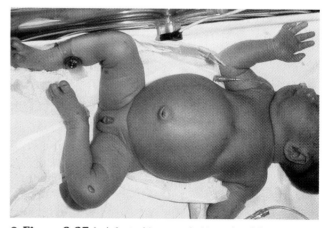

● **Figure 9.27** An infant with congenital hypothyroidism; note the short, thick neck and enlarged abdomen.

autosomal recessive in inheritance. It is rapidly progressive and often fatal.

Clinical Manifestations and Diagnosis. The onset of MSUD occurs very early in infancy. In the first week of life, these infants often have feeding problems and neurologic signs such as seizures, spasticity, and opisthotonos. The urine has a distinctive odor of maple syrup. Diagnosis is made through a blood test for the amino acids leucine, isoleucine, and valine. This is easily done at the same time as the heel stick for PKU is performed.

Treatment. Treatment of MSUD is dietary and must be initiated within 12 days of birth to be successful. The special formula is low in the branched chain amino acids. The special diet must be continued indefinitely.

Homocystinuria

In homocystinuria, a relatively rare inborn error of metabolism, there is a deficiency of the enzyme cystathionine B synthase. This enzyme blocks the conversion of methionine to cystine. Mental retardation, early-onset thrombosis, seizures, and behavioral disorders result from high levels of serum methionine.

Clinical Manifestations and Diagnosis. The newborn with this deficiency may have skeletal abnormalities, mental retardation, dislocation of ocular lenses, or intravascular thromboses as the result of methionine and homocystine in the blood. Diagnosis can be made through screening when newborn screening is performed.

Treatment. Homocystinuria is treated with a special diet low in methionine and is supplemented with cystine and pyridoxine (vitamin B_6). With prompt, early diagnosis and treatment, the long-term prognosis for the prevention of mental retardation is good.

KEY POINTS

● Many infants injured during birth or born with a congenital anomaly have long-term effects from their conditions.

● Advances in medical technology have improved the outlook for many infants who have sustained damage during intrauterine development or birth. The advances give infants a better chance for an improved quality of life, but many conditions still inflict overwhelming consequences and cause lifelong disabilities.

● Care of the newborn with special needs is a challenging aspect of nursing.

● All available resources must be used to deliver quality nursing care to infants with congenital anomalies or birth injuries and to the families of these infants.

● Nursing care must stimulate the infant's optimal growth and development as well as meeting his or her immediate physical needs.

● The nurse must prepare the family for infant home care and guide the family to support services that will enable them to manage their child's care for many years.

REFERENCES

1. Scott GB, Parks WP. (1999) Pediatric human immunodeficiency virus 1 infection. In *Oski's pediatrics: Principles and practice* (3rd ed). Philadelphia: Lippincott Williams & Wilkins.

BIBLIOGRAPHY

Fishman MA. (1999) Developmental defects. In *Oski's pediatrics: Principles and practice* (3rd ed). Philadelphia: Lippincott Williams & Wilkins.

Goldberg MJ. (2001) Early detection of developmental hip dysplasia. *Pediatrics in Review*, 22(4), 131–34.

Gorlin RJ. (1999) Craniofacial defects. In *Oski's pediatrics: Principles and practice* (3rd ed). Philadelphia: Lippincott Williams & Wilkins.

McDaniel NL. (2001) Heart ventricular and atrial septal defects. *Pediatrics in Review*, 22(8), 265.

NANDA Nursing diagnoses: Definitions and classification 2001–2002 (2001). Philadelphia: North American Nursing Diagnosis Association.

Oxley J. (2001) Are arm splints required following cleft lip/palate repair? *Pediatric Nursing*, 13(1) 27–30.

Pillitteri A. (1999) *Maternal and child health nursing* (3rd ed). Philadelphia: Lippincott Williams & Wilkins.

Robinson D, Drumm L. (2001) Maple syrup disease: A standard of nursing care. *Pediatric Nursing*, 27(3), 255.

Sommerlad BC. (2002) The management of cleft lip and palate. *Current Pediatrics*, 12(1), 36–42.

(2000) *Springhouse nurse's drug guide* (3rd ed). Springhouse, PA: Springhouse Corporation.

Sparks S, Taylor C. (2001) *Nursing diagnosis reference manual* (5th ed). Springhouse, PA: Springhouse Corporation.

Suddaby EC. (2001) Contemporary thinking for congenital heart disease. *Pediatric Nursing*, 27(3), 233.

Wedge JH, et. al. (2001) Congenital clubfoot. *Current Pediatrics*, 11(5), 332–40.

Wong DL. (1998) *Whaley and Wong's nursing care of infants and children* (6th ed). St. Louis: Mosby.

Wong DL, Perry S, Hockenberry M. (2002) *Maternal child nursing care* (2nd ed). St. Louis: Mosby.

Wong DL, Hess C. (2000) *Wong and Whaley's clinical manual of pediatric nursing* (5th ed). St. Louis: Mosby.

Websites
Spina Bifida http://www.sbaa.org
Cleft Lip and Cleft Palate www.cleft.org

Workbook

NCLEX-STYLE REVIEW QUESTIONS

1. The nurse is doing an admission exam on an infant with a diagnosis of hydrocephalus. If the following data were collected, which might indicate a common symptom of this diagnosis?

   a. Sac protruding on the lower back

   b. Respiratory rate of 30 breaths a minute

   c. Gluteal folds higher on one side than the other

   d. Head circumference of 18 inches

2. When collecting data during an admission interview and exam on an infant, the nurse finds the infant has cyanosis, dyspnea, tachycardia, and feeding difficulties. These symptoms might indicate the infant has which of the following conditions?

   a. Spina bifida

   b. Tetralogy of Fallot

   c. Congenital rubella

   d. Hip dysplasia

3. An infant diagnosed with congestive heart failure has a decreased caloric intake. Which of the following nursing interventions would be appropriate for this infant?

   a. Offer 8 to 10 ounces of formula every 4 hours.

   b. Feed with nipples that have large openings.

   c. Encourage infant to nurse for at least 1 hour each feeding.

   d. Offer formula that is high in potassium.

4. In caring for an infant who has had a cleft lip/cleft palate repair, the HIGHEST priority for the nurse is to

   a. document the time period the restraints are on and off

   b. observe the incision for redness or drainage

   c. teach the caregivers about dental care and hygiene

   d. provide sensory stimulation and age-appropriate toys

5. In planning care for an infant who had a spica cast applied to treat a congenital hip dysplasia, which of the following nursing interventions would be included in this infant's plan of care?

   a. Inspect skin for redness and irritation.

   b. Change bedding and clothing every 4 hours.

   c. Weigh every morning and evening using same scale.

   d. Monitor temperature and pulse every 2 hours.

STUDY ACTIVITIES

1. Using the table below, list the common types of congenital heart defects. Include the description of the defect (chambers and parts of the heart involved), the blood flow characteristics, symptoms, and treatment.

2. Make a list of the maternal risk factors that may cause congenital heart defects. For each of these risk factors, state what could be done to decrease the occurrence of these risks.

3. Develop a teaching project by creating a mobile or gathering a collection of appropriate toys and activities that could be used for sensory stimulation with an infant who is in an orthopedic cast. Present your project to your classmates and explain why and how these items would be appropriate to use for developmental stimulation.

Defect	Description of Defect	Blood Flow Characteristics	Symptoms	Treatment

CRITICAL THINKING

1. Diane's baby was born with a bilateral cleft lip and cleft palate. When you bring the baby to her for feeding, she breaks down and sobs uncontrollably. Describe your immediate response. What feelings and emotions do you think Diane is experiencing? Write out an example of a therapeutic response you could make?

2. Identify the reason that infection control is of utmost importance in care of the infant with myelomeningocele. Make a list of the infection control measures that you would follow when caring for an infant with myelomeningocele.

3. Explain what happens as fluid builds up in the cranial cavity in an infant with hydrocephalus a) before the suture lines close and b) after the sutures line close. Identify the symptoms that an infant would display if fluid buildup in the brain were not relieved.

4. *Dosage calculation:* A newborn with a diagnosis of congestive heart failure is being treated with Digoxin. The child weighs 6.5 pounds. The usual dosage range of this medication is 4 to 8 mcg per kg per day in divided doses every 12 hours. Answer the following:
   a. How many mcg (micrograms) are in a mg (milligram)?
   b. How many kg does the child weigh?
   c. What is the low dose of Digoxin (in mcg) that this child could be given in a 24-hour-time period?
   d. What is the high dose of Digoxin (in mcg) that this child could be given in a 24-hour-time period?
   e. How many doses will the child receive in a day?
   f. How many mcg will the child receive in each dose?

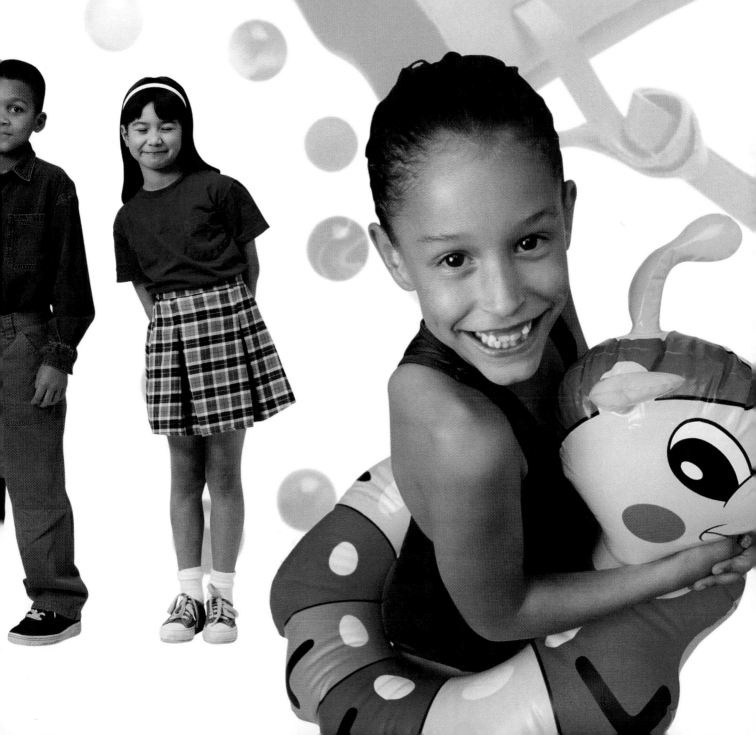

Care of the Child

Growth and Development of the Infant: 28 Days to 1 Year

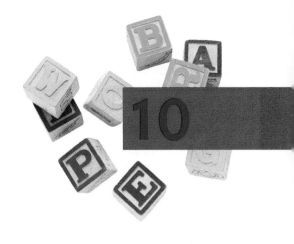

10

PHYSICAL DEVELOPMENT
Head and Skull
Skeletal Growth and Maturation
Eruption of Deciduous Teeth
Circulatory System
Body Temperature and Respiratory Rate
Neuromuscular Development

PSYCHOSOCIAL DEVELOPMENT
NUTRITION
Addition of Solid Foods
Weaning the Infant

Women, Infants, Children Food Program

HEALTH PROMOTION AND MAINTENANCE
Routine Checkups
Immunizations
Family Teaching
Accident Prevention

THE INFANT IN THE HEALTH CARE FACILITY
Parent-Nurse Relationship

The infant who has lived through the first month of life has a busy year ahead. During this year, the infant grows and develops skills more rapidly than he or she ever will again. In the brief span of a single year, this tiny, helpless bit of humanity becomes a person with strong emotions of love, fear, jealousy, and anger and gains the ability to rise from a supine to an upright position and move about purposefully.

In the first year, both weight and height increase rapidly. During the first 6 months, the infant's birth weight doubles and height increases about 6 inches. Growth slows slightly during the second 6 months but is still rapid. By 1 year of age, the infant has tripled his or her birth weight and has grown 10 inches to 12 inches.

Thinking in terms of the "average" child is misleading. To determine if an infant is reaching acceptable levels of development, birth weight and height must be the standard to which later measurements are compared. A baby weighing 6 lb at birth cannot be expected to weigh as much at 5 or 6 months of age as the baby who weighed 9 lb at birth, but each is expected to double his or her birth weight at about this time. A growth graph is helpful to the nurse, pediatrician, or caregiver for charting a child's progress (Fig. 10–1).

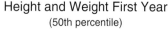

PHYSICAL DEVELOPMENT

Despite the many factors such as genetic background, environment, health, gender, and race, that affect growth in the first year of life, the healthy infant pro-gresses in a predictable pattern. By the end of the year, the dependent infant who at 1 month of age had no teeth and could not roll over, sit, or stand blossoms into an emerging toddler with teeth who can sit alone, stand, and begin to walk alone. The growth, seen in the prenatal development of the fetus, continues.

Head and Skull

At birth, an infant's head circumference averages about 13.75 inches (35 cm) and is usually slightly larger than the chest circumference. The chest measures about the same as the abdomen at birth. At about 1 year of age, the head circumference has grown to about 18 inches (47 cm). The chest also grows rapidly, catching up to the head circumference at about 5 to 7 months of age. From then on, the chest can be expected to exceed the head in circumference.

Fontanelles and Cranial Sutures

The posterior fontanelle is usually closed by the second or third month of life. The anterior fontanelle may increase slightly in size during the first few months of life. After the sixth month it begins to decrease in size, closing between the 12th and the 18th months. The sutures between the cranial bones do not ossify until later childhood.

Skeletal Growth and Maturation

During fetal life, the skeletal system is completely formed in cartilage at the end of 3 months' gestation. Bone ossification and growth occur during the

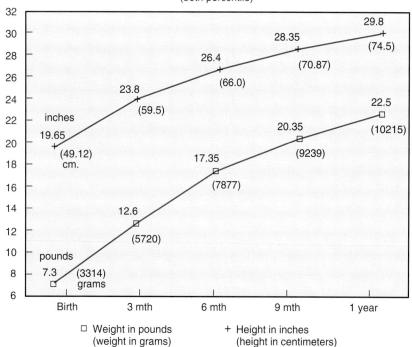

Height and Weight First Year
(50th percentile)

□ Weight in pounds
(weight in grams)

+ Height in inches
(height in centimeters)

● **Figure 10.1** Chart of infant growth representing an infant in the mid-range birthweight 7.3 lb (3314 g) and birth length 19.65 inches (49.12 cm). Infants of different races vary in average size. Asian infants tend to be smaller, African American infants larger.

remainder of fetal life and throughout childhood. The pattern of maturation is so regular that the "bone age" can be determined by radiologic examination. When the bone age matches the child's chronologic age, the skeletal structure is maturing at a normal rate. To avoid unnecessary exposure to radiation, radiologic examination is performed *only* if a problem is suspected.

Eruption of Deciduous Teeth

Calcification of the primary or **deciduous teeth** starts early in fetal life. Shortly before birth, calcification begins in the permanent teeth, which are the first to erupt in later childhood. The first deciduous teeth, usually the lower central incisors, usually erupt between 6 and 8 months of age (Fig. 10–2).

Babies in good health who show normal development may differ in the timing of tooth eruption. Some families show a tendency toward very early or very late eruption without having other signs of early or late development. Some infants may become restless or fussy from swollen, inflamed gums during teething. A cold teething ring may be helpful in soothing the baby's discomfort. Teething is a normal process of development and does not cause high fever or upper respiratory conditions.

Nutritional deficiency or prolonged illness in infancy may interfere with calcification of both the deciduous and the permanent teeth. The role of fluoride in strengthening calcification of teeth has been well documented. The American Dental Association recommends administration of fluoride to infants and children in areas where the fluoride content of drinking water is inadequate or absent.

Circulatory System

In the first year of life, the circulatory system undergoes several changes. During fetal life, high levels of hemoglobin and red blood cells are necessary for adequate oxygenation. After birth when oxygen is supplied through the respiratory system, hemoglobin decreases in volume, and red blood cells gradually decrease in number until the third month of life. Thereafter, the count gradually increases until adult levels are reached.

Obtaining an accurate blood-pressure measurement in an infant is difficult. Electronic or ultrasonographic monitoring equipment is often used (see Chap. 5). The average blood pressure during the first year of life is 85/60 mm Hg. However, variability is expected among children of the same age and body build.

An accurate determination of the infant's heartbeat requires an apical pulse count. A pediatric stethoscope with a small-diameter diaphragm is placed over the left side of the chest in a position where the heart beat can be clearly heard. A count is then taken for 1 full minute (see Chap. 5). During the first year of life, the average apical rate ranges from 70 (asleep) to 150 (awake) beats per minute and as high as 180 beats per minute while the infant is crying.

Body Temperature and Respiratory Rate

Body temperature follows the average normal range after the initial adjustment to postnatal living. Respirations average 30 breaths per minute with a wide range (20–50 breaths per minute) according to the infant's activity.

Neuromuscular Development

As the infant grows, nerve cells mature and fine muscles begin to coordinate in an orderly pattern of development. Naturally the family caregivers are full of pride in the infant who learns to sit or stand before the neighbor's baby does, but accomplishing such milestones early means little. Each child follows a unique rhythm of progress within reasonable limits.

Average rates of growth and development are useful for purposes of making comparisons. Few landmarks call for special attention, and their absence may indicate the need for additional environmental stimulation. Do not emphasize routine developmental

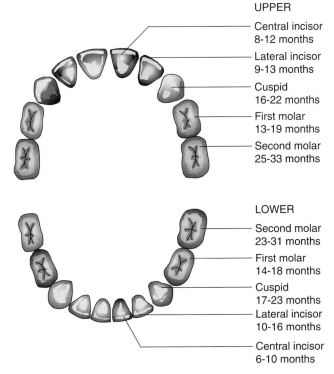

UPPER

Central incisor
8-12 months

Lateral incisor
9-13 months

Cuspid
16-22 months

First molar
13-19 months

Second molar
25-33 months

LOWER

Second molar
23-31 months

First molar
14-18 months

Cuspid
17-23 months

Lateral incisor
10-16 months

Central incisor
6-10 months

● *Figure 10.2* Approximate ages for the eruption of deciduous teeth.

tables with family caregivers; a small time lag may be insignificant. A large time lag may require greater stimulation from the environment or a watchful attitude to discover how overall development is proceeding.

Table 10–1 summarizes the accepted norms in physical, psychosocial, motor, language, and cognitive growth and development in the first year of life (Fig. 10–3).

TABLE 10.1	Growth and Development Chart: Birth to 1 Year					
Age	**Physical**	**Psychosocial**	**Fine Motor**	**Gross Motor**	**Language**	**Cognition**
Birth–4 wk	Weight gain of 5–7 oz (150–270 g) per wk Height gain of 1″ per mo first 6 mo Head circumference increase ½″ per mo Moro, Babinski, rooting, and tonic neck reflexes present	Some smiling Begins Erikson's stage of "trust vs. mistrust"	Grasp reflex very strong Hands flexed	Catches and holds objects in sight that cross visual field Can turn head from side to side when lying in a prone position (see Fig. 10–3A) When prone, body in a flexed position When prone, moves extremities in a crawling fashion	Cries when upset Makes enjoyment sounds during mealtimes	At 1 mo, sucking activity associated with pleasurable sensations
6 wk	Tears appear	Smiling in response to familiar stimuli	Hands open Less flexion noted	Tries to raise shoulders and arms when stimulated Holds head up when prone Less flexion of entire body when prone	Cooing predominant Smiles to familiar voices Babbling	**Primary Circular Reactions** Begins to repeat actions
10–12 wk	Posterior fontanelle closes	Aware of new environment Less crying Smiles at significant others	No longer has grasp reflex Pulls on clothes, blanket, but does not reach for them	No longer has Moro reflex Symmetric body positioning Pumps arms, shoulders, and head from prone position (see Fig. 10–3B)	Makes noises when spoken to	Beginning of coordinated responses to different kinds of stimuli
16 wk	Moro, rooting, and tonic neck reflexes disappear; drooling begins	Responds to stimulus Sees bottle, squeals, laughs Aware of new environment and shows interest	Grasps objects with two hands Grasps objects in crib voluntarily and brings them to mouth Eye–hand coordination beginning	Plays with hands Brings objects to mouth Balances head and body for short periods in sitting position	Laughs aloud Sounds "n," "k," "g," and "b"	Likes social situations Defiant, bored if unattended
20 wk	May show signs of teething	Smiles at self in mirror Cries when limits are set or when objects are taken away	Holds one object while looking for another one Grasps objects wanted	Able to sit up (see Fig. 10–3C) Can roll over Can bear weight on legs when held in a standing position	Cooing noises Squeals with delight	Visually looks for an object that has fallen

TABLE 10.1 (continued)	Growth and Development Chart: Birth to 1 Year					
Age	Physical	Psychosocial	Fine Motor	Gross Motor	Language	Cognition
24 wk	Birth weight doubles; weight gain slows to 3–5 oz (90–150 g) per wk Height slows to ½" per mo Teething begins with lower central incisors	Likes to be picked up Knows family from strangers Plays "Peek-a-Boo" Knows likes and dislikes Fear of strangers	Holds a bottle fairly well Tries to retrieve a dropped article	Able to control head movements Tonic neck reflex disappears Sits alone in high chair, back erect Rolls over and back to abdomen	Makes sounds "guh," "bah" Sounds "p," "m," "b," and "t" are pronounced Bubbling sounds	**Secondary Circular Reactions** Repeats actions that affect an object Beginning of object permanence
28 wk	Lower lateral incisors are followed in the next month by upper central incisors	Imitates simple acts Responds to "no" Shows preferences and dislikes for food	Holds cup Transfers objects from one hand to the other	Reaches without visual guidance Can lift head up when in a supine position	Babbling decreases Duplicates "ma-ma" and "pa-pa" sounds	
32 wk	Teething continues	Dislikes diaper and clothing change Afraid of strangers Fear of separating from mother	Adjusts body position to be able to reach for an object May stand up while holding on	Crawls around (see Fig. 10-3D) Pulls toy toward self	Combines syllables but has trouble attributing meaning to them	
40 wk– 1 yr	Birth weight tripled; has six teeth; Babinski reflex disappears Anterior fontanelle closes between now and 18 mo	Does things to attract attention Tries to follow when being read to Imitates parents Looks for objects not in sight	Holds tools with one hand and works on it with another Puts toy in box after demonstration Starts blocks Holds crayon to scribble on paper	Stands alone; begins to walk alone Can change self from prone to sitting to standing position	Words emerge Says "da-da" and "ma-ma" with meaning	Coordination of secondary schemes; masters barrier to reach goal, symbolic meanings

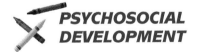

PSYCHOSOCIAL DEVELOPMENT

The give-and-take of life is experienced by the infant who actively seeks food to fulfill feelings of hunger. The infant begins to develop a sense of trust when fed on demand. However, the infant eventually learns that not every need is met immediately on demand. Slowly the infant becomes aware that something or someone separate from oneself fulfills one's needs. Gradually as a result of the loving care of family caregivers, the infant learns that the environment responds to desires expressed through one's own efforts and signals. The infant is now aware that the environment is separate from self.

Caregivers who expect too much too soon from the infant are not encouraging optimal development. Rather than teaching the rules of life before the infant has learned to trust the environment, the caregivers

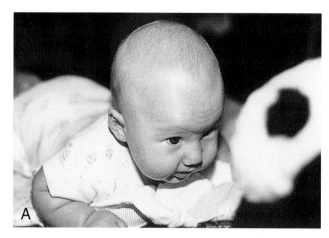

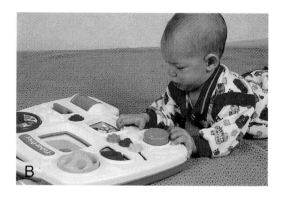

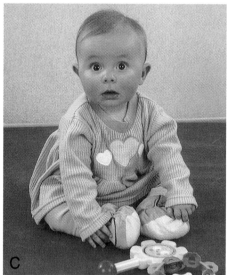

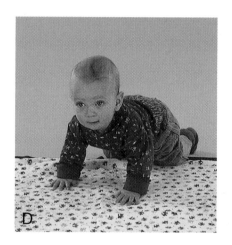

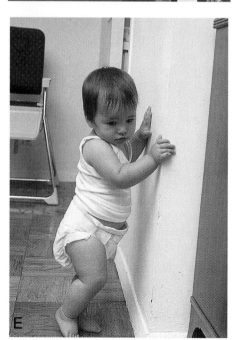

● **Figure 10.3** Growth and development of the infant. **(A)** At 4 weeks, this infant turns her head when lying in a prone position. **(B)** At 12 weeks, this infant pushes up from a prone position to look at his toy. **(C)** At 21 weeks, the infant sits up but tilts forward for balance. **(D)** At 30 weeks, this infant is crawling around and on the go. **(E)** At 43 weeks, this infant is getting ready to walk.

FAMILY TEACHING TIPS

Infants from Birth to 1 Year

First 6 weeks: Frequent holding of infant gives infant feeling of being loved and cared for. Rocking and soothing baby are important.

6 weeks to 3½ months: Continue to give infant feeling of being loved and cared for; respond to cries; provide visual stimulation with toys, pictures, mobiles, and auditory stimulation by talking and singing to baby; repeat sounds that infant makes to encourage vocal stimulation.

3½ to 5 months: Play regularly with baby; give child variety of things to look at; talk to baby; offer a variety of items to touch—soft, fuzzy, smooth, and rough—to provide tactile stimulation; continue to respond to infant's cries; move baby around home to provide additional visual and auditory stimulation; begin placing infant on floor to provide freedom of movement.

5 to 8 months: Continue to give infant feeling of being loved and cared for by holding, cuddling, and responding to needs; talk to infant; put infant on floor more often to roll and move about; fear of strangers is common at this age.

8 to 12 months: Accident-proof the house; give the infant maximum access to living area: supply infant with toys; stay close by to support infant in difficult situations; continue to talk to infant to provide language stimulation. The baby at this age loves surprise toys like jack-in-the-box and separation games like "Peek-a-Boo"; loves putting-in and taking-out activities. The child is developing independence, and temper tantrums may begin.

are actually teaching that nothing is gained by one's own activity and that the world does not respond to one's needs.

Conversely, caregivers who rush to anticipate every need give the infant no opportunity to test the environment. The opportunity to discover that through one's own actions the environment may be manipulated to suit one's own desires is withheld from the infant by these "smothering" caregivers. The box on Family Teaching Tips for infants in the first year of life suggests healthy childrearing patterns during infancy.

No one is perfect, and every family caregiver misinterprets the infant's signals at times. The caregiver may be tired, preoccupied, and responding momentarily to his or her own needs. The caregiver may not be able to ease the infant's pain or soothe the restlessness, but this also is a learning experience for the baby.

As mentioned earlier, the infant's development depends on a mutual relationship with give and take between the infant and the environment in which the family caregivers play the most important role. Table 10–2 summarizes significant caregiver-infant interactions indicating positive behaviors.

During the first few weeks of life, actions such as kicking and sucking are simple reflex activities. In the next sequential stage, reflexes are coordinated and elaborated. For example, the eyes follow random hand movements (Fig. 10–4A). The infant finds that repetition of chance movements brings interesting changes, and in the latter part of the first year these

TABLE 10.2	Criteria of Positive Caregiver-Infant Interactions	
Area of Interaction	**Positive Caregiver Response**
Feeding	Offers infant adequate amounts and proper types of food and prepares food appropriately
	Holds infant in comfortable, secure position during feeding
	Burps infant during or after feeding
	Offers food at a comfortable pace for infant
Stimulation	Provides appropriate nonaggressive verbal stimulation to infant
	Provides a variety of tactile experiences and touches infant in caring ways other than during feeding times or when moving infants away from danger
	Provides appropriate toys and interacts with infant in a way satisfying to infant
Rest and sleep	Provides a quiet, relaxed environment and a regular, scheduled sleep time for infant
	Makes certain infant is adequately fed, warm and dry before putting down to sleep
Understanding of infant	Has realistic expectations of infant and recognizes infant's developing skills and behavior
	Has realistic view of own parenting skills
	View of infant's health condition similar to the view of medical or nursing diagnosis
Problem-solving initiative	Motivated to manage infant's problems; diligently seeks information about infant; follows through on plans involving infant
Interaction with other children	Demonstrates positive interaction with other children in home without aggression or hostility
Caregiver's recreation	Seeks positive outlets for own recreation and relaxation
Parenting role	Expresses satisfaction with parenting role; expresses positive attitudes

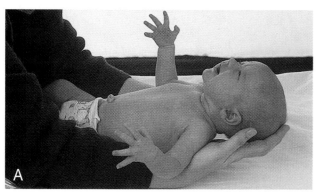
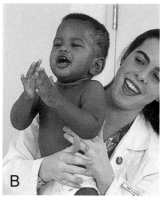

● *Figure 10.4* **(A)** In the early stages of infancy, hand movements are random. **(B)** Later in infancy, hand movements are coordinated and intentional.

acts become clearly intentional (see Fig. 10–4*B*). The infant expects that certain results follow certain actions.

The smiling face looking down is soon connected by the infant with the pleasure of being picked up, fed, or bathed. Anyone who smiles and talks softly to the infant may make that small face light up and cause squirming of anticipation. In only a few weeks, however, the infant learns that one particular person is the main source of comfort and pleasure.

An infant cannot apply abstract reasoning but understands only through the five senses. As the infant matures enough to recognize the mother or primary caregiver, the infant becomes fearful when this person disappears. To the infant, out of sight means out of existence, and the infant cannot tolerate this. For the infant, self-assurance is necessary to confirm that objects and people do not cease to exist when out of sight. This is a learning experience on which the infant's entire attitude toward life depends.

The ancient game of "Peek-a-Boo" is a universal example of this learning technique. It is also one of the joys of infancy as the child affirms the ability to control the disappearance and reappearance of self. In the same manner by which the infant affirms self-existence, the existence of others is confirmed even when temporarily out of sight.

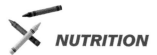

NUTRITION

During the first year of life, the infant's rapid growth creates a need for nutrients greater than at any other time of life. The Academy of Pediatrics Committee on Nutrition has endorsed breast-feeding as the best method of feeding infants.

Most of the infant's requirements for the first 4 to 6 months of life are supplied by either breast milk or commercial infant formulas. Nutrients that may need to be supplemented are vitamins C and D, iron, and fluoride. Breast-fed infants need supplements of iron

as well as vitamin D, which can be supplied as vitamin drops. Most commercial infant formulas are enriched with vitamins C and D. Some infant formulas are fortified with iron. Infants who are fed home-prepared formulas (based on evaporated milk) need supplemental vitamin C and iron; however, evaporated milk has adequate amounts of vitamin D, which is unaffected by heating in the preparation of formula. Vitamin C can be supplied in orange juice or juices fortified with vitamin C.

Fluoride is needed in small amounts (0.25 mg/day) for strengthening calcification of the teeth and preventing tooth decay. A supplement is recommended for breast-fed and commercial formula-fed babies and for those whose home-prepared formulas are made with water that is deficient in fluoride. Vitamin preparations are available combined with fluoride.

Addition of Solid Foods

The time or order requirement for starting foods is not exact. However, at about 4 to 6 months of age the infant's iron supply becomes low and supplements of iron-rich foods are needed. Guidelines for introducing new foods into an infant's diet are provided in Table 10–3.

Infant Feeding

The infant knows only one way to take food: namely, to thrust the tongue forward as if to suck. This is called the **extrusion** (protrusion) **reflex** (Fig. 10–5) and has the effect of pushing solid food out of the infant's mouth. The process of transferring food from the front of the mouth to the throat for swallowing is a complicated skill that must be learned. The eager, hungry baby is puzzled over this new turn of events and is apt to become frustrated and annoyed, protesting loudly and clearly. Taking the edge off the very hungry infant's appetite by giving part of the formula is best before proceeding with this new experience. If the family caregivers understand that pushing food

TABLE 10.3	Suggested Feeding Schedule for the First Year of Life		
Age	**Food Item**	**Amount***	**Rationale**
Birth–6 mo	Human milk or iron-fortified formula	Daily totals 0–1 mo 18–24 oz 1–2 mo 22–28 oz 2–3 mo 25–32 oz 3–4 mo 28–32 oz 4–5 mo 27–39 oz 5–6 mo 27–45 oz	Infants' well-developed sucking and rooting reflexes allow them to take in milk and formula. Infants do not accept semisolid food because their tongues protrude when a spoon is put in their mouths. They cannot transfer food to the back of the mouth. Human milk needs supplementation.
	Water	Not routinely recommended	Small amounts may be offered under special circumstances (eg, hot weather, elevated bilirubin level, or diarrhea).
4–6 mo	*Iron-fortified infant cereal;† begin with rice cereal (delay adding barley, oats, and wheat until 6th mo)	4–8 tbsp after mixing	At this age, there is a decrease of the extrusion reflex, the infant can depress the tongue and transfer semisolid food from a spoon to the back of the pharynx to swallow it.
	*Unsweetened fruit juices;†‡ plain, vitamin C-fortified	2–4 oz	Cereal adds a source of iron and B vitamins; fruit juices introduce a source of vitamin C.
	Dilute juices with equal parts of water		Delay orange, pineapple, grapefruit, or tomato juice until 6th mo.
	Human milk or iron-fortified formula	Daily totals 4–5 mo 27–39 oz 5–6 mo 27–45 oz	Do not offer water as a substitute for formula or breast milk, but rather as a source of additional fluids.
	Water	As desired	
7–8 mo	*Fruits, plain strained; avoid fruit desserts	1–2 tbsp	Teething is beginning; thus, there is an increased ability to bite and chew.
	*Yogurt†		
	*Vegetables,† plain strained; avoid combination meat and vegetable dinners	5–7 tbsp	Vegetables introduce new flavors and textures.
	*Meats,† plain strained; avoid combination or high-protein, dinners	1–2 tbsp	Meat provides additional iron, protein, and B vitamins.
	*Crackers, toast, zwieback†	1 small serving	
	Iron-fortified infant cereal or enriched cream of wheat	4–6 tbsp	
	Fruit juices‡	4 oz	
	Human milk or iron-fortified formula	24–32 oz	Iron-fortified formula or iron supplementation with human milk is still needed because the infant is not consuming significant amounts of meat.
	Water	As desired	May introduce a cup to the infant.
9–10 mo	*Finger foods†—well-cooked, mashed, soft, bite-sized pieces of meat and vegetables	In small servings	Rhythmic biting movements begin; enhance this development with foods that require chewing.
	Iron-fortified infant cereal or enriched cream of wheat	4–6 tbsp	Decrease amounts of mashed foods as amounts of finger foods increase.
	Fruit juices‡	4 oz	
	Fruits	6–8 tbsp	
	Vegetables	6–8 tbsp	
	Meat, fish, poultry, yogurt, cottage cheese	4–6 tbsp	Formula or breast milk consumption may begin to decrease; thus, add other sources of calcium, riboflavin, and protein (eg, cheese, yogurt, and cottage cheese).
	Human milk or iron-fortified formula	24–32 oz	
	Water	As desired	

(table continues on page 180)

TABLE 10.3 (continued)	Suggested Feeding Schedule for the First Year of Life		
Age	Food Item	Amount*	Rationale
11–12 mo	Soft table foods† as follows: Cereal; iron-fortified infant cereal; may introduce dry, unsweetened cereal as a finger food	4–6 tbsp	Motor skills are developing; enhance this development with more finger foods.
	Breads; crackers, toast, zwieback	1 or 2 small servings	Rotary chewing motion develops; thus, child can handle whole foods that require more chewing.
	Fruit juice‡	4 oz	
	Fruit: soft, canned fruits or ripe banana, cut up, peeled raw fruit as the infant approaches 12 mo	½ cup	Infant is relying less on breast milk or formula for nutrients; a proper variety of solid foods (fruits, vegetables, starches, protein sources, and dairy products) will continue to meet the young child's needs.
	Vegetables: soft cooked, cut into bite-sized pieces	½ cup	
	Meats and other protein sources: strips of tender, lean meat, cheese strips, peanut butter	2 oz or ½ cup chopped	Delay peanut butter until 12th month.
	Mashed potatoes, noodles		
	Human milk or iron-fortified infant formula	24–30 oz	
	Water	As desired	

*Amounts listed are daily totals and goals to be achieved gradually. Intake varies depending on the infant's appetite.

†New food items for age group.

(Adapted from Twin Cities District Dietetic Association. *Manual of clinical nutrition,* with permission from its publisher, Chronimed Publishing, 13911 Ridgedale Dr, Minneapolis, MN 55343, 1994 54–56.)

‡The Committee on Nutrition of the American Academy of Pediatrics recommends that fruit juices be introduced when infant can drink from a cup.

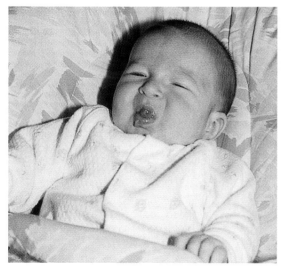

● *Figure 10.5* A baby thrusts the tongue forward using the extrusion reflex. This causes food to be pushed out of the mouth.

out with the tongue does not mean rejection, their patience will be rewarded.

The baby's clothing (and the caregiver's as well) needs protection when the baby is held for a feeding. A small spoon fits the infant's mouth better than a large one and makes it easier to put food further back on the tongue—but not far enough to make the baby gag. If the food is pushed out, the caregiver must catch it and offer it again. The baby soon learns to manipulate the tongue and comes to enjoy this novel way of eating. To avoid the danger of aspiration, the caregiver must quiet an upset or crying baby before proceeding with feeding.

Foods are started in small amounts, 1 or 2 tsp daily. Babies like their food smooth, thin, lukewarm, and bland. The choice of mealtime does not matter. It works best, at first, to offer one new food at a time, allowing 4 or 5 days before introducing another so that the baby becomes accustomed to it. This method also helps determine which food is responsible if the baby has a reaction to a new food.

When teeth start erupting anytime between 4 and 7 months of age, the infant appreciates a piece of zwieback or hard toast to practice chewing. At about 9 or 10 months of age, after a few teeth have erupted, chopped foods can be substituted for pureed foods. Breast milk or formula gradually is replaced with whole milk as the infant learns to drink from a cup. This change takes some time because the infant continues to derive comfort from sucking at the breast or bottle. Infants need fat and should not be given reduced-fat milk (skim, 1%, or 2%).

Preparation of Foods

Various pureed baby foods, chopped junior foods, and prepared milk formulas are available on the market. These products save caregivers much preparation time, but many families cannot afford them. No matter which type of food is used, family caregivers should read food labels carefully to avoid foods that have undesirable additives, especially sugar and salt.

The nurse can point out that vegetables and fruits can be cooked and strained or pureed in a blender and are as acceptable to the baby as commercially prepared baby foods. Baby foods prepared at home should be made from freshly prepared foods, not canned, to avoid commercial additives. Labels of frozen foods used should be checked for added sugar, salt, or other unnecessary ingredients. Excess blended food can be stored in the freezer in ice cube trays for future use. Cereals may be cooked and formulas may be prepared at home as well. Instead of purchasing junior foods, the caregiver can substitute well-cooked, unseasoned table foods that have been mashed or ground.

Preparation and storage of baby food at home require careful sanitary practices. All equipment used in the preparation of the infant's food must be carefully cleaned with hot, soapy water and rinsed thoroughly.

Some families prefer to spend more money for convenience and economize elsewhere, but no one should be made to feel that a baby's health or well-being depends on commercially prepared foods.

The healthy baby's appetite is the best index of the proper amount of food. Healthy babies enjoy eating and accept most foods, but they do not like strongly flavored or bitter foods. If the baby shows a definite dislike for any particular food, forcing it may develop into a battle of wills. A dislike for a certain food is not always permanent, and the rejected food may be offered again later. The important point is to avoid making an issue of likes or dislikes. The caregiver also should avoid introducing any personal attitudes about food preferences.

Self-Feeding

The infant has an overpowering urge to investigate and to learn. At around 7 or 8 months of age, the baby may grab the spoon from the caregiver, examine it, and mouth it. The baby also sticks fingers in the food to feel the texture and to bring it to the mouth for tasting (Fig. 10–6). This is an essential, although messy, part of the learning experience.

After preliminary testing, the infant's next task is to try self-feeding. The baby soon finds that the motions involved in getting a spoon right side up into the mouth are too complex, so fingers become favored over the spoon. However, the infant returns to the spoon again until he or she eventually succeeds in getting some food from spoon to mouth at least part of the time. The nurse can help family caregivers understand that all this is not deliberate messiness to be forbidden but rather a necessary part of the infant's learning.

Weaning the Infant

Weaning, either from the breast or bottle, must be attempted gradually without fuss or strain. The infant is still testing the environment. The abrupt removal of a main source of satisfaction—sucking—before basic distrust of the environment has been conquered may prove detrimental to normal development. The speed with which weaning is accomplished must be suited to each infant's readiness to give up this form of pleasure for a more mature way of life.

At the age of 5 or 6 months, the infant who has watched others drink from a cup usually is ready to try a sip when it is offered. The infant seldom is ready at this point, however, to give up the pleasures of sucking altogether. Forcing the child to give up

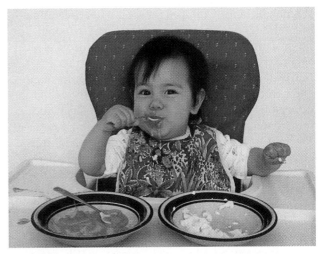

● **Figure 10.6** Eating by yourself is a messy business but so much fun!

sucking creates resistance and suspicion. Letting the infant set the pace is best.

An infant who takes food from a dish and milk from a cup during the day may still be reluctant to give up a bedtime bottle. However, the infant must never be permitted to take a bottle of formula, milk, or juice along to bed. **Pedodontists** (dentists who specialize in the care and treatment of children's teeth) discourage the bedtime bottle because the sugar from formula or sweetened juice coats the infant's teeth for long periods and causes erosion of the enamel on the deciduous teeth, resulting in a condition known as **"bottle mouth"** or **"nursing bottle" caries.** This condition can also occur in infants who sleep with their mother and nurse intermittently throughout the night. In addition to the caries, liquid from milk, formula, or juice can pool in the mouth and flow into the eustachian tube, causing otitis media (ear infection) if the infant falls asleep with the bottle. A bottle of plain water or a pacifier can be used if the infant needs the comfort of sucking at bedtime.

A few babies resist drinking from a cup. Milk needs (calcium, vitamin D) may be met by offering yogurt, custard, cottage cheese, and other milk products until the infant becomes accustomed to the cup. The caregiver should be cautioned not to use honey or corn syrup to sweeten milk because of the danger of botulism, which the infant's system is not strong enough to combat.

During the second half of the first year, the infant's milk consumption alone is not likely to be sufficient to meet caloric, protein, mineral, and vitamin needs.

Women, Infants, Children Food Program

Women, Infants, Children (WIC) is a special supplemental food program for pregnant, breast-feeding, or postpartum women and infants and children as old as 5 years of age. This federal program provides nutritious supplemental foods, nutrition information, and health care referrals. It is available free of charge to persons who are eligible based on financial and nutritional needs and who live in a WIC service area. The family's food stamp benefits or schoolchildren's breakfast and lunch program benefits are unaffected. The foods prescribed by the program include iron-fortified infant formula and cereal, milk, dry beans, peanut butter, cheese, juice, and eggs. These foods may be purchased with vouchers or distributed through clinics. To encourage the use of WIC services, many health care facilities give WIC information to eligible mothers during prenatal visits or at the time of delivery.

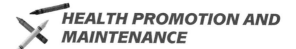

HEALTH PROMOTION AND MAINTENANCE

Routine checkups, immunizations, family teaching, and education about accident prevention are important aspects of health promotion and maintenance. Immunizations and frequent well-baby visits help ensure good health. Family teaching and accident prevention help caregivers provide the best care for their rapidly growing child.

Routine Checkups

During the first year of life, at least six visits to the health care facility are recommended. These are essentially considered well-baby visits and usually occur at 2 weeks, 2 months, 4 months, 6 months, 9 months, and 12 months. During these visits, the nurse collects data regarding the infant's growth and development, nutrition, and sleep, the caregiver-infant relationship, and any potential problems. The infant's

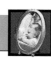

A PERSONAL GLIMPSE

Prepped as we were by those "over-the-counter" baby books, our first out-of-the-hospital visit to the pediatrician seemed daunting beforehead. We had many questions. The staff answered all our questions in a respectful and unhurried way and we felt more at ease. For our second visit, we were less apprehensive. Natty received his immunization shots and all went well. But that night he was unusually fussy and he had a slight fever. We were alarmed. Was this a bad reaction to the immunization? Could he develop a seizure disorder (our neighbor had once told us that her niece developed a seizure disorder after her immunizations)? We knew that we were probably overreacting, but still we worried all night. In the morning, Natty was still sick. We immediately called the doctor's office. The nurse understood our concern and assured us that it is not uncommon for babies to have a slight fever and become irritable after an immunization. We appreciated her support but wished we had known ahead of time. That's one sleepless night we could have done without.

John and Coco

> **LEARNING OPPORTUNITY:** During the child's second visit, what could the nurse have discussed with these parents to prepare them for the common reactions that occurred following this child's immunizations?

weight, height, and head circumference are documented and the infant receives immunizations to guard against disease. Family teaching, particularly for first-time caregivers, is an integral part of health promotion and maintenance.

Immunizations

Every infant is entitled to the best possible protection against disease. Obviously infants cannot take proper precautions, so family caregivers and health professionals must be responsible for them. This care extends beyond the daily needs for food, sleep, cleanliness, love, and security to a concern for the infant's future health and well-being. Protection is available against a number of serious or disabling diseases such as diphtheria, tetanus, pertussis, hepatitis A and B, polio, measles, mumps, German measles (rubella), Varicella (chickenpox), *Haemophilus influenzae* meningitis and pneumococcal disease, making it unnecessary to take chances with a child's health due to inadequate immunization.

Immunization Schedule

The Academy of Pediatrics, through its committee on the control of infectious diseases, has recommended a schedule of immunizations for healthy children living in normal conditions (Table 10–4). Additional recommendations are made for children who live in certain regions and areas or who have certain risk factors. Immunizations should be given within the prescribed timetable unless the child's physical condition makes this impossible. An immunization need not be postponed if the child has a cold but should be postponed if the child has an acute febrile condition or a condition causing immunosuppression or if he or she is receiving corticosteroids, radiation, or antimetabolites.

Side effects vary with the type of immunization. The most common side effect is a fever within the first 24 to 48 hours and possibly a local reaction at the injection site. These reactions are treated symptomatically with acetaminophen for the fever and warm compresses to the injection site.

Many children do not get their initial immunizations in infancy and may not get them until they reach school age, when immunizations are required for school entrance. Health care personnel should make every effort to encourage parents to have their children immunized in infancy to avoid the danger of possible epidemic outbreaks. For instance, measles outbreaks resulting in the deaths of children have been increasing at an alarming rate because of inadequate immunization. Serious illnesses, permanent disability, and deaths from inadequate immunizations are senseless and tragic. Answer any questions the caregiver may have about immunizations. Remember, however, that the caregiver has a right to refuse immunization if he or she has been fully informed about immunizations and any possible reactions. Maintain a nonjudgmental viewpoint throughout the discussion.

INTERNET EXERCISE 10.1

http://www.cdc.gov

Centers for Disease Control
Click on Health Topics A–Z.
Click on Immunization.
Vaccines
Go to: "Are your child's shots up to date?" (children's schedule).
Go to: Childhood Immunization Schedule, click on the current immunization schedule and answer the following questions:

1. What is the date of this Immunization Schedule?

2. Compare the information on this site to Table 10–4. What is the same? What are the differences?

3. Why do you think these changes in the immunization schedule have been made?

Family Teaching

Because mothers are discharged so early after giving birth, every opportunity to perform teaching and promote healthy baby care should be used. Well-baby visits provide an opportunity to ask the caregiver about concerns and to provide teaching. During well visits, offer guidance to help caregivers prepare for the many changes that occur with each developmental level. Discuss normal growth and development milestones but emphasize that these milestones vary from infant to infant. The infant's overall progress is the most important concern, not when he or she accomplishes a given task as compared to another infant or a developmental table. Discuss any infant sleep and activity concerns that the caregiver has. Encourage the caregiver to seek information about any other problems, worries, or anxieties he or she has. Provide ample time and opportunity for the caregivers to ask questions and gain information. A perceptive nurse not only asks if the caregiver has concerns but also suggests possible topics that may need to be reinforced. Some of those topics are discussed here.

Bathing the Infant

A daily bath is unnecessary but is desirable and soothing in very hot weather. Placing the baby into a small tub for a bath rather than giving a sponge bath

TABLE 10.4	Recommended Childhood Immunization Schedule

		Range of recommended ages				Catch-up vaccination			Preadolescent assessment			
Age ▶ Vaccine ▼	Birth	1 mo	2 mos	4 mos	6 mos	12 mos	15 mos	18 mos	24 mos	4–6 yrs	11–12 yrs	13–18 yrs
Hepatitis B	Hep B #1	Hep B #2			Hep B #3					Hep B series		
Diphtheria, Tetanus, Pertussis			DTaP	DTaP	DTaP		DTaP			DTaP	Td	
Haemophilus influenzae Type b			Hib	Hib	Hib	Hib						
Inactivated Polio			IPV	IPV	IPV					IPV		
Measles, Mumps, Rubella						MMR #1				MMR #2	MMR #2	
Varicella						Varicella					Varicella	
Pneumococcal			PCV	PCV	PCV	PCV				PCV	PPV	
Hepatitis A										Hepatitis A series		
Influenza					Influenza (yearly)							

-------------- Vaccines below this line are for selected populations ------

This schedule indicates the recommended ages for routine administration of currently licensed childhood vaccines, as of December 1, 2001, for children through age 18 years. Any dose not given at the recommended age should be given at any subsequent visit when indicated and feasible. Indicates age groups that warrant special effort to administer those vaccines not previously given. Additional vaccines may be licensed and recommended during the year. Licensed combination vaccines may be used whenever any components of the combination are indicated and the vaccine's other components are not contraindicated. Providers should consult the manufacturer's package inserts for detailed recommendations.

Approved by the Advisory Committee on Immunization Practices (www.cdc.gov/nip/acip) the American Academy of Pediatrics (www.aap.org), and the American Academy of Family Physicians (www.aafp.org).

may have a soothing and comforting effect as long as the baby is healthy and has no open skin areas (Fig. 10–7). The small tub or large basin bath is described in the Family Teaching Tips display.

The bathing procedure is essentially the same for the older infant. When old enough to sit and move about freely, the infant may enjoy the regular bathtub, but often this is frightening to him or her. Splashing about in a small tub may be more fun especially with a floating toy. An infant in a tub should always be held securely. If possible, time should be scheduled so that bathing is a leisurely process, a time for the caregiver and baby to enjoy. The procedure for sponge baths is discussed in Chapter 8. As noted in Chapter 8, regular shampooing is important to prevent seborrheic dermatitis (cradle cap), which is caused by a collection of **seborrhea,** yellow crusty patches of lesions on the scalp.

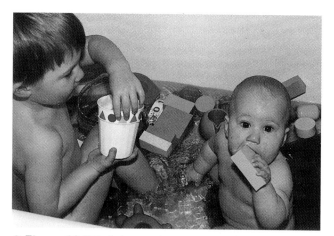

● *Figure 10.7* Bath time can be an enjoyable experience for the infant.

FAMILY TEACHING TIPS

Small Tub Bath

Make sure room is warm and draft-free. Wash hands, put on protective covering, and assemble the following equipment:
- Large basin or small tub
- Mild soap
- Nonsterile protective gloves
- Clean cotton balls
- Soft washcloth
- Large soft towel or small cotton blanket
- Clean diaper and clothes for infant

Fill tub with several inches of warm water (95–100°F [35–37°C]). This is comfortably warm to the elbow. Place basin or tub in crib or other protected surface. *Never* turn from the baby during bathing. *Always* keep at least one hand holding the infant.

PROCEDURE
Wash the infant's head and face at the beginning of the bath, following the procedure for a sponge bath (see Chap. 8). A mild shampoo may be used for the infant over 1 month old, but soap is adequate.

After drying the head, undress the infant and examine for skin rashes or excoriations. Wearing protective gloves, remove diaper and wipe any feces from diaper area.

Place infant in tub and soap the body while supporting infant's head and shoulders on your arm. If infant's skin is dry, soap may be eliminated or a prescribed soap substitute used.

If the baby is enjoying the experience, make it a leisurely one by engaging the infant in talk, paddling in the water, and playing for a few extra minutes. When finished, lift infant from tub, place on dry towel and pat dry with careful attention to folds and creases (underarms, neck, perineal area).

After the bath, gently separate the female infant's labia and cleanse with moistened cotton balls and clean water, wiping from *front to back* to avoid bacterial contamination from the anal region. Circumcised male infants need only be inspected for cleanliness. Uncircumcised males may have the foreskin gently retracted to remove smegma and accumulated debris. The foreskin is gently replaced. Do not force foreskin if not easily retracted, but document and report this occurrence.

Scented or talcum powder should not be used after the bath; powder tends to cake in creases causing irritation and may cause respiratory problems when inhaled by the infant. Scented powders and lotions cause allergic reactions in some babies. In any case, a clean baby has a sweet smell without the use of additional fragrances. Excessively dry skin may benefit from the application of lanolin or A and D Ointment, but oils are believed to block pores and cause infection. Various medicated ointments are available for excoriated skin areas.

After the bath, the baby's fingernails need to be inspected and cut, if long. Otherwise, the baby may scratch his or her face during random arm movements. The nails should be cut straight across with great care. While cutting, hold the arm securely and the hand firmly.

Caring for the Diaper Area

To prevent diaper rash, soiled diapers should be changed frequently. Check every 2 to 4 hours while the infant is awake to see if the diaper is soiled. Waking the baby to change the diaper is not necessary. Cleanse the diaper area with water and a mild soap if needed (see Family Teaching Tips to Prevent Diaper Rash in Chap. 11). Commercial diaper wipes also may be used, but they are an added expense (Fig. 10–8).

Diapers are available in various sizes and shapes. The choice of cloth versus disposable diapers is controversial: disposable diapers have an environmental impact, but cloth diapers are inconvenient and associated with a higher risk of infection. Whatever the type, size, and folding method used, there should be no bunched material between the thighs. Two popular cloth diaper styles are the oblong strip pinned at the sides or the square diaper folded kite-fashion. The latter has the advantage of being useful for different ages and sizes. When folding a cloth diaper for a boy, the excess material is folded in the front; for a girl, it is folded to the back. Safety pins must *always* be closed when they are used to fasten the diaper. When removed, they must be closed and placed out of the infant's reach.

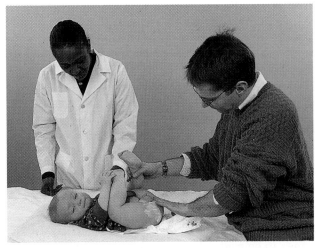

● **Figure 10.8** Noting that the dad has used an overly generous amount of Desitin cream, the nurse takes this opportunity to provide teaching on care of the diaper area.

For the older infant, the diaper must be fastened snugly at the hips and legs to prevent feces from running out the open spaces. Cleaning a soiled crib and a smeared baby once or twice serves as an effective reminder!

Dressing the Infant

Dressing an infant can sometimes create a dilemma especially for the first-time caregiver. Sometimes merely getting clothes on the baby is difficult. For instance, babies tend to spread their hands when the caregiver is trying to put on a top with long sleeves. The easiest way to put an infant's arm into a sleeve is to work the sleeve so that the armhole and the opening are held together, then to reach through the armhole and pull the arm through the opening. Clothing should not bind but should allow freedom of movement and be appropriate for the weather.

One rule of thumb is to dress the infant with the same amount of clothing that the adult finds comfortable. Overdressing in hot weather can cause overheating and prickly heat (miliaria rubra; see Chap. 11). In very hot weather, a diaper may be sufficient. When the infant begins to crawl, long pants help protect the knees from becoming chafed from the rug or flooring. When dressing the infant to go outdoors in cold weather, a head covering is important because infants lose a large amount of heat through their heads. In hot, sunny weather, the infant should not spend much time in the direct sun because the infant's skin is tender and burns easily.

Choosing shoes for the infant can be a problem for the new caregiver. Infants do not need hard-soled shoes; in fact, health care providers often recommend that infants be allowed to go barefoot and wear shoes only to protect them from harsh surfaces. Shoes with stiff soles actually hamper the development of the infant's foot. Sneakers made with a smooth lining with no rough surfaces to irritate the infant's foot are a good choice. They should be durable and flexible and have ample room in the toe. Properly made moccasins also are a good choice. High-topped shoes are unnecessary. Socks should provide plenty of toe room. Shoes should be replaced frequently as the infant's feet grow.

Dental Care

When teething begins in the second half of the first year, the caregiver can start practicing good dental hygiene with the infant. Initially the caregiver can rub the gums and newly erupting teeth with a clean, damp cloth while holding the infant in the lap. This time can be made pleasant by talking or singing to the infant. Brushing the teeth with a small, soft brush usually is not started until several teeth have erupted. Gentle cleansing with plain water is adequate. Tooth-

paste is not recommended at this stage because the infant will swallow too much of it.

Accident Prevention

Discussing safety issues with caregivers is important. Provide information about car safety and childproofing and preventing aspiration, falls, burns, poisoning, and bathing accidents. Remind caregivers that the infant is developing rapidly and safety precautions should stay one step ahead of the infant's developmental abilities. Older children in the family should be taught to be watchful for possible dangers to the infant, and caregivers must be alert to potential dangers that may be introduced by the sibling such as unsafe toys, rough play, or jealous harmful behavior (see Family Teaching Tips: Infant Safety).

FAMILY TEACHING TIPS

Infant Safety

1. The infant should always be placed in an approved infant car carrier when in the car.
2. Crib and playpen bars should be spaced less than 2½ inches apart.
3. Never leave infant unattended on a high surface.
4. Always close safety pins and keep out of infant's reach.
5. Choose toys carefully:
   a. Watch for loose or sharp parts.
   b. Avoid small buttons or parts that can come off and choke infant.
   c. Check for nontoxic material.
5. Never leave infant unattended in a car.
6. Baby proof your home:
   a. Cover unused plugs with plastic covers.
   b. Keep electrical cords out of sight.
   c. Move all toxic substances (cleaning fluids, detergents, insecticides) out of reach and keep them locked up.
   d. Keep small articles (such as buttons and marbles) off the floor and out of infant's reach.
   e. Remove tablecloths or dresser scarves that infant might grasp and pull.
   f. Remove any houseplants that may be poisonous.
   g. Pad sharp corners of low furniture or remove them from infant's living area.
7. Never leave infant alone in the bath.
8. Turn household hot water to a safe temperature— 120°F (48.8°C)—to avoid burns.
9. Protect infant from inhaling lead paint dust (from remodeling) or chewing on surfaces painted with lead paint.
10. Place medicines in locked cupboards; remind family and friends (especially those with grown children or no children) to do the same.
11. Be one step ahead of baby's development and prepared for the next stage.

THE INFANT IN THE HEALTH CARE FACILITY

Hospitalization, however brief, hampers the infant's normal pattern of living. Disruption occurs even if a family caregiver stays with the infant during hospitalization. All or most of the sick infant's energies may be needed to cope with the illness. If given sufficient affection and loving care and if promptly restored to the family, however, the infant is not likely to suffer any serious psychological problems. Long-term hospitalization, though, may present serious problems, even with the best of care.

Illness itself is frustrating; it causes pain and discomfort and limits normal activity, none of which the infant can understand. If the hospital atmosphere is emotionally unresponsive and offers little if any cuddling or rocking, the infant may fail to respond to treatment despite cleanliness and proper hygiene. Touching, rocking, and cuddling a child are essential elements of nursing care (Fig. 10–9).

Hospitalization may have other adverse effects. The small infant matures largely as a result of physical development. If hindered from reaching out and responding to the environment, the infant becomes apathetic and ceases to learn. This situation is particularly apparent when restraints are necessary to keep the child from undoing surgical procedures or dressings or to prevent injury. The child in restraints needs an extra measure of love and attention and the use of every possible method to provide comfort. Spending time, playing music in the room, or encouraging someone to stay with the infant might help to make the infant more comfortable.

Parent-Nurse Relationship

The nurse's relationship with family caregivers is extremely important. The hospitalized infant needs continued stimulation, empathetic care, and loving attention from family caregivers. Encourage caregivers to feed, hold, diaper, and participate in their infant's care as much as they can. Through conscientious use of the nursing process, collect data regarding the needs of the caregivers and the infant and plan care with these needs in mind. Identify and acknowledge the caregivers' apprehensions and develop plans to resolve or eliminate them. Make arrangements for rooming-in for the family caregiver, if possible. Family caregivers often are sensitive to changes in their infant that may help to identify discomfort, pain, or fear. Caregivers may sometimes assist during treatments and other procedures by stroking, talking to, and looking directly at the infant, thus helping to provide comfort during a time of stress. After the procedure, the infant may benefit from rocking, cuddling, singing, stroking, and other comfort measures that the family caregivers may provide. If the family caregivers are unavailable or can spend only limited time with the infant, the nursing staff must meet these emotional needs.

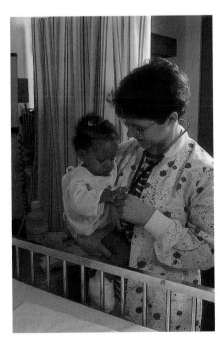

● **Figure 10.9** Holding and cuddling can ease the discomfort and fear of the hospital experience.

KEY POINTS

▶ During the first year of life, the infant grows and develops skills more quickly than at any other time of life.

▶ During the first year of life, the infant progresses from a totally dependent being to one who is ready to "take off and cruise solo."

▶ The infant whose world is secure develops the basic sense of trust that will enable progression to the next stage of development.

▶ The infant's development depends on a mutual relationship with give and take between the infant and the environment. Family caregivers play the most significant role in this interaction.

▶ The infant's nutrition needs are met during the first 4 to 6 months of life by breast milk or formula. Additional vitamins A and C, iron, and fluoride may be needed.

▶ During the second 6 months of life, the infant is introduced to solid foods and learns to drink from a cup.

- Routine immunizations scheduled in the first year of life include those for hepatitis B virus, diphtheria, tetanus, pertussis, *Haemophilus influenzae* type b, polio, and pneumococcal disease. Measles, mumps and rubella, and varicella (chickenpox) vaccines are scheduled between 12 and 18 months of age.
- The nurse has a primary responsibility to provide infant care health teaching during every contact with the caregiver.
- Safety, important in all stages of life, becomes critical as the infant becomes more independent.

BIBLIOGRAPHY

Brazelton TB, Greenspan S. (2001) *The irreducible needs of children: What every child must have to grow, learn, and flourish.* Cambridge, MA: Perseus Publishing.

Craven RF, Hirnle CJ. (1999) *Fundamentals of nursing* (3rd ed). Philadelphia: Lippincott Williams & Wilkins.

Dudek SG. (2000) *Nutrition essentials for nursing practice* (4th ed). Philadelphia: Lippincott Williams & Wilkins.

Halsey NA, Asturias EJ. (1999) Immunization. In *Oski's pediatrics: Principles and practice* (3rd ed). Philadelphia: Lippincott Williams & Wilkins.

Niederhauser V, et. al. (2001) Parental decision-making for the varicella vaccine. *Journal of Pediatric Health Care,* 15(5), 236.

Pillitteri A. (1999) *Maternal and child health nursing* (3rd ed). Philadelphia: Lippincott Williams & Wilkins.

Spock B, et. al. (1998) *Dr. Spock's baby and child care.* New York: Pocket Books.

Wong DL, Perry S, Hockenberry M. (2002) *Maternal child nursing care* (2nd ed). St. Louis: Mosby.

Wong DL, Hess C. (2000) *Wong and Whaley's clinical manual of pediatric nursing* (5th ed). St. Louis: Mosby.

Websites
www.cdc.gov
www.kidshealth.org/parent/growth
www.drspock.com

Workbook

NCLEX-STYLE REVIEW QUESTIONS

1. The nurse would expect an infant who weighs 7 pounds, 2 ounces at birth to weigh approximately how many pounds at 6 months of age?

   a. 10 pounds

   b. 14 pounds

   c. 17 pounds

   d. 21 pounds

2. In caring for a 4-month-old infant, which of the following actions by the infant would the nurse note as appropriate for a 4-month-old infant? The infant

   a. grasps objects with two hands

   b. holds a bottle well

   c. tries to pick up a dropped object

   d. transfers an object from one hand to the other

3. When assisting with a physical exam on an infant, the nurse would expect to find the posterior fontanelle closed by what age?

   a. 3 months

   b. 5 months

   c. 8 months

   d. 10 months

4. In teaching a group of parents of infants, the nurse would teach the caregiver that between 6 and 8 months of age, which of the following teeth usually erupt?

   a. first molars

   b. upper lateral incisors

   c. lower central incisors

   d. cuspid

5. To obtain an accurate heart rate in an infant, which of the following would be the MOST important for the nurse to do?

   a. Take an apical pulse.

   b. Count the pulse rate for 30 seconds.

   c. Use a regular stethoscope.

   d. Check when infant is quiet.

STUDY ACTIVITIES

1. List and compare the fine motor and gross motor skills in each of the following ages:

	4 week old	24 week old	32 week old
Fine motor skills			
Gross motor skills			

2. Answer the following regarding immunizations.

   a. By the time the infant is 1 year old, immunizations will have been given to prevent which diseases?

   b. How many doses of the Hepatitis B vaccine are recommended?

   c. What are the two most common side effects of immunizations? How are these treated?

3. List five safety tips important in the infant stage of growth and development.

CRITICAL THINKING

1. Tony Ricardo brings 6-month-old Essie for a routine checkup. Formulate a plan for the visit. Identify the characteristics to observe during the physical examination, immunizations she will need at this visit (assuming she is up to date), nutritional factors to cover, and other age-appropriate teaching. As you review nutrition with Mr. Ricardo, he states that Essie loves her bedtime bottle. Explain to him your concerns about this practice, and propose a plan to avoid the problems that often result from bedtime bottles.

2. At Nicole's 6-month checkup, her mother tells you that Nicole doesn't like baby food because she spits it out. What will you tell Nicole's mother to help her understand what is happening? What other information about feeding infants will you provide for this mother?

Health Problems of the Infant

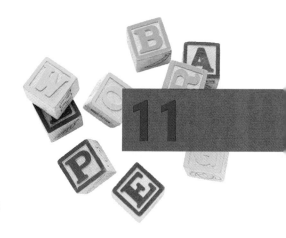

11

SPECIAL NURSING CONSIDERATIONS
PSYCHOLOGICAL PROBLEMS
  Nonorganic Failure to Thrive
  Nursing Process for the Infant with Nonorganic Failure to Thrive
GASTROINTESTINAL DISORDERS
  Malnutrition
  Food Allergies
  Nursing Process for the Nutritionally Deprived Infant
  Diarrhea and Gastroenteritis
  Nursing Process for the Infant with Diarrhea and Gastroenteritis
  Colic
  Pyloric Stenosis
  Nursing Process for the Infant with Pyloric Stenosis
  Congenital Aganglionic Megacolon
  Nursing Process for the Infant Undergoing Surgery for Congenital Megacolon
  Intussusception
CIRCULATORY SYSTEM DISORDERS
  Iron Deficiency Anemia
  Sickle Cell Disease
  Nursing Process for the Child with Sickle Cell Crisis
RESPIRATORY SYSTEM DISORDERS
  Acute Nasopharyngitis (Common Cold)

Otitis Media
Acute Bronchiolitis
Bacterial Pneumonia
Nursing Process for the Infant With a Respiratory Disorder
Sudden Infant Death Syndrome
GENITOURINARY DISORDERS
  Hydrocele
  Cryptorchidism
  Urinary Tract Infections
  Nursing Process for the Child With a Urinary Tract Infection
  Wilms' Tumor (Nephroblastoma)
NERVOUS SYSTEM DISORDERS
  Acute or Nonrecurrent Seizures
  Nursing Process for the Child at Risk for Seizures
  Haemophilus influenzae Meningitis
  Nursing Process for the Child With Meningitis
SKIN AND MUCOUS MEMBRANE DISORDERS
  Miliaria Rubra
  Diaper Rash
  Candidiasis
  Seborrheic Dermatitis
  Impetigo
  Acute Infantile Eczema
  Nursing Process for the Infant/Child With Infantile Eczema

STUDENT OBJECTIVES

On completion of this chapter, the student will be able to

1. Identify seven ways the infant's respiratory system differs from the adult's system.
2. Describe the characteristics of the child with nonorganic failure to thrive.
3. Differentiate between mild diarrhea and severe diarrhea.
4. Identify the symptoms of pyloric stenosis.
5. State another name for congenital megacolon and list its common symptoms.
6. Describe the diagnosis and treatment of intussusception.
7. Identify the common causes of iron deficiency anemia.
8. Explain how (a) sickle cell trait and (b) sickle cell anemia are inherited.
9. Describe the behavior of the infant with acute otitis media.
10. Describe the effect sudden infant death syndrome has on the infant's family.
11. Describe the nursing care specific to a child at high risk for seizures.
12. List four complications of *Haemophilus influenzae* meningitis.
13. Identify the causative organism of thrush.

KEY TERMS

colic
craniotabes
currant jelly stools
febrile seizure
gastroenteritis
invagination
kwashiorkor
lactose
lactose intolerance
marasmus
myringotomy
nuchal rigidity
opisthotonos
orchiopexy
pruritus
purpuric rash
rumination
teratogenicity
urticaria

nfancy is a period of continuing adjustment for the child and the family. The infant is adjusting to physical life outside the uterus and social life within the family. Family members are adjusting to their new roles as parents or siblings and to the presence of this new person in their midst. Although the adjustment is more gradual than the abrupt transition required at birth, it can still involve sufficient physiologic and psychosocial stresses to create health problems during the first year of life.

Three factors that help determine how health problems are manifested in the infant are

1. The pathogenic agent: how virulent the organism or how great the stress
2. The environment: how favorable or unfavorable external conditions are including nutrition and hygiene
3. The infant: his or her resistance to stress and ability to adapt to it and body responses to biological, chemical, and physical injuries.

All three factors need to be considered when planning nursing care for the infant and family.

Remember that even a minor health problem can create great anxiety for concerned caregivers.

Infants can rapidly become very ill often with a high fever (102° to 104° F [38.9° to 40° C] or more). Fortunately with prompt intervention, they usually recover just as quickly. Diagnosis of an infant's health problem is no simple matter, partly because the infant cannot say where it hurts and partly because the clinical manifestations are similar for many different minor or serious disorders.

Most acute health problems result from a respiratory or gastrointestinal (GI) infection or from an uncorrected, even undetected, congenital deviation. Respiratory problems occur more often and with greater severity in infants because of their immature body defenses and small, undeveloped anatomic structures (Fig. 11–1). Sometimes these problems require hospitalization, which interrupts development of the infant-family relationship and the infant's patterns of sleeping, eating, and stimulation. Although the illness may be acute, if recovery is rapid and the hospitalization brief, the infant probably will experience few if any long-term effects. If, however, the condition is chronic or so serious that it requires

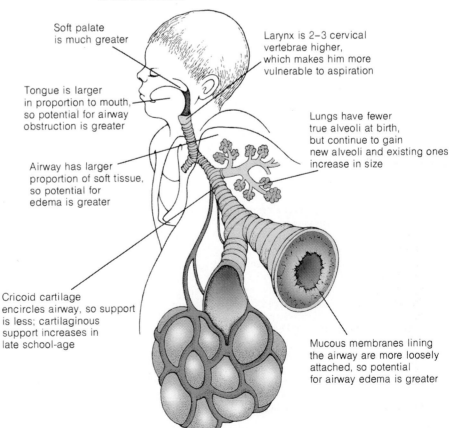

The infant's respiratory system differs from the adult's in that the infant's:

Soft palate is much greater

Larynx is 2–3 cervical vertebrae higher, which makes him more vulnerable to aspiration

Tongue is larger in proportion to mouth, so potential for airway obstruction is greater

Airway has larger proportion of soft tissue, so potential for edema is greater

Lungs have fewer true alveoli at birth, but continue to gain new alveoli and existing ones increase in size

Cricoid cartilage encircles airway, so support is less; cartilaginous support increases in late school-age

Mucous membranes lining the airway are more loosely attached, so potential for airway edema is greater

● *Figure 11.1* The infant or young child is at greater risk than the adult for airway obstruction due to anatomic differences in the respiratory tract. Alveolar damage in infancy is often not permanent, but airway damage remains throughout life.

long-term care, both infant and family may suffer serious consequences.

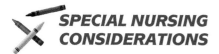

SPECIAL NURSING CONSIDERATIONS

Some special nursing considerations are evident in most nursing plans of care for the ill infant. They include infection control, promotion of normal growth and development, and safety precautions. General nursing diagnoses and interventions are discussed below.

A common nursing diagnosis for the infant with a health problem is *Risk for Infection*. The infant may be especially susceptible to infectious diseases because the immature immune system can easily become weakened. Malnutrition, dehydration, and surgery are typical conditions that place the infant at risk. To protect the infant, the guidelines shown in Box 11–1 should be carefully followed.

Delayed Growth and Development related to inadequate environmental stimulation or a chronic condition is another common nursing diagnosis for the ill infant. In the first weeks and months of life, the infant is developing quickly. Illness can slow this developmental process.

Provide age-appropriate sensory stimulation within the constraints of the infant's condition. Coo to and cuddle the infant, talk to him or her in warm and soft tones, and provide opportunities to fulfill sucking needs. Engage the infant in play. Singing songs, looking at picture books, reading stories, reciting rhymes, playing "Peek-a-Boo," and other activities are strongly recommended. Toys should be introduced that are safe and age-appropriate and that stimulate interest and responsiveness. Balloons are not safe if kept within the infant's reach. Provide family caregivers with information about normal developmental activities appropriate for the infant and encourage them to provide sensory and cognitive stimulation. This approach helps the infant build trust in the caregiver, which is a major developmental task, according to Erikson. It also helps caregivers feel needed and useful.

Risk for Injury related to the infant's developmental age is a nursing diagnosis relevant to the nursing process for all illnesses. Follow safety practices conscientiously. Keep side rails completely up, except when directly attending the infant. Infant seats are recommended instead of high chairs. Never leave equipment within the reach of an infant. Restraints should be used with extreme caution only if necessary to keep the infant or child from interfering with treatments. Teach the family caregivers safety practices and reinforce good safety rules at every opportunity. Always consider these nursing diagnoses when developing a nursing care plan.

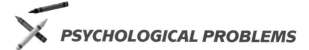

PSYCHOLOGICAL PROBLEMS

Nonorganic Failure to Thrive

Four principal factors are necessary for human growth: food, rest and activity, adequate secretions of hormones, and a satisfactory relationship with a caregiver or nurturing person who provides consistent, loving human contact, and stimulation. Growth is disturbed and development can be delayed when one of these four factors is missing or when the infant has a major birth defect such as congenital heart disease or a metabolic disorder.

Infants who fail to gain weight and who show signs of delayed development are classified as failure-to-thrive infants. Failure to thrive can be divided into two classifications: organic failure to thrive, which is a result of a disease condition, and nonorganic failure to thrive (NFTT), which has no apparent physical cause. The section below discusses NFTT; organic failure to thrive is covered under specific diseases.

Clinical Manifestations

Infants with NFTT are often listless, seriously below average weight and height, have poor muscle tone, a loss of subcutaneous fat, and are immobile for long periods of time (Fig 11–2). They may be unresponsive to (or actually try to avoid) cuddling and vocalization. Examination of the infant is likely to reveal no organic cause for this condition. Examination of the family relationship, particularly the mother-infant relationship, however, often provides important insights into the problem.

BOX 11.1	Guidelines to Prevent Infection

- Follow good handwashing procedures.
- Follow aseptic technique and transmission precautions.
- Teach good handwashing and aseptic techniques to family and all who come in contact with the infant.
- Keep anyone with viral or respiratory infections from contact with the infant.
- Report any signs of systemic infection—for example, fever, pulse or respiratory changes, pain, swelling, tenderness, lethargy, elevated white cell count.
- Observe neurologic signs—for example, nuchal rigidity, irritability, behavior changes.

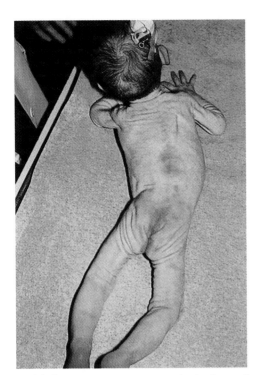

● **Figure 11.2** The child with failure to thrive is often seriously below average weight.

The family relationships of these infants are often so disrupted that there is no warm, close relationship with a family caregiver. For some reason, proper attachment has not occurred. Often the father is absent or emotionally unavailable, adding to the mother's feelings of isolation and inadequacy and leading to an atmosphere of additional stress and conflict.

The problem is not with the caregiver alone or with the infant but instead with their interaction and mutual lack of responsiveness. They are not in harmony. The caregiver does not stimulate the infant; therefore, the infant has no one to respond to and fails to do the "cute baby" things that would gain attention and stimulation. The infant cannot accomplish the developmental task of establishing basic trust.

Infants with NFTT often fall into the classification of "difficult" or irritable babies, but others may be listless and passive and do not seem to care about feedings. A common characteristic is **rumination** (voluntary regurgitation), perhaps as a means of self-satisfaction when the desired response is not received from the caregiver. When rumination occurs, a chain of events is activated that further strains the caregiver-infant relationship. The infant loses weight, sometimes becomes severely emaciated, grows increasingly listless and irritable, and smells "sour" because of frequent vomiting. None of this makes for an attractive baby to love, cuddle, and show off.

Diagnosis

The infant must be thoroughly evaluated by the physician to rule out a systemic or congenital disorder. Signs of deprivation are important elements in the diagnosis. When the infant begins to improve in a nurturing atmosphere, the diagnosis is confirmed.

Treatment

Treatment initially depends almost entirely on good nursing care. By teaching child care skills, acting as a role model, and supporting caregiver-infant interactions, the nurse can help reverse the infant's growth failure and begin an improved caregiver-infant relationship.

Prognosis is uncertain; much depends on the support and counseling the family receives. Long-term care is almost certainly necessary and may require several members of the health care team such as a family therapist, clergy, social worker, and public health nurse. Avoid judgmental, stereotyped feelings when dealing with the family of such an infant. A positive, nonjudgmental attitude on the part of the nurse can have a direct and lasting effect on the family's interaction with their infant.

● Nursing Process for the Infant With Nonorganic Failure to Thrive

ASSESSMENT

Conduct a careful physical exam of the infant including observing skin turgor, anterior fontanelle, signs of emaciation, weight, temperature, apical pulse, respirations, responsiveness, listlessness, and irritability. Observe for rumination or odor of vomitus.

When interviewing the family caregiver, carefully observe the interaction between the caregiver and the infant and note the caregiver's responsiveness to the infant's needs and the infant's response to the caregiver. Listen carefully for underlying problems while talking with the family caregivers. Note if other supportive, involved people are present or if the caregiver is a single parent with no support system. Take a careful history of feeding and sleeping patterns or problems. Determine the caregiver's confidence in handling the infant and note any apparent indication of feelings of stress or inadequacy.

NURSING DIAGNOSES

In caring for the infant with NFTT, the nurse needs to closely interact with the family caregivers, thus nursing diagnoses selected by the healthcare team include those that relate to the family. Careful data collection, assessment, diagnosis, and planning provide for sensory stimulation, adequate food intake (140 cal/kg) for weight gain, and tender loving care for the infant. As the infant becomes less fretful, more responsive, and gains weight, the caregiver will find the infant much more appealing. In addition to the nursing diagnoses identified under special considerations, some nursing diagnoses might include

- Disturbed Sensory Perception related to insufficient nurturing
- Imbalanced Nutrition: Less than Body Requirements related to inadequate intake of calories
- Deficient Fluid Volume related to inadequate oral intake
- Impaired Urinary Elimination related to decreased fluid intake
- Constipation related to dehydration
- Risk for Impaired Skin Integrity related to malnourishment
- Impaired Parenting related to lack of knowledge and confidence in parenting skills

OUTCOME IDENTIFICATION AND PLANNING

The major goals for the NFTT infant focus on improving alertness and responsiveness, increasing caloric and oral fluid intake, maintaining normal urinary and bowel elimination, and maintaining skin integrity. Other goals for the infant and family include improving parenting skills and building parental confidence. The caregiver's participation in the infant's care is essential. Plan individualized nursing according to these goals.

IMPLEMENTATION

Providing Sensory Stimulation. The nurse plays a critical role in reversing the infant's growth failure and improving the caregiver-infant relationship. Providing sensory stimulation is vital in the care of the NFTT infant. Therefore, it is especially important to follow the guidelines detailed in the beginning of this chapter.

Maintaining Adequate Nutrition and Fluid Intake. Feed the infant slowly and carefully in a quiet environment. During feeding, the infant might be closely snuggled and gently rocked. It may be necessary to feed the infant every 2 or 3 hours initially. Burp the infant frequently during and at the end of each feeding, then place him or her on the side with the head slightly elevated or held in a chest-to-chest position. Feed the infant until good eating habits are established. Extra fluids of unsweetened juices are encouraged. If a family caregiver is present, encourage him or her to become involved in the infant's feedings. Demonstrate the importance of talking encouragingly as the baby eats. An older child can sit at a low table facing the feeder while eating. Make the feeding time pleasant and comforting. Carefully document food intake with caloric intake and strict intake and output records.

Monitoring Elimination Patterns. As food and fluids are gradually increased and the infant becomes hydrated, bowel activity and urine production return to normal. Daily stools are of a soft consistency, and the hourly urinary output is 2 to 3 mL/kg.

Promoting Skin Integrity. Protect the infant's skin to prevent irritation. Lanolin or A and D Ointment can be used to lubricate dry skin. Apply the ointment at least once each shift and turn the infant at least every 2 hours.

Providing Family Teaching. While caring for the infant, point out to the caregiver the infant's development and responsiveness, noting and praising any positive parenting behaviors the caregiver displays. The caregiver who has not had a close, warm childhood relationship may not understand the infant's needs for cuddling and stimulation. Teaching about these needs must be done carefully and in a manner that doesn't further damage the caregiver's self-esteem. Many of these family caregivers are overly concerned about spoiling the infant: it is important to dispel these fears. Explain the need for the infant to develop trust, and teach the caregiver about the developmental tasks appropriate for infants. Involve other health care team members as needed.

EVALUATION: GOALS AND OUTCOME CRITERIA

- *Goal:* The infant will be more alert and responsive.
  Criteria: The infant visually follows the caregiver around the room.

- *Goal:* The infant's caloric intake will be adequate for age.
  Criteria: The infant's weight increases at a predetermined goal of 1 oz or more per day.
- *Goal:* The infant will have adequate fluid intake and urine output for age.
  Criteria: The infant's urine output will be 2–3 ml/kg/hr.
- *Goal:* The infant will have normal bowel elimination.
  Criteria: The infant will have a bowel elimination pattern and the stools will be soft.
- *Goal:* The infant's skin integrity will be maintained.
  Criteria: The infant's skin shows no signs of redness or irritation and remains intact.
- *Goal:* The family caregivers will demonstrate positive signs of good parenting.
  Criteria: The family caregivers feed the infant successfully and exhibit an appropriate response to the child.

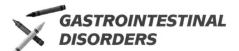

GASTROINTESTINAL DISORDERS

The GI system is responsible for taking in and processing nutrients that nourish all parts of the body. As a result, any problem of the GI system, whether a lack of nutrients, an infectious disease, or a congenital disorder, can quickly affect other parts of the body and ultimately affect general health and growth and development.

Malnutrition

The World Health Organization has widely publicized the malnutrition and hunger that affect more than half the world's population. In the United States, malnutrition contributes to the high death rate of the children of migrant workers and Native Americans. Malnourished children grow at a slower rate, have a higher rate of illness and infection, and have more difficulty concentrating and achieving in school. Appendix D lists foods that are good sources of the nutrients that a child needs for healthy growth.

Protein Malnutrition

Protein malnutrition results from an insufficient intake of high-quality protein or from conditions in which protein absorption is impaired or a loss of protein increases. Clinical evidence of protein malnutrition may not be apparent until the condition is well advanced.

Kwashiorkor results from severe deficiency of protein with an adequate caloric intake. It accounts for most of the malnutrition in the world's children today. The highest incidence is in children 4 months to 5 years of age. The affected child develops a swollen abdomen, edema, and GI changes; the hair is thin and dry with patchy alopecia; and the child becomes apathetic and irritable and has retarded growth with muscle wasting. In untreated patients, mortality rates are 30% or higher. Although strenuous efforts are being made around the world to prevent this condition, its causes are complex.

Traditionally these babies have been breast-fed until the age of 2 or 3 years. The child is weaned abruptly when the next child is born. The term *kwashiorkor* means "the sickness the older baby gets when the new baby comes." The older child is then given the regular family diet, which consists mostly of starchy foods with little meat or vegetable protein. Cow's milk generally is unavailable; in many places where goats are kept, their milk is not considered fit for human consumption (Fig 11–3).

Marasmus is a deficiency in calories as well as protein. The child with marasmus is seriously ill. The condition is common in children in Third World countries because of severe drought conditions. Not enough food is available to supply everyone in these countries, and the children are not fed until adults are fed. The child is severely malnourished and highly susceptible to disease. This syndrome may be seen in the child with NFTT.

Vitamin Deficiency Diseases

Rickets, a disease affecting the growth and calcification of bones, is caused by a lack of vitamin D. The

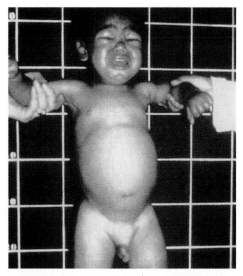

● **Figure 11.3** A child with kwashiorkor often has been abruptly weaned and may have a distended abdomen and muscle wasting.

absorption of calcium and phosphorus is diminished due to the lack of vitamin D, which is needed to regulate the use of these minerals. Early manifestations include **craniotabes** (softening of the occipital bones) and delayed closure of the fontanelles. There is delayed dentition, with defects in tooth enamel and a tendency to develop caries. As the disease advances, thoracic deformities, softening of the shafts of long bones, and spinal and pelvic bone deformities develop. The muscles are poorly developed and lacking in tone, so standing and walking are delayed. Deformities occur during periods of rapid growth. Although rickets itself is not a fatal disease, complications such as tetany, pneumonia, and enteritis are more likely to cause death in children with rickets than in healthy children.

Infants and children require an estimated 400 U of vitamin D daily to prevent rickets. Because a small child living in a temperate climate may not receive sufficient exposure to ultraviolet light, vitamin D is administered orally in the form of fish liver oil or synthetic vitamin. Whole milk and evaporated milk fortified with 400 U of vitamin D per quart are available throughout the United States. Breast-fed infants should receive vitamin D supplements, especially if the mother's intake of vitamin D is poor.

Scurvy is caused by inadequate dietary intake of vitamin C (ascorbic acid). Early inclusion of vitamin C in the diet, in the form of orange or tomato juice or a vitamin preparation, prevents the development of this disease. Febrile diseases seem to increase the need for vitamin C. A variety of fresh vegetables and fruits supply vitamin C for the older infant and child. Because much of the vitamin C content is destroyed by boiling or by exposure to air for long periods, the family caregivers should be taught to cook vegetables with minimal water in a covered pot and to store juices in a tightly covered opaque container. Vegetables cooked in a microwave oven retain more vitamin C because little water is added in the cooking process.

Early clinical manifestations of scurvy are irritability, loss of appetite, and digestive disturbances. A general tenderness in the legs severe enough to cause a pseudoparalysis develops. The infant is apprehensive about being handled and assumes a frog position, with the hips and knees semiflexed and the feet rotated outward. The gums become red and swollen, and hemorrhage occurs in various tissues. Characteristic hemorrhages in the long bones are subperiosteal, especially at the ends of the femur and tibia.

Recovery is rapid with adequate treatment, but death may occur from malnutrition or exhaustion in untreated cases. Treatment consists of therapeutic daily doses of ascorbic acid.

Thiamine is one of the major components of the vitamin B complex. Children whose diets are deficient in thiamine exhibit irritability, listlessness, loss of appetite, and vomiting. A severe lack of thiamine in the diet causes *beriberi*, a disease characterized by cardiac and neurologic symptoms. Beriberi does not occur when balanced diets that include whole grains are eaten.

Riboflavin deficiency usually occurs in association with thiamine and niacin deficiencies. Mainly skin lesions manifest it. The primary source of riboflavin is milk. Riboflavin is destroyed by ultraviolet light; thus opaque milk cartons are best for storage. Whole grains are also a good source of riboflavin.

Niacin insufficiency in the diet causes a disease known as *pellagra*, which presents with GI and neurologic symptoms. Pellagra does not occur in children who ingest adequate whole milk or who eat a well-balanced diet.

Mineral Insufficiency

Iron deficiency results in anemia. This condition is the most common cause of nutritional deficiency in children older than 4 to 6 months of age whose diets lack iron-rich foods. Anemia is often found in poor children younger than 6 years of age in the United States. Iron deficiency anemia is discussed more fully later in this chapter in the section on circulatory system disorders.

Calcium is necessary for bone and tooth formation and is also needed for proper nerve and muscle function. *Hypocalcemia* (insufficient calcium) causes neurologic damage including mental retardation. Rich sources of calcium include milk and milk products. Children with milk allergies are at an increased risk for hypocalcemia.

Food Allergies

The symptoms of food allergies vary from one child to another. Common symptoms are **urticaria** (hives), **pruritus** (itching), stomach pains, and respiratory symptoms. Some of the symptoms may appear quickly after the child has eaten the offending food, but other foods may cause a delayed reaction. Thus the investigation needed to find the cause can be frustrating.

Milk

Milk allergy is the most common food allergy in the young child. Symptoms that may indicate an allergy to milk are diarrhea, vomiting, colic, irritability, respiratory symptoms, or eczema. Infants who are breast-fed for the first 6 months or more may avoid developing milk allergies entirely unless a strong family history of

TABLE 11.1	Some Foods That May Cause Allergies and Possible Sources

Food	Sources
Milk	Yogurt, cheese, ice cream, puddings, butter, hot dogs, foods made with nonfat dry milk, lunch meat, chocolate candies
Eggs	Baked goods, ice cream, puddings, meringues, candies, mayonnaise, salad dressings, custards
Wheat	Breads, baked goods, hot dogs, lunch meats, cereals, cream soups. Oat, rye, and cornmeal products may have wheat added.
Corn	Products made with cornstarch, corn syrup, or vegetable starch; many children's juices, popcorn, cornbreads or muffins, tortillas
Legumes	Soybean products, peanut butter and peanut products
Citrus fruits	Oranges, lemons, limes, grapefruit, gelatins, children's juices, some pediatric suspensions (medications)
Strawberries	Gelatins, some pediatric suspensions
Chocolate	Cocoa, candies, chocolate drinks or desserts, colas

allergies exists. Infants with severe allergic reactions to milk are given commercial formulas that are soybean- or meat-based and formulated to be similar in nutrients to other infant formulas. If the infant has a severe milk allergy, the caregiver must learn to carefully read the labels on prepared foods to avoid lactose or lactic acid ingredients.

Other Food Allergies

Foods should be introduced to the infant one at a time with an interval of 4 or 5 days between each new food. If any GI or respiratory reaction occurs, the food should be eliminated. Among the foods most likely to cause allergic reactions are eggs, wheat, corn, legumes (including peanuts and soybeans), oranges, strawberries, and chocolate (Table 11–1). If a food has been eliminated because of a suspected allergy or reaction, it can be reintroduced at a later time in small amounts to test again for the child's response. This testing should be done in a carefully controlled manner to avoid serious or life-threatening reactions. Many allergies disappear as the child's GI tract matures.

Lactose Intolerance

Congenital lactose intolerance is seen in some infants of African-American, Native American, Eskimo, Asian, and Mediterranean heritage. Infants with **lactose intolerance** cannot digest **lactose,** the primary carbohydrate in milk, because of an inborn deficiency of the enzyme lactase. Symptoms include cramping, abdominal distention, flatus, and diarrhea after ingesting milk. Commercially available formulas such as Isomil, Nursoy, Nutramigen, and Prosobee are made from soybean, meat-based, or protein mixtures and contain no lactose. The infant needs supplemental vitamin D. Yogurt is tolerated by these infants.

● Nursing Process for the Nutritionally Deprived Infant

ASSESSMENT

Carefully interview the family caregiver to determine the underlying cause. If the difficulty lies in the caregiver's inability to give proper care, try to determine if this can be attributed to lack of information, financial problems, indifference, or other reasons. Do not make assumptions until the interview is completed. Cases of malnutrition have been reported in infants of families who believed it was better for their infants to eat vegetables only; this severely limits fat intake, which the infant needs. If food allergies are suspected as the cause of malnourishment, include a careful history of food intake. Obtain a history of stools and voiding from the caregiver.

The physical exam of the infant includes observing skin turgor and skin condition, the anterior fontanelle, signs of emaciation, weight, temperature, apical pulse, respirations, responsiveness, listlessness, and irritability.

NURSING DIAGNOSES

The malnourished infant is often seriously ill. The nursing diagnoses depend on the physical as well as the sociocultural causes of the condition. Some specific nursing diagnoses that may be used include

- Imbalanced Nutrition: Less than Body Requirements related to inadequate intake of nutrients secondary to poor sucking ability, lack of interest in food, lack of adequate food sources, or lack of knowledge of caregiver

- Deficient Fluid Volume related to insufficient fluid intake
- Constipation related to insufficient fluid intake
- Impaired Skin Integrity related to malnourishment
- Deficient Knowledge of caregivers related to understanding of infant nutritional requirements

OUTCOME IDENTIFICATION AND PLANNING

The major goals for the nutritionally deprived infant focus on increasing nutritional intake, improving hydration, monitoring elimination, and maintaining skin integrity. Other goals concentrate on improving caregiver knowledge and understanding of nutrition and facilitating the infant's ability to suck. Even with focused and individualized goals, developing a plan of care for the malnourished infant may be challenging. It may be necessary to try a variety of tactics to feed the child successfully. Include the family caregiver in the plan of care, as this is in the best interest of both the infant and the caregiver.

IMPLEMENTATION

Maintaining Adequate Nutrition. One primary nursing care problem may be persuading the infant to take more nourishment than he or she wants. Inexperienced nurses may find it difficult to persuade an uninterested infant to take formula, and this can become frustrating. Perhaps the nurse's insecurity and uncertainty communicate themselves to the infant in the way he or she handles the child. An experienced nurse may succeed in feeding an infant 3 or 4 oz in a short period, whereas the inexperienced nurse who seems to be going through the same motions persuades the infant to take only 1 oz or less. As the nurse and the infant become accustomed to each other, however, they both relax, and feeding becomes easier. In addition to having a lack of interest, the infant often is weak and debilitated with little strength to suck.

The baby who is held snugly, wrapped closely, and rocked gently finds it easier to relax and take in a little more feeding. An impatient, hurried attitude nearly always communicates tension to the child. Ask for help if the need to attend to other feedings causes tension. Never prop the bottle in the crib.

Gavage feedings or intravenous (IV) fluids may be needed to improve the infant's nutritional status, but it is important for the infant to develop an interest in food and in the process of sucking. A hard or small-holed nipple may completely discourage the infant. The nipple should be soft with holes large enough to allow the formula to drip without pressure. However, it should not be so soft that it offers no resistance and collapses when sucked on. The holes should not be so large that milk pours out, causing the infant to choke. This situation can frustrate a weak infant, who then no longer attempts to nurse.

Scheduling feedings every 2 or 3 hours is best because most weak babies can handle frequent, small feedings better than feedings every 4 hours. With more frequent feedings, promptness is important. Feedings should be limited to 20 to 30 minutes so that the infant does not tire. Demand schedules are not wise because the infant has probably lost the power to regulate the supply-and-demand schedule.

Improving Fluid Intake. Improved nutritional status is evidenced by improved hydration, which is noted by monitoring skin turgor, fontanelle tension, and intake and output. Check the fontanelles each shift and weigh the infant daily in the early morning. Oral mucous membranes should be moist and pink. Intravenous fluids may be needed initially to build up the infant's energy so that he or she can take more oral nourishment and to correct the fluid and electrolyte imbalance. During IV therapy, restraints should be adequate but kept to a minimum. Accurately document intake and output. At least every 2 hours, monitor the IV infusion placement, its patency, and the site for redness and induration. Report any unusual signs immediately.

Monitoring Elimination Patterns. Carefully document intake and output as well as the character, frequency, and amount of stools. Report any unusual characteristics of the stools or urine at once.

Promoting Skin Integrity. Closely observe the skin condition. Use A and D Ointment or lanolin for dry or reddened skin, and promptly change soiled diapers to prevent skin breakdown in weakened infants.

Providing Family Teaching. If malnutrition is related to economic factors or inadequate caregiver knowledge of the infant's needs, teach the family caregivers the essential facts of infant and child nutrition and make referrals for social services. Be alert to the possibility that the caregiver cannot read or understand English, and be certain that the teaching materials used are understood. Simply asking the family caregivers if they have questions is not sufficient to determine if the material has been understood.

Family caregivers may need information regarding assistance in obtaining nutritious food for the infant. Infant formulas and baby food can be expensive, and economic factors may be the actual cause of the infant's malnutrition. A referral to social services or the Women, Infant, Children (WIC) program may be appropriate (see Chap. 10).

EVALUATION: GOALS AND OUTCOME CRITERIA

- *Goal:* The infant's nutritional intake will be adequate for normal growth.
  Criteria: The infant gains 0.75 to 1 oz (22 to 30 g) per day if under 6 months of age and 0.5 to 0.75 oz (13 to 22 g) per day if over 6 months of age.
- *Goal:* The infant will show interest in feedings.
  Criteria: The infant shows evidence of adequate sucking and the ability to extend the amount of time feeding without showing signs of tiring.
- *Goal:* The infant's fluid intake will improve.
  Criteria: The infant's fontanelles are of normal tension, skin turgor is good, mucous membranes are pink and moist.
- *Goal:* The infant's parenteral fluid administration site will remain intact.
  Criteria: The infant's skin at IV infusion site shows no signs of redness or induration.
- *Goal:* The infant's urine and bowel outputs will be normal for age.
  Criteria: The infant's hourly urine output is 2 to 3 ml/kg; stool is soft and of normal character.
- *Goal:* The infant's skin will remain intact.
  Criteria: The infant's skin shows no signs of redness, breakdown.
- *Goal:* The family caregivers will verbalize a beginning knowledge of appropriate nutrition for a growing infant.
  Criteria: The family caregivers state five essential facts about infant nutrition.

Diarrhea and Gastroenteritis

Diarrhea in infants is a fairly common symptom of a variety of conditions. It may be mild with a small amount of dehydration or it may be extremely severe, requiring prompt and effective treatment. Simple diarrhea that does not respond to treatment can quickly turn into severe, life-threatening diarrhea.

Chronically malnourished infants with diarrheal symptoms are a common problem in many areas of the world. This condition is prevalent in areas where adequate clean water and sanitary facilities are lacking. Certain metabolic diseases, such as cystic fibrosis, have diarrhea as a symptom. Diarrhea also may be caused by antibiotic therapy.

Some conditions that cause diarrhea require readjustment of the infant's diet. Allergic reactions to food are not uncommon and can be controlled by avoiding the offending food. Overfeeding as well as underfeeding or an unbalanced diet may also be the cause of diarrhea in an infant. Adjusting the infant's diet, adding less sugar to formula, or reducing bulk or fat in the diet may be necessary.

Many diarrheal disturbances in infants are caused by contaminated food or from human or animal fecal waste through the oral-fecal route. Infectious diarrhea is commonly referred to as **gastroenteritis.** The infectious organisms may be salmonella, *Escherichia coli*, dysentery bacilli, and various viruses, most notably rotaviruses. It is difficult to determine the causative factor in many instances. Because of the seriousness of infectious diarrhea in infants and the danger of spreading diarrhea, the child with moderate or severe diarrhea is often isolated until the causative factor has been proved to be noninfectious.

Clinical Manifestations

Mild diarrhea may present as little more than loose stools; the frequency of defecation may be two to 12 per day. The infant may be irritable and have a loss of appetite. Vomiting and gastric distention are not significant factors, and dehydration is minimal.

Mild or moderate diarrhea can rather quickly become severe diarrhea in an infant. Vomiting usually accompanies the diarrhea; together, they cause large losses of body water and electrolytes. The infant becomes severely dehydrated and is gravely ill. The skin becomes extremely dry and loses its turgor. The fontanelle becomes sunken, and the pulse is weak and rapid. The stools become greenish liquid and may be blood-tinged.

Diagnosis

Stool specimens may be collected for culture and sensitivity testing to determine the causative infectious organism, if there is one; subsequently, effective antibiotics can be prescribed as indicated.

Treatment

Treatment to stop the diarrhea must be initiated immediately. Establishing normal fluid and electrolyte balance is the primary concern in treating gastroenteritis. The infant with acute dehydration may be given oral feedings of commercial electrolyte solutions, such as Pedialyte, Rehydralyte, and Infalyte unless there is shock or severe dehydration. This treatment is called *oral rehydration therapy.* As the diarrhea clears, food may be offered. Once commonly used, the BRAT diet (ripe *b*anana, *r*ice cereal, *a*pplesauce, and *t*oast) has become somewhat controversial because it is high in calories, low in energy and protein, and does not provide adequate nutrition. Salty broths should be avoided. Infants can return to breast-feeding if they have been NPO; formula-fed infants are given their formula. Foods can be added as the infant's condition improves, returning to a regular diet. Early return to the usual diet has been shown to reduce the number of stools and to decrease weight loss and the length of the illness.

In severe diarrhea with shock and severe dehydration, oral feedings are discontinued completely. Fluids to be given IV must be carefully calculated to replace the lost electrolytes. Frequent laboratory determinations of the infant's blood chemistries are necessary to guide the physician in this replacement therapy. For the infant who has had a serious bout of diarrhea, the physician may prescribe soybean formula for a few weeks to avoid a possible reaction to milk proteins.

● Nursing Process for the Infant With Diarrhea and Gastroenteritis

ASSESSMENT

In addition to basic information about the infant, the interview with the family caregiver must include specific information about the history of bowel patterns and the onset of diarrheal stools with details on number and type of stools per day. Suggest terms to describe the color and odor of stools to assist the caregiver with descriptions. Inquire about recent feeding patterns, nausea, and vomiting. Ask the caregiver about fever and other signs of illness in the infant and signs of illness in any other family members.

The physical exam of the infant includes observation of skin turgor and condition including excoriated diaper area, temperature, anterior fontanelle (depressed, normal, or bulging), apical pulse rate (observing for weak pulse), stools (character, frequency, amount, color and presence of blood), irritability,

lethargy, vomiting, urine (amount and concentration), lips and mucous membranes of the mouth (dry, cracked), eyes (bright, glassy, sunken, dark circles), and any other notable physical signs.

NURSING DIAGNOSES

A primary nursing diagnosis is "Diarrhea related to (whatever the cause is)." Other nursing diagnoses vary with the intensity of the diarrhea (mild or severe) as determined by the physical exam and caregiver interview. In addition to the nursing diagnoses suggested earlier in this chapter, some appropriate nursing diagnoses are

- Risk for Infection related to inadequate secondary defenses or insufficient knowledge to avoid exposure to pathogens.
- Impaired Skin Integrity related to constant presence of diarrheal stools
- Deficient Fluid Volume related to diarrheal stools
- Imbalanced Nutrition: Less than Body Requirements related to malabsorption of nutrients
- Hyperthermia related to dehydration
- Risk for Delayed Development related to decreased sucking when infant is NPO
- Compromised Family Coping related to the seriousness of the infant's illness
- Deficient Knowledge of caregivers related to understanding of treatment for diarrhea

OUTCOME IDENTIFICATION AND PLANNING

The major goal for the family with an infant who has diarrhea or gastroenteritis is eliminating the risk of infection transmission. Other important goals for the ill infant include maintaining good skin condition, improving hydration and nutritional intake, and satisfying sucking needs. Plan individualized nursing care according to these goals. Remember that stopping the diarrhea is a vital aspect of nursing care. The family should also be supported and educated regarding the disease and treatment for the infant.

IMPLEMENTATION

Preventing Infection. To prevent the spread of possibly infectious organisms to other pediatric patients, follow standard precautions issued by the Centers for Disease Control. All caregivers must wear gowns and gloves when handling articles contaminated with feces, but masks are unnecessary. Place contaminated linens and clothing in specially marked containers to be processed according to the policy of the health care facility. Place disposable diapers and other disposable items in specially marked bags and dispose of them according to policy. Visitors are limited to family only.

Teach the family caregivers the principles of aseptic technique and observe them to ensure understanding and compliance. Good hand-washing must be carried out and also taught to the family caregivers. Stress that gloves are needed for added protection, but careful hand-washing is also necessary.

Promoting Skin Integrity. To reduce irritation and excoriation of the buttocks and genital area, cleanse those areas frequently and apply a soothing protective preparation such as lanolin or A and D Ointment. Change diapers as quickly as possible after soiling. Some infants may be sensitive to disposable diapers, and others may be sensitive to cloth diapers, so it may be necessary to try both types. Leaving the diaper off and exposing the buttocks and genital area to the air is often helpful. Placing disposable pads under the infant can facilitate easy and frequent changing. Teach caregivers that waterproof diaper covers hold moisture in and do not allow air circulation, which increases irritation and excoriation of the diaper area.

Preventing Dehydration. An infant can dehydrate quickly and can get into serious trouble after less than 3 days of diarrhea. Carefully count diapers and weigh them to determine the infant's output accurately. Closely observe all stools. Document the number and character of the stools, as well as the amount and character of any vomitus.

Maintaining Adequate Nutrition. Weigh the infant daily on the same scale. Take measurements in the early morning before the morning feeding if infant is on oral feedings. Maintain precautions to prevent contamination of equipment while the infant is weighed. Monitor intake and output strictly.

In severe dehydration, IV fluids are given to rest the GI tract, restore hydration, and maintain nutritional requirements. Monitor the placement, patency, and site of the IV infusion at least every 2 hours. The use of restraints, with relevant nursing interventions, may be

necessary. Good mouth care is essential while the infant is NPO.

When oral fluids are started, the infant is given oral replacement solutions such as those listed earlier. After the infant tolerates these solutions, half-strength formula may be introduced. After the infant tolerates this formula for several days, full-strength formula is given (possibly lactose-free or soy formula to avoid disaccharide intolerance or reaction to milk proteins). The breast-fed infant can continue breast-feeding. Give the mother of a breast-fed infant access to a breast pump if her infant is NPO. Breast milk may be frozen for later use, if desired. The infant who is NPO needs to have his or her sucking needs fulfilled. To accomplish this, offer the infant a pacifier.

Maintaining Body Temperature. Monitor vital signs at least every 2 hours if there is fever. Do *not* take the temperature rectally, as insertion of a thermometer into the rectum can cause stimulation of stools as well as trauma and tissue injury to sensitive mucosa. Follow the appropriate procedures for fever reduction, and administer antipyretics and antibiotics as prescribed. Take the temperature with a thermometer that is used only for that infant.

Supporting Family Coping. Being the family caregiver of an infant who has become so ill in such a short time is frightening. Meeting the infant's emotional needs is difficult but very important. Suggest to the caregiver ways that the infant might be consoled without interfering with care. Soothing, gentle stroking of the head, and speaking softly help the infant bear the frustrations of the illness and its treatment. The infant can be picked up and rocked, as long as this can be done without jeopardizing the IV infusion site. If the IV infusion is in a position that may be displaced, this is not permitted. Threading a needle into the small veins of a dehydrated infant is difficult and replacement may be nearly impossible, but the infant's life may depend on receiving the proper parenteral fluids. Help fulfill the infant's emotional needs, and encourage the family caregiver to have some time away from the infant's room without feeling guilty about leaving.

Promoting Family Teaching. Explain to the family caregivers the importance of GI rest for the infant. The family caregivers (especially if young or poorly educated) may not understand the necessity for NPO status. Cooperation of the caregiver is improved with increased understanding. See the Family Teaching Tips on Diarrhea and Vomiting.

EVALUATION: GOALS AND OUTCOME CRITERIA

- *Goal:* The family caregivers will follow infection control measures.
  Criteria: The family caregivers verbalize standard precautions for infection control and follow those measures.
- *Goal:* The infant's skin integrity will be maintained.
  Criteria: The infant's diaper area shows no evidence of redness or excoriation.
- *Goal:* The infant will be well hydrated.
  Criteria: The infant's intake is sufficient to produce hourly urine output of 2 to 3 mL/kg; skin turgor is good; mucous membranes are moist and pink; and fontanelles exhibit normal tension.
- *Goal:* The infant will consume adequate caloric intake.
  Criteria: The infant consumes an age-appropriate amount of full-strength formula or breast milk 3 days after therapy with oral replacement solution.
- *Goal:* The infant will satisfy nonnutritive sucking needs.
  Criteria: The infant uses a pacifier to satisfy sucking needs.
- *Goal:* The infant will maintain a temperature within normal limits.
  Criteria: The infant's temperature is 98.6° to 100° F (37° to 37.8° C).
- *Goal:* The family caregivers anxiety will be reduced.
  Criteria: The family caregivers participate in the care and soothing of the infant.
- *Goal:* The family caregivers will verbalize an understanding of the infant's treatment.
  Criteria: The family caregivers describe three methods to increase hydration and list the warning signs of dehydration.

Colic

Colic consists of recurrent paroxysmal bouts of abdominal pain and is fairly common in young infants. It often disappears around the age of 3 months, but this is small comfort to the caregiver vainly trying to soothe a colicky infant. Although many theories have been proposed, none has been accepted as the causative factor.

FAMILY TEACHING TIPS

Diarrhea

The danger in diarrhea is dehydration (drying out). If the child becomes dehydrated, he or she can become very sick. Increasing the amount of liquid the child drinks is helpful. Solid foods may need to be decreased so the child will drink more.

SUGGESTIONS
1. Give liquids in small amounts (3 or 4 tbsp) about every half hour. If this goes well, increase the amount a little each half hour. Don't force the child to drink, because he or she may vomit.
2. Give solid foods in small amounts. Do not give milk for a day or two, because this can make diarrhea worse.
3. Give only non-salty soups or broths.
4. Liquids recommended for vomiting also may be given for diarrhea.
5. Soft foods to give in small amounts: applesauce, fine chopped or scraped apple without peel, bananas, toast, rice cereal, plain unsalted crackers or cookies, any meats.

CALL THE PHYSICIAN IF
1. Child develops sudden high fever.
2. Stomach pain becomes severe.
3. Diarrhea becomes bloody (more than a streak of blood)
4. Diarrhea becomes more frequent or severe.
5. Child becomes dehydrated (dried out).

SIGNS OF DEHYDRATION
1. Child has not urinated for 6 hours or more.
2. Child has no tears when crying.
3. Child's mouth is dry or sticky to touch.
4. Child's eyes are sunken.
5. Child is less active than usual.
6. Child has dark circles under eyes.

WARNING
Do not use medicines to stop diarrhea for children younger than 6 years of age unless specifically directed by the physician. These medicines can be dangerous if not used properly.

DIAPER AREA SKIN CARE
1. Change diaper as soon as it is soiled.
2. Wash area with mild soap, rinse, and dry well.
3. Use soothing, protective lotion recommended by your physician or hospital.
4. Do not use waterproof diapers or diaper covers; they increase diaper area irritation.
5. Wash hands with soap and water after changing diapers or wiping the child.

Clinical Manifestations and Diagnosis

Attacks occur suddenly, usually late in the day or evening. The infant cries loudly and continuously. The infant appears to be in considerable pain but otherwise seems healthy, nurses or takes formula

FAMILY TEACHING TIPS

Vomiting

Vomiting will usually stop in a couple days and can be treated at home as long as the child is getting some fluids.

WARNING

Some medications used to stop vomiting in older children or adults are dangerous in infants or young children. DO NOT use any medicine unless your physician has told you to use it for *this child.*
Give child clear liquids to drink in small amounts.

SUGGESTIONS

1. Pedialyte, Lytren, Rehydralyte, Infalyte
2. Flat soda (no fizz). Use caffeine-free type; do not use diet soda.
3. Jello water—double the amount of water, let stand to room temperature.
4. Ice popsicles
5. Gatorade
6. Tea
7. Solid Jell-O
8. Broth (not salty)

HOW TO GIVE

Give small amounts often. One tbsp every 20 minutes for the first few hours is a good rule of thumb. If this is kept down without vomiting, increase to 2 tbsp every 20 minutes for the next couple of hours. If there is no vomiting, increase the amount the child may have. If the child vomits, wait for 1 hour before offering more liquids.

FAMILY TEACHING TIPS

Colic

1. Pick up and rock the baby in a rocker or, with baby's tummy down across your knees, swing your legs side to side. (Be sure baby's head is supported.)
2. Walk around the room while rocking baby in your arms or in a front carrier. Hum or sing to baby.
3. Try a bottle, but don't overfeed. Give a pacifier if baby has eaten well within 2 hours.
4. Baby may like the rhythmic movements of a baby swing.
5. Try taking baby outside or for a car ride.
6. When feeding baby, try methods to decrease gas formation: frequent burping, giving smaller feedings more frequently; position baby in infant seat after eating.
7. Try doing something to entertain but not overexcite baby.
8. Gently rub baby's abdomen if it is rigid.
9. Sit with baby resting on your lap with legs toward you; gently move baby's legs in pumping motion.
10. Try putting baby down to sleep in a darkened room.
11. Keep remembering that it's temporary. Try to stay as calm and relaxed as possible.

well, and gains weight as expected. The baby may be momentarily soothed only by rocking or holding but eventually falls asleep, exhausted from crying. The infant with colic is often considered a "difficult" baby.

Differential diagnosis should be made to rule out an allergic reaction to milk or certain foods. Changing to a nonallergenic formula helps determine if there is an allergic factor or if the infant has lactose intolerance. If the baby is breast-fed, the mother's diet should be studied to determine if anything she is eating might be affecting the baby. Intestinal obstruction or infection also must be ruled out.

Treatment and Nursing Care

No single treatment is consistently successful. A number of measures may be employed, one or more of which might work. Medications such as sedatives, antispasmodics, and antiflatulents are sometimes prescribed, but their effectiveness is inconsistent. The family must remember that the condition will pass, even though at the time it seems it will last forever. Family caregivers need to be reassured that their parenting skills are not inadequate. The nurse can

support the family and promote coping skills by providing family teaching. See Family Teaching Tips for Colic.

Pyloric Stenosis

Pyloric stenosis is rarely symptomatic during the first days of life. It has occasionally been recognized shortly after birth, but the average affected infant does not show symptoms until about the third week of life. Symptoms rarely appear after the second month. Although symptoms appear late, pyloric stenosis is classified as a congenital defect. Its cause is unknown, but it occurs more frequently in white males and has a familial tendency.

The pylorus is the muscle that controls the flow of food from the stomach to the duodenum. Pyloric stenosis is characterized by hypertrophy of the circular muscle fibers of the pylorus, with a severe narrowing of its lumen. The pylorus is thickened to as much as twice its size, is elongated, and has a consistency resembling cartilage. As a result of this obstruction at the distal end of the stomach, the stomach becomes dilated (Fig. 11–4).

Clinical Manifestations

During the first weeks of life, the infant with pyloric stenosis often eats well and gains weight, then starts

COMMUNICATIONS BOX 11.1

Conversation with first-time mother of 10-week-old infant with colic:

LESS EFFECTIVE COMMUNICATION	MORE EFFECTIVE COMMUNICATION
Mother: I can't stand it! Joey cries for hours every evening. **Nurse:** Can't figure out what's making him cry? **Mother:** Well, not really; he pulls up his legs and just screams. **Nurse:** He must have colic. Don't let that upset you. A lot of babies have that. **Mother:** It makes me fell helpless. **Nurse:** Don't worry. It will only last a few months and then he'll outgrow it. **Mother:** I'm not sure I can take it. **Nurse:** Oh, it won't last forever; just keep hanging in there.	**Mother:** I can't stand it! Joey cries for hours every evening. **Nurse:** You are really frustrated by Joey's crying. **Mother:** Yeah. I feel like screaming. **Nurse:** It makes you feel like you are losing control, and this is upsetting to you. **Mother:** I just feel like shaking him. **Nurse:** You want to make him stop, but you really don't know what to do. You know that shaking him is dangerous and won't really do any good. **Mother:** That's right. I feel so helpless. What can I do? **Nurse:** Having a baby crying from colic is very upsetting to a parent. I have a handout with tips on caring for a baby with colic. Let me go over it with you. Some of these suggestions may help you cope with Joey's crying.
▶ *During this conversation, the nurse just continues to offer answers without acknowledging the mother's feelings. At the end of the conversation, the mother still feels helpless and perhaps out of control.*	▶ *From the beginning of this conversation, the nurse recognizes the mother's feelings and validates them. The nurse concludes the conversation by telling the mother this is a common problem and provides support by offering her some concrete solutions.*

vomiting occasionally after meals. Within a few days, the vomiting increases in frequency and force, becoming projectile. The vomited material is sour, undigested food; it may contain mucus but never bile, because it has not progressed beyond the stomach.

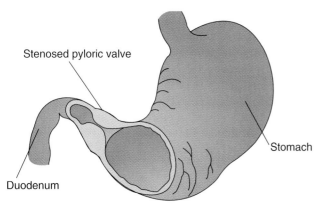

● **Figure 11.4** Pyloric stenosis (narrowed lumen of the pylorus).

Because the obstruction is a mechanical one, the baby does not feel ill, is ravenously hungry, and is eager to try again and again, but the food invariably comes back. As the condition progresses, the baby becomes irritable, loses weight rapidly, and becomes dehydrated. Alkalosis develops from the loss of potassium and hydrochloric acid, and the baby becomes seriously ill.

Constipation becomes progressive because little food gets into the intestine, and urine is scanty. Gastric peristaltic waves passing from left to right across the abdomen usually can be seen during or after feedings.

Diagnosis

Diagnosis is usually made on the clinical evidence. The nature, type, and times of vomiting are documented. When the infant drinks, gastric peristaltic waves are observed. The infant may have a history of weight loss with hunger and irritability. An experienced physician often can feel the olive-sized pyloric mass through deep palpation. Ultrasonographic or radiographic studies with barium swallow show an abnormal retention of barium in the stomach and increased peristalsis.

Treatment

A surgical procedure called a pyloromyotomy (also known as Fredet-Ramstedt operation) is the treatment of choice. This procedure simply splits the hypertrophic pyloric muscle down to the submucosa, allowing the pylorus to expand so that food may pass. Prognosis is excellent if surgery is performed before the infant is severely dehydrated.

● Nursing Process for the Infant With Pyloric Stenosis

ASSESSMENT

When the infant of 1 or 2 months of age has a history of projectile vomiting, pyloric stenosis is suspected. Carefully interview the family caregivers. Ask when the vomiting started and determine the character of the vomiting (undigested formula with no bile, vomitus progressively more projectile). The caregiver will relate a story of a baby who is an eager eater but cannot retain food. Ask the caregiver about constipation and scanty urine.

Physical exam reveals an infant who may show signs of dehydration. Obtain the infant's weight and observe skin turgor and skin condition (including excoriated diaper area), anterior fontanelle (depressed, normal, or bulging), temperature, apical pulse rate (observing for weak pulse and tachycardia), irritability, lethargy, urine (amount and concentration), lips and mucous membranes of the mouth (dry, cracked), and eyes (bright, glassy, sunken, dark circles). Observe for visible gastric peristalsis when the infant is eating. Document and report signs of severe dehydration to help determine the need for fluid and electrolyte replacement.

NURSING DIAGNOSES

The severity of dehydration and malnutrition determines to some extent the appropriate nursing diagnoses for this infant. Some diagnoses that may be used are

Preoperative
- Imbalanced Nutrition: Less than Body Requirements related to inability to retain food

- Deficient Fluid Volume related to frequent vomiting
- Impaired Oral Mucous Membrane related to NPO status
- Risk for Delayed Development related to decreased sucking
- Risk for Impaired Skin Integrity related to fluid and nutritional deficit
- Compromised Family Coping related to seriousness of illness and impending surgery

Postoperative
- Risk for Aspiration related to postoperative vomiting
- Acute Pain related to surgical trauma
- Imbalanced Nutrition: Less than Body Requirements related to postoperative condition
- Risk for Impaired Skin Integrity related to surgical incision
- Compromised Family Coping related to postoperative condition

OUTCOME IDENTIFICATION AND PLANNING: PREOPERATIVE

Preoperatively the major goals for the infant with pyloric stenosis include improving nutrition and hydration, maintaining mouth and skin integrity, comforting infant and relieving family anxiety. Plan individualized nursing care according to these goals including interventions to prepare the infant for surgery.

IMPLEMENTATION: PREOPERATIVE

Maintaining Adequate Nutrition and Fluid Intake. The pylorus is hypertrophied, and food (breast milk or formula) cannot pass through because of the narrow passage from the stomach into the duodenum. As a result, the infant loses weight and becomes dehydrated. If the infant is severely dehydrated and malnourished, IV fluids and electrolytes are necessary for rehydration to prepare for surgery and to correct hypokalemia and alkalosis. Carefully monitor the IV site for redness and induration. Improved skin turgor, weight gain, correction of hypokalemia and alkalosis, adequate intake of fluids, and no evidence of gastric distention are signs of improved nutrition and hydration.

Feedings of formula thickened with infant cereal and fed through a large-holed nipple may be given to improve nutrition before surgery. A smooth muscle relaxant may be ordered before feedings. Feed the infant slowly while he or she is sitting in an infant seat or being held upright. During the feeding, burp the infant frequently to avoid gastric distention. Document the feeding given and the approximate amount retained. Also record the frequency and type of emesis.

The infant must be prepared for surgery. Oral fluids are omitted for a specified time before the procedure, and the infant is placed on an IV infusion. Fluid and electrolyte balance must be restored and the stomach emptied. The physician may order placement of a nasogastric (NG) tube with saline lavage to empty the stomach after the barium swallow. The NG tube is left in place when the infant goes to surgery.

Providing Mouth Care and Nonnutritive Sucking. The infant needs good mouth care because the mucous membranes of the mouth may be dry because of dehydration, and the omission of oral fluids before surgery. A pacifier can satisfy the baby's need for sucking due to the interruption in normal feeding and sucking habits.

Promoting Skin Integrity. Depending on the severity of dehydration, the skin may easily break down and become irritated. The infant is repositioned, the diaper is changed, and lanolin or A and D Ointment is applied to dry skin areas. Intravenous therapy may also affect skin integrity. Closely observe and document the infant's skin condition.

Promoting Family Coping. The family caregivers are anxious because their infant is obviously seriously ill, and when they learn that the infant is to undergo surgery, their apprehensions increase. Include the caregivers in the preparation for surgery and explain

- The importance of added IV fluids preoperatively to improve electrolyte balance and rehydrate the infant
- The reason for ultrasonographic or barium swallow examination
- The function of the NG tube and saline lavage

Explain the location of the pylorus (at the distal end of the stomach) and what happens when the circular muscle fibers hypertrophy. You can liken it to a doughnut that thickens, so that the opening closes and very little food gets through. Describe the surgical procedure to be performed. During the procedure, the muscle is simply split down to, but not through, the submucosa, allowing it to balloon and let food pass.

Direct the family caregivers to the appropriate waiting area during surgery so that the surgeon can find them immediately after surgery. Explain to the caregivers what to expect and about how long the operation will last. Describe the procedure for the post-anesthesia care unit so that the caregivers know the infant will be under close observation postoperatively until fully recovered.

OUTCOME IDENTIFICATION AND PLANNING: POSTOPERATIVE

Postoperatively, the major goals for the infant include keeping airway clear, maintaining comfort, improving nutrition status, preserving skin integrity, and reducing family anxiety. Individualize the nursing plan of care according to these goals.

IMPLEMENTATION: POSTOPERATIVE

Preventing Aspiration. Postoperatively, position the infant on the side and prevent aspiration of mucus or vomitus particularly during the anesthesia recovery period. After fully waking from surgery, the infant may be held by a family caregiver. Help the caregiver find a position that does not interfere with IV infusions and that is comforting to both caregiver and child.

Relieving Pain. The infant's behavior is observed to evaluate discomfort and pain. Excessive crying, restlessness, listlessness, resistance to being held and cuddled, rigidity, and increased pulse and respiratory rates can indicate pain. Administer analgesics as ordered. Nursing interventions that may provide comfort include rocking, holding, cuddling, and offering a pacifier. Include the family caregivers in helping to comfort the infant.

Providing Nutrition. The first feeding, given 4 to 6 hours postoperatively, is usually an electrolyte replacement such as Lytren or Pedialyte. Give feedings slowly in small amounts with frequent burping. Intravenous fluid is necessary until the infant is taking sufficient oral feedings. Continue to use all nursing measures for IV care that were followed preoperatively. Accurate intake and output and daily weight determinations are required.

Promoting Skin Integrity. Closely observe the surgical site for blood, drainage, and secretions.

Make observations at least every 4 hours. Record and report any odor. Care for the incision and dressings as ordered by the physician.

Promoting Family Coping. The family caregivers will be anxious if the infant vomits after surgery, but reassure them that this is not uncommon in the first 24 hours after surgery. The caregivers should be involved in postoperative care. Reassure them that the care they gave at home did not cause the condition. Offer them support and understanding and encourage them in feeding and providing for the infant's needs. They can be told that the likelihood of a satisfactory recovery in a few weeks, with steady progression to complete recovery, is excellent. The operative fatality rate under these conditions has become less than 1%.

EVALUATION: GOALS AND OUTCOME CRITERIA

Preoperative

- *Goal:* The infant's nutritional status will be adequate for normal growth.
  Criteria: The infants weight is maintained.
- *Goal:* The infant will be hydrated.
  Criteria: The infant's skin turgor improves, mucous membranes are moist and pink, and the hourly urine output is 2 to 3 mL/kg.
- *Goal:* The infant's IV infusion site will remain intact.
  Criteria: The infant's skin shows no signs of redness or induration.
- *Goal:* The infant's mucous membranes of the mouth will remain intact.
  Criteria: The infant's mucous membranes are moist and pink and saliva is sufficient, as evidenced by typical drooling.
- *Goal:* The infant's sucking needs will be satisfied.
  Criteria: The infant uses a pacifier sufficiently to meet sucking needs.
- *Goal:* The infant's skin integrity will be maintained.
  Criteria: The infant shows no signs of skin irritation or breakdown.
- *Goal:* The family caregiver anxiety will be reduced.
  Criteria: The family caregivers verbalize an understanding of the procedures and treatments, cooperate with the nursing staff, ask appropriate questions, and express confidence in the treatment plan.

Postoperative

- *Goal:* The infant will not aspirate vomitus or mucus.
  Criteria: The infant rests quietly in a side-lying position without choking or coughing.
- *Goal:* The infant will show signs of being comfortable.
  Criteria: The infant sleeps and rests in a relaxed manner, cuddles with caregivers and nurses, and does not cry excessively.
- *Goal:* The infant's nutrition status and fluid intake will improve.
  Criteria: The infant's daily weight gain is 0.75 to 1 oz (22 to 30 g). Oral fluids are retained with minimal vomiting. Hourly urine output is 2 to 3 mL/kg.
- *Goal:* The infant's skin integrity will be maintained.
  Criteria: The infant's surgical site shows no signs of infection as evidenced by absence of redness, foul odor, or drainage.
- *Goal:* The family caregivers anxiety will be reduced.
  Criteria: The family caregivers are involved in the postoperative feeding of the infant and demonstrate an understanding of feeding technique.

Congenital Aganglionic Megacolon

Congenital aganglionic megacolon, also called Hirschsprung disease, is characterized by persistent constipation resulting from partial or complete intestinal obstruction of mechanical origin. In some cases, the condition may be severe enough to be recognized during the neonatal period; in other cases the blockage may not be diagnosed until later infancy or early childhood.

Parasympathetic nerve cells regulate peristalsis in the intestine. The name *aganglionic megacolon* actually describes the condition because there is an absence of parasympathetic ganglion cells within the muscular wall of the distal colon and the rectum. As a result, the affected portion of the lower bowel has no peristaltic action. Thus, it narrows, and the portion directly proximal to (above) the affected area becomes greatly dilated and filled with feces and gas (Fig. 11–5).

Clinical Manifestations

Accurate reporting of the first meconium stool in the newborn is vital. Failure of the newborn to have a stool in the first 24 hours may indicate a number of conditions, one of which is megacolon. Other

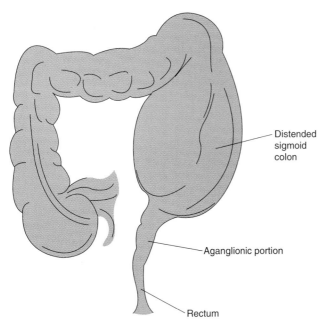

● **Figure 11.5** Dilated colon in Hirschsprung disease.

Distended
sigmoid
colon

Aganglionic portion

Rectum

neonatal symptoms are suggestive of complete or partial intestinal obstruction such as bile-stained emesis and generalized abdominal distention. Gastroenteritis with diarrheal stools may be present, and ulceration of the colon may occur.

The affected older infant or young child has obstinate, severe constipation dating back to early infancy. Stools are ribbon-like or consist of hard pellets. Formed bowel movements do not occur except with the use of enemas, and soiling does not occur. The rectum is usually empty because the impaction occurs above the aganglionic segment.

As the child grows older, the abdomen becomes progressively enlarged and hard. General debilitation and chronic anemia are usually present. Differentiation must be made between this condition and psychogenic megacolon due to coercive toileting or other emotional problems. The child with aganglionic megacolon does not withhold stools or defecate in inappropriate places, and no soiling occurs.

Diagnosis

In the newborn, the absence of a meconium stool within the first 24 hours, and in the older infant or young child, a history of obstinate, severe constipation may indicate the need for further evaluation. Definitive diagnosis is made through barium studies and must be confirmed by rectal biopsy.

Treatment

Treatment involves surgery with the ultimate resection of the aganglionic portion of the bowel. A colostomy is often performed to relieve the obstruc-

tion. This allows the infant to regain any weight lost and also gives the bowel a period of rest to return to a more normal state. Resection is deferred until later in infancy.

● Nursing Process for the Infant Undergoing Surgery for Congenital Megacolon

ASSESSMENT

Carefully gather a history from the family caregivers, noting especially the history of stooling. If the child is not a young infant, ask about the onset of constipation, the character and odor of stools, the frequency of bowel movements, and the presence of poor feeding habits, anorexia, and irritability.

During the physical exam, observe for a distended abdomen and signs of poor nutrition (see the earlier section on the malnourished infant). Record weight and vital signs. Observe the infant for developmental milestones.

NURSING DIAGNOSES

Many of the nursing diagnoses for pyloric stenosis also may be appropriate for congenital megacolon with some adjustment. The following are some specific diagnoses that may apply:

Preoperative
- Constipation related to decreased bowel motility
- Imbalanced Nutrition: Less than Body Requirements related to anorexia
- Fear (in the older child) related to impending surgery
- Compromised Family Coping related to the serious condition of the infant and lack of knowledge about impending surgery

Postoperative
- Risk for Impaired Skin Integrity related to irritation from the colostomy
- Acute Pain related to the surgical procedure
- Deficient Fluid Volume related to postoperative condition
- Impaired Oral and Nasal Mucous Membranes related to NPO status and irritation from NG tube
- Deficient Knowledge of caregivers related to understanding of postoperative care of the colostomy

OUTCOME IDENTIFICATION AND PLANNING: PREOPERATIVE CARE

The preoperative goals for the infant undergoing surgery for congenital megacolon include preventing constipation, improving nutritional status, and relieving fear (in the older child). The major goal for the family is reducing anxiety. Base the preoperative nursing plan of care on these goals. Plan interventions that prepare the infant for surgery.

IMPLEMENTATION: PREOPERATIVE CARE

Preventing Constipation. Decreased bowel motility may lead to constipation, which in turn may result in injury. Enemas may be given to achieve bowel elimination and also before diagnostic and surgical procedures are performed. Administer colonic irrigations with saline solutions. Neomycin or other antibiotic solutions are used to cleanse the bowel and prepare the GI tract. Never administer soapsuds or tap water enemas, because the lack of peristaltic action causes the enemas to be retained and absorbed into the tissues, causing water intoxication. This could cause syncope, shock, or even death after only one or two irrigations.

Maintaining Adequate Nutrition. Parenteral nutrition may be needed to improve nutritional status because the constipation and distended abdomen cause loss of appetite. The infant or child does not want to eat and they have a poor nutritional status. In older children a low residue diet is given.

Reducing Fear. Children who are preschool-age and older are more aware of the approaching surgery and have a number of fears reflective of the developmental stage. Preschoolers are still in the age of magical thinking. They may overhear a word or two that they misinterpret and exaggerate; this can lead to imagined pain and danger. Careful explanations must be provided for the preschooler to reduce any fears about mutilation. Talk about the surgery, reassure the child that the "insides won't come out," and answer questions seriously and sincerely. Encourage family caregivers to stay with the young child if possible to increase the child's feelings of security.

The older school-age child may have a more realistic view of what is going to happen but may still fear the impending surgery. Peer contact may help comfort the school-age child. For more information on reducing preoperative fears and anxiety, see Chapters 4 and 17.

Promoting Family Coping. Family caregivers are apprehensive about the preliminary procedures as well as the impending surgery. Explain all aspects of the preoperative care including examinations, colonic irrigations, and IV fluid therapy. As with other surgical procedures, inform the caregivers about the waiting area, the post-anesthesia care unit, and the approximate length of the operation, and answer any questions. Building good rapport preoperatively is an essential aspect of good nursing care. Answer the family caregivers' questions about the later resection of the aganglionic portion. With successful surgery, these children will grow and develop normally.

OUTCOME IDENTIFICATION AND PLANNING: POSTOPERATIVE CARE

The major postoperative goals for the infant include maintaining skin integrity, preventing intense pain, maintaining fluid intake, and maintaining moist, clean nasal mucous membrane. Goals for the family include reducing caregiver anxiety and preparing for home care of the infant. Develop the individualized nursing plan of care according to these goals.

IMPLEMENTATION: POSTOPERATIVE CARE

Promoting Skin Integrity. Skin integrity of the surgical site, especially around the colostomy stoma, is very important. When routine colostomy care is performed, give careful attention to the area around the colostomy. Record and report redness, irritation, and rashy appearances of the skin around the stoma. Prepare the skin with skin-toughening preparations that strengthen it and provide better adhesion of the appliance.

Relieving Pain. The child may have abdominal pain postoperatively. Observe for signs of pain such as crying, pulse and respiration rate increase, restlessness, guarding of the abdomen, or drawing up the legs. Administer analgesics promptly as ordered. Additional nursing measures that can be used are changing the child's position, holding the child when possible, stroking, cuddling, and engaging in age-appropriate activities. Observe for abdominal distention, which must be documented and reported promptly.

Maintaining Fluid Intake. The NG tube is left in place after surgery and IV fluids are given until bowel function is established. Accurate intake and output determinations and reporting the character, amount, and consistency of stools help determine when the child may have oral feedings. To monitor fluid loss, record and report the drainage from the NG tube every 8 hours. Immediately report any unusual drainage such as bright-red bleeding.

Providing Oral and Nasal Care. Perform good mouth care at least every 4 hours. At the same time, gently clean the nares to relieve any irritation from the NG tube. If the infant is young, sucking needs can be satisfied with a pacifier.

Providing Family Teaching. Show the family caregiver how to care for the colostomy at home. If available, an ostomy nurse may be consulted to help teach the family caregivers. Discuss topics such as devices and their use, daily irrigation, and skin care. The caregivers should demonstrate their understanding by caring for the colostomy under the supervision of nursing personnel several days before discharge. Family caregivers also need referrals to support personnel.

EVALUATION: GOALS AND OUTCOME CRITERIA

Preoperative
- *Goal:* The infant will have adequate bowel elimination and constipation will be avoided.
  Criteria: The infant has bowel elimination daily and the colon is clean and well prepared for surgery.
- *Goal:* The infant's nutritional status will be maintained preoperatively.
  Criteria: The infant ingests diet adequate to maintain weight and promote growth.
- *Goal:* The older child will display minimal fear of bodily injury.
  Criteria: The older child realistically describes what will happen in surgery and interacts with family, peers, and nursing staff in a positive manner.
- *Goal:* The family caregivers will demonstrate an understanding of preoperative procedures.

Criteria: The family caregivers cooperate with care, ask relevant questions, and accurately explain procedures when asked to repeat information.

Postoperative
- *Goal:* The infant's skin integrity will be maintained.
  Criteria: The infant has no skin irritation at the colostomy site; no redness, foul odor, or purulent drainage is noted at the surgical site.
- *Goal:* The infant's behavior will indicate minimal pain.
  Criteria: The infant rests quietly without signs of restlessness; he or she verbalizes comfort if old enough to communicate.
- *Goal:* The infant's fluid intake will be adequate.
  Criteria: The infant's hourly urine output is 2 to 3 mL/kg, indicating adequate hydration.
- *Goal:* The infant's oral and nasal mucous membranes will remain intact.
  Criteria: The infant's oral and nasal mucous membranes are moist and pink; the infant uses a pacifier to meet sucking needs.
- *Goal:* The family caregivers will demonstrate skill and knowledge in caring for the colostomy.
  Criteria: The family caregivers irrigate the colostomy and clean the surrounding skin under the supervision of nursing personnel.

Intussusception

Intussusception is the **invagination,** or telescoping, of one portion of the bowel into a distal portion. It occurs most commonly at the juncture of the ileum and the colon, although it can appear elsewhere in the intestinal tract. The invagination is from above downward, the upper portion slipping over the lower portion and pulling the mesentery along with it (Fig. 11–6).

This condition occurs more often in boys than in girls and is the most common cause of intestinal obstruction in childhood. The highest incidence occurs in infants between the ages of 4 and 10 months. The condition usually appears in healthy babies without any demonstrable cause. Possible contributing factors may be the hyperperistalsis and unusual mobility of the cecum and ileum normally present in early life. Occasionally a lesion such as Meckel's diverticulum or a polyp is present.

Clinical Manifestations
The infant who previously appeared healthy and happy suddenly becomes pale, cries out sharply, and

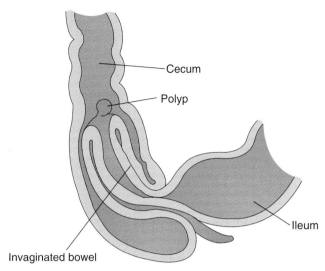

● **Figure 11.6** In this drawing of intussusception, note the telescoping of a portion of the bowel into the distal portion.

Cecum

Polyp

Ileum

Invaginated bowel

draws up the legs in a severe colicky spasm of pain. This spasm may last for several minutes after which the infant relaxes and appears well until the next episode, which may occur 5, 10, or 20 minutes later.

Most of these infants start vomiting early. Vomiting becomes progressively more severe and eventually is bile-stained. The infant strains with each paroxysm, emptying the bowels of fecal contents. The stools consist of blood and mucus, thereby earning the name **currant jelly stools.**

Signs of shock appear quickly and characteristically include a rapid, weak pulse, increased temperature, shallow, grunting respirations, pallor, and marked sweating. Shock, vomiting, and currant jelly stools are the cardinal symptoms of this condition. Because these signs coupled with the paroxysmal pain are quite severe, professional health care is often initiated early.

The nurse, who is often consulted by neighbors, friends, and relatives when things go wrong, needs to be informed and alert; therefore, a word of caution is needed. The nurse needs to be aware that on rare occasions a more chronic form of the condition appears, particularly during an episode of severe diarrheal disturbance. The onset is more gradual and the infant may not show all the classic symptoms, but the danger of sudden, complete strangulation is present. Such an infant should already be in the care of a physician because of the diarrhea.

Diagnosis

The physician usually can make a diagnosis from the clinical symptoms, rectal examination, and palpation of the abdomen during a calm interval when it is soft. A baby is often unwilling to tolerate this palpation, and sedation may be ordered. A sausage-shaped mass can often be felt through the abdominal wall.

Treatment and Nursing Care

Unlike pyloric stenosis, this condition is an emergency in the sense that prolonged delay is dangerous. The telescoped bowel rapidly becomes gangrenous, thus markedly reducing the possibility of a simple reduction. Adequate treatment during the first 12 to 24 hours should have a good outcome with complete recovery. The outcome becomes more uncertain as the bowel deteriorates, making resection necessary.

Immediate treatment consists of IV fluids, NPO status, and a diagnostic barium enema. The barium enema can often reduce the invagination simply by the pressure of the barium fluid pushing against the telescoped portion. The barium enema should not be done if signs of bowel perforation or peritonitis are evident. Abdominal surgery is performed if the barium enema does not correct the problem. Surgery may consist of manual reduction of the invagination or resection with anastomosis, or possible colostomy if the intestine is gangrenous.

If the invagination was reduced, the infant is returned to normal feedings within 24 hours and discharged in about 48 hours. Carefully observe for recurrence during this period. If surgery is necessary, many of the same preoperative and postoperative nursing diagnoses can be used as for congenital aganglionic megacolon.

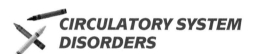

CIRCULATORY SYSTEM DISORDERS

Anemia is a common childhood blood disorder. It may result from inadequate production or excessive loss of red blood cells or hemoglobin. The following are examples of the more common types of anemia found in childhood, but there are many others:

- Inadequate production of erythrocytes or of hemoglobin as in iron deficiency anemia and in anemia of chronic infection
- Excessive loss of red cells, as in hemorrhage
- Hemolytic anemia associated with congenital abnormalities of erythrocytes or hemoglobin as in thalassemia or sickle cell disease
- Hemolytic anemia associated with acquired abnormalities of erythrocytes or hemoglobin from drugs, chemicals, or bacterial reaction

Iron Deficiency Anemia

Iron deficiency anemia is a common nutritional deficiency in young children. It is a hypochromic, microcytic anemia—in other words, the blood cells are deficient in hemoglobin and smaller than normal—

and is common between the ages of 9 and 24 months. The full-term newborn has a high hemoglobin level (needed during fetal life to provide adequate oxygenation) that decreases during the first 2 or 3 months of life. Considerable iron is reclaimed and stored, however, usually in sufficient quantity to last for 4 to 9 months of life.

A child needs to absorb 0.8 to 1.5 mg of iron per day. Because only 10% of dietary iron is absorbed, a diet containing 8 to 10 mg of iron is needed for good health. During the first years of life, obtaining this quantity of iron from food is often difficult for a child. If the diet is inadequate, anemia quickly results. (In addition, adolescent girls may have iron deficiency anemia because of improper dieting to lose weight.)

Babies with an inordinate fondness for milk can take in an astonishing amount and, with their appetites satisfied, show little interest in solid foods. These babies are prime candidates for iron deficiency anemia. They may have a history of consuming 2 or 3 quarts of milk daily while not accepting any other foods or at best only foods with a high carbohydrate content. Many caregivers believe, incorrectly, that milk is a perfect food and that they should let the baby have all the milk desired. These infants are commonly known as milk babies. They have pale, almost translucent (porcelain-like) skin, and are chubby and susceptible to infections.

Many children with iron deficiency anemia, however, are undernourished because of the family's economic problems. Along with the economic factor, a caregiver knowledge deficit about nutrition is often present. The WIC program, discussed in Chapter 10, does much to alleviate this problem.

Clinical Manifestations

The signs of iron deficiency anemia include below-average body weight, pale mucous membranes, anorexia, growth retardation, and listlessness, in addition to the characteristics of milk babies described earlier.

Diagnosis

In blood tests that measure hemoglobin, a level lower than 11 g/dL or a hematocrit lower than 33% is highly suspect. Stool is tested for occult blood to rule out low GI bleeding as a cause for the depleted hemoglobin and hematocrit.

Treatment and Nursing Care

Treatment consists of improved nutrition with ferrous sulfate administered between meals with juice (preferably orange juice, because vitamin C aids in iron absorption). For best results, iron should not be given with meals. To prevent staining, teach the family caregivers to brush the child's teeth after administering ferrous sulfate. Tell the caregivers that ferrous sulfate can cause constipation or turn the child's stools black.

A few children have a hemoglobin level so low or anorexia so acute that they need additional therapy. An iron/dextran mixture for intramuscular use (Imferon) is administered. This medication should be administered in the vastus lateralis by the Z-track method to avoid leakage into the subcutaneous tissues because of its irritating nature. For infants who are seriously ill, refer to the nursing process for the nutritionally deprived infant.

For most infants with iron deficiency anemia, teaching for home care is needed. When teaching caregivers, remember that attitudes and food choices are often influenced by cultural differences. See Family Teaching Tips: Iron Deficiency Anemia.

Sickle Cell Disease

Sickle cell disease is a hereditary trait occurring most commonly in blacks. It is characterized by the production of abnormal hemoglobin that causes the red blood cells to assume a sickle shape. It appears as an

FAMILY TEACHING TIPS

Iron Deficiency Anemia

FOODS HIGH IN IRON

1. One of the most important things you can do for your baby and family is to learn about the foods that will help them stay healthy.
2. Milk is good for your baby, but no more than a quart a day (four 8-oz bottles).
3. Shop for baby cereals fortified with iron.
4. Some baby formulas are iron-fortified.
5. Egg yolks are rich in iron. Avoid egg whites for young babies because of allergies.
6. Green leafy vegetables are good sources of iron.
7. Dried beans, dried peas, canned refried beans, and peanut butter provide good iron sources for toddlers and older children.
8. Fruits that are iron-rich include peaches, prune juice, and raisins (don't give to child younger than 3 years of age because of danger of choking).
9. For older children, fortified instant oatmeal and cream of wheat are good sources of iron.
10. Read labels to check for iron content of processed foods.
11. Organ meat, poultry, and fish are good iron sources.
12. Orange juice helps the body absorb iron.
13. Liquid iron preparations should be taken through a straw to prevent staining of teeth.

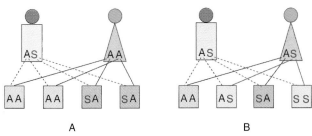

● *Figure 11.7* Inheritance patterns. **(A)** Heterozygous type. One parent carries a hemoglobin S gene, and one does not. Two children will be free of the gene (AA), and two will be carriers (AS). **(B)** Homozygous type. Each parent is carrying one hemoglobin A gene and one hemoglobin S gene. One child is free of the gene (AA), two are carriers (AS), and one has sickle cell disease (SS).

asymptomatic trait when the sickling trait is inherited from one parent alone (heterozygous state). There is a 50% probability that each child born to one parent carrying the sickle cell trait will inherit the trait from that parent. When the trait is inherited from both parents (homozygous state), the child has sickle cell disease, and anemia develops (Fig. 11–7). A rapid breakdown of red blood cells carrying hemoglobin S, the abnormal hemoglobin, causes a severe hemolytic anemia. Persons who inherit the gene for the sickle cell trait from only one parent are asymptomatic with normal hemoglobin levels and red blood cell counts.

The sickling trait occurs in about 10% of African-Americans; there is a much higher incidence in parts of Africa. In African-Americans, the disease itself, sickle cell anemia, has an incidence of 0.3% to 1.3%. The tendency to sickle can be demonstrated by a laboratory test.

Clinical Manifestations

Clinical symptoms of the disease usually do not appear before the latter half of the first year of life because sufficient fetal hemoglobin is still present to prevent sickling. Sickle cell disease causes a chronic anemia with a hemoglobin level of 6 to 9 g/dL (the normal level in an infant is 11 to 15 g/dL). The chronic anemia causes the child to be tired and have a poor appetite and pale mucous membranes.

Sickle cell crisis is the most severe manifestation of the condition. Normal red blood cells, which carry oxygen to the tissues, are disc-shaped and normally move through the blood vessels while bending and flexing to flow through smoothly. The smooth, uniform shape of the red blood cells and the low viscosity (thickness) of the blood is such that these cells split relatively easily at Y-intersections and go single file through the capillaries with little or no clustering. The affected red blood cells (hemoglobin S) do much the same thing until an episode

causes sickling. An episode (sickle cell crises) can be precipitated by low oxygen levels, which can be caused by a respiratory infection or extremely strenuous exercise, dehydration, acidosis, or stress. When sickling occurs, the affected red blood cells become crescent-shaped and, therefore, do not slip through as easily as do the disc-shaped cells. The viscosity of the blood increases (becomes thicker), causing slowdown and sludging of the red blood cells. The impaired circulation results in tissue damage and infarction.

A sickle cell crisis may be the first clinical manifestation of the disease and may recur frequently during early childhood. This disturbance presents a variety of symptoms. The most common symptom is severe, acute abdominal pain (caused by sludging, which leads to enlargement of the spleen) together with muscle spasm, fever, and severe leg pain that may be muscular, osseous (bony), or localized in the joints that become hot and swollen. The abdomen becomes boardlike with an absence of bowel sounds. This makes it extremely difficult to distinguish the condition from an abdominal condition requiring surgery. Several days after a crisis, the child will be jaundiced, evidenced by yellow sclera as a result of the hemolysis. The crisis may have a fatal outcome caused by cerebral, cardiac, or hemolytic complications.

Diagnosis

Screening for the presence of hemoglobin S may be done with a test called Sickledex, a finger stick screening test that gives results in 3 minutes. Definite diagnosis is made through hemoglobin electrophoresis ("fingerprinting"). If the Sickledex screening results are positive, diagnosis can be done to determine if the child is carrying the trait or has sickle cell disease.

Treatment

Prevention of crises is the goal between episodes. Adequate hydration is vital; fluid intake of 1,500 to 2,000 mL daily is desirable for a child weighing 20 kg and should be increased to 3,000 mL during the crisis. Extremely strenuous activities that may cause oxygen depletion are to be avoided. These children should also avoid visiting areas of high altitude. Small blood transfusions help bring the hemoglobin to a near-normal level temporarily. Iron preparations have no effect in sickle cell disease.

Treatment for a crisis is supportive for each presenting symptom, and bed rest is indicated. Oxygen may be administered. Analgesics are given for pain. Dehydration and acidosis are vigorously treated. Prognosis is guarded, depending on the severity of the disease.

● Nursing Process for the Child With Sickle Cell Crisis

ASSESSMENT

The parents who have a child with sickle cell disease may suffer a great deal of guilt for having passed the disease to their child. Take care not to increase this guilt, but help them cope with it. During the interview with the family caregivers, ask about activities or events that led to this crisis, obtain a history of the child's health and any previous episodes, and evaluate the caregivers' knowledge about the condition.

Data collection techniques vary somewhat depending on the child's age. Record vital signs particularly noting fever, abdominal pain, presence of bowel sounds, pain or swelling and warmth in the joints, and muscle spasms. Observe the young child for dactylitis (hand-foot syndrome), which results from soft-tissue swelling caused by interference with circulation. This swelling further impairs circulation.

NURSING DIAGNOSES

Nursing diagnoses vary somewhat with the child's age and the stage of advancement of the disease. Some diagnoses that may be used, in addition to those suggested early in this chapter, are
* Acute Pain related to disease condition affecting abdominal organs or joints and muscles
* Deficient Fluid Volume related to low fluid intake, impaired renal function, or both
* Activity Intolerance related to oxygen depletion and pain
* Impaired Physical Mobility related to muscle and joint involvement
* Risk for Impaired Skin Integrity related to altered circulation
* Compromised Family Coping related to child's condition
* Deficient Knowledge of caregivers related to understanding of disorder and appropriate care measures

OUTCOME IDENTIFICATION AND PLANNING

Maintaining comfort and relieving pain, increasing fluid intake, and conserving energy are major goals for the child with sickle cell disease. Other goals include improving physical mobility, maintaining skin integrity, and reducing the caregivers' anxiety. Another important goal is decreasing the number of future episodes by increasing the caregiver's knowledge about the causes of crisis episodes. Plan individualized nursing care according to these goals.

IMPLEMENTATION

Relieving Pain. The child in sickle cell crisis often has severe pain. Enlargement of the spleen (splenomegaly) causes severe abdominal pain. Joint and muscle pain are also common due to poor perfusion of the tissues. Monitoring the child's pain level, nursing measures to relieve pain, and prompt administration of analgesics are essential. The family caregivers can be involved, if they wish, in helping administer comfort measures to the child. Sometimes diverting activities can help alleviate perceived pain, but be assured that these children are in pain and need analgesics promptly.

Maintaining Fluid Intake. The child is prone to dehydration because of the kidney's inability to concentrate urine. Observe for signs of dehydration such as dry mucous membranes, weight loss, or, in the case of infants, sunken fontanelles. Strict intake and output measurements and daily weights are necessary. In sickle cell crisis, urine specific gravity is not a good indicator of dehydration. Teach the family caregivers that fluid intake is important, and intake should be maintained at 1,500 to 2,000 mL when the child is not in crisis. Offer the child appealing fluids such as juices, popsicles, noncaffeinated soda, and favorite flavored gelatins. Teach family caregivers that increasing fluid intake as the child ages will help to avoid a crisis during the child's activities such as hiking, swimming, and sports. The child also needs increased fluids during episodes of infections.

Promoting Energy Conservation. The child may become dyspneic doing any kind of activity. Plan nursing care so that the child is disturbed as little as possible and can rest. Bed rest is necessary to decrease the demands on oxygen supply. Oxygen may be administered by mask or nasal cannula to improve tissue perfusion.

Improving Physical Mobility. Sickling that affects the muscles and joints causes a great deal of pain for the child. The child needs careful handling and should be moved slowly and gently. Joints can be supported with pillows.

Warm soaks and massages may help relieve some of the discomfort. Administer analgesics before exercise and as needed. Passive exercises help prevent contractures and wasting of muscles.

Promoting Skin Integrity. Increased fluid intake and improved nutrition are important. Observe the child's skin regularly each shift and provide good skin care consisting of lotion, massage, and skin-toughening agents especially over bony prominences. Additional padding in the form of foam protectors and egg-crate pads or mattresses may be helpful where there is irritation from bedding.

Promoting Family Coping. Guilt plays an important part in the anxiety that the family caregivers experience. Explain procedures, planned treatments, and care to help the caregivers feel that they are being included in the care. Caregivers need to feel that they have some control over the disease.

Providing Family Teaching. Teach measures that may help alleviate pain or encourage fluid intake. Also emphasize the importance of protecting the child from situations that may cause over exhaustion or that may otherwise deplete the child's oxygen supplies or lead to dehydration. This knowledge may give the family caregivers a feeling of control. In addition, caregivers may need more information concerning the disorder. If the child has been previously diagnosed, the caregivers should already have had information presented to them. In this instance, determine their knowledge level and supplement and reinforce that information.

EVALUATION: GOALS AND OUTCOME CRITERIA

- *Goal:* The child's pain will be reduced or eliminated.
  Criteria: The child rests quietly and, if possible, reports his or her comfort.
- *Goal:* The child's fluid intake will improve.
  Criteria: The child has an intake of at least 3,000 mL/day.
- *Goal:* The child's energy will be conserved.
  Criteria: The child's activities are restricted to conserve energy. The oxygen saturation is greater than 90%.
- *Goal:* The child's muscles and joints will remain flexible.

  Criteria: The child cooperates with daily passive exercises.
- *Goal:* The child's skin integrity will be maintained.
  Criteria: The child's skin shows no signs of redness, irritation, or breakdown.
- *Goal:* The family caregivers' anxiety will be reduced.
  Criteria: The family caregivers are more self-confident and cooperate with nursing personnel.
- *Goal:* The family caregivers express understanding of disease process.
  Criteria: The family caregivers verbalize an understanding of the disease process and state ways to prevent a crisis from occurring.

INTERNET EXERCISES 11.1

http://www.emory.edu/PEDS/SICKLE

The Sickle Cell Information Center
Go to section entitled "How May We Serve You."
Click on "Patients and Families Online Resources."

1. What are some of the topics available that you might share with your peers?

2. What are some of the topics available that you might suggest to a family who has a child with sickle cell anemia?

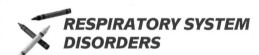

RESPIRATORY SYSTEM DISORDERS

Acute Nasopharyngitis (Common Cold)

The common cold is one of the most common infectious conditions of childhood. The young infant is as susceptible as the older child but is generally not as frequently exposed.

The illness is of viral origin such as rhinoviruses, respiratory syncytial virus (RSV), influenza virus, parainfluenza virus, or adenovirus. Bacterial invasion of the tissues may cause complications such as ear, mastoid, and lung infections. The young child appears to be more susceptible to complications than an adult. The infant should be protected from people who have colds because complications in the infant can be serious.

Clinical Manifestations

The infant older than the age of 3 months usually develops fever early in the course of the infection, often as high as 102° to 104° F (38.9° to 40° C).

Younger infants usually are afebrile. The infant sneezes and becomes irritable and restless. The congested nasal passages interfere with nursing, increasing the infant's irritability. The infant may have vomiting or diarrhea, which may be caused by mucous drainage into the digestive system.

Diagnosis

This nasopharyngeal condition may appear as the first symptom of many childhood contagious diseases, such as measles, and must be observed carefully. The common cold also needs to be differentiated from allergic rhinitis.

Treatment

The child with an uncomplicated cold may not need any treatment in addition to rest, increased fluids and adequate nutrition, normal saline nose drops, suction with a bulb syringe, and a humidified environment. In the older child, acetaminophen can be administered as an analgesic and antipyretic. Aspirin is best avoided. If the nares or upper lip become irritated, cold cream or petrolatum (Vaseline) can be used. The infant needs to be comforted by holding, rocking, and soothing. If the symptoms persist for several days, the child must be seen by a physician to rule out complications such as otitis media.

Otitis Media

Otitis media is one of the most common infectious diseases of childhood. Two out of three children have at least one episode of otitis media by the time they are 1 year old.[1] The eustachian tube in an infant is shorter and wider than in the older child or adult (Fig. 11–8). The tube is also straighter, thereby allowing nasopharyngeal secretions to enter the middle ear more easily. *Haemophilus influenzae* is an important causative agent of otitis media in infants.

Clinical Manifestations

A restless infant who repeatedly shakes the head and rubs or pulls at one ear should be checked for an ear infection. These behaviors often indicate that the infant is having pain in the ears. Symptoms include fever, irritability, and hearing impairment. Vomiting or diarrhea may occur.

Diagnosis

Examination of the ear with an otoscope is done in the infant by pulling the ear down and back to straighten the ear canal. In the older child the ear is pulled up and back. The exam reveals a bright-red, bulging eardrum in otitis media. Spontaneous rupture of the eardrum may occur, in which case there will be purulent drainage, and the pain caused

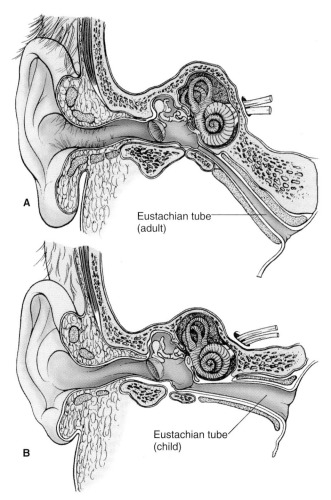

● *Figure 11.8* Comparison of the eustachian tube in the adult (**A**) and the infant (**B**).

by the pressure build-up in the ear will be relieved. If present, purulent drainage is cultured to determine the causative organism and appropriate antibiotic.

Treatment

Antibiotics are used during the period of infection and for several days following to prevent mastoiditis or chronic infection. A 10-day course of amoxicillin is a common treatment. Most infants respond well to antibiotics.

Some infants and young children have repeated episodes of otitis media. Children with chronic otitis media may be put on a prophylactic course of an oral penicillin or sulfonamide drug. **Myringotomy** (incision of the eardrum) may be performed to establish drainage and to insert tiny tubes into the tympanic membrane to facilitate drainage. In most cases, the tubes eventually fall out spontaneously. Attention to chronic otitis media is essential because permanent hearing loss can result from frequent occurrences.

Mastoiditis (infection of the mastoid sinus) is a possible complication of untreated acute otitis media. Mastoiditis was much more common before the advent of antibiotics. Currently it is seen only in children who have an untreated ruptured eardrum or inadequate treatment (through noncompliance of caregivers or improper care) of an acute episode.

Most infants and young children with otitis media are cared for at home; therefore, a primary responsibility of the nurse is to teach the family caregivers about prevention and the care of the child (see Family Teaching Tips: Otitis Media).

Acute Bronchiolitis

Acute bronchiolitis (acute interstitial pneumonia) is most common during the first 6 months of life and is rarely seen after the age of 2 years. Most cases occur in infants who have been in contact with older children or adults with upper respiratory viral infections. It usually occurs in the winter and early spring.

Acute bronchiolitis is caused by a viral infection. The causative agent in more than 50% of cases has been shown to be RSV. Other viruses associated with the disease are parainfluenza virus, adenoviruses, and other viruses not always identified.

The bronchi and bronchioles become plugged with thick, viscid mucus, causing air to be trapped in the lungs. The infant can breathe air in but has difficulty expelling it. This hinders the exchange of gases, and cyanosis appears.

Clinical Manifestations

The onset of dyspnea is abrupt, sometimes preceded by a cough or nasal discharge. There are a dry and persistent cough, extremely shallow respirations, air hunger, and often marked cyanosis. Suprasternal and subcostal retractions are present. The chest becomes barrel-shaped from the trapped air. Respirations are 60 to 80 breaths per minute.

Fever is not extreme, seldom higher than 101° to 102° F (38.3° to 38.9° C). Dehydration may become a serious factor if competent care is not given. The infant appears apprehensive, irritable, and restless.

Diagnosis

Diagnosis is made from clinical findings and can be confirmed by laboratory testing (enzyme-linked immunosorbent assay) of the mucus obtained by direct nasal aspiration or nasopharyngeal washing.

Treatment

The infant is usually hospitalized and treated with high humidity by mist tent (see Chap. 6, Figure 6–8), rest, and increased fluids. Oxygen may be adminis-

FAMILY TEACHING TIPS

Otitis Media

The eustachian is a connection between the nasal passages and the middle ear. The eustachian tube is wider, shorter, and straighter in the infant, allowing organisms from respiratory infections to travel into the middle ear to cause infection (otitis media).

PREVENTION
1. Hold infant in an upright position or with head slightly elevated while feeding to prevent formula from draining into the middle ear through the wide eustachian tube.
2. Never prop a bottle.
3. Do not give infant a bottle in bed. This allows fluid to pool in the middle ear, encouraging organisms to grow.
4. Protect infant from exposure to others with upper respiratory infections.
5. Protect infant from passive smoke; don't permit smoking in baby's presence.
6. Remove sources of allergies from home.
7. Observe for clues to ear infection: shaking head, rubbing or pulling at ears, fever, combined with restlessness or screaming and crying.
8. Be alert to signs of hearing difficulty in toddlers and preschoolers. This may be the first sign of an ear infection.
9. Teach toddler or preschooler gentle nose blowing.

CARE OF CHILD WITH OTITIS MEDIA
1. Have child with upper respiratory infection who shows symptoms of ear discomfort checked by a health care professional.
2. Complete the entire amount of antibiotic prescribed, even though the child seems better.
3. Heat (such as a heating pad on low setting) may provide comfort, but an adult must stay with the child.
4. Soothe, rock, and comfort child to help relieve discomfort. The child is more comfortable sleeping on side of infected ear.
5. Give pain medications (such as acetaminophen) as directed. Never give aspirin.
6. Provide liquid or soft foods; chewing causes pain.
7. Hearing loss may last up to 6 months after infection.
8. Follow-up with hearing test should be scheduled as advised.

tered in addition to the mist tent. Monitoring of oxygenation may be done by means of capillary gases or pulse oximetry. Antibiotics are not prescribed because the causative organism is a virus. Intravenous fluids often are administered to ensure an adequate intake and to permit the infant to rest. The hospitalized infant is placed on contact transmission precautions to prevent the spread of infection.

Ribavirin (Virazole) is an antiviral drug that may be used to treat certain infants with RSV. It is administered as an inhalant by hood, mask, or tent. The American Academy of Pediatrics states that the use of ribavirin must be limited to infants at high risk for severe or complicated RSV such as infants with chronic lung disease, premature infants, transplant recipients, and infants receiving chemotherapy. Ribavirin is classified as a category X drug, signifying a high risk for **teratogenicity** (causing damage to a fetus). Health care personnel and others may inhale the mist that escapes into the room, so women who might be pregnant should stay out of the room where ribavirin is being administered.

Bacterial Pneumonia

Pneumococcal pneumonia is the most common form of bacterial pneumonia in infants and children. Its incidence has decreased during the last several years. This disease occurs mainly during the late winter and early spring, principally in children younger than 4 years of age.

In the infant, pneumococcal pneumonia is generally of the bronchial type rather than the lobar type seen in older children. It is usually secondary to an upper respiratory viral infection. The most common finding in infants is a patchy infiltration of one or several lobes of the lung. Pleural effusion is often present.

H influenzae pneumonia also occurs in infants and young children. Its clinical manifestations are similar to those of pneumococcal pneumonia, but its onset is more insidious, its clinical course is longer and less acute, and it is usually seen in the lobe of the lung. Complications in the young infant are common—usually bacteremia, pericarditis, and empyema (pus in the lungs). The treatment is the same. Immunization with *H influenzae* type B conjugate vaccine (Hib) is currently recommended beginning at 2 months of age.

Clinical Manifestations

The onset of the pneumonic process is usually abrupt, following a mild upper respiratory illness. Temperature increases rapidly to 103° to 105° F (39.4° to 40.6° C). Respiratory distress is marked with obvious air hunger, flaring of the nostrils, circumoral cyanosis, and chest retractions. Tachycardia and tachypnea are present with a pulse rate frequently as high as 140 to 180 beats per minute and respirations as high as 80 breaths per minute.

Generalized convulsions may occur during the period of high fever. Cough may not be noticeable at the onset but may appear later. Abdominal distention due to swallowed air or paralytic ileus commonly occurs.

Diagnosis

Diagnosis is made based on clinical symptoms, chest radiograph, and culture of the organism from secretions. The white blood cell count may be elevated. The antistreptolysin titer (ASO titer) is usually elevated in children with staphylococcal pneumonia.

Treatment

The use of antibiotics early in the disease gives a prompt and favorable response. Penicillin or ampicillin has proved to be the most effective treatment and is generally used unless the infant has a penicillin allergy. Oxygen started early in the disease process is important. Infants are sometimes placed in a croupette or mist tent. The use of mist tents without constant observation is considered unsafe by some nurses. Children have become cyanotic in mist tents, with subsequent arrest, due to the difficulty seeing the child; therefore, a mask or hood is thought to be the better choice. Intravenous fluids are often necessary to supply the needed amount of fluids. Prognosis for recovery is excellent.

A PERSONAL GLIMPSE

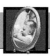

The first time I put Bobbie in the hospital it was very scary. I knew the nurses, but still I was afraid for him. I felt like someone was punishing me. I couldn't leave him for a minute. I was afraid he wouldn't be alive when I came back. I was also afraid he would be frightened. He was so small he needed me to protect him, but I couldn't help him. We were in the hospital every couple of weeks. He would get better then have another attack. It got to the point where I would call the doctor and say that Bobbie was having another attack and they would just send us to admitting. After a few times, I got used to caring for him in the hospital. The nurses taught me how to keep his tent humidified and I could just take care of it myself. Finally I was able to go back to work during the day and care for him on my breaks and time off. It was very difficult each and every time, but we adjusted to hospital life. Although I was afraid for him, I knew he was a fighter and I had to be too. I feel this experience made him a stronger person. He is now 8 years old and has had no severe attacks since he was about 2 years old. He has had a few mild attacks but it doesn't affect him or myself.

Tracee

> **LEARNING OPPORTUNITY:** Give specific examples of what the nurse could do to support this mother and to help decrease the fear she had when her child was hospitalized.

● Nursing Process for the Infant With a Respiratory Disorder

ASSESSMENT

Conduct a thorough interview with the caregiver including the standard information as well as specific information such as when the caregiver first noticed the symptoms; the course of the fever thus far; the caregiver's description of respiratory difficulties; how well the infant was taking nourishment and fluids; nausea; vomiting; urinary and bowel output; and history of exposure to other family members with respiratory infections.

Conduct a physical exam including measurement of temperature, apical pulse, respirations (rate, respiratory effort, retractions [costal, intercostal, sternal, suprasternal, substernal], and flaring of nares). Also note breath sounds (crackles, wheezing), cough (dry, productive, hacking), irritability, restlessness, skin color (pallor, cyanosis), circumoral (around the mouth) cyanosis, skin turgor, anterior fontanelle (depressed or bulging), nasal passage congestion (color, consistency), mucous membranes (mouth dry, lips dry or cracked), and eyes (bright, glassy, sunken, moist, crusted).

NURSING DIAGNOSES

Nursing diagnoses are based on the interview with the family caregivers and the physical findings and should be reasonable and realistic. Some nursing diagnoses that may be used for the infant with a respiratory condition are

- Impaired Gas Exchange related to inflammatory process
- Ineffective Airway Clearance related to nasal and chest congestion and obstructed airway
- Hyperthermia related to infection process
- Imbalanced Nutrition: Less than Body Requirements related to inability to nurse, suck, or swallow adequately with congested nasal passages
- Activity Intolerance related to inadequate gas exchange
- Risk for further infection related to location and anatomic structure of the eustachian tubes
- Compromised Family Coping related to child's illness

OUTCOME IDENTIFICATION AND PLANNING

The major goals for the infant with a respiratory disorder include maintaining respiratory function, maintaining body temperature, adequate nutrition and fluid intake, conserving energy, preventing otitis media, and reducing family anxiety. Plan nursing plan care according to these goals and the infant's status.

The infant may need to be placed on respiratory precautions according to the policy of the health care facility to prevent nosocomial spread of infection. Many infants with a respiratory condition need to be placed in a croupette or mist tent. Plan additional nursing interventions for the infant in a mist tent. If IV fluids are ordered, interventions that promote tissue and skin integrity are needed. To ensure that the infant does not interfere with the IV infusion site, it may be necessary to prepare restraints. Intravenous administration and the use of restraints are discussed in Chapter 6.

IMPLEMENTATION

Monitoring Respiratory Function. Monitor respirations by observing for tachypnea and retractions and listening to breath sounds at least every 4 hours. If deep retractions are noted, make observations more frequently. Oxygen saturation may be monitored by pulse oximeter. Oxygen can be administered by hood or mist tent if the physician desires, especially in cases of pneumococcal pneumonia.

Maintaining Airway Clearance. A moisturized atmosphere is provided with an ice-cooled mist tent or cool vaporizer. The moisturized air helps thin the mucus in the respiratory tract to ease respirations. Suction or clear secretions as needed to keep the airway open. Position the child to provide maximum ventilation. Use pillows and padding to maintain the infant's position. Observe frequently for slumping, which causes crowding of the infant's diaphragm. Avoid use of constricting clothes and bedding. Stuffed toys are not recommended in mist tents, as they become saturated and provide an environment in which organisms flourish.

Maintaining Body Temperature. Monitor the infant's temperature frequently, at least every 2 hours if it is higher than 101.3° F (38.58 C). If the infant has a fever, remove excess clothing and covering. Antipyretic medications may be ordered.

Maintaining Adequate Nutrition and Fluid Intake. Clear the infant's nasal passages with a bulb syringe. Be certain to clear the passages immediately before feeding. Administer normal saline nose drops to thin secretions about 10 to 15 minutes before feedings and at bedtime. Feed the infant slowly allowing frequent stops with suctioning during feeding as needed. Avoid overtiring the infant during feeding. Offer juices and water appropriate for the infant's age between meals. Use a relatively small-holed nipple so that the infant does not choke, but be careful not to make the infant work too hard. Maintain accurate intake and output measurements. Observe the infant for dehydration: Skin turgor, anterior fontanelle, and urine output are good indicators. Maintain diaper counts and weigh diapers to determine the amount of urine output (1 mL urine weighs 1 g).

The infant may be so exhausted by respiratory effort that IV fluids are necessary. Observe patency, placement, site integrity, and flow rate at least hourly.

Promoting Energy Conservation. During an acute stage, allow the infant to rest as much as possible. Plan work so that rest and sleep are interrupted no more than necessary. See Nursing Care Plan: The Infant With Respiratory Infection.

Preventing Otitis Media. Turn the infant from side to side every hour so that mucus is less likely to drain into the eustachian tubes. An infant seat may help facilitate breathing and prevent the complication of otitis media. Observe the infant for irritability, shaking of the head, or pulling at the ears. Do not give the infant a bottle while he or she is lying in bed. The best position for feeding is upright to avoid excessive drainage into the eustachian tubes.

Promoting Family Coping. Family caregivers need teaching and reassurance. Talk to the caregivers while working with the infant, explaining what is happening and why. Explain equipment and treatments to caregivers so that their questions (both spoken and unspoken) are answered. Actively listen to caregivers and use communication skills to respond to their worries. Teach the family caregivers

- To clear the nasal passage with a bulb syringe
- To feed the infant slowly and allow the infant to nurse without tiring; burp frequently to prompt infant to expel swallowed air
- The importance of a croup tent and the need to leave the infant in it except for feedings and bathing (unless otherwise indicated)
- How to soothe the infant in the tent
- The need for respiratory precautions and good handwashing technique
- The importance of extra fluids for the infant
- The desirability of using a humidifier at home after discharge
- How to clean a humidifier properly
- The importance of preventing people who have infections from visiting the infant

EVALUATION: GOALS AND OUTCOME CRITERIA

- *Goal:* The infant's respiratory function will be normal.
  Criteria: The infant's respiratory rate is 25 to 35/min, regular, with breath sounds clear; the infant no longer uses respiratory accessory muscles to aid in breathing.
- *Goal:* The infant's airway will remain patent.
  Criteria: The infant's mucous secretions are thin and scant; airway remains clear.
- *Goal:* The infant will maintain a temperature within normal limits.
  Criteria: The infant's temperature is 98.6° to 100° F (37° to 37.8° C).
- *Goal:* The infant will have an adequate intake.
  Criteria: The infant consumes an amount of oral nutrition appropriate for age with no signs of tiring; skin turgor is good; fontanelles are of normal tension; and hourly urine output is 2 to 3 mL/kg.
- *Goal:* The infant's energy will be conserved.
  Criteria: The infant has extended periods of uninterrupted rest and tolerates increased activity.
- *Goal:* The infant will be free from complications of otitis media.
  Criteria: The infant shows no signs of ear pain such as irritability, shaking of the head, and pulling on the ears.
- *Goal:* The family caregivers' anxiety will be reduced.
  Criteria: The family caregivers verbalize methods to care for the infant with a respiratory disorder.

NURSING CARE PLAN

The Infant With Respiratory Infection

CW, a 6-month-old infant with a respiratory infection, has been brought to the hospital from the doctor's office by his mother. He has a copious amount of thick nasal discharge and has rapid, shallow respirations with substernal and intercostal retractions. His temperature is 101.5°F (39.1°C). His young mother appears very anxious.

NURSING DIAGNOSIS
Ineffective Airway Clearance related to infectious process

GOAL: *The infant's respiratory function will improve and airway will be patent.*

OUTCOME CRITERIA
• The infant no longer uses respiratory accessory muscles to aid in breathing.
• The infant's breath sounds are clear and respirations are regular.
• Mucous secretions become thin and scant; nasal passages are clear.

NURSING INTERVENTIONS	*RATIONALE*
Provide moist atmosphere by placing him in ice-cooled mist tent.	Moisture helps liquefy and thin secretions for easier respirations.
Keep nasal passages clear, using bulb syringe.	Open passages increase air flow.
Monitor respiratory function by observing for retractions, respiratory rate, and listening to breath sounds at least every 4 hours. Monitor more frequently if tachypnea or deep retractions are noted.	Changes in the infant's breathing may be early indicators of respiratory distress.
Monitor infant's bedding and clothing every 4 hours.	Clothing and bedding can become very wet from mist. Dry clothing and bedding helps to prevent chilling.

NURSING DIAGNOSIS
Imbalanced Nutrition: Less than Body Requirements related to inability to suck or swallow because of congested nasal passages or fatigue from difficulty breathing

GOAL: *The infant will have adequate food and fluid intake to maintain normal growth and development.*

OUTCOME CRITERIA
• The infant has an adequate caloric intake as evidenced by appropriate weight gain of 1 oz or more a day.
• The infant is able to suck and swallow easily without tiring.
• Skin turgor returns to normal.

NURSING INTERVENTIONS	*RATIONALE*
Clear nasal passages immediately before feeding. Teach family caregiver to use bulb syringe.	Infants are obligatory nasal breathers. Clearing eases infant's breathing to permit adequate feeding. Family caregiver can use this technique at home as needed.
Administer normal saline nose drops before feedings and at bedtime.	Normal saline nose drops help thin mucous secretions.
Weigh infant daily in morning before first feeding.	Infant will maintain weight with gain of 1 to 2 oz a day.

NURSING DIAGNOSIS
Risk for further infection (Otitis Media) related to current respiratory infection and the size and location of infant's eustachian tube

GOAL: *The infant will remain free from further infection and complications of Otitis Media.*

OUTCOME CRITERIA
• The infant shows no signs of ear pain such as irritability, shaking head, pulling on ears.

NURSING INTERVENTIONS	*RATIONALE*
Change infant's position, turning from side to side every hour.	Turning infant prevents mucus from pooling in the eustachian tubes.

nursing care plan continues on page 222

NURSING CARE PLAN continued

The Infant With Respiratory Infection

CW, a 6-month-old infant with a respiratory infection, has been brought to the hospital from the doctor's office by his mother. He has a copious amount of thick nasal discharge and has rapid, shallow respirations with substernal and intercostal retractions. His temperature is 101.5°F (39.1°C). His young mother appears very anxious.

NURSING INTERVENTIONS	RATIONALE
Feed infant in upright position.	Improves drainage and helps open nasal passages.
Observe for irritability, shaking of head, or pulling at ears.	Early recognition of signs of otitis media promotes early diagnosis and treatment.

NURSING DIAGNOSIS
Compromised Family Coping related to infant's illness

GOAL: *The caregiver's anxiety will be reduced.*

OUTCOME CRITERIA
• The family caregivers verbalize understanding of infant's condition and treatments.
• The family caregivers reflect confidence in the staff evidenced by cooperation and appropriate questions.

NURSING INTERVENTIONS	RATIONALE
Actively listen to caregivers' concern.	Family members gain confidence when they feel their concerns are being heard.
Provide reassurance and explain what you are doing and why you are doing it when working with infant.	Understanding the disease and treatment methods helps family to feel that infant's illness is under control.
Involve caregivers in caring for infant. Teach techniques of care that can be used at home.	Family caregivers feel valued and benefit from nursing care tips that they can use at home.

Sudden Infant Death Syndrome

Sudden infant death syndrome (SIDS) has caused much grief and anxiety among many families for centuries. One of the leading causes of infant mortality worldwide, SIDS claims an estimated 2,500 lives annually in the United States alone. Although this is a dramatic drop in incidence of deaths over the past 20 years, it is still the leading cause of death in infants between 7 and 365 days.[2]

Throughout history, this syndrome has presented a most exasperating problem. Commonly called "crib death," it is the sudden, unexpected death of an apparently healthy infant in whom the postmortem fails to reveal an adequate cause. The term SIDS is not a diagnosis, but rather a description of a syndrome.

Varying theories have been suggested about the cause of SIDS. In ancient writings, it was attributed to "overlaying" by the infant's mother or nurse. The adult supposedly rolled over onto the infant during sleep. This cause was eventually ruled out particularly because many affected infants were alone in their cribs when they ceased breathing. Over the years much research has been done but no single cause has been identified; physicians can neither prevent nor predict the event.

Infants who die of SIDS are usually 2 to 4 months of age, although some deaths have occurred during the first and second weeks of life. Few infants older than 6 months of age die of SIDS. It is a greater threat to low-birth weight infants than to term infants. It occurs more often in winter and affects more male infants than female infants as well as more infants from minority and lower socioeconomic groups. Babies born to mothers younger than 20 years of age, infants who are not firstborn, and infants whose mothers smoked during pregnancy also have been found to be at greater risk. Research has revealed that a greater number of infants with SIDS have been sleeping in a prone (face down) position than in a supine (lying on the back with face up) position. As a result of these studies, the American Academy of Pediatrics recommends that infants must *not* be placed in a prone position to sleep. Infants must be placed in a supine position until they are 6 months old.

Sudden infant death syndrome is rapid and silent. Previous studies had suggested that nighttime was the peak time of death, but recent studies reveal that about half the attacks occur during the day. The history reveals that no cry has been heard nor is there any evidence of a struggle. People who have been sleeping nearby claim to have heard nothing unusual before the death was discovered. It is not uncommon for the infant to have been recently examined by a physician and found to be in excellent health. The autopsy often reveals a mild respiratory disorder, but nothing considered serious enough to have caused the death.

Emergency personnel must be observant for clues that may indicate child abuse, but they must be careful not to cast any suspicion on the family caregivers. The guilt feelings of the caregivers are overwhelming, and any suggestion from medical personnel that the cause of death is questionable is inexcusable and may be more than the caregivers can handle.

A closely related syndrome is apparent life-threatening events (ALTE). These are episodes in which the infant is found in distress but, when quickly stimulated, recovers with no lasting problems. These were formerly called "near-miss SIDS." These infants are placed on home apnea monitors. The apnea monitor is set to sound an alarm if the infant has not taken a breath within a given number of seconds. Family caregivers are taught infant cardiopulmonary resuscitation so that they can respond quickly if the alarm sounds. Infants who have had an episode of ALTE are at risk for additional episodes and may be at risk for SIDS. Infants are usually kept on home apnea monitors until they are 1 year old. This is a stressful time for the family because someone who is trained in infant cardiopulmonary resuscitation must be with the infant at all times (Fig. 11–9).

Emotional Support for Caregivers and Families

The effects of SIDS on caregivers and families are devastating. Grief is coupled with guilt, even though SIDS cannot be predicted or prevented. Disbelief, hostility, and anger are common reactions that families exhibit. An autopsy must be done and the results promptly made known to the family. Even though the family caregivers are told that they are not to blame for the infant's death, it is difficult for most caregivers not to keep searching for evidence of some possible neglect on their part. Prolonged depression usually follows the initial shock and anguish over the infant's death.

The immediate response of the emergency department staff should be to allow the family to express their grief, encouraging them to say goodbye

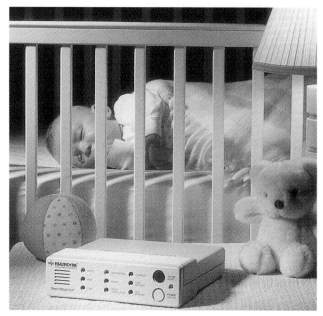

● *Figure 11.9* An apnea monitor for home monitoring.

to their baby and providing a quiet, private place for them to do so. Compassionate care of the family caregivers includes helping to find someone to accompany them home or to meet them there. Referrals should be made to the local chapter of the National SIDS Foundation immediately. Sudden Infant Death Alliance is another resource for help. In some states, specially trained community health nurses who are knowledgeable about SIDS are available. These nurses are prepared to help families and can provide written materials as well as information, guidance, and support in the family's home. They maintain contact with the family as long as necessary and will provide support in a subsequent pregnancy.

One concern of the caregivers is how to tell other children in the family what has happened and how to help them deal with their grief and anger. Many books and booklets have been written to help caregivers and siblings learn to cope with the feelings and emotions that occur when a child dies from SIDS.

Caregivers are particularly concerned about subsequent infants. Data previously had suggested that these infants were at greater risk, but more recent studies have indicated that this risk is no greater than in the general population. Many physicians, however, continue to recommend monitoring these infants for the first few months of life to help reduce the family's stress. This is a decision that each physician and family must make together after looking at all the pros and cons. Monitoring is usually maintained until the new infant is past the age of the SIDS infant's death.

Grief waxes and wanes for months and years for these caregivers. Having another child does not cause them to forget the one they lost. Mothers often relate that they think they are healing, only to have some small incident set them off again. Friends and acquaintances must be sensitive to their needs. Comments such as "You are young; you can always have more children," "God must have needed a little angel," and "Well, you have the other children" are inappropriate. The best way to interact with these caregivers is by actively listening and showing compassionate concern.

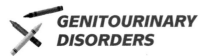

GENITOURINARY DISORDERS

A few conditions may affect the genitourinary system of the infant in the first year of life. Two structural defects, hydrocele (fluid in the saclike cavity around the testes) and cryptorchidism (undescended testes), occur in a few male infants. Urinary tract infections (UTIs) may occur when poor hygiene exists in infants wearing diapers. The most common type of renal cancer, Wilms' tumor (nephroblastoma), may first be seen in infancy. Each of these conditions is briefly discussed in this section.

Hydrocele

Hydrocele is a collection of peritoneal fluid that accumulates in the scrotum through a small passage called the processus vaginalis. This processus is a fingerlike projection in the inguinal canal through which the testes descend. Usually the processus closes soon after birth; if the processus does not close, fluid from the peritoneal cavity passes through causing hydrocele. This is the same passage through which intestines may slip causing an inguinal hernia. If the hydrocele remains by the end of the first year, corrective surgery is performed.

Cryptorchidism

Shortly before or soon after birth, the male gonads (testes) descend from the abdominal cavity into their normal position in the scrotum. Occasionally one or both of the testes do not descend, which is a condition called cryptorchidism. The testes are usually normal in size; the cause for failure to descend is not clearly understood.

In most infants with cryptorchidism, the testes descend by the time the infant is 1 year old. If one or both testes have not descended by this age, treatment is recommended. If both testes remain undescended, the male will be sterile.

A surgical procedure called **orchiopexy** is used to bring the testis down into the scrotum and anchor them there. Some physicians prefer to try medical treatment—injections of human chorionic gonadotropic hormone—before doing surgery. If this is unsuccessful in bringing the testis down, orchiopexy is performed. Surgery usually is performed when the child is 1 to 2 years of age. Prognosis for a normal functioning testicle is good when the surgery is performed at this young age and no degenerative action has taken place before treatment.

Urinary Tract Infections

Infections of the urinary tract are fairly common in the "diaper age," in infancy, and again between the ages of 2 and 6 years. The condition is more common in girls than in boys except in the first 4 months of life, when it is more common in boys. Although many different bacteria may infect the urinary tract, intestinal bacteria, particularly *Escherichia coli*, account for about 80% of acute episodes. The female urethra is shorter and straighter than the male urethra, so it is more easily contaminated with feces. Inflammation may extend into the bladder, ureters, and kidney.

Clinical Manifestations

In infants, the symptoms may be fever, nausea, vomiting, foul-smelling urine, weight loss, and increased urination. Occasionally there is little or no fever. Vomiting is common, and diarrhea may occur. The infant is irritable. In acute pyelonephritis (inflammation of the kidney and renal pelvis), the onset is abrupt with a high fever for 1 or 2 days. Convulsions may occur during the period of high fever. In preschool children, bedwetting may be a symptom.

Diagnosis

Diagnosis is based on the finding of pus in the urine under microscopic examination. The urine specimen must be fresh and uncontaminated. A "clean catch" voided urine, properly performed, is essential for microscopic examination (see Chap. 6). If a culture is needed, the infant may be catheterized, but this is usually avoided if possible. A suprapubic aspiration also may be done to obtain a sterile specimen. In the cooperative, toilet-trained child, a clean midstream urine may be used successfully.

Treatment

Simple UTIs may be treated with antibiotics (usually sulfisoxazole or ampicillin) at home. The child with acute pyelonephritis is hospitalized. Fluids are given freely. The symptoms usually subside within a few days after antibiotic therapy has been initiated, but this is not an indication that the infection is completely cleared. Medication must be continued after symptoms disappear. An intravenous pyelogram or ultrasonographic study may be performed to assess the possibility of structural defects if the child has recurring infections.

● Nursing Process for the Infant/Child With a Urinary Tract Infection

ASSESSMENT

During the interview with the family caregiver, include basic information about the child such as feeding and sleeping patterns and history of other illnesses. Gather information about the present illness: when the fever started and its course thus far, signs of pain or discomfort on voiding, recent change in feeding pattern, presence of vomiting or diarrhea, irritability, lethargy, abdominal pain, unusual odor to urine, chronic diaper rash, and signs of febrile convulsions. If the child is toilet-trained, ask the caregivers about toileting habits (how does the child wipe? does the child wash the hands when toileting?). Also ask about the use of bubble baths and the type of soap used, especially for girls.

Collecting data regarding the child includes temperature; pulse (be alert for tachycardia) and respiration rates; weight and height; observation of a wet diaper or the urine in an older child; inspection of the perineal area for rash; presence of irritability and lethargy; and general skin condition, color, and turgor. A urine specimen is needed on admission. A midstream urine collection method is desirable, and catheterization is avoided if possible. Record and report any indications of urinary burning, frequency, urgency, or pain.

In the child who has repeated UTIs, observe the interaction between the child and the family caregivers to detect any indications that the infection may be caused by sexual abuse. Look for possible indications of sexual abuse, such as bruising, bleeding, and lacerations of the external genitalia, especially in the child who is extremely shy and frightened.

NURSING DIAGNOSES

Nursing diagnoses vary with the child's age and condition. Nursing diagnoses concerning development and safety are common to most nursing care plans for infants and children. Some specific nursing diagnoses that may be used are
- Hyperthermia related to infection
- Impaired Urinary Elimination related to pain and burning on urination and decreased fluid intake
- Deficient Knowledge of caregivers related to understanding of UTI

OUTCOME IDENTIFICATION AND PLANNING

Major goals for the infant with a UTI include reducing temperature, maintaining normal urinary elimination and increasing fluid intake. An important family goal is improving knowledge about infection control to help prevent recurrent infections. Base the nursing plan of care on these goals with adjustments appropriate for the child's age. To promote normal elimination, plan nursing care that helps relieve pain and increase fluid intake. Be sure to include family teaching that focuses on infection prevention at home.

IMPLEMENTATION

Maintaining Body Temperature. Monitor the infant's temperature frequently, at least every 2 hours if it is higher than 101.3° F (3°.5° C). If the infant has a fever, follow the procedures to reduce elevated temperatures. Administer antibiotics as ordered and observe the child for signs of any reactions to the antibiotics. Antipyretic medications may be ordered. Increasing oral fluids also will help to reduce body temperature.

Maintaining Normal Elimination. Because of pain and burning on urination, the toilet-trained child may try to hold urine and not void. Encourage the child to void every 3 or 4 hours to prevent recurrent infection. Observe the child for signs of burning, pain, and frequency. If possible, observe the voiding pattern to note trickling or other signs that the bladder is not being emptied completely. Carefully monitor and measure urine output. An infant's diaper should be weighed for accuracy. Accurate intake and output measurements are important.

Increasing the child's fluid intake is necessary to help dilute the urine and flush the bladder. An increase in fluid intake also helps decrease the pain experienced on urination. Although getting the infant to accept fluids is often difficult, frequent, small amounts of glucose water or liquid gelatin may be accepted. Enlisting the aid of family caregivers may be helpful, but if they are unsuccessful, the nurse must persevere. Most infants and children like apple juice, which helps acidify the urine. Cranberry juice is a good choice for the older child, if he or she tolerates it. Administer analgesics and antispasmodics as ordered.

Providing Family Teaching. The family caregivers are the key people in helping prevent recurring infections. See Family Teaching Tips: Urinary Tract Infection. Prepare the family caregivers and the child for any other procedures that may be ordered, and give appropriate explanations.

EVALUATION: GOALS AND OUTCOME CRITERIA

- *Goal:* The infant will maintain a temperature within normal limits.
  Criteria: The infant's temperature is 98.6° to 100° F (37° to 37.8° C).
- *Goal:* The infant's normal urinary elimination will be maintained.
  Criteria: The infant produces 2 to 3 mL/kg of urine per hour; the older child voids every 3 to 4 hours, emptying the bladder each time without apprehension.
- *Goal:* The family caregivers will verbalize an understanding of the genitourinary system and good hygiene habits.
  Criteria: The family caregivers list signs and symptoms of a UTI, methods to prevent a recurrence, and state when to contact a health practitioner.

Wilms' Tumor (Nephroblastoma)

Wilms' tumor, an adenosarcoma in the kidney region, is one of the most common abdominal neoplasms of early childhood. The tumor arises from bits of embryonic tissue that remain after birth. This tissue can spark rapid cancerous growth in the area of the kidney. The tumor is rarely discovered until it is large enough to be palpated through the abdominal wall. As the tumor grows, it invades the kidney or the renal vein and disseminates to other parts of the

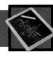

FAMILY TEACHING TIPS

Urinary Tract Infection

1. Change infant's diaper when soiled, and clean baby with mild soap and water. Dry completely.
2. Teach girls to wipe from front to back.
3. Teach child to wash hands before and after going to the toilet.
4. Bubble baths create a climate that encourages bacteria to grow, especially in young girls.
5. Teach young girls to take showers. Avoid using water softeners in tub baths.
6. Encourage child to try to urinate every 3 or 4 hours and to empty the bladder.
7. Girls should wear cotton underpants to provide air circulation to perineal area.
8. Encourage child to drink fluids especially cranberry juice.
9. Older girls should avoid whirlpools or hot tubs.

body. When the child is being evaluated and treated, a sign must be visibly posted stating that abdominal palpation should be avoided because cells may break loose and spread the tumor. Treatment consists of surgical removal as soon as possible after the growth is discovered, combined with radiation and chemotherapy.

Prognosis is best for the child younger than 2 years of age but has improved markedly for others with improved chemotherapy. Follow up consists of regular evaluation for metastasis to the lungs or other sites. All long-term implications for chemotherapy apply to this child.

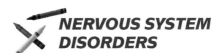

NERVOUS SYSTEM DISORDERS

Acute or Nonrecurrent Seizures

A seizure (convulsion) may be a symptom of a wide variety of disorders. In infants and children between the age of 6 months and 3 years, **febrile seizures** are the most common. Febrile seizures usually occur in the form of a generalized seizure early in the course of a fever. Although commonly associated with high fever (102° to 106° F [38.9° to 41.1° C]), some children appear to have a low seizure threshold and convulse when a fever of 100° to 102° F (37.8° to 38.9° C) is present. These seizures are often one of the initial symptoms of an acute infection somewhere in the body.

Less common causes of convulsions are intracranial infections such as meningitis, toxic reactions to certain drugs or minerals such as lead, metabolic disorders, and various brain disorders.

Clinical Manifestations

A seizure may occur suddenly without warning; however, restlessness and irritability may precede an episode. The body stiffens and the infant loses consciousness. In a few seconds, clonic movements occur. These movements are quick, jerking movements of the arms, legs, and facial muscles. Breathing is irregular and the child cannot swallow saliva.

Diagnosis

Immediate treatment is based on the presenting symptoms. Further evaluation is made after the urgency of the seizure has passed.

Treatment

Emergency care to protect the child during the seizure is the primary concern. If the seizure activity continues, Diazepam (Valium) may be administered IV to control the seizure. Acetaminophen is administered to reduce the temperature.

● Nursing Process for the Child at Risk for Seizures

ASSESSMENT

During the family caregiver interview, ask about any history of seizure activity. Have the caregivers describe any previous episodes including the infant's temperature, how the infant behaved immediately before the seizure, movements during the seizure, and any other information they believe to be relevant. Ask about the presence of any fever during the present illness and any indications of seizure activity before this admission. Promptly institute seizure precautions. An infant or child whose fever or other symptoms indicate that a seizure may be anticipated should be placed under constant observation.

During the physical exam, obtain a baseline temperature. Using a neurologic tool, observe the child's neurologic status, and make other observations appropriate for the present illness.

NURSING DIAGNOSES

In addition to nursing diagnoses related to the presenting symptoms, those specific to anticipated seizure activity are suggested in this section. If the seizure is preceded by fever, nursing diagnoses and measures for fever reduction also are included. Some of the diagnoses specific to possible seizure activity are

- Risk for Aspiration during seizure related to decreased level of consciousness
- Risk for Injury related to uncontrolled muscular activity during seizure
- Compromised Family Coping related to the child's seizure activity
- Deficient Knowledge of caregivers related to seizure prevention and precautions during seizures

OUTCOME IDENTIFICATION AND PLANNING

The immediate goals for the infant during a seizure are maintaining a clear and patent airway and preventing injury. Goals for the family include relieving anxiety and increasing knowledge about seizures. With safety in mind, develop the nursing plan of care according to these goals.

IMPLEMENTATION

Preventing Aspiration. When convulsions begin, position the infant to one side to prevent aspiration of saliva or vomitus. Do not put *anything* in the child's mouth. Remove blankets, pillows, or other items that may block the child's airway. Oxygen and suction equipment must be readily available for emergency use.

Promoting Safety Practices. Keep the child who has a history of seizures under close observation. Pad the crib sides, and keep sharp or hard items out of the crib. Do not, however, completely hide the view of the surroundings outside the crib as this could make the child feel isolated. During the seizure, stay with the child to protect but not restrain him or her. Loosen any tight clothing. If the child is not in bed when the seizure starts, move him or her to a flat surface.

Document the seizure completely after the episode. Document the type of movements (rigidity, jerking, twitching), the body parts involved, the duration of the seizure, pulse and respirations, the child's color, and any deviant eye movements or other notable signs.

Promoting Family Coping. A convulsion or seizure is very frightening to family caregivers.

With a calm, confident attitude, reassure caregivers that the child is in good hands. Explain that febrile seizures are not uncommon in small children. Reassure caregivers that the physician will evaluate the child to determine if the seizure has any cause other than nervous system irritation resulting from the high fever.

Providing Family Teaching. Teach family caregivers seizure precautions so that they can handle a seizure that occurs at home. Also instruct them on what observations to make during a seizure so that they can report these to the physician to help in evaluating the child. Explain methods to control fever, cautioning caregivers to avoid using aspirin for fever reduction. Refer to Chapter 6, Family Teaching Tips for Reducing Fever, when teaching caregivers how to reduce fevers at home.

EVALUATION: GOALS AND OUTCOME CRITERIA

- *Goal:* The child's airway will remain patent throughout the seizure.
  Criteria: The child's airway remains patent with no aspiration of saliva or vomitus.
- *Goal:* The child will remain free from injury during the seizure.
  Criteria: The child is free from bruises, abrasions, concussions, or fractures after the seizure.
- *Goal:* The family caregivers anxiety will be reduced.
  Criteria: The family caregivers verbalize their concerns and relate an understanding of febrile seizures.
- *Goal:* The family caregivers will verbalize an understanding of seizure precautions.
  Criteria: The family caregivers state methods to reduce fevers and handle seizures at home.

Haemophilus influenzae *Meningitis*

Purulent meningitis in infancy and childhood is caused by a variety of agents including meningococci, the tubercle bacillus, and the *Haemophilus influenzae* type B bacillus. The most common form is *H influenzae* meningitis. Meningococcal meningitis is spread by means of droplet infection from an infected person; all other forms are contracted by invasion of the meninges via the bloodstream from an infection elsewhere.

Peak occurrence of *H influenzae* meningitis is between the ages of 6 and 12 months. It is rare during the first 2 months of life and is seldom seen after the fourth year. Purulent meningitis is an infectious disease. In addition to standard precautions, droplet transmission precautions should be observed for 24 hours after the start of effective antimicrobial therapy or until pathogens can no longer be cultured from nasopharyngeal secretions. Current immunizations include the Hib, which is given at 2 months and repeated at 4, 6, and 12 months (see Table 10–4 in Chap. 10).

Clinical Manifestations

The onset may be either gradual or abrupt following an upper respiratory infection. Young infants with meningitis may have a characteristic high-pitched cry, fever, and irritability. Other symptoms include headache, **nuchal rigidity** (stiff neck) that may progress to **opisthotonos** (arching of the back), and delirium. Projectile vomiting may be present. Generalized convulsions are common in infants. Coma may occur early, particularly in the older child. Meningococcal meningitis, which tends to occur as epidemics in older children, produces a **purpuric rash** (caused by bleeding under the skin) in addition to the other symptoms.

Diagnosis

Early diagnosis and treatment are essential for uncomplicated recovery. A spinal tap is performed promptly whenever symptoms raise a suspicion of meningitis. For accurate results, the spinal tap is done before antibiotics are administered. The nurse assists by holding the infant during the spinal tap (Fig. 11–10). The spinal fluid is under increased pressure, and laboratory examination of the fluid reveals increased protein and decreased glucose content. Early in the disease, the spinal fluid may be clear but it rapidly becomes purulent. The causative organism usually can be determined from stained smears of the spinal fluid, enabling specific medication to be started early without waiting for growths of organisms on culture media.

Treatment

The child is initially isolated and treatment is started using IV administration of antibiotics. Third-generation cephalosporins, such as ceftriaxone (Rocephin), are commonly used often in combination with other antibiotics. Antibiotics chosen for treatment depend on sensitivity studies. Later in the disease, medications may be given orally. Treatment depends on the progress of the condition and continues as long as there is fever or signs of subdural effusion or otitis media. The administration of IV steroids early in the course has decreased the incidence of deafness as a complication. If seizures occur, anticonvulsants are often given.

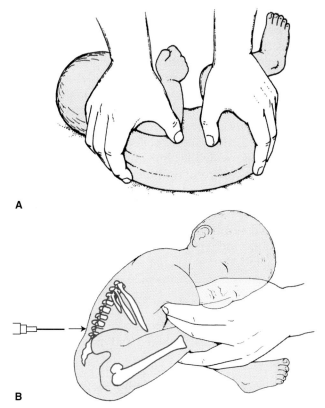

A

B

● *Figure 11.10* Two positions for a spinal tap. **(A)** Knee–chest position for a young infant. The nurse can hold the infant securely. **(B)** Sitting position. A small infant is held in a sitting position, with the knees flexed on the abdomen, and the nurse holds the elbow and knee in each hand, flexing the spine.

Subdural effusion may complicate the condition in infants during the course of the disease. Fluid accumulates in the subdural space between the dura and the brain. Needle aspiration through the infant's open suture lines or bur holes (in the skull of the older child) is used to remove the fluid. Repeated aspirations may be required.

Complications of *H influenzae* meningitis with long-term implications are hydrocephalus, nerve deafness, mental retardation, and paralysis. The risk of complications is lessened when appropriate medication is started early in the disease.

● Nursing Process for the Child With Meningitis

ASSESSMENT

The infant or child with meningitis is obviously extremely sick, and the anxiety level of the family caregivers is understandably high. Be patient and sensitive to their feelings when doing an interview. Obtain a complete history with partic-

ular emphasis on the present illness, including any recent upper respiratory infection or middle ear infection. Information on other children in the family and their ages is also important.

The physical exam of the infant includes obtaining temperature, pulse, and respirations; use a neurologic evaluation tool to monitor neurologic status including the child's level of consciousness (see the section on neurologic evaluation, Chap. 5). Examine the young infant for a bulging fontanelle, and measure the head circumference for a baseline. Perform this exam after the spinal tap is completed and IV fluids and antibiotics are initiated because these procedures take precedence over everything else.

NURSING DIAGNOSES

The following nursing diagnoses are some that may be used in planning the care of the child with meningitis:
- Decreased Intracranial Adaptive Capacity related to infection and seizure activity
- Risk for Aspiration related to decreased level of consciousness
- Risk for Injury related to Seizure Activity
- Risk for Deficient Fluid Volume related to vomiting, fever, and fluid restrictions
- Excess Fluid Volume related to syndrome of inappropriate antidiuretic hormone
- Deficient Knowledge of family caregivers related to airborne transmission exposure to others
- Compromised Family Coping related to the child's condition and prognosis

OUTCOME IDENTIFICATION AND PLANNING

The goals for the infant with meningitis include monitoring for changes in vital signs and neurologic status, maintaining a clear and patent airway, keeping the child safe from injury during a seizure, and maintaining fluid balance. The goals for the family include teaching ways of preventing the transmission of infection and reducing anxiety. Plan the nursing care according to these goals. Include interventions such as eliminating the infection by administering antibiotics and observing for signs of increased intracranial pressure.

IMPLEMENTATION

Monitoring for Complications. The child is closely monitored for signs of increased intracranial pressure including increased head size, headache, bulging fontanelle, decreased pulse, vomiting, seizures, high-pitched cry, increased blood pressure, change in level of consciousness or in eyes, and irritability or other behavioral changes. An increase in blood pressure, decrease in pulse, change in neurologic signs, or signs of respiratory distress must be reported at once. Measure the infant's head circumference at least every 4 hours to detect complications of subdural effusion or obstructive hydrocephalus. The child's room should be quiet and darkened to decrease stimulation that may cause seizures. While in the room, speak softly, avoid sudden movements, move quietly, and raise and lower side rails carefully. The head of the bed can be elevated.

Preventing Aspiration. Position the child in a side-lying position with the neck supported for comfort and the head elevated. Remove pillows, blankets, and soft toys that might obstruct the airway. Watch for and remove excessive mucus as much as possible. Use suction sparingly.

Promoting Safety Practices. Keep the child under close observation. Implement seizure precautions. Every 2 hours observe the child for seizure activity, vital signs, neurologic changes, and change in level of consciousness. Pad the crib sides, and keep sharp or hard items out of the crib. During a seizure, stay with the child to protect but not restrain him or her. Loosen any tight clothing (see Nursing Process for the Child at Risk for Seizures, page 227).

Maintaining Fluid Intake. Fluid balance is an important aspect of this child's care. Strict intake and output measurements are critical. Methods of reducing fever may be used as needed. Administer IV fluids while observing and monitoring the IV infusion site and following safety precautions to maintain the site.

Monitoring Fluid Volume. The infectious process may increase secretion of the antidiuretic hormone produced by the posterior pituitary gland. As a result, the child may not excrete urine adequately, and a body fluid volume excess will occur. Strictly measure intake and output, and monitor daily weight and electrolytes. Signs for concern that must be reported immediately are decreased urinary output, hyponatremia, increased weight, nausea, and irritability. The child is placed on fluid restrictions if these signs occur.

Providing Family Teaching Regarding Spread of Infection. H influenzae is a highly contagious organism that may spread to other people by means of droplet transmission. Droplet transmission precautions must be maintained for the first 24 hours after the antibiotic is administered. Staff members and family caregivers must follow proper precautions. Other children in the family may need to be examined to determine if they should receive prophylactic antibiotics.

Promoting Family Coping. Teach the caregivers isolation and good handwashing technique and encourage them to stay with their child, if possible. Support family caregivers through every step of the process. Their anxiety about procedures, the child's seizures and condition, and the possible complications are all serious concerns. Family caregivers must be included and made to feel useful. If they are not too apprehensive, help them find small things they can do for their child. Keep them advised about the child's progress at all times.

EVALUATION: GOALS AND OUTCOME CRITERIA

- *Goal:* The child's will have a normal neurologic status.
  Criteria: The child's vital signs are within normal limits and neurologic status is stable.
- *Goal:* The child's airway will remain patent and clear.
  Criteria: The child's position is side-lying with neck supported and head elevated; airway remains patent with no aspiration of saliva or vomitus.
- *Goal:* The child will remain free from injury.
  Criteria: The child is free from bruises, abrasions, concussions, or fractures during seizure activity.
- *Goal:* The child will maintain normal fluid balance.
  Criteria: The child's intake and output are within normal limits; temperature is 98.6° to 100° F (37° to 37.8° C); there are no signs of dehydration.
- *Goal:* The child will maintain normal weight and have adequate urinary output.
  Criteria: The child's weight and electrolyte levels are within normal limits; hourly urine output is 2 to 3 mL/kg.

- *Goal:* The family caregivers follow measures to prevent the transmission of *H influenzae* bacteria to others.
  Criteria: The family caregivers identify measures for preventing the spread of bacteria and discuss the need for isolation of the ill child.
- *Goal:* The family caregivers' anxiety will decrease.
  Criteria: The family caregivers verbalize understanding of the disease process and relate the child's progress throughout the crisis.

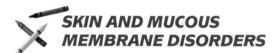

SKIN AND MUCOUS MEMBRANE DISORDERS

Miliaria Rubra

Miliaria rubra, often called prickly heat, is common in infants who are exposed to summer heat or are over-dressed. It also may appear in febrile illnesses and may be mistaken for the rash of one of the communicable diseases. The rash appears as pinhead-sized erythematous (reddened) papules. It is most noticeable in areas where sweat glands are concentrated such as folds of the skin, the chest, and about the neck. It usually causes itching, making the infant uncomfortable and fretful.

Treatment primarily should be preventive. Family caregivers should be taught to avoid bundling their infants in layers of clothing in hot weather—a diaper may be all the child needs. Tepid baths without soap help control the itching. A small amount of baking soda may be added to the bath water to help relieve discomfort.

Diaper Rash

Diaper rash is common in infancy, causing the baby discomfort and fretfulness. Bacterial decomposition of urine produces ammonia, which is irritating to an infant's tender skin. Diarrheal stools also produce a burning erythematous area in the anal region. Some infants seem to be more susceptible than others, possibly due to inherited sensitive skin. Prolonged exposure to wet or soiled diapers, use of plastic or rubber pants, infrequently changed disposable diapers, inadequate cleansing of the diaper area (especially after bowel movements), sensitivity to some soaps or disposable diaper perfumes, and the use of strong laundry detergents without thorough rinsing are considered to be causes. Yeast infections, notably candidiasis, are also causative factors.

Treatment and Nursing Care

Caregivers should be taught that the primary treatment is prevention. Diapers must be changed frequently without waiting for obvious leaking. Regular checking is necessary. Manufacturers of disposable diapers are constantly trying to improve the ability of disposable diapers to wick the wetness away from the infant's skin. Diapers washed at commercial laundries are sterilized, preventing the growth of ammonia-forming bacteria. Caregivers may be unable, however, to afford disposable diapers or a commercial diaper service. Diapers washed at home should be presoaked (good commercial products are available), washed in hot water with a mild soap, and rinsed thoroughly with an antiseptic added to the final rinse. Drying diapers in the sun or in a dryer also helps destroy bacteria.

Exposing the diaper area to the air helps clear up the dermatitis. The use of baby powder when diapering is discouraged, as caked powder helps create an environment in which organisms thrive. Cleaning the diaper area from front to back with warm water and drying thoroughly with each diaper change helps improve or prevent the condition. If soap is necessary when cleaning stool from the infant's buttocks and rectal area, be certain that the soap is completely rinsed before diapering. The use of commercial wet wipes may aggravate the condition. If the area becomes excoriated and sore, the health care provider may prescribe an ointment. See Family Teaching Tips: Diaper Rash.

Candidiasis

Calbicans is the causative agent for thrush and some cases of diaper rash. Newborns can be exposed to a candidiasis vaginal infection in the mother during delivery. Thrush appears in the infant's mouth as a white coating that looks like milk curds. Poor hand-washing practices and inadequate washing of bottles and nipples are contributing factors. In addition, infants and toddlers may experience episodes of thrush or diaper rash after antibiotic therapy caused by the upset of the normal intestinal flora that allows an overgrowth of *Candida*.

Treatment for diaper rash caused by *Candida* (Fig. 11-11) is the application of nystatin ointment or cream to the affected area. Application of nystatin (Mycostatin, Nilstat) to the oral lesions every 6 hours is an effective treatment. Good hygiene practices should be reinforced.

FAMILY TEACHING TIPS

Diaper Rash

1. Rinse all baby's clothes thoroughly to eliminate soap or detergent residue that may irritate baby's skin.
2. Rinse cloth diapers in clear water. Do not use fabric softeners because they can cause a skin reaction.
3. Use plastic or rubber diaper covers only when necessary. They hold moisture, which makes rash worse.
4. Change diapers as soon as wet or soiled. Disposable diapers hold moisture the same as plastic or rubber covers.
5. Avoid fastening diaper too tightly, which irritates baby's skin.
6. Expose baby's bottom to air without diapers as much as possible to help rash heal.
7. Do not overdress or overcover baby. Sweating makes rash worse.
8. Wash baby's bottom with lukewarm water only, using wet cotton balls or pouring over bath basin or sink. Pat dry with soft cloth. Do not use commercial baby wipes. Do not rub rash.
9. A cool, wet cloth placed over red diaper rash is very soothing. Try this for 5 minutes three or four times a day.
10. Use ointment only as recommended by health care provider. Apply very thin layer only. Wash off at each diaper change.
11. Dry diaper area thoroughly before rediapering. A hair dryer on low warm setting used after patting dry may help.

Seborrheic Dermatitis

Seborrheic dermatitis (cradle cap) usually can be prevented by daily washing of the infant's hair and scalp. Characterized by yellowish, scaly, or crusted patches on the scalp, it occurs in newborns and in older infants possibly as a result of excessive sebaceous gland activity. Family caregivers may be afraid to wash vigorously over the "soft spot." However, they need to understand that this is where cradle cap often begins and that careful but vigorous washing of the area with a washcloth can prevent this disorder. Using a fine-toothed baby comb after shampooing is also a helpful preventive measure. These principles are stressed during teaching about care of the newborn.

Once the condition exists, daily application of mineral oil helps loosen the crust. No attempt should be made to loosen it all at once, however, as the delicate skin on the scalp may break and bleed and can easily become infected.

Impetigo

Impetigo is a superficial bacterial skin infection (Fig. 11–12). In the newborn, the primary causative organism is *Staphylococcus aureus.* In the older child, the most common causative organism is group A beta-hemolytic streptococci. Impetigo in the newborn is usually bullous (blister-like); in the older child, the lesions are nonbullous.

Impetigo in the newborn nursery is cause for immediate concern, as the condition is highly contagious and can spread through a nursery quickly. The nurse caring for an infant who has impetigo must follow contact (skin and wound) precautions,

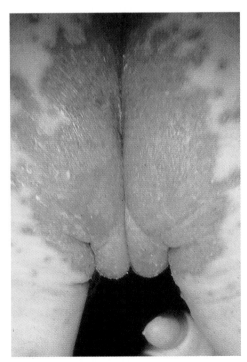

● **Figure 11.11** Diaper rash caused by *Candida.*

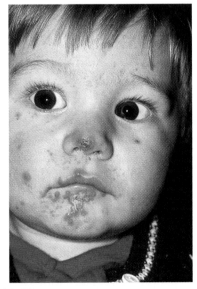

● **Figure 11.12** Typical lesion of impetigo.

including wearing a cover gown and gloves. The infant should be segregated from other infants in the nursery to deter spread of the disease. Crusts can be soaked off with warm water followed by an application of topical antibiotics such as Bacitracin and Neosporin. The infant's hands must be covered or elbow restraints applied to prevent scratching of lesions. Careful handwashing by nursing personnel and family members is essential.

The older child with impetigo is treated at home. The family caregivers must be taught hygiene practices to prevent the spread of impetigo to other children in the household or other contacts of the child in the day care center, nursery school, or elementary school. Lesions occur primarily on the face but may spread to any part of the body. The crusts and drainage are contagious. Because the lesions are pruritic (itchy), the child must learn to keep his or her fingers and hands away from the lesions. Nails should be trimmed to prevent scratching of lesions. Family members should be taught not to share towels and washcloths. Medical treatment includes oral penicillin or erythromycin for 10 days. Daily washing of the crusts helps speed the healing process. Mupirocin (Bactroban) ointment may be used.

Because this is commonly a streptococcal infection in the older child, rheumatic fever or acute glomerulonephritis may follow. Family caregivers should be alerted to this rare possibility.

Acute Infantile Eczema

Infantile eczema is an atopic dermatitis considered at least in part an allergic reaction to an irritant. It is fairly common during the first year of life after the age of 3 months. It is uncommon in breast-fed babies before they are given additional foods.

Infantile eczema is characterized by three factors:

- Hereditary predisposition
- Hypersensitivity of the deeper layers of the skin to protein or protein-like allergens
- Allergens to which the child is sensitive that may be inhaled, ingested, or absorbed through direct contact such as house dust, egg white, and wool

Infants who have eczema tend to have hay fever or asthma later in life.

Clinical Manifestations

Eczema usually starts on the cheeks and spreads to the extensor surfaces of the arms and legs (Fig. 11–13). Eventually the entire trunk may become affected. The initial reddening of the skin is quickly followed by papule and vesicle formation. Itching is intense, and the infant's scratching makes the skin

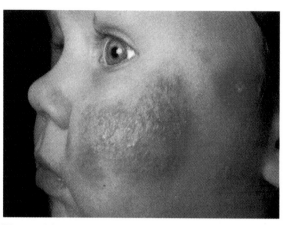
● **Figure 11.13** Infant with infantile eczema (atopic dermatitis).

weep and crust. The areas easily become infected by hemolytic streptococci or by staphylococci.

Diagnosis

The most common allergens involved in eczema are

- Foods: egg white, cow's milk, wheat products, orange juice, tomato juice
- Inhalants: house dust, pollens, animal dander
- Materials: wool, nylon, plastic

Diagnosis, however, is not simple. Often trial by elimination is as effective as any other diagnostic tool. Skin testing on a young infant generally is not considered valid, so it is discouraged as a means of diagnosis.

Diagnostic Diet. An elimination diet may be helpful in ruling out offending foods. A hypoallergenic diet consisting of a milk substitute such as soy formula, vitamin supplement, and other foods known to be hypoallergenic is given. If the skin condition shows improvement, other foods are added one at a time at an interval of about 1 week; note effects and eliminate any foods that cause a reaction. The protein of egg white is such a common offender that most pediatricians advise against feeding whole eggs to infants until late in the first year of life (see Table 11–1).

Great care must be taken to prevent the child from becoming undernourished. An elimination program must always be initiated under the supervision of a competent pediatric nurse practitioner, dietitian, or physician.

Treatment

Smallpox vaccination is *definitely contraindicated* for the child with eczema. In fact, such a child must be kept away from anyone who has recently been vaccinated. A serious condition called *eczema vaccinatum* results when an infant with eczema is vaccinated or is exposed to the vaccination of another person. The infant becomes seriously ill, and mortality rates have been high. Fortunately because smallpox vaccination is no longer required, this is not a major concern; the reaction could occur if the child is exposed to someone who's been vaccinated in preparation for travel.

Of greater current concern is protecting the child from anyone with a herpes simplex infection (cold sore). If the lesions become infected with herpes simplex, a generalized reaction may occur. In the child with severe eczema with many lesions, body fluid loss from oozing through the lesions can be serious. The infant may have severe pain and be gravely ill with this complication.

Oral antibiotics may be ordered for a coexistent infection such as staphylococci, streptococci, or viral infections. Oral antihistamines and sedatives may help relieve the itching and allow rest. If no infection exists, topical hydrocortisone ointments may be used to relieve inflammation. Wet soaks or colloidal baths also may be prescribed for their soothing effects. The water should be tepid for further soothing, and soap may not be used because of its drying effect. Some physicians recommend the use of a mild soap, such as Dove or Neutrogena, or a soap substitute. Lubrication is essential to retain moisture and prevent evaporation after the bath. Emollients containing lanolin or petrolatum, such as Eucerin, may be prescribed.

Inhalant and contact allergens should be avoided as far as possible. In the infant's bedroom, window drapes or curtains, dresser scarves, and rugs should be removed or made of washable fabric that can be frequently laundered. Furniture should be washed off frequently. The crib mattress should have a nonallergenic covering and be washed frequently with careful cleaning along the binding. Feather pillows must be eliminated, and stuffed toys should be washable. It may be necessary to provide new homes for household pets. However, dander from the pets can remain in carpets, crevices, and overstuffed furniture for a long time. Carpets and area rugs may need to be removed. A home, especially an older one with a damp basement, may be harboring molds that shed allergenic spores. Bathrooms are also places for molds and mildews to hide especially in warm, humid climates.

● Nursing Process for the Infant/Child With Infantile Eczema

ASSESSMENT

The family caregivers of the child with infantile eczema are often frustrated and exhausted.

Although the caregiver can be assured that most cases of infant eczema clear up by the age of 2, this does little to relieve the present situation. Hospitalization is avoided whenever possible because these infants are highly susceptible to infections. Sometimes, however, admission seems to be the only answer to provide more intensive therapy or to relieve an exhausted caregiver.

During the interview with the family caregivers, cover the history of the condition including treatments that have been tried and foods that have been ruled out as allergens. Include a thorough review of the home environment. Evaluate the caregivers' knowledge of the condition.

The data collection about the infant includes obtaining vital signs, observing general nutritional state, and doing a complete examination of all body parts with careful documentation of the eruptions and their location and size. Unaffected areas as well as those that are weeping and crusted should be indicated.

NURSING DIAGNOSES

Regardless of the severity of the eczema, the nursing diagnoses are much the same. Some nursing diagnoses that may be used are

- Impaired Skin Integrity related to lesions and inflammatory process
- Disturbed Sleep Pattern related to itching and discomfort
- Imbalanced Nutrition: Less than Body Requirements related to elimination diet
- Risk for Infection related to broken skin and lesions
- Deficient Knowledge of caregivers related to disease condition and treatment

OUTCOME IDENTIFICATION AND PLANNING

The major goals for the infant with eczema are preserving skin integrity, maintaining comfort, improving sleep patterns, maintaining good nutrition (within the constraints of allergens), and preventing infection of skin lesions. A family goal is increasing knowledge about the disease process. Base the nursing plan of care on these goals.

IMPLEMENTATION

Maintaining Skin Integrity. Cover the lesions with light clothing. Especially appropriate are the one-piece, loose-fitting terry pajamas, or one-piece cotton underwear known as "onesies." This type of clothing helps keep the infant from scratching. In addition, the nails must be kept closely cut, and mitten-like hand coverings can be used. Use restraints only if necessary. Elbow restraints may sometimes be used. Remove restraints at least every 4 hours—more often, if feasible—but do not allow the child to rub or scratch while the restraints are off. If ointments or wet dressings must be kept in place on the infant's face, a mask may be made by cutting holes into a cotton stockinette-type material to correspond to eyes, nose, and mouth. Wet dressings on the rest of the body can be kept in place by wrapping the infant "mummy" fashion. Dressings may be left on for an extended period but should not be allowed to dry, because that can create open areas when they are removed.

Providing Comfort Measures. Plan soothing baths, such as a colloidal bath (Aveeno), just before naptime or bedtime. Time medications such as sedatives or antihistamines so that they will be effective immediately after the bath when the infant is most relaxed.

Maintaining Adequate Nutrition. Weigh the child on admission and daily thereafter. This procedure gives some indication of weight gain. If an elimination diet is being used, the diet should be carefully balanced within the framework of the foods permitted and supplemented with vitamin and mineral preparations as needed. Fluids are encouraged to prevent dehydration.

Preventing Infection. As stated earlier, usually these children are kept out of the health care facility because of the concern about infection. However, they can also become infected at home. Whether in the health care facility or at home, the infant should be placed in a room alone or in a room where there is no other child with any type of infection. Administer antibiotics as ordered. For open lesions, aseptic techniques are necessary to prevent infection.

Providing Family Teaching. Help the family caregivers understand the condition and possible food, contact, or inhalant allergens. Teach them ways to soothe the infant. They should avoid overdressing and overheating the infant, because perspiration causes itching. Explain that they should use a mild detergent to launder the infant's clothing and bedding. Help them determine ways to encourage normal growth and development. Teach them to read labels of prepared foods, watching carefully for hidden allergens. Family caregivers may feel apprehensive or repulsed by this unsightly infant. Support them in expressing their feelings, and help them view this as a distressing but temporary skin condition.

Children with eczema are frequently active and "behaviorally itchy." Assist caregivers in handling challenging behavior. Help caregivers develop a strong self-image in the child to protect against strangers' openly negative reactions.

EVALUATION: GOALS AND OUTCOME CRITERIA

- *Goal:* The child's skin integrity will be maintained or will improve.
  Criteria: The child has decreased scratching and the skin will have fewer breakdowns.
- *Goal:* The child's sleep pattern will not be disturbed.
  Criteria: The child sleeps an adequate amount for his or her age after comfort measures are provided.
- *Goal:* The child's nutritional intake will meet the needs for growth and development.
  Criteria: The child has no weight loss and has weight gain appropriate for age.
- *Goal:* The child will be free of infected skin lesions.
  Criteria: The child does not scratch lesions; lesions do not become infected.
- *Goal:* The family caregivers understand the disease and its treatment.
  Criteria: The family caregivers demonstrate an acceptance of the infant and the condition by interacting in a positive fashion with the child.

KEY POINTS

- Small anatomic structures and immature systems contribute to the vulnerability of the infant in the first year of life.
- Infants need adequate nutrition for healthy development.
- Infants can quickly become seriously dehydrated from a bout of vomiting or diarrhea.

- Iron deficiency anemia occurs in infants who have an inadequate iron intake.
- Otitis media is a common complication of upper respiratory infections in infants.
- Immunizations can now eliminate the danger of *H influenzae*, a bacteria that can cause serious respiratory illnesses and complications in infants.
- Safety precautions must be included in any nursing care plan for infants.
- Sudden infant death syndrome, the leading cause of death in infants over 1 month of age, is devastating to the infant's family.
- Febrile seizures commonly occur in infants and children between 6 months and 3 years of age.
- Many infant skin conditions can be avoided with good preventive care.

REFERENCES

1. Kline MK. (1999) Otitis media. In *Oski's pediatrics: Principles and practices* (3rd ed). Philadelphia: Lippincott Williams & Wilkins.
2. Carroll JL, Loughlin GM. (1999) Sudden infant death syndrome. In *Oski's pediatrics: Principles and practices* (3rd ed). Philadelphia: Lippincott Williams & Wilkins.

BIBLIOGRAPHY

Cooper KE. (2001) The effectiveness of ribavirin in the treatment of RSV. *Pediatric Nursing*, 27(1).

Demmler GJ. (1999) Rotaviruses. In *Oski's pediatrics: Principles and practice* (3rd ed). Philadelphia: Lippincott Williams & Wilkins.

Kirkland RT. (1999) Failure to thrive. In *Oski's pediatrics: Principles and practice* (3rd ed). Philadelphia: Lippincott Williams & Wilkins.

Malhotra A, Krilow L. (2001) Viral Croup. *Pediatrics in Review*, 22(1), 5.

NANDA nursing diagnoses: Definitions and classification 2001–2002 (2001) Philadelphia: North American Nursing Diagnosis Association.

Parini S. (2001) Eight faces of meningitis. *Nursing*, 31(8), 51.

Pillitteri A. (1999) *Maternal and child health nursing* (3rd ed). Philadelphia: Lippincott Williams & Wilkins.

Sparks S, Taylor C. (2001) *Nursing diagnosis reference mannual* (5th ed). Springhouse, PA: Springhouse Corporation.

(2000) *Springhouse nurse's drug guide* (3rd ed). Springhouse, PA: Springhouse Corporation.

Wong DL, Perry S, Hockenberry M. (2002) *Maternal child nursing care* (2nd ed). St. Louis: Mosby.

Wong DL, Hess C. (2000) *Wong and Whaley's clinical manual of pediatric nursing* (5th ed). St. Louis: Mosby.

Websites
Sickle Cell Disease www.sicklecelldisease.org
Colic www.answer-for-colic.com
Failure to Thrive
    http://kidshealth.org/parent/nutrition/failure_thrive.html

Workbook

NCLEX-STYLE REVIEW QUESTIONS

1. An infant with a diagnosis of Failure to Thrive has had an inadequate intake of calories. In planning care for this child, which of the following goals would be MOST appropriate for this infant? The infant's

   a. current weight will be maintained

   b. fluid intake will be increased by 10cc per hour

   c. urinary output will be 2 to 3 ml/kg/hour

   d. caloric intake will be appropriate for weight gain

2. If an infant has been diagnosed with pyloric stenosis, the child will likely have a history of which of the following?

   a. Iron deficiency

   b. Projectile vomiting

   c. Muscle spasms

   d. Nasal congestion

3. When developing a plan of care for a child with sickle cell disease, which of the following nursing interventions would be MOST important to include?

   a. Provide support for family caregivers.

   b. Observe skin for any breakdown.

   c. Move the extremities gently.

   d. Administer analgesics promptly.

4. If an infant has a febrile seizure, the HIGHEST priority for the nurse is to

   a. Document the infant's behavior during the seizure

   b. Teach the caregivers about fever reduction methods

   c. Protect the infant during the seizure activity

   d. Reassure the caregivers that seizures are common

5. After discussing ways to lower a fever with the caregiver of an infant, the caregiver makes the following statements. Which statement requires further teaching?

   a. "I won't give my child baby aspirin when she has a fever."

   b. "I know I need to dress my baby lightly if she has a fever."

   c. "When my baby has a fever, I will sponge her in cool water for 20 minutes."

   d. "I need to recheck my baby's temperature until it is below 101."

STUDY ACTIVITIES

1. Using the table below, make a list of foods that may cause allergies in infants and children. List some sources of these food-causing allergies.

Food That May Cause Allergies	Sources of Foods That May Cause Allergies

2. Describe the most important procedure to follow to prevent the spread of infection. Explain the reasons that the spread of infection is especially a concern in infants.

3. Adequate nutrition is important for healthy development in the infant. Describe important factors to assure that nutritional needs are meet in the infant.

CRITICAL THINKING

1. Nine-month-old Tina has severe diarrhea. What symptoms and physical characteristics would you look for in her? What documentation is especially important in her care?

2. James, a 6-month-old infant, has a fever of 102.8° F. While you are with the child, he begins to have a seizure. Describe your actions and appropriate teaching for his caregivers.

3. Identify the relation between *Candida albicans* and some cases of diaper rash. Detail the teaching that you would provide for a mother about diaper rash.

4. *Dosage Calculation:* An infant with a diagnosis of otitis media is being treated with Amoxicillin. The child weighs 13.2 pounds. The usual dosage of this medication is 40 mg per kg per day in divided doses every 8 hours. Answer the following:

a. How many kg does the child's weigh?
b. How much Amoxicillin will be given in a 24-hour time period?
c. How many mg per dose will be given?
d. How many doses will the child receive in a day?

Growth and Development of the Toddler: 1 to 3 Years

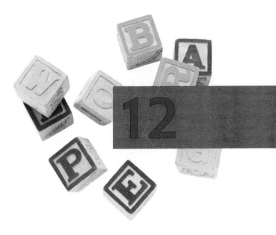

12

PHYSICAL DEVELOPMENT
PSYCHOSOCIAL DEVELOPMENT
  Play
  Discipline
  Sharing With a Sibling
NUTRITION
HEALTH PROMOTION AND MAINTENANCE

Routine Checkups
Family Teaching
Accident Prevention
THE TODDLER IN THE HEALTH CARE FACILITY
  Special Considerations

STUDENT OBJECTIVES

On completion of this chapter, the student will be able to

1. Identify characteristics of the age group known as the toddler.
2. State why parenting a toddler is often frustrating.
3. Describe physical growth that occurs during toddlerhood.
4. Define the following terms as they relate to the psychosocial development of the toddler: a) negativism, b) ritualism, c) dawdling.
5. List three reasons why eating problems often appear in this age group.
6. Describe the progression of the toddler's self-feeding skills.
7. State the age when a child should be taught tooth brushing, and explain why this is an appropriate age.
8. Describe the relationship between sweet foods and plaque formation on the teeth.
9. Discuss the purpose of the toddler's first dental visit and the ideal age for it.
10. Describe the elements in timing the beginning of toilet training.
11. Identify six suggestions to aid in bowel training.
12. State the physiological development required for complete bowel and bladder control and the typical age when this development occurs.
13. State why accident prevention is a primary concern when caring for a toddler.
14. State the four leading causes of accidental death of toddlers.
15. List preventive measures for each of the leading causes of accidental death of toddlers.
16. List eight types of medications most commonly involved in childhood poisonings.
17. List information that should be gathered in a social assessment when a toddler is admitted to the hospital.

KEY TERMS

autonomy
dawdling
discipline
negativism
parallel play
punishment
ritualism
temper tantrum

Soon after a child's first birthday, important and sometimes dramatic changes take place. Physical growth slows considerably; mobility and communication skills improve rapidly; and a determined, often stubborn little person begins to create a new set of challenges for the caregivers. "No" and "want" are favorite words. Temper tantrums appear.

During this transition from infancy to early childhood, the child learns many new physical and social skills. With additional teeth and better motor skills, the toddler's self-feeding abilities improve and include the addition of a new assortment of foods. Left unsupervised, the toddler also may taste many nonfood items that may be harmful, even fatal.

This transition is a time of unpredictability: one moment, the toddler insists on "me do it;" the next moment, the child reverts to dependence on the mother or other caregiver. While seeking to assert independence and achieve autonomy, the toddler develops a fear of separation. The toddler's curiosity about the world increases, as does his or her ability to explore. Family caregivers soon discover that this exploration can wreak havoc on orderly routine and a well-kept house and that the toddler requires close supervision to prevent injury to self or objects in the environment (Fig. 12–1). The toddler justly earns the title of "explorer."

Toddlerhood can be a difficult time for family caregivers. Just as parents are beginning to feel confident in their ability to care for and understand their infant, the toddler changes into a walking, talking person whose attitudes and behaviors disrupt the entire family. Accident-proofing, safety measures, and firm but gentle discipline are primary tasks for caregivers of toddlers. Learning to discipline with patience and understanding is difficult but eventually rewarding. At the end of the toddlerhood stage, the child's behavior generally becomes more acceptable and predictable.

Erikson's psychosocial developmental task for this age group is **autonomy** (independence) while overcoming doubt and shame. In contrast to the infant's task of building trust, the toddler seeks independence, wavers between dependence and freedom, and gains self-awareness. This behavior is so common that the stage is commonly referred to as the "terrible twos," but it is just as often referred to as the "terrific twos" because of the toddler's exciting language development, the exuberance with which he or she greets the world, and a newfound sense of accomplishment. Both aspects of being 2 years old are essential to the child's development, and caregivers must learn how to manage the fast-paced switching between anxiety and enthusiasm.

PHYSICAL DEVELOPMENT

Toddlerhood is a time of slowed growth and rapid development. Each year the toddler gains 5 to 10 lb (2.26 to 4.53 kg) and about 3 inches (7.62 cm). Continued eruption of teeth, particularly the molars, helps the toddler learn to chew food. The toddler learns to stand alone (Fig. 12–2) and to walk between

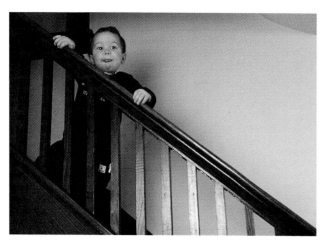

● **Figure 12.1** Playing on the stairs is a daring and fun activity for the toddler. It can also get him into big trouble.

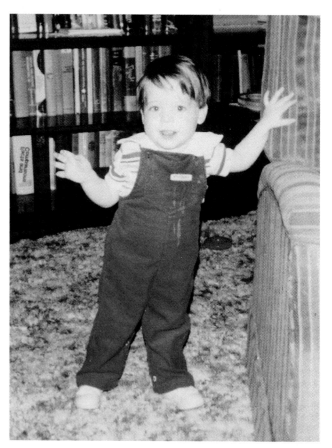

● **Figure 12.2** The toddler is proud of his ability to stand.

the ages of 1 and 2 years. During this time, most children say their first words and continue to improve and refine their language skills. By the end of this period, the toddler may have learned partial or total toilet training.

The rate of development varies with each child, depending on the individual personality and the opportunities available to test, explore, and learn. Significant landmarks in the toddler's growth and development are summarized in Table 12–1.

TABLE 12.1	**Growth and Development: The Toddler**				
Age (months)	**Personal–Social**	**Fine Motor**	**Gross Motor**	**Language**	**Cognition**
12–15	Begins Erikson's stage of "autonomy versus shame and doubt" Seeks novel ways to pursue new experiences Imitations of people are more advanced	Builds with blocks; finger paints Able to reach out with hands and bring food to mouth Holds a spoon Drinks from a cup	Movements become more voluntary Postural control improves; able to stand and may take few independent steps	First words are not generally classified as true language. They are generally associated with the concrete and are usually activity-oriented.	Begins to accommodate to the environment, and the adaptive process evolves
18	Extremely curious Becomes a communicative social being Parallel play Fleeting contacts with other children "Make-believe" play begins	Better control of spoon; good control when drinking from cup Turns page of a book Places objects in holes or slots	Walks alone; gait may still be a bit unsteady Begins to walk sideways and backward	Begins to use language in a symbolic form to represent images or ideas that reflect the thinking process Uses some meaningful words such as "hi," "bye-bye," and "all gone" Comprehension is significantly greater	Demonstrates foresight and can discover solutions to problems without excessive trial-and-error procedures Can imitate without the presence of a model (deferred imitation)
24	Language facilitates autonomy Sense of power from saying "no" and "mine" Increased independence from mother	Turns pages of a book singly Adept at building a tower of six or seven cubes When drawing, attempts to enclose a space	Runs well with little falling Throws and kicks a ball Walks up and down stairs one step at a time	Begins to use words to explain past events or to discuss objects not observably present Rapidly expands vocabulary to about 300 words; uses plurals	Enters preconceptual phase of cognitive development State of continuous investigations Primary focus is egocentric
36	Basic concepts of sexuality are established Separates from mother more easily Attends to toilet needs	Copies a circle and a straight line Grasps spoon between thumb and index finger Holds cup by handle	Balances on one foot; jumps in place; pedals tricycles	Quest for information furthered by questions like "why," "when," "where," and "how" Has acquired the language that will be used in the course of simple conversation during adult years	Preconceptual phase continues; can think of only one idea at a time; cannot think of all parts in terms of the whole

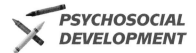

PSYCHOSOCIAL DEVELOPMENT

The toddler develops a growing awareness of self as a being, separate from other people or objects. Intoxicated with newly discovered powers and lacking experience, the child tends to test personal independence to the limit. This age has been called an age of **negativism.** Certainly the toddler's response to nearly everything is a firm "no," but this is more an assertion of individuality than of an intention to disobey.

Ritualism, dawdling, and temper tantrums also characterize this age. **Ritualism,** employed by the young child to help develop security, involves following routines that make rituals of even simple tasks. At bedtime, all toys must be in accustomed places, and the caregiver must follow a habitual practice. This passion for a set routine is not found in every child to the same degree, but it does provide a comfortable base from which to step out into new and potentially dangerous paths. These practices often become more evident when a sitter is in the home especially at bedtime. This gives the child some measure of security when the primary caregiver is absent.

Dawdling serves much the same purpose. The young child must decide between following the wishes and routines of the caregiver and asserting independence by following personal desires. Because he or she is incapable of making such a choice, the toddler compromises and tries both. If the task to be done is an important one, the caregiver with a firm and friendly manner should help the child to follow along the way he or she should go; otherwise, dawdling can be ignored within reasonable limits.

Temper tantrums spring from the many frustrations that are natural results of a child's urge to be independent. Add to this a child's reluctance to leave the scene for necessary rest and frequently the frustrations become too great. Even the best of caregivers may lose patience and show a temporary lack of understanding. The child reacts with enthusiastic rebellion, but this, too, is a phase that must be lived through while the child works toward becoming a person.

Reasoning, scolding, or punishing during a tantrum is useless. A trusted person who remains calm and patient needs to be nearby until the child gains self-control. After the tantrum is over, help the child relax by diverting attention with a toy or some other interesting distraction. However, do not yield the point or give in to the child's whim. That would tell the child that to get whatever her or she wants, a person need only throw oneself on the floor and scream. The child would have to learn painfully later in life that people cannot be controlled in this manner.

Admittedly it is not easy to handle a small child who drops to the floor screaming and kicking in rage in the middle of the supermarket or the sidewalk, nor are comments from onlookers at all helpful. The best a caregiver can do is pick up the out-of-control child as calmly as possible and carry him or her to a quiet, neutral place to regain self-control. These tantrums can be accompanied by head-banging and breath-holding. Breath-holding can be frightening to the caregiver, but the child will shortly lose consciousness and begin breathing. Head-banging can cause injury to the child, so the caregiver needs to provide protection.

The caregiver should try to be calm when dealing with a toddler having a tantrum. The child is out of control and needs help to regain control; the adult must maintain self-control to reassure the child and provide security.

Play

The toddler's play moves from the solitary play of the infant to **parallel play** in which the toddler plays alongside other children but not with them (Fig. 12–3). Much of the playtime is filled with imitation of the people the child sees as role models: adults around him or her, siblings, and other children. Toys that involve the toddler's new gross motor skills, such as push-pull toys, rocking horses, large blocks, and balls, are popular. Fine motor skills are developed by use of thick crayons, Play-Dough, finger paints, wooden puzzles with large pieces, toys that fit pieces into shaped holes, and cloth books. Toddlers enjoy talking on a play telephone and like pots, pans, and toys such as brooms, dishes, and lawnmowers that help them imitate the adults in

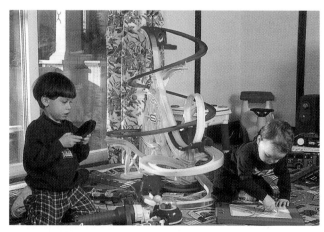

● *Figure 12.3* Toddlers engaged in parallel play.

their environment and promote socialization. The toddler cannot share toys until the later stage of toddlerhood, and adults should not make an issue of sharing at this early stage.

Toys should be carefully checked for loose pieces and sharp edges to ensure the toddler's safety. Toddlers still put a lot of things into their mouths; therefore, small pieces that may come loose, such as small beads and buttons, must be avoided.

For an adult, staying quietly on the sidelines and observing the toddler play can be a fascinating revelation of what is going on in the child's world. However, the adult must intervene if necessary to avoid injury.

Discipline

The word "discipline" has come to mean punishment to many people, but the concepts are not the same. To **discipline** means to train or instruct to produce a particular behavior pattern, especially moral or mental improvement, and self-control. **Punishment** means penalizing someone for wrongdoing. Although all small children need discipline, the need for punishment occurs much less frequently.

The toddler learns self-control gradually. The development from an egotistic being, whose world exists only to give self-satisfaction, into a person who understands and respects the rights of others is a long, involved process. The child cannot do this alone but must be taught.

Two-year-old children begin to show some signs of accepting responsibility for their own actions, but they lack inner controls because of their egocentricity. The toddler still wants the forbidden thing but may repeat "no, no, no" while reaching for a desired treasure, recognizing that the act is not approved. Although the child understands the act is not approved, the desire is too strong to resist. Even at this age, children want and need limits. When no limits are set, the child develops a feeling of insecurity and fear. With proper guidance, the child gradually absorbs the restraints and develops self-control or conscience.

Consistency and timing are important in the approach that the caregiver uses when disciplining the child. The toddler needs a lot of help during this time. People caring for the child should agree on the methods of discipline and should all operate by the same rules, so that the child knows what is expected. This need for consistency can cause disagreement for family caregivers who have experienced different types of childrearing themselves. The caregivers may be confused by this child who had been a sweet, loving baby and now has turned into a belligerent little being who throws tantrums at will.

This period can be challenging to adults. The child needs to learn that the adults are in control and will help the child to gain self-control while learning to be independent. When the toddler hits or bites another child, calmly remove the offender from the situation. Negative messages such as "You are a bad boy for hitting Jamal" or "Bad girl! You don't bite people" are not helpful. Instead, use messages that do not label the child as bad but label the act as unacceptable such as "Biting hurts—be gentle."

Another useful method for a child who is not cooperating or who is out of control is to send the child to a "time out" chair. This should be a place where the child can be alone but observed without other distractions. The duration of the isolation should be limited—1 minute per year of age is usually adequate. Warn the child in advance of this possibility, but only one warning per event is necessary. Praise children for good behavior and, when possible, ignore negative behavior.

"Extinction" is another discipline technique effective with this age group. If the child has certain undesirable behaviors that occur frequently, ignore the behavior. Do not react to the child as long as the behavior is not harmful to the child or others. Be consistent, and never react in any way to that particular behavior. Act as though you do not hear the child. However, when the child responds acceptably in a situation in which the undesirable behavior was the usual response, be sure to compliment the child. Suppose, for example that the child screams or makes a scene when you won't buy cookies in the grocery store. If, after you have practiced extinction, the child talks in a normal voice on another visit to the grocery store, compliment the child's "grown-up" behavior.

Spanking or other physical punishment usually does not work well because the child is merely taught that hitting or other physical violence is acceptable, and the child who is spanked frequently becomes immune to it.

Sharing With a Sibling

The first child has the caregivers' undivided attention until a new baby arrives, often when the first child is a toddler. Preparing a child just emerging from babyhood for this arrival is difficult. Although the toddler can feel the mother's abdomen and understand that this is where the new baby lives, this alone does not give adequate preparation for the baby's arrival. This real baby represents a rival for the mother's affection.

As in many stressful situations, the toddler frequently regresses to more infantile behavior. The toddler who no longer takes milk from a bottle may need or want a bottle when the new baby is being fed.

Toilet training, which may have been moving along well, may regress with the toddler having episodes of soiling and wetting.

The new infant creates considerable change in the home, whether he or she is the first child or the fifth. In homes where the previous baby is displaced by the newcomer, however, some special preparation is necessary. Moving the older child to a larger bed some time before the new baby appears lets the toddler take pride in being "grown up" now.

Preparation of the toddler for a new brother or sister is helpful but should not be intense until just before the expected birth. Many hospitals have sibling classes for new siblings-to-be that are scheduled shortly before the anticipated delivery. These classes, geared to the young child, give the child some tasks to do for the new baby and discuss both negative and positive aspects of having a new baby in the home. Many books are available to help prepare the young child for the birth and that explore sibling rivalry.

Probably the greatest help in preparing the child of any age to accept the new baby is to help the child feel that this is "our baby" not just "mommy's baby" (Fig. 12–4). Helping to care for the baby, according to the child's ability, contributes to a feeling of continuing importance and self-worth.

The displaced toddler almost certainly will feel some jealousy. With careful planning, however, the mother can reserve some time for cuddling and playing with the toddler just as before. Perhaps the toddler may profit from a little extra parental attention for a time. The toddler needs to feel that parental love is just as great as ever and that there is plenty of room in the parents' lives for both children.

The child should not be made to grow up too soon. The toddler should not be shamed or reproved for reverting to babyish behavior but should receive understanding and a bit more love and attention.

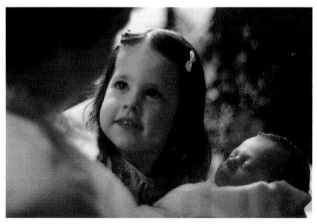

● *Figure 12.4* The toddler is meeting her new baby brother.

Perhaps the father or other family member can occasionally take over the care of the new baby while the mother devotes herself to the toddler. The mother also may plan special times with the toddler when the new infant is sleeping and mother has no interruptions. This approach helps the toddler feel special.

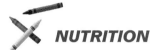

NUTRITION

Eating problems commonly appear between the ages of 1 and 3 years. These problems occur for a number of reasons such as

1. The child's growth rate has slowed; therefore, he or she may want and need less food than before. Family caregivers need to know that this is normal.
2. The child's strong drive for independence and autonomy compels an assertion of will to prove his or her individuality both to self and others.
3. A child's appetite varies according to the kind of foods offered. "Food jags," the desire for only one kind of food for a while, are common.

To minimize these eating problems and ensure that the child gets a balanced diet with all the proteins, carbohydrates, minerals, and vitamins essential for health and well-being, meals should be planned with an understanding of the toddler's developing feeding skills. Family Teaching Tips for Feeding Toddlers offers guidance for toddler mealtimes. Messiness is to be expected and prepared for when learning begins; it gradually diminishes as the child gains skill in self-feeding. At 15 months, the toddler can sit through meals, prefers finger feeding, and wants to self-feed. He or she tries to use a spoon but has difficulty with scooping and spilling. The 15-month-old grasps the cup with the thumb and forefinger but tilts the cup instead of the head. By 18 months, the toddler's appetite decreases. The 18-month-old has improved control of the spoon, puts spilled food back on the spoon, holds the cup with both hands, spills less often, and may throw the cup when finished if no one is there to take it. At 24 months, the toddler's appetite is fair to moderate. The toddler at this age has clearly defined likes and dislikes and food jags. The 24-month-old grasps the spoon between the thumb and forefinger, can put food on the spoon with one hand, continues to spill, and accepts no help ("Me do!"). By 30 months, refusals and preferences are less evident. Some toddlers at this age hold the spoon like an adult, with the palm turned inward. The cup, too, may be handled in an adult manner. The 30-month-old tilts the head back to get the very last drop. A sample daily food plan is provided in Table 12–2.

TABLE 12.2	Suggested Daily Food Guidelines for the Toddler	
Food Items	Daily Amounts*	Comments/Rationale
Cooked eggs	3–5/wk	Good source of protein. Moderate use is recommended because of high cholesterol content in egg yolk.
Breads, cereal, rice, pasta: whole-grain or enriched	6 or more servings (eg, ½ slice bread, ¼ cup cereal, ¼ cup rice, 2 crackers, ¼ cup noodles)	Provide thiamine, niacin, and, if enriched, riboflavin and iron. Encourage child to identify and appreciate a wide variety of foods.
Fruit juices; fruit—canned or small pieces	2–4 child-sized servings (eg, ½ cup juice, ¼–½ cup fruit pieces)	Use those rich in vitamins A and C; also source of iron and calcium. Self-feeding enhances the child's sense of independence.
Vegetables	3–5 child-sized servings (eg, ¼–⅓ cup)	Include at least one dark-green or yellow vegetable every other day for vitamin A.
Meat, fish, poultry, cottage cheese, peanut butter, dried peas and beans	2–3 child-sized servings (eg, 1 oz meat, ¼ cup cottage cheese, 1–2 tbsp peanut butter)	Source of complete protein, iron, thiamine, riboflavin, niacin, and vitamin B_{12} Nuts and seeds should not be offered until after age 3 when risk of choking is minimal.
Milk, yogurt, cheese	4–6 child-sized servings (eg, 4–6 oz milk, ½ cup yogurt, 1 oz cheese)	Cheese, cottage cheese, and yogurt are good calcium and riboflavin sources. Also sources of calcium, phosphorus, complete protein, riboflavin, and niacin and vitamin D if milk is fortified
Fats and sweets	In moderation	May interfere with consumption of nutrient-rich foods. Chocolate should be delayed until the child is 1 year old.
Salt and other seasonings	In moderation	Children's taste buds are more sensitive than those of adults. Salt is a learned taste, and high intakes are related to hypertension.

*Amounts are daily totals and goals to be achieved gradually.

Adapted from Dudek, SG. (2000) *Nutrition essentials for nursing practice* (4th ed). Philadelphia: Lippincott Williams & Wilkins.

FAMILY TEACHING TIPS

Feeding Toddlers

1. Serve small portions, and provide a second serving when the first has been eaten. One or 2 teaspoonfuls is an adequate serving for the toddler. Too much food on the dish may overwhelm the child.
2. There is no *one* food essential to health. Allow substitution for a disliked food. Food jags where toddlers prefer one food for days on end are common and not harmful. If the child refuses a particular food such as milk, use appropriate substitutes such as pudding, cheese, yogurt, and cottage cheese. Avoid a battle of wills at mealtime.
3. Toddlers like simply prepared foods served warm or cool, *not* hot or cold.
4. Provide a social atmosphere at mealtimes; allow the toddler to eat with others in the family. Toddlers learn by imitating the acceptance or rejection of foods by other family members.
5. Toddlers prefer foods that they can pick up with their fingers; however, they should be allowed to use a spoon or fork when they want to try.

6. Try to plan regular mealtimes with small nutritious snacks between meals. Do not attach too much importance to food by urging the child to choose what to eat.
7. Dawdling at mealtime is common with this age group and can be ignored unless it stretches to unreasonable lengths or becomes a play for power. Mealtime for the toddler should not exceed 20 minutes. Calmly remove food without comment.
8. Do not make desserts a reward for good eating habits. It gives unfair value to the dessert and makes vegetables or other foods seem less desirable.
9. Offer regularly planned nutritious snacks such as milk, crackers and peanut butter, cheese cubes, and pieces of fruit. Plan snacks midway between meals and at bedtime.
10. Remember that the total amount eaten each day is more important than the amount eaten at a specific meal.

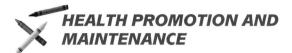

HEALTH PROMOTION AND MAINTENANCE

Two important aspects of health promotion and maintenance for the toddler are routine checkups and accident prevention. Routine checkups help protect the toddler's health and ensure continuing growth and development. The nurse can encourage good health through family teaching, support of positive parenting behaviors, and reinforcement of the toddler's achievements. Toddlers need a stimulating environment and the opportunity to explore it. This environment, however, must be safe to help prevent accidents and infection. Give caregivers information regarding accident prevention and home safety.

Routine Checkups

The child is seen at 15 months for immunization boosters and at least annually thereafter. Routine physical checkups include assessment of growth and development, oral hygiene, toilet training, daily health care, the caregiver-toddler relationship, and parenting skills. Interviews with caregivers, observations of the toddler, observations of the caregiver-toddler interaction, and communication with the toddler are all effective means to elicit this information. Remember that caregiver interpretations may not be completely accurate. Communicate with the toddler on his or her level and offer only realistic options.

Current immunizations should be administered (see Figure 10–8 in Chap. 10). Table 12–3 details nursing measures that may be implemented to ensure optimal health practices.

Family Teaching

The toddler is learning rapidly about the world in which she or he lives. As part of that process, the toddler learns about everyday care needed for healthy growth and development. The toddler's urge for independence and the caregiver's response to that urge play an important part in everyday life with the

TABLE 12.3 | Guidelines for Health Promotion in the Toddler

Developmental Characteristics of Toddler (2–3 Yr)	Possible Deviations From Health	Nursing Measures to Ensure Optimal Health Practices
Self-feeding (foods and objects more accessible for mouthing, handling, and eating)	Inadequate nutritional intake Accidental poisoning Gastrointestinal disturbances: Instability of gastrointestinal tract Infection from parasites (pinworm)	Diet teaching Childproofing the home Careful handwashing (before meals, after toileting) Avoidance of rich foods Observe for perianal itching (Scotch tape test, administer anthelmintic)
Toilet training	Constipation (if training procedures are too rigid) Urinary tract infection (especially prevalent in girls due to anatomic structure and poor toilet habits)	Teaching toileting procedures Urinalysis when indicated (eg, burning) Teaching hygiene (at the onset of training, instruct girls to wipe from front to back, and wash hands to prevent cross-infection)
Increased socialization	Increased prevalence of upper respiratory infections (immune levels still at immature levels)	Hygienic practices (eg, use of tissue or handkerchief, not drinking from same glass) Immunizations for passive immunity against communicable disease
Primary dentition	Caries with resultant infection or loss of primary as well as beginning permanent teeth	Oral hygiene, regular tooth brushing, dental examination at 2½–3 years Proper nutrition to ensure dentition
Sleep disturbances	Lack of sleep may cause irritability, lethargy, decreased resistance to infection	Teaching regarding recommended amounts of sleep (12–14 h in first year, decreasing to 10–12 h by age 3); need for rituals to enhance transition process to bedtime; possibility of need for nap; setting bedtime limits

toddler. Some of these activities are included in the following discussion.

Bathing

Toddlers generally love to take a tub bath. Setting a regular time each day for the bath helps give the toddler a sense of security about what to expect. Although the toddler can sit well in the tub, he or she should never be left alone. An adult must supervise the bath continuously to prevent an accident. The toddler enjoys having tub toys to play with. Avoid using bubble bath, especially for little girls, because it can create an environment that encourages the growth of organisms that cause bladder infections. A bath often is relaxing and may help the toddler quiet down before bedtime.

Dressing

By their second birthday, toddlers take an active interest in helping to put on their clothes. They often begin around 18 months by removing their socks and shoes whenever they choose. This behavior can be frustrating to the caregiver but if accepted as another small step in development, the caretaker may feel less frustration. Between the ages of 2 and 3 years, the toddler can begin by putting on underpants, shirts, or socks (Fig. 12–5). Often the clothing ends up backwards, but the important thing is that the toddler accomplished the task. Encourage the caregiver to take a relaxed attitude as the toddler learns to dress him or herself. If clothes must be put on correctly, the caregiver should try to do it without criticizing the toddler's job. The caregiver should warmly acknowledge the toddler's accomplishment of putting on a piece of clothing that he or she may have struggled with for some time. Roomy clothing with easy buttons, large, smooth-running zippers, or Velcro is easier for the toddler to handle.

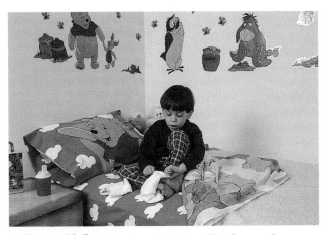

● **Figure 12.5** Getting dressed by himself is a fun morning activity for this 3-year-old.

As in late infancy, shoes need to be worn primarily to protect the toddler's feet from harsh surfaces. Sneakers are still a good choice. Avoid hard-soled shoes. High-topped shoes are unnecessary.

Dental Care

Dental caries (cavities) are a major health problem in children and young adults. Sound teeth depend in part on sound nutrition. The development of dental caries is linked to the effect the diet has on the oral environment.

Bacteria that act in the presence of sugar and form a film, or dental plaque, on the teeth cause tooth decay. People who eat sweet foods frequently accumulate plaque easily and are prone to dental caries. Sugars eaten at mealtime appear to be neutralized by the presence of other foods and, therefore, are not as damaging as between-meal sweets and bedtime bottles. Foods consisting of hard or sticky sugars, such as lollipops and caramels that remain in the mouth for longer periods, tend to cause more dental caries than those eaten quickly. Sugarless gum or candies are not as harmful.

When the child is about 2 years of age, he or she should be taught to brush the teeth or at least to rinse the mouth after each meal or snack. Because this is the period when the toddler likes to imitate others, the child is best taught by example. Plain water should be used until the child has learned how to spit out toothpaste. An adult should also brush the toddler's teeth until the child becomes experienced. One good method is to stand behind the child in front of a mirror and brush the child's teeth. In addition to cleaning adequately, this also helps the child learn how it feels to have the teeth thoroughly brushed.

The use of fluoride toothpaste strengthens tooth enamel and helps to prevent tooth decay, particularly in communities with unfluoridated water. An adult should supervise the use of fluoride toothpaste; the child should use only a small pea-sized amount. The physician may recommend supplemental fluoride, but families on limited incomes may find this difficult to afford. A fluoride supplement is a medication and should be treated and stored as such. Fluoride also can be applied during regular visits to the dentist, but the greatest benefit to the tooth enamel occurs before the eruption of the teeth.

The first visit to the dentist should occur at about 2 years of age just so the child gets acquainted with the dentist, staff, and office. A second visit might be a good time for a preliminary examination, and subsequent visits twice a year for checkups are recommended. If there are older siblings, the toddler can go along on a visit with them to help overcome the fears of a strange setting. Some clinics are recommending earlier visits to check the child and give dietary guidance. Children of low-income families often have poor dental hygiene and care, both because of the cost of care and parental lack of knowledge about proper care and nutrition. Some caregivers may believe it is unnecessary to take proper care of baby teeth because "they fall out anyway." The care and condition of the baby teeth affect the normal growth of permanent teeth, which are forming in the jaw under the baby teeth. It is important for the nurse to teach the caregivers the importance of proper care of the child's baby teeth.

Toilet Training

Learning bowel and bladder control is an important part of the socialization process. In Western culture, a great sense of shame and disgust has been associated with body waste products. To function successfully in this culture, one must learn to dispose of body waste products in a place considered proper by society.

The toddler has been operating on the pleasure principle by simply emptying the bowel and bladder when the urge is present without thinking of anything but personal comfort. During toilet training, the child, who is just learning about control of the personal environment, finds that some of that control must be given up to please those most important people, the caregivers. The toddler now must learn to conform not only to please those special loved ones; to preserve self-integrity, the toddler must persuade himself or herself that this acceptance of the dictates of society is voluntary. These new routines make little sense to the child.

Timing. To be able to cooperate in toilet training, the child's sphincter muscles must have developed to the stage when the child can control them. Control of the rectal sphincter develops first. The child also must be able to postpone the urge to defecate until reaching the toilet or potty and must be able to signal the need *before* the event. This level of maturation seldom takes place before the age of 18 to 24 months.

Bowel Training. At the start of training, the child has no understanding of the uses of the potty chair, but to please the caregiver the child will sit there for a short time (Fig. 12–6). If the child's bowel movements occur at about the same time every day, one day a bowel movement will occur while sitting on the potty. Although there is no sense of special achievement as yet, the child does like the praise and approval. Eventually the child will connect this approval with the bowel movement in the potty, and the child will be happy that the caregiver is pleased.

Suggestions for bowel training include

1. A potty chair in which a child can comfortably sit with the feet on the floor is preferable. Most small children are afraid of a flush toilet.
2. The child should be left on the potty chair for only

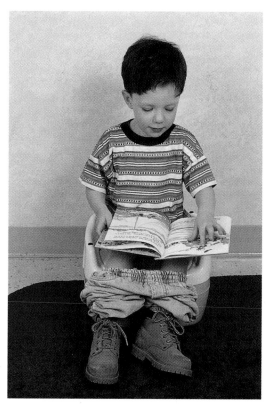

● *Figure 12.6* Toddlers will sit on the potty chair to please a caregiver.

a short time. The caregiver should be readily available but should not hover anxiously over the child. If a bowel movement occurs, approval is in order; if not, no comment is necessary.
3. During the beginning stages of training, the child is likely to have a movement soon after leaving the potty. This is not willful defiance and need not be mentioned.
4. The potty should be emptied unobtrusively after the child has resumed playing. The child has cooperated and produced the product desired. If it is immediately thrown away, the child may be confused and not so eager to please the next time.
5. The ability to feel shame and self-doubt appears at this age. Therefore, the child should not be teased about reluctance or inability to conform. This teasing can shake the child's confidence and cause feelings of doubt in self-worth.
6. The caregiver should not expect perfection, even after control has been achieved. Lapses inevitably occur perhaps because the child is completely absorbed in play or because of a temporary episode of loose stools. Occasionally a child feels aggression, frustration, or anger and may use this method to "get even." As long as the lapses are occasional, they should be ignored. If the lapses are frequent and persistent, however, the cause should be sought.

COMMUNICATIONS BOX 12-1

Conversation about toilet training with Mike (father of 2-year-old Josh):

LESS EFFECTIVE COMMUNICATION	*MORE EFFECTIVE COMMUNICATION*
Mike: I don't get it. Josh doesn't let me know when he has to pee. He just goes off to a corner and wets himself.	*Mike:* I don't get it. Josh doesn't let me know when he has to pee. He just goes off to a corner and wets himself.
Nurse: Why don't you just pick him up and run for the bathroom when he does that?	*Nurse:* You get disgusted with Josh because he doesn't let you know when he has to urinate.
Mike: It's already too late. He's wet and I just get mad.	*Mike:* Well, yeah. I mean, if he knows enough to go off to the corner, why doesn't he just tell me?
Nurse: Don't get mad at him. He's just a little guy. He's not doing it to be mean.	*Nurse:* You are puzzled that he doesn't let you know ahead of time.
Mike: Well, it seems to me like he is. I know he knows better.	*Mike:* Yeah. I think he's just being stubborn.
Nurse: Maybe he does, but he's not just doing it to be mean. Sooner or later he'll learn what he's supposed to do. You just have to be patient with him.	*Nurse:* When Josh goes to the corner, he is indicating that he knows he is going to urinate. Perhaps you could quickly take him to his potty chair at that time, if you notice him.
	Mike: Well, I suppose so. But how long is this going to go on?
	Nurse: You feel like he will never learn. Toilet training can be a rather long and frustrating experience with some children. Josh needs continued positive support and praise when he "gets it right." Try to use a positive approach. Avoid punishing him for his mistakes. Eventually he will be successful and be very proud of himself.
	Mike: Well, OK. I'll give that a try.
	Nurse: Good. And if you continue to have problems, don't hesitate to seek guidance. Toddlers are challenging but amazing when you think of all they accomplish in that period of their development.

▶ *During this conversation, the nurse does not acknowledge Mike's feelings. Telling him not to get mad does not help him ventilate his own feelings. Telling him he must just be patient with Josh contributes to Mike's feelings of inadequacy.*

▶ *By acknowledging to Mike that toilet training is one of the frustrating aspects of parenting a toddler, the nurse helps him to understand that his feelings are not unusual and that Josh is behaving like a normal toddler. Offering him concrete ideas to help and further support if needed are positive ways to communicate.*

Bladder Training. Generally the first indication of readiness for bladder training is when the child makes a connection between the puddle on the floor and something he or she did. In the next stage, the child runs to the caregiver and indicates a need to urinate, but only after it has happened. Not much benefit is gained from a serious program of training until the child is sufficiently mature to control the bladder sphincter and reach the desired place. When the child stays dry for about 2 hours at a time during the day, sufficient maturity may be indicated.

Each child follows an individual pattern of development, so no caregiver should feel embarrassed or ashamed because a child is still having accidents. No one should expect the child to accomplish self-training, and family caregivers should be alert to the signs of readiness. Patience and understanding by the caregivers are essential. Complete control, especially at night, may not be achieved until the fourth or fifth year of age. Each child should be taught a term or phrase to use for toileting that is recognizable to others, clearly understood, and socially acceptable. This is especially true for children who are cared for outside the home.

INTERNET EXERCISE 12.1

http://www.lee-bee.com

Lee-Bee Motivational Charts
Click on "Need help potty training your child?"
Click on "When to start potty training" on left hand side of screen.

1. What are the 15 common signs of toilet training readiness?

2. After reading this section, what could you share with the caregivers of a toddler regarding potty training?

3. What else is available on this site for caregivers of a toddler?

Sleep

The toddler's sleep needs change gradually between the ages of 1 and 3 years. A total daily need for 12 to 14 hours of sleep is to be expected in the first year of toddlerhood, decreasing to 10 to 12 hours by 3 years. The toddler soon gives up a morning nap, but most continue to need an afternoon nap until sometime near the third birthday.

Rituals are a common part of bedtime procedures. A bedtime ritual provides structure and a feeling of security because the toddler knows what to expect and what is expected of him or her. The separation anxiety common in the toddler may contribute to some of the toddler's reluctance to go to bed. Family caregivers must be careful that the toddler does not use this to manipulate them and delay bedtime. Gentle, firm consistency by caregivers is ultimately reassuring to the toddler. Regular schedules with set bedtimes and a story time or quiet time beforehand often help the toddler settle for the night. Many wonderful stories are available to read to the toddler and can provide a calming end to a busy day.

Accident Prevention

Toddlers are explorers who require constant supervision in a controlled environment to encourage autonomy and prevent injury. When supervision is inadequate or the environment is unsafe, tragedy often results; accidents are the leading cause of death for children between the ages of 1 and 4 years.

A PERSONAL GLIMPSE

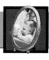

One day I came home from work and my wife told me an amazing (and frightening) story about our 2-year-old son. I have a rifle cabinet in our living room. It is always locked, and only my wife and I know where the key is, or so we thought. My wife was at the sink doing dishes. While she has busy, Richie pulled a chair up to the wall and somehow reached up to the shelves where the keys were kept. By the time Becky noticed what he was up to, Richie was putting the key in the lock of the drawer where the pistols are kept. Of course, none of them are ever loaded, and the bullets are nowhere near where the weapons are kept. Anyway, she took the key from him and figured that was that. Well, he had other ideas! Somehow, without her knowing it, he had gotten two keys and gave her the wrong one on purpose (or maybe not, we'll never know). Luckily, his second attempt was also unsuccessful. We don't know how 2-year-olds think, but I wonder what comes after 2. I guess 3.

Max

▶ **LEARNING OPPORTUNITY:** What behaviors seen in toddlers would be important to review with the caregivers of this child? What are some important safety measures to take with all children but especially with toddlers?

Accidents involving motor vehicles, drowning, burns, poisoning, and falls are the most common causes of death. The number of motor vehicle deaths in this age group is more than three times greater than the numbers of deaths caused by burns or drowning. Family teaching can help minimize the risk for accident and injury.

Motor Vehicle Accidents

Many childhood deaths or injuries resulting from motor vehicle accidents can be prevented by proper use of restraints. Federally approved child safety seats are designed to give the child maximum protection if used correctly (Fig. 12–7). Adults must be responsible for teaching the child that seat belts are required for safe car travel and that he or she must be securely fastened in the car seat before the car starts. Adults in the car with a child should set the example by also using seat belts. Many toddlers are killed or injured by moving vehicles while playing in their own driveways or garages. Caregivers need to be aware that these tragedies can occur and must take proper precautions at all times. See Family Teaching Tips: Preventing Motor Vehicle Accidents.

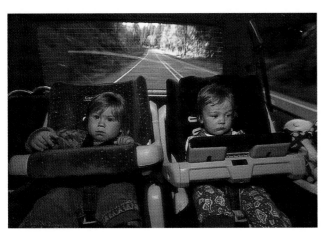

● *Figure 12.7* Car seats are used for safety when toddlers ride in a vehicle.

Drowning

Although drowning of young children is often associated with bathtubs, the increased number of home swimming pools has added significantly to the number of accidental drownings. Often these pools are fenced on three sides to keep out nonresidents but are bordered on one side by the family home, making the pool accessible to infants and toddlers. Even small plastic wading pools hold enough water

to drown an unsupervised toddler. Any family living near a body of water, no matter how small, must not leave a mobile infant or toddler unattended even for a moment. Even a small amount of water, such as that in a bucket, may be enough to drown a small child.

Burns

Burn accidents occur most often as scalds from immersions and spills and from exposure to uninsulated electrical wires or live extension-cord plugs. Children also are burned while playing with matches or while left unattended in a home where a fire breaks out. Whether the fire results from a child's mischief, an adult's carelessness, or some unforeseeable event, the injuries, even if not fatal, can have long-term or permanent effects. Often burns can be prevented by following simple safety practices (see Family Teaching Tips: Preventing Burns).

Ingestion of Toxic Substances

The curious toddler wants to touch and taste everything. Left unsupervised, the toddler may sample household cleaners, prescription or over-the-counter drugs, kerosene, gasoline, peeling lead-based paint chips, or dust particles. Poisoning is still the most common medical emergency in children with the highest incidence between the ages of 1 and 4 years.

Caregivers need continual reminders about the possibility of childhood poisoning. Even with

---

FAMILY TEACHING TIPS

Preventing Motor Vehicle Accidents

1. Never start the car until the child is securely in the car seat.
2. If the child manages to get out of the car seat or unfasten it, pull over to the curb or side of the road as soon as possible, turn off the car, and tell the child that the car will not go until he or she is safely in the seat. Children love to go in the car, and they will comply if they learn that they cannot go unless in the car seat.
3. Never permit a child to stand in a car that is in motion.
4. Teach the toddler to stop at a curb and wait for an adult escort to cross the street. An older child should be taught to look both ways for traffic. Start this as a game with toddlers, and continually reinforce it.
5. Teach the child to cross only at corners.
6. Begin in toddlerhood to teach awareness of traffic signals and their meanings. As soon as the child recognizes color, he or she can tell you when it is all right to cross.
7. Never let a child run into the street after a ball.
8. Teach a child never to walk between parked cars to cross.
9. As a driver, always be on the alert for children running into the street when in a residential area.

FAMILY TEACHING TIPS

Preventing Burns

1. Do not let electrical cords dangle over a counter or table. Repair frayed cords. Newer small appliances have shorter cords to prevent dangling.
2. Cover electrical wall outlets with safety caps.
3. Turn handles of pans on the stove toward the back of the stove. If possible, place pans on back burners out of the toddler's reach.
4. Place cups of hot liquid out of reach. Do not use overhanging tablecloths that toddlers can pull.
5. Use caution when serving foods heated in the microwave; they can be hotter than is apparent.
6. Supervise small children at all times in the bathtub so they cannot turn on the hot water tap.
7. Turn thermostat on home water heater down so that the water temperature is no higher than 120°F.
8. Place matches in metal containers and out of reach of small children. Keep lighters out of reach of children.
9. Never leave small children unattended by an adult or responsible teenager.

FAMILY TEACHING TIPS

Preventing Poisoning

1. Keep medicines in their original containers in a locked cupboard. Do not rely on a high shelf being out of a child's reach.
2. Never refer to medicines as candy.
3. Discard unused medicines by a method that eliminates any possibility of access by children, other persons, or animals (e.g., flush them down the toilet).
4. Replace safety caps properly, but do not depend on them to be childproof. Children can sometimes open them more easily than adults can.
5. Keep a bottle of syrup of ipecac in a locked cupboard to induce vomiting if recommended by the poison control center.
6. Keep the telephone number of the nearest poison control center posted near the telephone.
7. Keep a chart with emergency treatment for poisoning in a handy permanent spot.
8. Store household cleaning and laundry products out of children's reach.
9. Never put kerosene or other household fluids in soda bottles or other drink containers.

precautionary labeling and "child-resistant" packaging of medication and household cleaners, children display amazing ingenuity in opening bottles and packages that catch their curiosity. Mr. Yuk labels are available from the nearest poison control center. The child can be taught that products are harmful if they have the Mr. Yuk label on them. However, labeling is not sufficient: all items that are in any way toxic to the child must be placed under lock and key or totally out of the child's reach.

Preventive measures that should be observed by all caregivers of small children are listed in Family Teaching Tips: Preventing Poisoning.

The following medications are most commonly involved in cases of childhood poisoning:

Acetaminophen
Salicylates (aspirin)
Laxatives
Sedatives
Tranquilizers
Analgesics
Antihistamines
Cold medicines
Birth-control pills

The importance of careful, continuous supervision of toddlers and other young children cannot be overemphasized.

THE TODDLER IN THE HEALTH CARE FACILITY

Although hospitalization is difficult and frightening for a child of any age, the developmental stage of the toddler intensifies these problems. When planning care, the nurse caring for the toddler must keep in mind the toddler's developmental tasks and needs. The toddler, engaged in trying to establish self-control and autonomy, finds that strangers seem to have total power; this eliminates any control on the toddler's part. Add these fears to the inability to communicate well, discomfort from pain, separation from family, the presence of unfamiliar people and surroundings, physical restraint, and uncomfortable or frightening procedures, and the toddler's reaction can be clearly understood.

As part of the child's admission procedure, a social assessment survey should be completed by interviewing the family caregiver who has accompanied the child to the facility. Usually part of the standard pediatric nursing assessment form, the social assessment covers eating habits and food preferences, toileting habits and terms used for toileting, family members and the names the child calls them, the name the child is called by family members, pets and their names, favorite toys, sleeping or napping patterns and rituals, and other significant information that helps the staff better plan care for the toddler (see Fig. 5–2 in Chap. 5). This information should become an indispensable part of the nursing care plan. Using this information, the nurse should develop a nursing care plan that provides opportunities for independence for the toddler whenever possible.

Separation anxiety is high during the toddler age. As discussed in detail in Chapter 2, the stages of protest and despair are common. Acknowledge these stages and communicate to the child that it is acceptable to feel angry and anxious at being separated from the primary family caregiver, the person foremost in the child's life. *Never* interpret the toddler's angry protest as a personal attack. Many facilities encourage family involvement in the child's care to minimize separation anxiety. The mother is often the family member who stays with the child, but in many families other members who are close to the child may take turns staying. Having a family caregiver with the toddler can be extremely helpful. Do not, however, neglect caring for the toddler who has a loved one present. In many families, it is impossible for the family caregiver to stay with the child for any of a number of reasons. These children need extra attention and care. All children should be assigned a constant caregiver while in the facility, but this is especially important for the toddler who is alone.

The nurse assigned to the toddler will become a surrogate parent while caring for the child. Maintaining as much as possible the pattern, schedule, and rituals that the toddler is used to helps to provide some measure of security to the child. This is a time when the toddler needs the security of a beloved thumb or other "lovey," a favorite stuffed animal or blanket. The nurse needs to recognize that the toddler uses this to provide self-comfort (Fig. 12–8). The lovey may be well worn and dirty, but the toddler finds great reassurance in having it to snuggle or cuddle. Do not ridicule the child for its unkempt appearance, and make every effort to allow the toddler to have it whenever desired.

When the family caregiver must leave the toddler, it may be helpful for the adult to give the child some personal item to keep until the adult returns. The caregiver can tell the child he or she will return "when the cartoons come on TV" or "when your lunch comes." These are concrete times that the toddler will probably understand.

Special Considerations

The busy toddler just learning to use the toilet, self-feed, and be disciplined presents a unique challenge to the staff nurse. The nurse must maintain control on the pediatric unit, promote safety, and help establish the toddler's sense of security while allowing the toddler's development to continue.

The toddler learning sphincter control is still dependent on familiar surroundings and the family caregiver's support. For this reason, some pediatric personnel automatically put toddlers back in diapers when they are admitted. This practice should be discouraged. Under the right circumstances and especially with the caregiver's help, many of these children can maintain control. They at least should be given a chance to try. Potty chairs can be provided for the child when appropriate. The nursing staff must know the method and times of accomplishing toilet training used at home and must try to comply with them as closely as possible in the hospital.

Some limits are needed for the toddler but be careful when setting them. Toddlers, like children of any age, need to feel that someone is in control and need limits set with love and understanding. A child who has been overindulged for a long time may need firm, calm statements of limits delivered in a no-nonsense but kind manner. Explaining what is going to be done, what is expected of the toddler, and what the toddler can expect from the nurse may be helpful. Sometimes the nurse may give some tactful guidance to the family caregiver to help set limits for the toddler. This is an area where experience helps the nurse to solve difficult problems. Discipline on the pediatric unit is discussed in Chapter 4.

A toddler's eating habits may loom large in the nurse's mind as a potential problem. In the hospital or clinic as at home, food can assume an importance out of proportion to its value and create unnecessary problems. Some helpful hints to minimize potential problems are

- View mealtime as a social event.
- Encourage self-feeding.
- Do not push the child to eat.
- Allow others to eat with the child.
- Offer familiar foods.
- Provide fluids in small but frequent amounts.

Eating concerns for the pediatric patient are fully discussed in Chapter 4.

Safety is a concern with all hospitalized children, but safety promotion for a toddler may be particularly challenging. The curious toddler needs to be watched with extra care but should not be unnecessarily prohibited from exploring and moving about freely. Safety in the hospital setting is discussed in detail in Chapter 4.

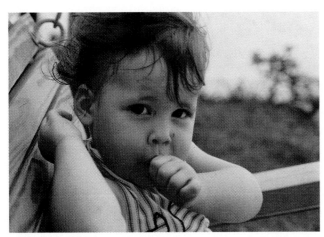

● *Figure 12.8* The toddler finds security and comfort in her "beloved" thumb.

KEY POINTS

▶ The toddler's physical growth slows while motor, social, and language development rapidly increase.

▶ Autonomy versus doubt and shame is the development task identified by Erikson for the toddler.

▶ During the toddler period, toilet training, ritualistic behavior, dawdling, negativism, temper tantrums, discipline, and separation anxiety are challenging issues. Caretakers who are understanding, patient, and consistent in their approach best meet these issues.

▶ As a result of the of the toddler's exploring nature, safety concerns are extremely important. Caregivers must provide a safe environment and protect the toddler from motor vehicle accidents, burns, and ingestion of poisonous substances.

▶ The toddler's language development proceeds from a few words to the ability to form short sentences by age 2. Verbal language increases rapidly between the toddler's second and third birthday.

▶ When caring for a toddler, the nurse provides for age-appropriate developmental tasks and encourages autonomy while protecting the toddler from harm.

BIBLIOGRAPHY

Banks M. (2001) Fluoridated water: Nature's cavity fighter. *Community Health Forum*, 2(6).

Brazelton TB, Greenspan S. (2001) *The irreducible needs of children: What every child must have to grow, learn, and flourish.* Cambridge, MA: Perseus Publishing.

Bufalini M. (2001) Dental health life cycle. *Community Health Forum*, 2(6).

Craven RF, Hirnle CJ. (1999) *Fundamentals of nursing* (3rd ed). Philadelphia: Lippincott Williams & Wilkins.

Dudek SG. (2000) *Nutrition essentials for nursing practice* (4th ed). Philadelphia: Lippincott Williams, and Wilkins.

Gaylord N. (2001) Parenting classes: From birth to 3 years. *Journal of Pediatric Health Care*, 15(4), 179.

Monsen R. (2001) Giving children control and toilet training. *Journal of Pediatric Nursing*, 16(5), 375.

Pillitteri A. (2003) *Maternal and child health nursing* (4th ed). Philadelphia: Lippincott Williams & Wilkins.

Spock B, et. al. (1998) *Dr. Spock's baby and child care.* New York: Pocket Books.

Starr N. (2001) Kids and car safety: Beyond car seats and seat belts. *Journal of Pediatric Health Care* 15(5), 257.

Wong DL, Perry S, Hockenberry M. (2002) *Maternal child nursing care* (2nd ed). St. Louis: Mosby.

Websites
www.babycenter.com/toddler
Poison Control: *www.aapcc.org*
Accident Prevention: *www.childrens.com*

Workbook

NCLEX-STYLE REVIEW QUESTIONS

1. The nurse is weighing a toddler who is three years old. If this child has had a typical pattern of growth and weighed 18 pounds at the age of 1 year, the nurse would expect this toddler to weigh approximately how many pounds?

   a. 22 pounds

   b. 30 pounds

   c. 36 pounds

   d. 42 pounds

2. The nurse is observing a group of two-year-olds. Which of the following actions by the toddlers would indicate a gross motor skill seen in children this age?

   a. turns pages of a book

   b. uses words to explain an object

   c. drinks from a cup

   d. runs with little falling

3. The toddler-aged child engages in "parallel play." The nurse observes the following behaviors in a room where children are playing with dolls and stuffed animals. Which of the following is an example of parallel play? Two children are

   a. sharing stuffed animals with each other

   b. sitting next each other, each playing with her or his own doll

   c. taking turns playing with the same stuffed animal

   d. feeding the first doll, then feeding the second doll

4. In preparing snacks for a 15-month-old toddler, which of the following would be the BEST choice for this age child?

   a. small cup of yogurt

   b. five or six green grapes

   c. handful of dry cereal

   d. three or four cookies

5. During the toddler years, the child attempts to become autonomous or independent. If the following statements were made by caregivers of three-year-olds, which observation reflects that the child is developing autonomy?

   a. "When my child falls down, he always wants me to pick him up."

   b. "My child has temper tantrums when we go to the store."

   c. "Every night my child follows the same routine at bedtime."

   d. "My child uses the potty chair and is dry all day long."

STUDY ACTIVITIES

1. List and compare the fine motor and gross motor skills in each of the following ages:

	15 Months	24 Months	36 Months
Fine motor skills			
Gross motor skills			

2. Discuss the development of language seen in toddlerhood. Compare the language development of the 15-month-old child to the language development of the 36-month-old child.

3. List the four leading causes of accidents in toddlers. For each of these causes state three prevention tips that you could share with family caregivers of toddlers.

CRITICAL THINKING

1. You are in the supermarket with your 2-year-old niece, Lauren. She is having a loud, screaming temper tantrum because you won't buy some expensive cookies she wants. Based on your knowledge of toddlers and tantrums, describe how you will handle the situation.

2. Marti complains to you that 2-year-old Tasha is very difficult to put to bed at night. Marti often just gives up and lets Tasha fall asleep in front of the television. Create a parent-teaching plan with suggestions to help Marti ease the bedtime scene.

3. Jed is a 26-month-old whose family caregivers work outside the home. He goes to a day care center 3 days a week and is kept by his grandmother the other 2 days. Explain the guidance you would give his family caregiver to assist in toilet training in this situation.

Health Problems of the Toddler

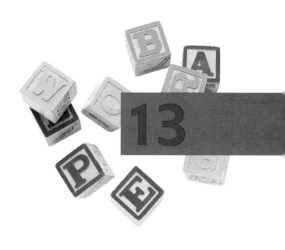

13

STUDENT OBJECTIVES

On completion of this chapter, the student will be able to

1. Describe four characteristics of infantile autism.
2. Identify four goals of treatment of infantile autism.
3. Describe treatment for bacterial conjunctivitis.
4. Explain the diagnosis of celiac disease.
5. Describe the usual treatment for spasmodic laryngitis.
6. Discuss acute laryngotracheobronchitis including the symptoms and treatment.
7. Identify the basic defect in cystic fibrosis.
8. State the major organs affected by cystic fibrosis.
9. Name the most common type of complication in cystic fibrosis.
10. List the diagnostic procedures used to diagnose cystic fibrosis.
11. Describe the dietary and pulmonary treatment of cystic fibrosis.
12. State the most common cause of poisoning in toddlers.
13. List five common substances that children ingest.
14. List seven sources of lead that may cause chronic lead poisoning.
15. Describe the symptoms, diagnosis, treatment, and prognosis of lead poisoning.
16. Discuss the incidence of burns in small children.
17. State the three major causes of burns in small children.
18. Differentiate between first-, second-, and third-degree burns.
19. Describe emergency treatment of a minor burn and of a moderate or severe burn.
20. List the reasons why hypovolemic shock occurs in the first 48 hours after a burn.
21. Describe the treatment of a child who has swallowed a foreign object.

KEY TERMS

achylia
allograft
amblyopia
autograft
binocular vision
cataract
celiac syndrome
chelating agent
circumoral pallor
conjunctivitis
contractures
coryza
croup
débridement
diplopia
dysphagia
echolalia
emetic
encephalopathy
eschar
esotropia
exotropia
external hordeolum
goniotomy
heterograft
homograft
hydrotherapy
hypervolemic
hypochylia
lacrimation
orthoptics
photophobia
pica
steatorrhea
strabismus
stridor

Children from ages 1 to 3 years are likely to have a number of minor health problems; many of them are caused by infection or environmental hazards. Most of these health problems can be managed at home after a visit to the pediatrician's office or clinic. Some problems, however, are serious enough to require hospitalization, thus separating the toddler from his or her family caregivers. This separation increases the seriousness of the health problem and the need for loving and understanding attention to the child's emotional needs as well as physical condition.

PSYCHOLOGICAL PROBLEMS

Autism

Although often called *infantile autism* because it is thought to be present from birth, autism usually is not conclusively diagnosed until after 12 months of age. The word *autism* comes from the Greek word *auto* meaning "self" and was first used by Dr. Leo Kanner in 1943 to describe a group of behavioral symptoms in children. The term *pervasive developmental disorder* was introduced in 1980 when the American Psychiatric Association revised the terminology. Disorders in this category are characterized by severe behavioral disturbance that affects the practical use of language as a means of communication, interpersonal interaction, attention, perception, and motor activity. Autistic children are totally self-centered and unable to relate to others; they often exhibit bizarre behaviors and often are destructive to themselves and others.

Autism occurs in about 2 to 5 of 10,000 births and four times as often in males as in females. Several theories exist about its cause as well as its treatment or management. Originally thought to result from an unsatisfactory early mother-child relationship (with emotionally cold, detached mothers sometimes described as "refrigerator mothers"), autism now appears to have organic and perhaps genetic causes instead. Researchers suggest that autism may result from a disturbance in language comprehension, a biochemical problem involving neurotransmitters or abnormalities in the central nervous system and probably brain metabolism. These children score poorly on intelligence tests but may have good memories and good intellectual potential.

Because the cause of autism is not understood, treatment attempts have met with limited success. These children experience the normal health problems of childhood in addition to those that result from their behaviors. Therefore, it is important that nurses understand this unexplained disorder and how it affects children and families.

Clinical Manifestations

The characteristics of autism are divided into three categories: inability to relate to others, inability to communicate with others, and obviously limited activities and interests. Children with autism do not develop a smiling response to others or an interest in being touched or cuddled. In fact, they can react violently at attempts to hold them. Their blank expressions and lack of response to verbal stimulation can suggest deafness. They do not show the normal fear of separation from parents that most toddlers exhibit. Often they seem not to notice when family caregivers are present.

During their second year, autistic children become completely absorbed in strange repetitive behaviors such as spinning an object, flipping an electrical switch on and off, or walking around the room feeling the walls. Their bodily movements are bizarre: rocking, twirling, flapping arms and hands, walking on tiptoe, twisting and turning fingers. If these movements are interrupted or if objects in the environment are moved, a violent temper tantrum may result. These tantrums may include self-destructive acts such as hand biting and head banging. Although infants and toddlers normally are self-centered, ritualistic, and prone to displays of temper, autistic children show these characteristics to an extreme degree coupled with an almost total lack of response to other people.

The autistic child is slow to develop speech, and any speech that develops is primitive and ineffective in its ability to communicate. **Echolalia** ("parrot speech") is typical of autistic children; they echo words they have heard, such as a television commercial, but offer no indication that they understand the words. Although autistic children are self-centered, their speech indicates that they seem to have no sense of self because they never use the pronouns "I" or "me."

Standard intelligence tests that count on verbal ability usually indicate that these children are mentally deficient. However, many of these children also demonstrate unusual memory and mathematic, artistic, and musical abilities.

Diagnosis

To confirm a diagnosis of autism, at least eight of 16 identified characteristics must be present and all three categories must be represented. The symptoms of autism can suggest other disorders such as lead poisoning, phenylketonuria, congenital rubella, and measles encephalitis. Therefore, a complete pediatric physical and neurologic examination is necessary including vision and hearing testing, electroen-cephalography, radiographic studies of the skull, urine screening, and other laboratory studies. In addition, the nurse usually takes a complete prenatal, natal, and postnatal history including development, nutrition, and family dynamics. Other members of the health team may be involved in the evaluation and treatment of the autistic child including audiologists, psychiatrists, psychologists, special education teachers, speech and language therapists, and social workers.

Treatment

The treatment of an autistic child is extremely challenging. The child is mentally retarded but may demonstrate exceptional talent in areas such as factual memory and art or music. Four goals toward which treatment is geared are

- Promotion of normal development
- Specific language development
- Social interaction
- Learning

The treatment of using behavioral modification, pharmacotherapeutics, and other techniques must be individually planned and is highly structured. Mixed results occur, and no one technique has met with resounding success. The family needs therapy to help relieve guilt and help them understand this puzzling child. The overall long-term prognosis for these children is not optimistic; however, the long-term outlook is better the earlier treatment is started. Facilitated communication involves working with language development of autistic children by helping them express themselves in language through use of a computer keyboard. This method, however, is viewed as controversial and is not proved by the American Psychological Association.

Nursing Care

Caring for the autistic child requires recognizing that autism creates great stresses for the entire family. The problems that cause family caregivers to seek diagnosis are difficult to live with; diagnosis itself is usually a lengthy and expensive process, and the hope for successful treatment is slight. Most caregivers of autistic children feel guilty despite the fact that current theories accept organic rather than psychological causes for this disorder. The possibility of genetic factors adds to this guilt. Often other children in the family who are normal suffer from a lack of attention because the caregivers' energies are almost totally directed to solving the autistic youngster's problems.

Nurses who care for these children should consider the family caregivers as their most valuable source of information about the child's habits and communication skills. To gain the child's cooperation, the nurse must learn which techniques the caregivers used to communicate with the child. Establishing a relationship of trust between the child and the nurse is essential. To provide consistency this child should be cared for by a constant primary nurse.

In the hospital setting, a private or semiprivate room is generally preferred; visual and auditory stimulation should be minimized. Familiar toys or other valued objects from home reduce the child's anxiety about the strange environment.

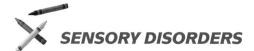

SENSORY DISORDERS

As toddlers explore their environment, they use all their senses to gather information; as toddlers grow, their senses become more fully developed. Vision screening is part of routine health maintenance; the following section discusses some eye conditions and injuries seen in toddlers.

Eye Conditions

Cataracts, congenital infantile glaucoma, and strabismus are disease conditions that may need to be dealt with during the toddler years. Eye injuries can occur in this exploring stage. In addition, eye infections may occur because exploring hands can easily carry infectious organisms to the eyes.

Cataracts

A **cataract** is a development of opacity in the crystalline lens that prevents light rays from entering the eye. Congenital cataracts may be hereditary or they may be complications of maternal rubella during the first trimester of pregnancy. Cataracts also may develop later in infancy or childhood from eye injury or from metabolic disturbances such as galactosemia and diabetes.

Surgical extraction of the cataracts is performed at an early age. With early removal, the prognosis for good vision is improved. The infant or child is fitted with a contact lens. If only one eye is affected, the "good" eye is patched to prevent amblyopia (see discussion in the section on strabismus). As the child gets older, numerous lens changes are needed to change the strength.

Glaucoma

Glaucoma may be of the congenital infantile type and occurs in children younger than age 3 years; juvenile glaucoma showing clinical manifestations after age 3; or secondary glaucoma resulting from injury or disease. Increased intraocular pressure due to over-production of aqueous fluid causes the eyeball to enlarge and the cornea to become large, thin, and sometimes cloudy. Untreated, the disease slowly progresses to blindness. Pain may be present. **Goniotomy** (surgical opening into Schlemm's canal) provides drainage of the aqueous humor and is often effective in relieving intraocular pressure. Goniotomy may need to be performed multiple times to control intraocular pressure. Surgery is performed as early as possible to prevent permanent damage.

Strabismus

Strabismus is the failure of the two eyes to direct their gaze at the same object simultaneously and is commonly called "squint" or "crossed eyes."(Fig. 13–1) **Binocular** (normal) **vision** is maintained through the muscular coordination of eye movements, so that a single vision results. In strabismus, the visual axes are not parallel and **diplopia** (double vision) results. In an effort to avoid seeing two images, the child's central nervous system suppresses vision in the deviant eye causing **amblyopia** (dimness of vision from disuse of the eye), which is sometimes called "lazy eye."

A wide variation in the manifestation of strabismus exists; there are lateral, vertical, and mixed lateral and vertical types. There may be monocular strabismus in which one eye deviates while the other eye is used, or alternating strabismus in which deviation alternates from one eye to the other. The term **esotropia** is used when the eye deviates toward the other eye; **exotropia** denotes a turning away from the other eye (Fig. 13–2).

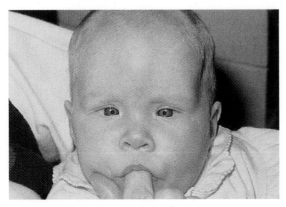

● *Figure 13.1* Strabismus in an infant.

Treatment depends on the type of strabismus present. In monocular strabismus, occlusion of the better eye by patching to force the use of the deviating eye should be initiated at an early age. Patching is continued for weeks or months. The younger the child is, the more rapid the improvement. The patching may be for set periods or continuous depending on the child's age. The older child needs continuous periods of patching, whereas the younger one may respond quickly to short periods of patching. The child should be stimulated to use the unpatched eye by occupations such as puzzles, drawing, sewing, and similar activities.

Glasses can correct a refractive error if amblyopia is not present. **Orthoptics** (therapeutic ocular muscle exercises) to improve the quality of vision may be prescribed to supplement the use of glasses or surgery.

Surgery on the eye muscle to correct the defect is necessary for children who do not respond to glasses and exercises. Many children need surgery after amblyopia has been corrected. Early detection and treatment of strabismus are essential for a successful outcome. The correction is believed to be necessary before the child reaches age 6 years or the visual damage may be permanent; however, some authorities believe that correction can be successful up to age 10 years.

Eye Injury and Foreign Objects in the Eye

Eye injuries are fairly common, particularly in older children. Ecchymosis of the eye (black eye) is of no great importance unless the eyeball is involved. A penetrating wound of the eyeball is potentially serious—BB shots in particular are dangerous—and requires the ophthalmologist's attention. With any history of an injury, a thorough examination of the entire eye is necessary.

Sympathetic ophthalmia may follow perforation wounds of the globe, even if the perforations are small. Sympathetic ophthalmia, an inflammatory reaction of the uninjured eye, often includes **photophobia** (intolerance to light), **lacrimation** (secretion of tears), pain, and some dimness of vision. The retina may finally become detached, and atrophy of the eyeball may occur. Prompt and skillful treatment at the time of the injury is essential to avoid involvement of the other eye.

Small foreign objects, such as specks of dust, that have lodged inside the eyelid may be removed by rolling the lid back and exposing the object. Cotton-tipped applicators should not be used for this purpose because of the danger of sudden movement and possible perforation of the eye. If the object cannot be easily removed with a small piece of

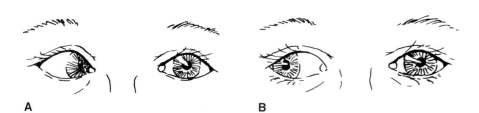

A   **B**

● *Figure 13.2* Strabismus. (*A*) Esotropia. (*B*) Exotropia.

moistened cotton or soft clean cloth or flushed out with saline solution, the child should be taken to the physician.

Eye Infections

External hordeolum, known commonly as a stye, is a purulent infection of the follicle of an eyelash generally caused by *Staphylococcus aureus.* Localized swelling, tenderness, pain, and a reddened lid edge are present. The maximal tenderness is over the infected site. The lesion progresses to suppuration with eventual discharge of the purulent material. Warm saline compresses applied for about 15 minutes three or four times daily give some relief and hasten resolution, but recurrence is common. The stye should never be squeezed. Antibiotic ointment may help prevent accompanying conjunctivitis and recurrence.

Conjunctivitis is an acute inflammation of the conjunctiva. In children, a virus, bacteria, allergy, or foreign body may cause conjunctivitis. Conjunctivitis caused by bacteria is the most common type. The purulent drainage, a common characteristic, can be cultured to determine the causative organism. Due to the danger of spreading infection, bacterial conjunctivitis is treated with ophthalmic antibacterial agents such as erythromycin, bacitracin, sulfacetamide, and polymyxin. Because ointments blur vision, eye drops are used during the day and ointments at night. Before applying medication, warm moist compresses can be used to remove the crusts that form on the eyes. The child who has bacterial conjunctivitis should be kept separate from other young children until the condition has been treated. The use of separate washcloths and towels and disposable tissues is important to prevent spread of infection among family members.

Nursing Care for the Child Undergoing Eye Surgery

Anyone experiencing sensory deprivation finds it difficult to stay in touch with reality, and a child whose eyes are covered is particularly vulnerable. Nurses who have not experienced this deprivation do not always appreciate the implications of not being able to see. A young child who wakens from

surgery to total darkness may go into a state of panic. Observation of the child returning from surgery may reveal panic and anxiety evidenced by trembling and nervousness. The child needs a family caregiver or loved one to stay during the time when vision is restricted.

The child should be as well prepared for the event as possible, but the small child has no experience to help in understanding what actually is going to happen. The darkness, pain, and total strangeness of the situation can be overwhelming. One preoperative preparation might be to play a game with a blindfold to help the child become used to having his or her eyes covered (Fig. 13–3).

Restraints should not be used indiscriminately, but most small children need some reminder to keep their hands away from the sore eye unless someone is beside them to prevent them from rubbing it or from removing eye dressings. Elbow restraints are useful, although they do not prevent rubbing the eye with the arm. Flannel strips applied to the wrists in clove-hitch fashion can be tied to the crib sides in such a manner as to allow freedom of arm movement but to prevent the child from causing damage to the operative site.

To alert the child, the nurse should speak when approaching. The child needs tactile stimulation; therefore, after speaking, the nurse would do well to

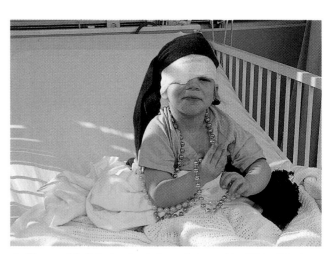

● *Figure 13.3* Pretending to be a pirate enables this toddler to find enjoyment in wearing an eye patch.

stroke or pat the child. If permitted, the nurse may hold the child for additional reassurance.

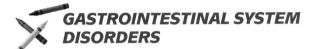

GASTROINTESTINAL SYSTEM DISORDERS

Celiac Syndrome

Intestinal malabsorption with **steatorrhea** (fatty stools) is a condition brought about by various causes, the most common being cystic fibrosis and gluten-induced enteropathy, the so-called idiopathic celiac disease. The term **celiac syndrome** is used to designate the complex of malabsorptive disorders.

Gluten-Induced Enteropathy

Idiopathic celiac disease is a basic defect of metabolism precipitated by the ingestion of wheat gluten or rye gluten, which leads to impaired fat absorption. The exact cause is not known; the most acceptable theory is that of an inborn error of metabolism with an allergic reaction to the gliadin fraction of gluten (a protein factor in wheat) as a contributing or possibly the sole factor.

Severe manifestations of the disorder have become rare in the United States and in western Europe, but mild disturbances in intestinal absorption of rye, wheat, and sometimes oat gluten are common, occurring in about 1 in 2,000 children in the United States.

Clinical Manifestations. Signs generally do not appear before age 6 months and may be delayed until age 1 year or later. Manifestations include chronic diarrhea with foul, bulky, greasy stools and progressive malnutrition. Anorexia and a fretful, unhappy disposition are typical. The onset is generally insidious with failure to thrive, bouts of diarrhea, and frequent respiratory infections. If the condition becomes severe, the effects of malnutrition are prominent. Retarded growth and development, a distended abdomen, and thin, wasted buttocks and legs are characteristic signs (Fig. 13–4).

The chronic course of this disease may be interrupted by a celiac crisis, an emergency situation. Frequently this is triggered by an upper respiratory infection. The child vomits copiously, has large, watery stools, and becomes severely dehydrated. As the child becomes drowsy and prostrate, an acute medical emergency develops. Parenteral fluid therapy is essential to combat acidosis and to achieve normal fluid balance.

Diagnosis and Treatment. One way to determine if a small child's failure to thrive is caused by celiac disease is to initiate a trial gluten-free diet

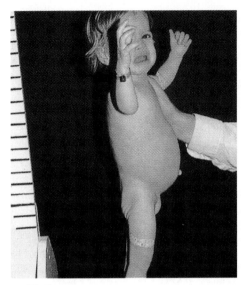

● **Figure 13.4** A child with celiac disease. Notice the protruding abdomen and wasted buttocks.

and observe the results. Improvement in the nature of the stools and general well-being with a gain in weight should follow, although several weeks may elapse before clear-cut manifestations can be confirmed. Conclusive diagnosis can be made by a biopsy of the jejunum through endoscopy that shows changes in the villi. Serum screening of IgG and IgA antigliaden antibodies shows the presence of the condition and also aids in monitoring the progress of therapy.

Response to a diet from which rye, wheat, and oats are excluded is generally good, although probably no cure can be expected and dietary indiscretions or respiratory infections may bring relapses. The omission of wheat products in particular should continue through adolescence because the ingestion of wheat appears to inhibit growth in these children.

Dietary Program. The young child is usually started on a starch-free, low-fat diet. If the condition is severe, this diet consists of skim milk, glucose, and banana flakes. Bananas contain invert sugar and are usually well tolerated. Lean meats, puréed vegetables, and fruits are gradually added to the diet. Eventually fats may be added, and the child can be maintained on a regular diet with the exception of all wheat, rye, and oat products.

Commercially canned creamed soups, cold cuts, frankfurters, and pudding mixes generally contain wheat products. The forbidden list also includes malted milk drinks, some candies, many baby foods, and breads, cakes, pastries, and biscuits unless they are made from corn flour or cornmeal. Vitamins A and D in water-miscible (able to be mixed with water) solutions are needed in double amounts to supplement the deficient diet.

262   UNIT 3 ● *Care of the Child*

Nursing Care. The primary focus of nursing care is to help caregivers maintain a restrictive diet for the child. Family teaching should include information regarding the disease and the need for long-term management as well as guidelines for a gluten-free diet. Caregivers must learn to read the list of ingredients on packaged foods carefully before purchasing anything. The diet of the young child may be monitored fairly easily, but when the child goes to school monitoring becomes a much greater challenge. As the child grows, caregivers and children might need additional nursing support to help them make dietary modifications.

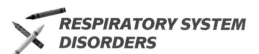

RESPIRATORY SYSTEM DISORDERS

Croup

Croup is not a disease but a group of disorders typically involving a barking cough, hoarseness, and inspiratory **stridor** (shrill, harsh respiratory sound). The disorders are named for the respiratory structures involved. Acute laryngotracheobronchitis, for instance, affects the larynx, trachea, and major bronchi.

Spasmodic Laryngitis

Spasmodic laryngitis occurs in children between ages 1 and 3 years. The cause is undetermined; it may be of infectious or allergic origin, but certain children seem to develop severe laryngospasm with little, if any, apparent cause. The attack may be preceded by **coryza** (runny nose) and hoarseness or by no apparent signs of respiratory irregularity during the evening. The child awakens after a few hours of sleep with a bark-like cough, increasing respiratory difficulty, and stridor. The child becomes anxious, restless, and markedly hoarse. A low-grade fever and mild upper respiratory infection may be present.

This condition is not serious but is frightening both to the child and the family. The episode subsides after a few hours; little evidence remains the next day when an anxious caregiver takes the child to the physician. Attacks frequently occur two or three nights in succession.

Treatment. Humidified air is helpful in reducing laryngospasm. Taking the child into the bathroom and opening the hot water taps with the door closed is a quick method for providing moist air, if the water runs hot enough. The physician may prescribe an **emetic** (an agent that causes vomiting), such as syrup of ipecac, in a dosage less than that needed to produce vomiting; this usually gives relief by helping

to reduce spasms of the larynx. Humidifiers may be used in the child's bedroom to provide high humidity. Cool humidifiers are recommended, but vaporizers also may be used. If a vaporizer is used, caution must be taken to place it out of the child's reach to protect the child from being burned. Cool-mist humidifiers provide safe humidity. Humidifiers and vaporizers must be cleaned regularly to prevent the growth of undesirable organisms. Sometimes the spasm is relieved by exposure to cold air—when, for instance, the child is taken out into the night to go to the emergency department or to see the physician.

Acute Laryngotracheobronchitis

Laryngeal infections are common in small children, and they often involve tracheobronchial areas as well. Acute laryngotracheobronchitis (bacterial tracheitis or laryngotracheobronchitis) may progress rapidly and become a serious problem within a matter of hours. The toddler is the most frequently affected member of the 1- to 4-year age group. This condition is usually of viral origin but bacterial invasion, usually staphylococcal, follows the original infection. It generally occurs after an upper respiratory infection with fairly mild rhinitis and pharyngitis.

The child develops hoarseness and a barking cough with a fever that may reach 104° to 105°F (40° to 40.6°C). As the disease progresses, marked laryngeal edema occurs and the child's breathing becomes difficult; the pulse is rapid and cyanosis may appear. Congestive heart failure and acute respiratory embarrassment can result.

Treatment. The major goal of treatment for acute laryngotracheobronchitis is to maintain an airway and adequate air exchange followed by antimicrobial therapy. The child is placed in a supersaturated atmosphere such as a croupette or some other kind of mist tent that also can include the administration of oxygen. To effect bronchodilation, racemic epinephrine may be administered by means of a nebulizer usually by a respiratory therapist. Rapid improvement may be seen because of vasoconstriction, but the child must be carefully watched for reappearance of symptoms. Nebulization is usually administered every 3 or 4 hours. Nebulization often produces relief, but if necessary intubation with a nasotracheal tube may be performed for a child with severe distress unrelieved by other measures. Tracheostomies, once performed frequently, are rarely performed today; intubation is preferred. Antibiotics are administered parenterally initially and continued after the temperature has normalized.

Close and careful observation of the child is important. Observation includes checking the pulse, respirations, and color, listening for hoarseness and stridor, and noting any restlessness that may indicate an impending respiratory crisis. Pulse oximetry is used to determine the degree of hypoxia.

Epiglottitis

Epiglottitis is acute inflammation of the epiglottis (the cartilaginous flap that protects the opening of the larynx). Commonly caused by *Haemophilus influenzae* type B, epiglottitis most often affects children ages 2 to 7 years. The epiglottis becomes inflamed and swollen with edema. The edema decreases the ability of the epiglottis to move freely, which results in blockage of the airway and creates an emergency.

The child may have been well or may have had a mild upper respiratory infection before the development of a sore throat, **dysphagia** (difficulty swallowing), and a high fever of 102.2° to 104°F (39° to 40°C). The dysphagia may cause drooling. A tongue blade should *never* be used to initiate a gag reflex because complete obstruction may occur. The child is very anxious and prefers to breathe by to sitting up and leaning forward with the mouth open and the tongue out. This is called the "tripod" position (Fig. 13–5). Immediate emergency attention is necessary.

The child may need endotracheal intubation or a tracheostomy if the epiglottis is so swollen that intubation cannot be performed. Moist air is necessary to help reduce the inflammation of the epiglottis. Pulse oximetry is required to monitor oxygen requirements. Antibiotics are administered intravenously (IV). After 24 to 48 hours of antibiotic therapy, the child may be extubated. Antibiotics are usually continued for 10 days. Although this condition is not common, it is extremely frightening for the child and the family.

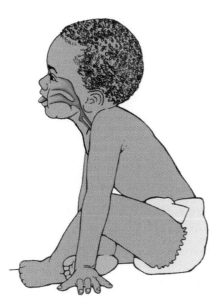

● *Figure 13.5* The "tripod" position of the child with epiglottis.

● Nursing Process for the Toddler With an Upper Respiratory Disorder

ASSESSMENT

Conduct a thorough interview with the caregiver. In addition to standard information, include specific data such as when the symptoms were first noticed, if the child has had a fever, a description of respiratory difficulties, signs of hoarseness, the character of any cough, and any other information that can be determined about the condition.

Conduct a physical exam including obtaining vital signs. Closely observe the child's respiratory effort. Inspect the accessory muscles; listen to lung sounds and note signs of impending respiratory obstruction; observe for **circumoral pallor,** cyanotic nail beds, irritability, or mental confusion. If the child is old enough to communicate verbally, ask questions to determine how the child feels.

NURSING DIAGNOSES

The nursing diagnoses depend on the data collected on the child and the severity of the respiratory distress. The following nursing diagnoses may be appropriate:

- Ineffective Airway Clearance related to obstruction associated with edema and mucous secretions of the upper airway
- Risk for Deficient Fluid Volume related to respiratory fluid loss, fever, and difficulty swallowing
- Anxiety related to dyspnea, invasive procedures, and separation from caregiver
- Compromised Family Coping related to child's respiratory symptoms
- Deficient Caregiver Knowledge related to child's condition and home care

OUTCOME IDENTIFICATION AND PLANNING

The major goals for the young child with an upper respiratory disorder are maintaining respiratory status, preventing fluid deficit, and relieving anxiety. Goals for the family include relieving anxiety and improving caregiver knowledge. The need for immediate intubation is always a possibility; thus vigilance is essential. The child's energy must be conserved to reduce oxygen requirements.

IMPLEMENTATION

Monitoring Respiratory Function. Be continuously alert for warning signs of airway obstruction. Monitor the child at least every hour; uncover the child's chest and observe the child's breathing efforts, noting the amount of chest movement, shallow breathing, and retractions. Listen with a stethoscope for breath sounds particularly noting the amount of stridor, which indicates difficult breathing. Increasing hoarseness should be reported. In addition, observe for pallor, listlessness, circumoral cyanosis, cyanotic nail beds, and restlessness; these are indications of impaired oxygenation and should be reported at once. Cool, high humidity provides relief. Oxygen may be administered. Pulse oximetry is used to monitor oxygen saturation.

Monitoring Adequate Fluid Intake. Adequate hydration helps reduce thick mucus. Maintaining adequate fluid intake may be a problem, as the child may be too ill to want to eat. Offer warm, clear fluids to encourage oral intake. Observe carefully for aspiration especially in severe respiratory distress. The child may need to be kept NPO to prevent this threat. Parenteral fluids may be administered to replace those lost through respiratory loss, fever, and anorexia. Follow all safety measures for administration of parenteral fluids. Fluid needs are determined by the amount needed to maintain body weight with sufficient amounts added to replace the additional losses. Monitor daily weights and accurately record intake and output. Monitor serum electrolyte levels to ensure they are within normal limits. At least once per shift, observe and record skin turgor and the condition of mucous membranes.

Reducing the Child's Anxiety. When frightened or upset and crying, the child with croup or a related upper respiratory condition may hyperventilate, which causes additional respiratory distress. For this reason, maintain a calm, soothing manner while caring for the child. When possible, the child should be cared for by a constant caregiver with whom a trusting relationship has been achieved. Offering support to the child during invasive procedures, such as when an IV is being started, will help decrease the child's anxiety. The family can provide the child with a favorite blanket or toy. The family caregiver is encouraged to stay with the child if possible to provide reassurance and avoid separation anxiety in the child. Plan care to minimize interrupting the child's much-needed rest. Give the child age-appropriate explanations of treatment and procedures. As the child improves, provide age-appropriate diversional activities to help relieve anxiety and boredom. Make extra efforts to relieve the child's feelings of loneliness while in respiratory isolation.

Promoting Family Coping. Watching a child with severe respiratory symptoms is frightening for the parent or family caregiver. The parent or caregiver may feel helpless, and these feelings of anxiety and helplessness may be exhibited in a variety of ways. To alleviate these feelings, encourage the caregiver to discuss them. Using easily understood terminology, explain procedures, treatments, the illness, and the prognosis to the caregiver. Include the caregiver in the child's care as much as possible and encourage him or her to soothe and comfort the child.

Providing Family Teaching. Provide the caregiver with thorough explanations of the condition's signs and symptoms. Explain which symptoms can be treated at home (hoarseness, croupy cough, and inspiratory stridor when disturbed) and which indicate that the child needs to be seen by the care provider (continuous stridor, use of accessory muscles, labored breathing, lower rib retractions, restlessness, pallor, and rapid respirations). The family must be aware that recurrence of these conditions is common. Teach the use of cool humidifiers or vaporizers including cleaning methods and safety measures to avoid burns when using a steam vaporizer. Explain the effects, administration, dosage, and side effects of medications. To be certain the information was understood, have the parent relate back specific facts. Write the information down in a simple way so that it can be clearly understood, and determine that the parent can read and understand the written material. When appropriate, observe the caregiver demonstrate care of equipment and any treatments to be done at home.

EVALUATION: GOALS AND OUTCOME CRITERIA

- *Goal:* The child's airway will remain clear. *Criteria:* The child's airway is clear with no evidence of retractions, stridor, hoarseness, or cyanosis.

- *Goal:* The child's fluid intake will be adequate for age and weight.
  Criteria: The child exhibits good skin turgor and moist, pink mucous membranes. Urine output is 1 mL/kg/hr.
- *Goal:* The child will experience a reduction in anxiety.
  Criteria: The child rests quietly with no evidence of hyperventilation, cooperates with care, cuddles a favorite toy for reassurance, smiles, and plays contentedly.
- *Goal:* The family caregiver anxiety will be reduced.
  Criteria: The caregiver cooperates with and participates in the child's care, appears more relaxed, verbalizes his or her feelings, and soothes the child.
- *Goal:* The family caregivers will verbalize an understanding of the child's condition and how to provide home care for the child.
  Criteria: The family caregiver accurately describes facts about the child's condition, asks appropriate questions, relates signs and symptoms to observe in the child, and names the effects, side effects, dosage, and administration of medications.

Cystic Fibrosis

When first described, cystic fibrosis (CF) was called "fibrocystic disease of the pancreas." Further research has revealed that this disorder represents a major dysfunction of all exocrine glands. The major organs affected are the lungs, pancreas, and liver. Because about half of all children with CF have pulmonary complications, this disorder is discussed here with other respiratory conditions.

Cystic fibrosis is hereditary and transmitted as an autosomal recessive trait. Both parents must be carriers of the gene for CF to appear. With each pregnancy, the chance is one in four that the child will have the disease. In the United States the incidence is about 1 in 3,300 in white children and 1 in 16,300 in black children.

Recent studies have determined that the gene involved in CF normally produces a protein, cystic fibrosis transmembrane conductance regulator, which serves as a channel through which chloride enters and leaves cells. When mutated, the gene blocks chloride movement, which brings on the apparent signs of CF. The blocking of chloride transport results in a change in sodium transport; this in turn results in abnormal secretions of the exocrine (mucus-producing) glands that produce thick, tenacious mucus rather than the thin, free-flowing secretion normally produced. This abnormal mucus leads to obstruction of the secretory ducts of the pancreas, liver, and reproductive organs. Thick mucus obstructs the respiratory passages, causing trapped air and overinflation of the lungs. In addition, the sweat and salivary glands excrete excessive electrolytes, specifically sodium and chloride.

Clinical Manifestations

Meconium ileus is the presenting symptom of CF in 5% to 10% of the newborns who later develop additional manifestations. Depletion or absence of pancreatic enzymes before birth results in impaired digestive activity, and the meconium becomes viscid (thick) and mucilaginous (sticky). The inspissated (thickened) meconium fills the small intestine, causing complete obstruction. Clinical manifestations are bile-stained emesis, a distended abdomen, and an absence of stool. Intestinal perforation with symptoms of shock may occur. These newborns taste salty when kissed because of the high sodium chloride concentration in their sweat.

Initial symptoms of CF may occur at varying ages during infancy, childhood, or adolescence. A hard, nonproductive chronic cough may be the first sign. Later, frequent bronchial infections occur. Development of a barrel chest and clubbing of fingers (Fig. 13–6) indicate chronic lack of oxygen. Despite an excellent appetite, malnutrition is apparent and

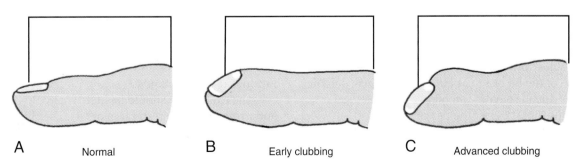

A   Normal   B   Early clubbing   C   Advanced clubbing

● *Figure 13.6* Clubbing of fingers indicates chronic lack of oxygen. **(A)** Normal angle; **(B)** early clubbing—flattened angle; **(C)** advanced clubbing—the nail is rounded over the end of the finger.

becomes increasingly severe. The abdomen becomes distended, and body muscles become flabby.

Pancreatic Involvement. Thick, tenacious mucus obstructs the pancreatic ducts, causing **hypochylia** (diminished flow of pancreatic enzymes) or **achylia** (absence of pancreatic enzymes). This achylia or hypochylia leads to intestinal malabsorption and severe malnutrition. The deficient pancreatic enzymes are lipase, trypsin, and amylase. Malabsorption of fats causes frequent steatorrhea. Anemia or rectal prolapse is common if the pancreatic condition remains untreated. The incidence of diabetes is greater in these children than in the general population possibly due to changes in the pancreas. The incidence of diabetes in patients with CF is expected to increase because of their increasing life expectancy.

Pulmonary Involvement. The degree of lung involvement determines the prognosis for survival. The severity of pulmonary involvement differs in individual children with a few showing only minor involvement. Now more than half of children with CF are expected to live beyond age 18 with increasing numbers living into adulthood.

Respiratory complications pose the greatest threat to children with CF. Abnormal amounts of thick, viscid mucus clog the bronchioles and provide an ideal medium for bacterial growth. *S aureus* coagulase can be cultured from the nasopharynx and sputum of most patients. *Pseudomonas aeruginosa* and *H influenzae* also are found frequently. The basic infection, however, appears most often to be caused by *S aureus*.

Numerous complications arise from severe respiratory infections. Atelectasis and small lung abscesses are common early complications. Bronchiectasis and emphysema may develop with pulmonary fibrosis and pneumonitis; this eventually leads to severe ventilatory insufficiency. In advanced disease, pneumothorax, right ventricular hypertrophy, and cor pulmonale are common complications. Cor pulmonale is a common cause of death.

Other Affected Organs. The tears, saliva, and sweat of children with CF contain abnormally high concentrations of electrolytes, and most have enlarged submaxillary salivary glands. In hot weather, the loss of sodium chloride and fluid through sweating produces frequent heat prostration. Additional fluid and salt should be given in the diet as a preventive measure. In addition, males with CF who reach adulthood will most likely be sterile because of the blockage or absence of the vas deferens or other ducts. Females often have thick cervical secretions that prohibit the passage of sperm.

Diagnosis

Diagnosis is based on family history, elevated sodium chloride levels in the sweat, analysis of duodenal secre-

tions (via a nasogastric [NG] tube) for trypsin content, a history of failure to thrive, chronic or recurrent respiratory infections, and radiologic findings of hyperinflation and bronchial wall thickening. In the event of a positive sodium chloride sweat test, at least one other criterion must be met to make a conclusive diagnosis.

The principal diagnostic test to confirm CF is a sweat chloride test using the pilocarpine iontophoresis method. This method induces sweating by using a small electric current that carries topically applied pilocarpine into a localized area of the skin. Elevations of 60 mEq/L or more are diagnostic with values of 50 to 60 mEq/L highly suspect. Although the test itself is fairly simple, conducting the test on an infant is difficult and false-positive results do occur.

Treatment

In the newborn, meconium ileus is treated nonoperatively with hyperosmolar enemas administered gently. If this does not resolve the blockage of thick, gummy meconium, surgery is necessary. During surgery, a mucolytic such as Mucomyst may be used to liquefy the meconium. If this procedure is successful, resection may not be necessary.

In the older child, treatment is aimed at correcting pancreatic deficiency, improving pulmonary function, and preventing respiratory infections. If bowel obstruction does occur (meconium ileus equivalent), the preferred management includes hyperosmolar enemas and an increase in fluids, dietary fiber, oral mucolytics, lactulose, and mineral oil.

The overall treatment goals are to improve the child's quality of life and to provide for long-term survival. A health care team is needed, including a primary care provider, a nurse, a respiratory therapist, a dietitian, and a social worker, to work together with the child and family. Treatment centers with a staff of specialists are becoming more common particularly in larger medical centers. With improved treatment, it is not unusual for a child with CF to grow into adulthood.

Dietary Treatment. Commercially prepared pancreatic enzymes given during meals or with snacks aid digestion and absorption of fat and protein. Because pancreatic enzymes are inactivated in the acidic environment of the stomach, microencapsulated capsules are used to deliver the enzymes to the duodenum where they are activated. These enzymes come in capsules that can be swallowed or opened and sprinkled on the child's food. A powdered preparation is used for infants.

The child's diet should be high in carbohydrates and protein with no restriction of fats. The child may need 1.5 to 2 times the normal caloric intake to promote growth. These children have large appetites unless they are acutely ill. Even with their large appetites, however, they can receive little nourishment without a pancreatic supplement. With proper diet and enzyme supplements, these children show evidence of improved nutrition and their stools become relatively normal. Enteric-coated pancreatic enzymes essentially eliminate the need for dietary restriction of fat.

Because of the increased loss of sodium chloride, these children are allowed to use as much salt as they wish even though onlookers may think it is too much. During hot weather, additional salt may be provided with pretzels, salted bread sticks, and saltine crackers.

Supplements of fat-soluble vitamins A, D, and E are necessary because of the poor digestion of fats. Vitamin K may be supplemented if the child has coagulation problems or is scheduled for surgery. Water-miscible preparations can be given to provide the needed supplement.

Pulmonary Treatment. The treatment goal is to prevent and treat respiratory infections. Respiratory drainage is provided by thinning the secretions and by mechanical means, such as postural drainage and clapping, to loosen and drain secretions from the lungs. Antibacterial drugs for the treatment of infection are necessary as indicated. Some physicians prescribe a prophylactic antibiotic regimen when the child is diagnosed. Antibiotics may be administered orally or parenterally even in the home. With home parenteral administration of antibiotic therapy, a central venous access device is used. Immunization against childhood communicable diseases is extremely important for these chronically ill children. All immunization measures may be used and should be maintained at appropriate intervals. Physical activity is essential because it improves mucous secretion and helps the child feel good. The child can be encouraged to participate in any aerobic activity he or she enjoys. Activity along with physical therapy should be limited only by the child's endurance.

Inhalation therapy can be preventive or therapeutic. Hand-held nebulizers are easy to use and convenient for the ambulatory child. A bronchodilator drug such as theophylline or a beta-adrenergic agonist (metaproterenol, terbutaline, or albuterol) may be administered either orally or through nebulization. Recombinant human DNA (DNase, Pulmozyme) breaks down DNA molecules in sputum, breaking up the thick mucus in the airways. A mucolytic such as Mucomyst may be prescribed during acute infection.

A humidified atmosphere can be provided with humidifiers. In summer, a room air conditioner can help provide comfort and controlled humidity.

Chest physical therapy, a combination of postural drainage and chest percussion, is performed routinely at least every morning and evening even if little drainage is apparent (Fig. 13–7). Performed correctly, chest percussion (clapping and vibrating of the affected areas) helps to loosen and move secretions

out of the lungs. The physical therapist usually performs this procedure in the hospital and teaches it to the family. Chest physical therapy, although time-consuming, is part of the ongoing, long term treatment and should be continued at home.

Home Care

The home care for a child with CF places a tremendous burden on the family. This is not a one-time hospital treatment, nor is there a prospect of cure to brighten the horizon. Each day, much time is spent performing treatments. Family caregivers must learn to perform chest physical therapy and how to operate respiratory equipment and administer IV antibiotics when necessary. The child's diet must be planned with additional enzymes regulated according to need. Great care is needed to prevent exposure to infections.

Family caregivers must guard against overprotection and against undue limitation of their child's physical activity. Somehow a good family relationship must be preserved with time and attention given to other members of the family.

Physical activity is an important adjunct to the child's well-being and is necessary to get rid of secretions. Capacity for exercise is soon learned, and the child can be trusted to become self-limiting as necessary especially if given an opportunity to learn the nature of the disease. The child may find postural drainage fun when a caregiver raises the child's feet in the air and walks the child around "wheelbarrow" fashion or if the older child can learn to hang from a monkey bar by the knees. Providing as much normalcy as possible is always desirable. Hot-weather activity should be watched a little more closely with additional attention to increased salt and fluid intake during exercise.

Caring for a child with CF places great stress on a family's financial resources. The expense of daily medications, frequent clinic or office visits, and sometimes lengthy hospitalizations can be devastating to an ordinary family budget even with medical insurance coverage. The Cystic Fibrosis Foundation with chapters throughout the United States is helpful in providing education and services. Some assistance may be available through local agencies or community groups.

● Nursing Process for the Child With Cystic Fibrosis

ASSESSMENT

The collection of data on the child with CF varies depending on the child's age and the

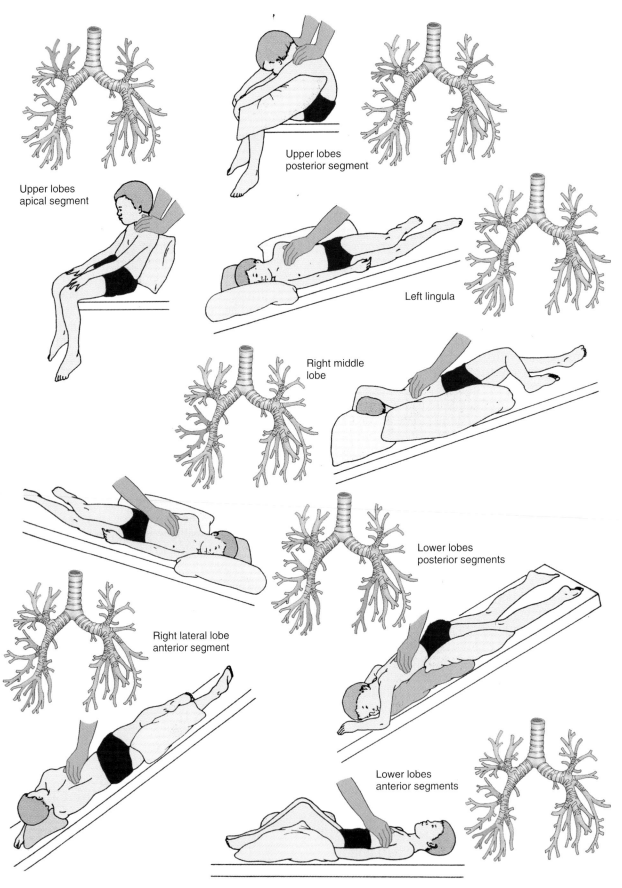

Upper lobes
apical segment

Upper lobes
posterior segment

Left lingula

Right middle
lobe

Right lateral lobe
anterior segment

Lower lobes
posterior segments

Lower lobes
anterior segments

● **Figure 13.7** Positions for postural drainage.

circumstances of the admission. Conduct a complete parent interview that includes the standard information as well as data concerning respiratory infections, the child's appetite and eating habits, stools, noticeable salty perspiration, history of bowel obstruction as an infant, and family history for CF, if known. Also determine the caregiver's knowledge of the condition.

When collecting data about vital signs, include observation of respirations such as cough, breath sounds, and barrel chest; respiratory effort such as retractions and nasal flaring; clubbing of the fingers; and signs of pancreatic involvement such as failure to thrive and steatorrhea. Examine the skin around the rectum for irritation and breakdown from frequent foul stools. Ask the child age-appropriate questions, involve the child in the interview process, and determine the child's perception of the disease and this current illness.

NURSING DIAGNOSES

The nursing diagnoses for CF may be many and varied. The reason for the present admission, the child's age, the progression of the condition, the level of understanding that the child and the caregiver have about the condition, and the current illness all merge to determine the pertinent nursing diagnoses for this admission. For the child who has just been diagnosed, the nursing diagnoses may be much more complex than for the child with complications of a long-standing condition. The family caregiver and the child (as suitable for age) should be included in the determination of current nursing diagnoses. Some diagnoses that may be appropriate include

- Ineffective Airway Clearance related to thick, tenacious mucous production
- Ineffective Breathing Pattern related to tracheobronchial obstruction
- Risk for Infection related to bacterial growth medium provided by pulmonary mucus and impaired body defenses
- Imbalanced Nutrition: Less Than Body Requirements related to impaired absorption of nutrients
- Anxiety related to hospitalization
- Compromised Family Coping related to child's chronic illness and its demands on caregivers
- Deficient Caregiver Knowledge related to illness, treatment and home care.

OUTCOME IDENTIFICATION AND PLANNING

As stated before, much depends on the reason for the specific admission and other factors discussed under the nursing diagnosis. The child's age and ability for self-expression affect any goal-setting the child can do. The major goals for the child include relieving immediate respiratory distress, maintaining adequate oxygenation, remaining free from infection, improving nutritional status, and relieving anxiety. The caregivers' primary goal may include relieving problems related to this admission. Other goals, however, may include concerns about stress on the family related to the illness, as well as a need for additional information about the disease, treatment, and prevention of complications.

IMPLEMENTATION

Improving Airway Clearance. Mucus causes obstruction of the airways and diminishes gas exchange. Monitor the child for signs of respiratory distress, while observing for dyspnea, tachypnea, labored respirations with or without activity, retractions, nasal flaring, and color of nail beds. Perform aerosol treatments. Teach the child to cough effectively. Examine and document the mucus produced, noting the color, consistency, and odor. Send cultures to the laboratory as appropriate. Increase fluid intake to help thin mucous secretions. Encourage the child to drink extra fluids and ask the child (or the caregiver if the child is too young) what favorite drinks might be appealing. Intravenous fluids may be necessary. Provide humidified air, either in the form of a cool mist humidifier or mist tent as prescribed.

Improving Breathing. Maintain the child in a semi-Fowler's or high Fowler's position to promote maximal lung expansion. Pulse oximetry may be used. Maintain oxygen saturation higher than 90%. Administer oxygen if the oxygen saturation falls below this level for an extended period. Administer mouth care every 2 to 4 hours especially when oxygen is administered. Perform chest physical therapy every 2 to 4 hours as ordered. If respiratory therapy technicians or physical therapists do these treatments, observe the child after the treatment to determine effectiveness and if more frequent treatments may be needed. Supervise the child who can self-administer nebulizer treatments to ensure correct use. Conserve the child's energy. Plan nursing and therapeutic activities so that maximal rest time is provided for the child. Note dyspnea and respiratory distress in relation to any activities. Plan quiet diversional activities as the child's physical condition warrants. Help the child and family to understand that activity is excellent for the child not in an acute situation. Teach them that exercise helps loosen the thick mucus and also improves the child's self-image.

Preventing Infection. The child with CF has low resistance especially to respiratory infections. For this reason, take care to protect the child from any exposure to infectious organisms. Good handwashing techniques should be practiced by all; teach the child and family the importance of this first line of defense. Practice and teach other good hygiene habits. Carefully follow medical asepsis when caring for the child and the equipment. Monitor vital signs every 4 hours for any indication of an infectious process. Restrict people with an infection such as staff, family members, other patients, and visitors, from contact with the child. Advise the family to keep the child's immunizations up to date. Administer antibiotics as prescribed, and teach the child or caregiver home administration as needed. Also teach the family the signs and symptoms of an impending infection so they can begin prophylactic measures at once.

Maintaining Adequate Nutrition. Adequate nutrition helps the child resist infections. Greatly increase the child's caloric intake to compensate for impaired absorption of nutrients and to provide adequate growth and development. In addition to increased caloric intake at meals, provide the child with high-calorie, high-protein snacks such as peanut butter and cheese. Newer low-fat products can be selected if desired. Administer pancreatic enzymes with all meals and snacks. In addition, multiple vitamins and iron may be prescribed. Reinforce the need for these supplements to both the child and the family. The child also may require additional salt in the diet. Encourage the child to eat salty snacks. If the child has bouts of diarrhea or constipation, the dosage of enzymes may need to be adjusted. Report any change in bowel movements. Weigh and measure the child. Plot growth on a chart so that progress can easily be visualized.

Reducing the Child's Anxiety. Provide age-appropriate activities to help alleviate anxiety and the boredom that can result from enforced hospitalization. Choose activities such as reading or arts and crafts according to age. Schoolwork may help ease some anxiety. Some older children may enjoy a video game, if available, but watch the child for overexcitement. Encourage the family caregiver to stay with the child to help diminish some of the child's anxiety. Allow the child to have familiar toys or mementos from home. Stay with the child during acute episodes of coughing and dyspnea to reduce anxiety. Give the child age-appropriate information about CF. Quiz the child in a relaxed, friendly manner to help determine what the child knows and what teaching may be needed. Learning about CF can be turned into a game for some children, making it much more enjoyable.

Providing Family Support. The family is faced with a long-term illness and may have already seen deterioration in the child's health. Give the family and the child opportunities to voice fears and anxieties. Respond with active-listening techniques to help authenticate their feelings. Provide emotional support throughout the entire hospital stay. Demonstrate an interest and willingness to talk to the family; do not make family members feel as though they are intruding on time needed to do other things. The nurse is the person who can best provide overall support.

Providing Family Teaching. Evaluate the family's knowledge about CF to determine their teaching needs. The family may need to have all the information repeated or may have just a few areas of need. Provide information for resources such as the Cystic Fibrosis Foundation, the American Lung Association, and other local organizations. The family may have questions about genetic counseling and may need referrals for counseling.

EVALUATION: GOALS AND OUTCOME CRITERIA

- *Goal:* The child's airway will be clear.
  Criteria: The child effectively clears mucus from the airway and the airway remains patent. The child cooperates with chest physical therapy
- *Goal:* The child will exhibit adequate respiratory function.

Criteria: The child rests quietly with no dyspnea; the respiratory rate is even and appropriate for age. The oxygen saturation remains above 90%.
- Goal: The child will remain free of signs and symptoms of infection.
Criteria: The child's vital signs are within normal limits for age. The child and family follow infection-control practices.
- Goal: The child's nutritional intake will be adequate to compensate for decreased absorption of nutrients and to provide for adequate growth and development.
Criteria: The child has weight gain appropriate for age and growth chart shows normal growth.
- Goal: The child's anxiety will subside.
Criteria: The child engages in age-appropriate activities and appears relaxed.
- Goal: The family caregivers will verbalize feelings related to the child's chronic illness.
Criteria: The family caregivers verbalize fears, anxieties, and other feelings related to child's illness.
- Goal: The family caregivers will verbalize an understanding of the child's illness and treatment.
Criteria: The family caregivers can explain CF, describe treatments and possible complications, and become involved in available support groups.

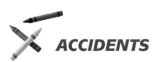

ACCIDENTS

Toddlers are natural explorers, examining their environment to learn all they can about it. As a result of their lack of experience and judgment, however, toddlers are prone to accidents, which are the leading cause of death in children over age 1 year. Nurses can contribute to safety education by providing information to families of young children pertaining to accident prevention and appropriate emergency responses.

Ingestion of Toxic Substances

One way in which toddlers find out about their environment is to taste the world around them. Toddlers and preschoolers are developing autonomy and initiative, which add to their tendency to examine their environment on their own. Because their senses of taste and smell are not yet refined, young children

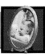

A PERSONAL GLIMPSE

While peeling apples, I stopped to get the ringing phone. My 3-year-old, Kasey, thought this was the perfect time to be a mother's helper. She managed to get on top of the table and tried to peel an apple herself.

I had to take her to the emergency room for a badly cut finger. The doctor on staff was not personable with children or with their parents! After going through a barrage of questions on why I would GIVE a child a knife to play with, things got worse. He did not want me in the room with her, which caused Kasey to become hysterical. He had to put her in a restraint. I had to assure her I was not leaving.

The doctor grabbed Kasey's hand and a small scissors. She was screaming that he was going to cut her fingers off. Of course I was questioned again. The doctor asked me if I often trimmed Kasey's fingers. I had to explain that she didn't even like to have her fingernails clipped and that he was what was making her more scared. I guess he was unaware that not all accidents are child abuse.

This entire experience made me angry and my daughter frightened.

Daria

> **LEARNING OPPORTUNITY:** What are some other ways this physician might have handled this situation? If you had been the ER nurse hearing this conversation, what would you say to this child and mother following this interaction?

ingest substances that would repel an adult because of their taste or smell. This makes these age groups prime targets for ingestion of poisonous substances. The ordinary household has an abundance of poisonous substances in almost every room. The kitchen, bathroom, bedroom, and garage are the most common sites harboring substances that are poisonous when ingested. Although most poisonings occur in the child's home, grandparents' homes offer many temptations to the young child as well. Grandparents tend to be less concerned about placing dangerous substances out of children's reach simply because the children are not part of the household, or the grandparents may place supplies where they are convenient, while never considering the young grandchild's developmental stage and exploratory nature.

When a child is found with a container whose contents he or she has obviously sampled, action should be taken immediately. When a child manifests symptoms that are difficult to pinpoint or that do not appear to relate specifically to any known cause, the possibility of poisoning should be suspected. Ingestion of a poisonous substance can produce symptoms that simulate an attack of an acute disease—vomiting, abdominal pain, diarrhea, shock, cyanosis, coma, and convulsions. If evidence of such a disease is lacking, acute poisoning should be suspected.

In instances of apparent poisoning where the substance is unknown, family caregivers are asked to consider all medications in their home. Is it possible that any medication could have been available to the child, or did an older child or other person possibly give the child the container to play with? Is it possible that a parent inadvertently gave a wrong dose or wrong medication to a child? All such possibilities need to be considered. In the meantime, the most important priority is treatment for the child who shows symptoms of poisoning.

Emergency Treatment

The first step the caregiver should take when poison ingestion is suspected is to call the poison control center. The caregiver should call the local poison control center; for areas without a local center, a toll-free number is available to access a poison control center. This number can be found in the local telephone directory; all homes with young children should have the poison control center number posted by every telephone for quick reference. The caregiver should remove any obvious poison from the child's mouth before calling. The poison control center evaluates the situation and tells the caller whether the child can be treated at home or needs to be transported to a hospital or treatment center.

Except when corrosive or highly irritant poisons have been swallowed, the first measure is to induce vomiting. If the child is convulsing or unconscious, however, vomiting should not be induced because of the danger of aspiration.

The approved method for producing vomiting is to have the child swallow 15 mL of syrup of ipecac. A second 15-mL dose can be given if vomiting does not occur within 15 to 30 minutes. Stimulating the child's posterior pharynx with the adult's finger also may induce vomiting. The child's head should be allowed to droop forward or should be turned to the side to avoid aspiration of the vomitus.

If the ingested substance is unknown, all material vomited at home or on the way to the hospital or treatment center should be saved for analysis. If the substance that the child swallowed is known, the container should be taken to the treatment facility. If

the container is left behind in the panic and confusion, someone will need to go to the home and retrieve it.

If the substance the child has swallowed is known, the ingredients can be found on the label and the poison control center can suggest an antidote. If the substance is a prescription drug, the pharmacist who filled the prescription or who is familiar with the drug also can be contacted for information. In some instances, it is necessary to analyze the residual stomach contents.

Specific antidotes are available for certain poisons but not for all. Some antidotes react chemically with the poison to render it harmless while others prevent absorption of the poison. Activated charcoal given after vomiting absorbs many poisons. A dose of 5 to 10 g per gram of ingested poison is given by mouth in 6 to 8 ounces of water or may be given through an NG tube if necessary.

Treatment Steps in Order of Importance. The treatment steps in order of importance are

1. Remove the obvious remnants of the poison.
2. Call the poison control center.
3. Prevent further absorption.
4. Administer appropriate antidote if known.
5. Administer general supportive and symptomatic care.

Further specific treatment is given according to the kind and amount of the toxic substance ingested. Common types of poisoning and general treatment are described in Table 13–1. Complete listings of poisonous substances with the specific treatment for each are available from poison control centers, clinics, and pharmacies.

Lead Poisoning (Plumbism)

Chronic lead poisoning has been a serious problem among children for many years. It is responsible for neurologic handicaps including mental retardation because of its effect on the central nervous system. Infants and toddlers are potential victims because of their tendency to put any object within their reach into their mouths. In some children, this habit leads to **pica** (the ingestion of nonfood substances such as laundry starch, clay, paper, and paint). The unborn fetus of a pregnant mother who is exposed to lead (such as lead dust from renovation of an older home) also can be affected by lead contamination. Screening for lead poisoning is part of a complete well-baby checkup between ages 6 months and 6 years.

Causes of Chronic Lead Poisoning. The most common causes of lead poisoning are

- Lead-containing paint used on the outside or the inside of older houses
- Furniture and toys painted with lead-containing paint; vinyl miniblinds

TABLE 13.1	**Commonly Ingested Toxic Substances**

Agent	Symptoms	Treatment
acetaminophen	Under 6 y—vomiting is the earliest sign Adolescents—vomiting, diaphoresis, general malaise. Liver damage can result in 48–96 hr if not treated	Induce vomiting with syrup of ipecac. Gastric lavage may be necessary. Administer acetylcysteine (Mucomyst) diluted with cola, fruit juice, or water if plasma level elevated. Mucomyst may be administered by gavage, especially because its odor of rotten eggs makes it objectionable.
acetylsalicyclic acid (aspirin)	Hyperpnea (abnormal increase in depth and rate of breathing), metabolic acidosis, hyperventilation, tinnitus, vertigo are initial symptoms. Dehydration, coma, convulsions, and death follow untreated heavy dosage.	Induce vomiting with syrup of ipecac. Gastric lavage may be necessary. Activated charcoal may be administered. IV fluids, sodium bicarbonate to combat acidosis, and dialysis for renal failure may be necessary when large amounts are ingested.
ibuprofen (Motrin, Advil)	Similar to aspirin; metabolic acidosis, GI bleeding, renal damage	Induce vomiting. Activated charcoal is administered in emergency department. Observe for and treat GI bleeding. Electrolyte determination is done to detect acidosis. IV fluids are given.
ferrous sulfate (iron)	Vomiting, lethargy, diarrhea, weak rapid pulse, hypotension are common symptoms. Massive dose may produce shock, erosion of small intestine, black, tarry stools, bronchial pneumonia.	Induce vomiting with syrup of ipecac. Deferoxamine, a chelating agent that combines with iron, may be used when child has ingested a toxic dose.
barbiturates	Respiratory, circulatory, and renal depression may occur. Child may become comatose.	Establish airway; administer oxygen if needed; perform gastric lavage. Close observation of level of consciousness is needed.

corrosives
  alkali: lye, bleaches
  acid: drain cleaners, toilet bowl cleaners, iodine, silver nitrate
	Intense burning and pain with first mouthful; severe burns of mouth and esophageal tract; shock, possible death.	*Never have child vomit.*
		  Alkali corrosives are treated initially with quantities of water, diluted acid fruit juices, or diluted vinegar.
		  Acid corrosives are treated with alkaline drinks such as milk, olive oil, mineral oil, or egg white.
		Lavage or emetics are never used.
		  Continuing treatment includes antidotes, gastrostomy or IV feedings, and specialized care. A tracheostomy may be needed.

hydrocarbons kerosene, gasoline, furniture polish, lighter fluid, turpentine	Damage to the respiratory system is the primary concern. Vomiting often occurs spontaneously, possibly causing additional damage to the respiratory system. Pneumonia, bronchopneumonia, or lipoid pneumonia may occur.	Emergency treatment and assessment are necessary. Vital signs are monitored; oxygen is administered as needed. Gastric lavage is performed only if the ingested substance contains other toxic chemicals that may threaten other body system such as the liver, kidneys, or cardiovascular system.

- Drinking water contaminated by lead pipes or copper pipes with lead-soldered joints
- Dust containing lead salts from lead paint; emission from lead smelters
- Storage of fruit juices or other food in improperly glazed earthenware
- Inhalation of motor fumes containing lead or from burning of storage batteries
- Exposure to industrial areas with smelteries or chemical plants
- Exposure to hobby materials containing lead, e.g., stained glass, solder, fishing sinkers, bullets

Lead poisoning has other causes but the most common cause has been the lead in paint. Children tend to nibble on fallen plaster, painted wooden furniture (including cribs), and painted toys because they have a sweet taste. Fine dust that results from removing lead paint in remodeling also can cause harm to the young children in the household without parents being aware of exposure. When the danger of lead poisoning became apparent, attempts were made to control the sale of lead-based paint. In 1973, federal regulations banned the sale of paint containing more than 0.5% lead for interior residential use or use on toys. This has not eliminated the problem, however, because many homes built before the 1960s were painted with lead-based paint, and they still exist in inner-city areas as well as small towns and suburbs. Older mansions where upper-income families may live also may have lead paint because of the building's age. Only contractors experienced in lead-based paint removal should do renovation.

Clinical Manifestations. The onset of chronic lead poisoning is insidious. Some early indications may be irritability, hyperactivity, aggression, impulsiveness, or disinterest in play. Short attention span, lethargy, learning difficulties, and distractibility also are signs of poisoning.

The condition may progress to **encephalopathy** (degenerative disease of the brain) because of intracranial pressure. Acute manifestations include convulsions, mental retardation, blindness, paralysis, coma, and death. Acute episodes sometimes develop sporadically and early in the condition.

Diagnosis. The nonspecific nature of the presenting symptoms makes it important to examine the child's environmental history. Testing blood lead levels is used as a screening method. Target screening is done in areas where the risk of lead poisoning is high. Finger sticks, or heel sticks for infants, can be used to collect samples for lead level screening. In 1997, the Centers for Disease Control in Atlanta modified the guidelines related to lead screening. The CDC continues to define elevated blood levels of lead as equal to or greater than 10 µg/dL. The CDC's emphasis is on primary prevention and screening.

Treatment. The most important aspect of treatment of a child with lead poisoning is to remove the lead from the child's system and environment. The use of a **chelating agent** (an agent that binds with metal) increases the urinary excretion of lead. Several chelating agents are available; individual circumstances and the physician's choice determine the particular drug used. Edetate calcium disodium, known as EDTA, is usually given IV because intramuscular administration is painful. Renal failure can occur with inappropriate dosage. Dimercaptopropanol (dimercaprol), also known as BAL, causes excretion of lead through bile and urine; it may be administered intramuscularly. Because of its peanut oil base, BAL should not be used in children allergic to peanuts. These two drugs may be used together in children with extremely high levels of lead.

The oral drug penicillamine (D-Penamine) can be used to treat children with blood lead levels lower than 45 µg/dL. The capsules can be opened and sprinkled on food or mixed in liquid for administration. This drug should not be administered to children who are allergic to penicillin. The drug succimer (Chemet) is an oral drug used for treating

children with blood lead levels higher than 45 µg/dL. Succimer comes in capsules that can be opened and mixed with applesauce or other soft foods or can be taken from a spoon followed by a flavored beverage.

All the chelating drugs may have toxic side effects, and children being treated must be carefully monitored with frequent urinalysis, blood cell counts, and renal function tests. Any child receiving chelation therapy should be under the care of an experienced health care team.

Outcome. The prognosis after lead poisoning is uncertain. Early detection of the condition and removal of the child from the lead-containing surroundings offer the best hope. Follow-up should include routine examinations to prevent recurrence and to observe for signs of any residual brain damage not immediately apparent.

Although the incidence of lead poisoning has decreased, it is still prevalent. Measures to educate the public on the importance of preventing this disorder are essential if the problem is to be eliminated. Education of the family caregivers is an essential aspect of the treatment (see Family Teaching Tips: Preventing Lead Poisoning).

FAMILY TEACHING TIPS

Preventing Lead Poisoning

1. If you live in an older home, make sure your child does not have access to any chips of paint or chew any surface painted with lead-based paint. Look for paint dust on window sills, and clean with a high-phosphate sodium cleaner (the phosphate content of automatic dishwashing detergent is usually high enough).
2. Wet-mop hard-surfaced floors and woodwork with cleaner at least once a week. Vacuuming hard surfaces scatters dust.
3. Wash child's hands and face before eating.
4. Wash toys and pacifiers frequently.
5. Prevent child from playing in dust near an old lead-painted house.
6. Prevent child from playing in soil or dust near a major highway.
7. If your water supply has a high lead content, fully flush faucets before using for cooking, drinking, or making formula.
8. Avoid contamination from hobbies or work.
9. Make sure your child eats regular meals. Food slows absorption of lead.
10. Encourage your child to eat foods high in iron and calcium.

From Centers for Disease Control and Prevention: Preventing lead poisoning in young children: a statement by The Centers for Disease Control. Atlanta, 2002. *http://www.cdc.gov*

Ingestion of Foreign Objects

Young children are apt to put any small objects into their mouths; they often swallow these objects. Normally many of these objects pass smoothly through the digestive tract and are expelled in the feces. Occasionally, however, something such as an open safety pin, a coin, a button, or a marble may lodge in the esophagus and need to be extracted. Foods such as hot dogs, peanuts, carrots, popcorn kernels, apple pieces, grapes, and round candy are frequent offenders.

Unless symptoms of choking, gagging, or pain are present, waiting and watching the feces carefully for 3 or 4 days is usually safe. Any object, however, may pass safely through the esophagus and stomach only to become fixed in one of the curves of the intestine, causing an obstruction or fever due to infection. Also, sharp objects present the danger of perforation somewhere in the digestive tract.

Diagnosis of a swallowed solid object is often, but not always, made from the history. If a foreign object in the digestive tract is suspected, fluoroscopic and radiographic studies may be required.

Treatment

If a caregiver has seen an infant swallow an object and begin choking, the caregiver should hold the infant along the rescuer's forearm with the infant's head lower than its chest and give the infant several back blows. After delivering the back blows, the caregiver should support the infant's back and head and turn the infant over onto the opposite thigh. The caregiver should deliver up to five quick downward chest thrusts and remove the foreign body if visualized. A child older than age 1 year can be encouraged to continue to cough as long as the cough remains forceful. If the cough becomes ineffective (no sound with cough) or respirations become more difficult and stridor is present, the caregiver can attempt the Heimlich maneuver (Fig. 13–8).

If the child is not having respiratory problems and coughing has not resulted in removal of the object, the child needs to be transported to an emergency depart-

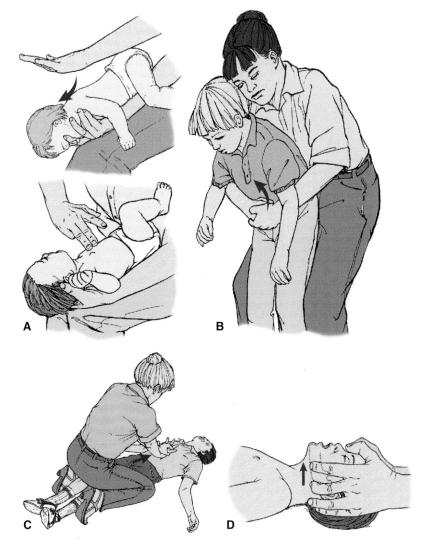

● *Figure 13.8* (*A*) Back blows (*top*) and chest thrusts (*bottom*) to relieve foreign-body airway obstruction in infant. Hold infant over arm as illustrated, supporting head by firmly holding jaw. Deliver up to five back blows. Turn infant over while supporting head, neck, jaw, and chest with one hand and back with other hand. Keep head lower than trunk. Give five quick chest thrusts with one finger below intermammary line. If foreign body is not removed and airway remains obstructed, attempt rescue breathing. Repeat these 2 steps until successful. (*B*) Abdominal thrusts with child standing or sitting can be performed when child is conscious. Standing behind child, place thumb side of one fist against child's abdomen in midline slightly above navel and well below xiphoid process. Grab fist with other hand and deliver five quick upward thrusts. Continue until successful or child loses consciousness. (*C*) Abdominal thrusts with child lying can be performed on a conscious or unconscious child. Place heel of hand on child's abdomen slightly above the navel and below the xiphoid process and rib cage. Place other hand on top of first hand. Deliver five separate, distinct thrusts. Open airway and attempt rescue breathing if object is not removed. Repeat until successful. (*D*) Combined jaw thrust-spine stabilization maneuver for a child trauma victim with possible head and neck injury. To protect from damage to cervical spine, the neck is maintained in a neutral position and traction on or movement of neck is avoided.

ment to be assessed by a physician. Objects in the esophagus are removed by direct vision through an esophagoscope. Attempts to push the object down into the stomach or to extract it blindly can be dangerous. Some objects may need to be removed surgically. If the object is small and the physician believes that there is little danger to the gastrointestinal tract, the caregiver may be advised to take the child home and watch the child's bowel movements over the next several days to confirm that the object has passed through the system.

Increasing respiratory difficulties indicate that the object has been aspirated rather than swallowed. Foreign objects aspirated into the larynx or bronchial tree may become lodged in the trachea or larynx. Back blows and chest thrusts or the Heimlich maneuver should be delivered as described. The child's airway should be opened and rescue breathing attempted. If the child's chest does not rise, the child should be repositioned and rescue breathing tried again. If the airway is still obstructed, these steps should be repeated until the object is removed and respirations are established. The child should be transported to the emergency department as quickly as possible. The caregiver should get emergency assistance while continuing to try to remove the offending object.

Adults must be aware of the power of example. A child who sees an adult holding pins or nails in his or her mouth may follow this example with disastrous and often fatal results.

Insertion of Foreign Bodies Into the Ear or Nose

Children also may insert small objects, such as peas or beans, crumpled paper, beads, and small toys, into their ears or noses. Irrigation of the ear may remove small objects, except paper, which becomes impacted as it absorbs moisture. The physician generally uses small forceps to remove objects not dislodged by irrigation.

The child may have placed a foreign body in the nose just inside the nares, but manipulation may push it in further. If the object remains in the nose for any length of time, infection may occur. When the object is discovered, a physician should inspect with a speculum and remove the object.

Drowning

Drowning is the second leading cause of accidental death in children. Toddlers and older adolescents have the highest actual rate of death from drowning. Drowning in young children occurs when the child has been left unattended in a body of water. Infants more commonly drown in a bathtub; toddlers and preschoolers drown in pools or small bodies of water. A pail of water may become something for the toddler to investigate, which could lead to accidental death. Many deaths in this age group occur in home pools including spas, hot tubs, and whirlpools.

A responsible adult must continuously supervise all infants and young children when they are near any source of water. Older children and adolescents should not play alone around any body of water. Swimming in undesignated swimming areas such as creeks, quarries, and rivers is hazardous for older children and adolescents.

When a drowning victim of any age is discovered, cardiopulmonary resuscitation (CPR) should be started immediately and continued until the victim can be transported to a medical facility for further care. Intensive care is carried out according to the patient's needs. All adults who care for children in any capacity must learn CPR and be ready to perform it immediately (Table 13–2, Fig. 13–9).

TABLE 13.2	**Summary of Basic Life Support Maneuvers in Infants and Children**	
Maneuver	Infant (<1 y)	Child (1 to 8 y)
Airway	Head tilt-chin lift (unless trauma present) Jaw thrust	Head tilt-chin lift (unless trauma present) Jaw thrust
Breathing		
Initial	2 breaths at 1 to 1½ s/breath	2 breaths at 1 to 1 ½ s/breath
Subsequent	20 breaths/min	20 breaths/min
Circulation		
Pulse check	Brachial/femoral	Carotid
Compression area	Lower half of sternum	Lower half of sternum
Compression width	2 or 3 fingers	Heel of 1 hand
Compression depth	About ½–1 inch	About 1–1 ½ inch
Rate	At least 100/min	100/min
Compression-ventilation ratio	5:1 (pause for ventilation)	5:1 (pause for ventilation)
Foreign body airway obstruction	Back blows/chest thrusts	Heimlich maneuver

Adapted from American Heart Association (2001) *Basic life support for healthcare providers.* Dallas, TX: AHA.

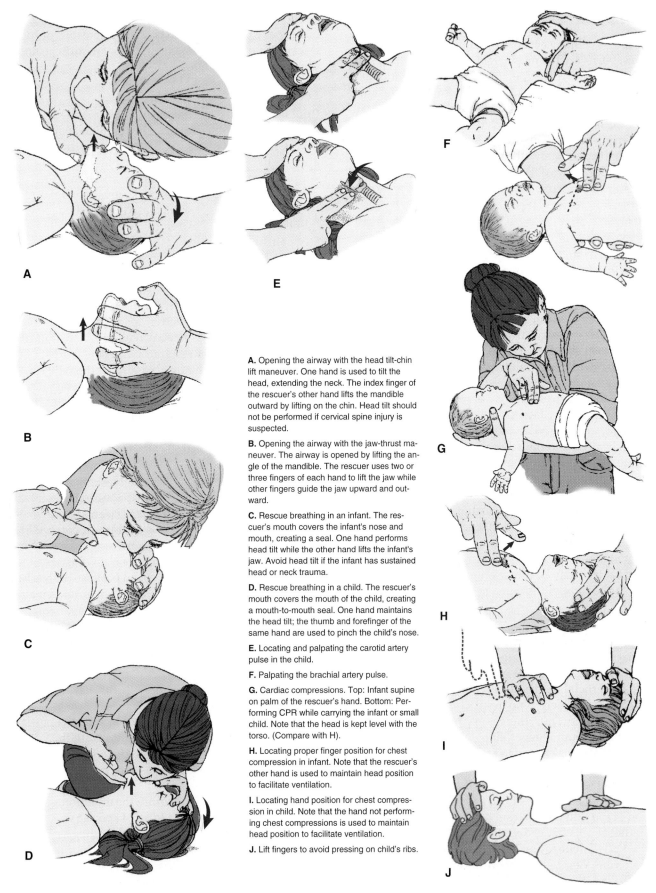

A. Opening the airway with the head tilt-chin lift maneuver. One hand is used to tilt the head, extending the neck. The index finger of the rescuer's other hand lifts the mandible outward by lifting on the chin. Head tilt should not be performed if cervical spine injury is suspected.

B. Opening the airway with the jaw-thrust maneuver. The airway is opened by lifting the angle of the mandible. The rescuer uses two or three fingers of each hand to lift the jaw while other fingers guide the jaw upward and outward.

C. Rescue breathing in an infant. The rescuer's mouth covers the infant's nose and mouth, creating a seal. One hand performs head tilt while the other hand lifts the infant's jaw. Avoid head tilt if the infant has sustained head or neck trauma.

D. Rescue breathing in a child. The rescuer's mouth covers the mouth of the child, creating a mouth-to-mouth seal. One hand maintains the head tilt; the thumb and forefinger of the same hand are used to pinch the child's nose.

E. Locating and palpating the carotid artery pulse in the child.

F. Palpating the brachial artery pulse.

G. Cardiac compressions. Top: Infant supine on palm of the rescuer's hand. Bottom: Performing CPR while carrying the infant or small child. Note that the head is kept level with the torso. (Compare with H).

H. Locating proper finger position for chest compression in infant. Note that the rescuer's other hand is used to maintain head position to facilitate ventilation.

I. Locating hand position for chest compression in child. Note that the hand not performing chest compressions is used to maintain head position to facilitate ventilation.

J. Lift fingers to avoid pressing on child's ribs.

● **Figure 13.9** Cardiopulmonary resuscitation. (Adapted from American Heart Association [2001] *Basic life support for healthcare providers.* Dallas, TX: AHA.)

Burns

Among the many accidents that occur in children's lives, burns are the most frightening. More than 70% of burn accidents happen to children younger than age 5 years. Nearly all childhood burns are preventable, and this causes considerable guilt for families and the child. Adult carelessness, the child's exploring and curious nature, and failure to supervise the child adequately all contribute to the high incidence of burns in children. In addition, burns are a common form of child abuse.

Causes

Scalds From Hot Liquids. This type of burn, common in small children, results from a dangling electric coffee-maker cord, pans of hot liquid on the stove with handles turned out, cups of hot tea or coffee, bowls of soup or other hot liquids, or small children left alone in bathtubs. Dangerous, sometimes fatal, burns can occur from these conditions.

Burns From Fire. The second most common kind of burn results from children playing with matches or being left alone in buildings that catch fire. Careless use of smoking materials is a common cause of house fires. Children are fascinated by fires and must be carefully supervised around fireplaces, campfires, room heaters, and outside barbecues. Cigarette lighters are currently being produced with a "child-safe" lighting mechanism, but they should still be kept away from children.

Electricity. Although uncommon in children, infants and toddlers can suffer severe facial or mouth burns from biting on electrical cords plugged into a socket; they may require extensive plastic surgery. These burns may be more serious than they first appear because of the damage to underlying tissues.

Types of Burns

Burns are divided into types according to the depth of tissue involvement: superficial, partial thickness, or total thickness (Table 13–3, Fig. 13–10).

Superficial or First-Degree Burns. The epidermis is injured, but there is no destruction of tissue or nerve endings. Thus, there is erythema, edema, and pain but prompt regeneration.

Partial-Thickness or Second-Degree Burns. The epidermis and underlying dermis are both injured and devitalized or destroyed. Blistering usually occurs with an escape of body plasma but regeneration of the skin occurs from the remaining viable epithelial cells in the dermis (Fig. 13–11).

Full-Thickness or Third-Degree Burns. The epidermis, dermis, and nerve endings are all destroyed (Fig. 13–12). Pain is minimal, and there is no longer any barrier to infection or any remaining viable epithelial cells. Fourth-, fifth-, and sixth-degree burns have been described that are extensions of full-thickness burns with involvement of fat, muscle, and bone respectively.

Emergency Treatment

Cool water is an excellent emergency treatment for burns involving small areas. The immediate application of cool compresses or cool water to burn areas appears to inhibit capillary permeability and thus suppress edema, blister formation, and tissue destruction. Ice water or ice packs must not be used because of the danger of increased tissue damage. Immersing a burned extremity in cool water alleviates pain and may prevent further thermal injury. This can be done after the airway, breathing, and circulation have been observed and restored if necessary but should not be done when large areas are involved because of the danger of hypothermia.

In the case of a fire victim, special attention should be given to the airway to observe for signs of smoke inhalation and respiratory passage burns. Clothing should be removed to inspect the whole body for burned areas; also clothing may retain heat, which can cause further tissue damage. The child should be transported to a medical facility for assessment. If transported to a special burn unit, the child may be wrapped in a sterile sheet and the burn treated on arrival.

Superficial Burns. Superficial burns can usually be treated on an outpatient basis because they heal readily unless infected. The area is cleaned, an anesthetic ointment is applied, and the burn is covered with a sterile gauze bandage or dressing. An analgesic may be needed to relieve pain. Blisters should not be intentionally broken because of the risk of infection, but blisters that are already broken may be débrided (cut away). The child is seen again in 2 days to inspect for infection. The caregiver is instructed to keep the area clean and dry (no bathing the area) until the burn is healed usually in about a week to 10 days.

Partial- and Full-Thickness Burns. Distinguishing between partial- and full-thickness burns is not always possible. In the presence of infection, a partial-thickness burn may be converted into a full thickness one; also with extensive burns, a greater amount of full-thickness burn often exists than had been estimated.

Full-thickness burns require the attention, skill, and conscientious care of a team of specialists. Children with mixed second- and third-degree burns or with third-degree burns involving 15% or more of the body surface require hospitalization. Burns are classified according to criteria of the American Burn Association (Table 13–4).

TABLE 13.3	Characteristics of Burns						
Degree	Cause	Surface Appearance	Color	Pain Level	Histologic Depth	Healing Time
First (superficial) All are considered minor unless under 18 mo, over 65 y, or with severe loss of fluids	Flash, flame, ultraviolet (sunburn)	Dry, no blisters, edema	Erythematous	Painful	Epidermal layers only	2 to 5 days with peeling, no scarring, may have discoloration
Second (partial-thickness) Minor—less than 15% in adults, less than 10% in children Moderate—15% to 30% in adults or less than 15% with involvement of face, hands, feet, or perineum; minor chemical or electrical; in children, 10% to 30% Severe—more than 30%	Contact with hot liquids or solids, flash flame to clothing, direct flame, chemical	Moist blebs, blisters	Mottled white to pink, cherry red	Very painful	Epidermis, papillary, and reticular layers of dermis; may include fat domes of subcutaneous layer	Superficial—5 to 21 days with no grafting Deep with no infection—21 to 35 days If infected, convert to full thickness.
Third (full-thickness) Minor—less than 2% Moderate—2% to 10%, any involvement of face, hands, feet, or perineum Severe—more than 10% and major chemical or electrical	Contact with hot liquids or solids, flame, chemical, electricity	Dry with leathery eschar until débridement; charred blood vessels visible under eschar	Mixed white (waxy or pearly), dark (khaki or mahogany), charred	Little or no pain; hair pulls out easily	Down to and including subcutaneous tissue; may include fascia, muscle, and bone	Large areas require grafting that may take many months. Small areas may heal from the edges after weeks.

Adapted from Wiebelhaus, P. (2001). Managing burn emergencies. *Nursing Management, 32*(7),29–36.

Treatment of Moderate to Severe Burns: First Phase—48 to 72 Hours

Hypovolemic shock is the major manifestation in the first 48 hours in massive burns. As extracellular fluid pours into the burned area, it collects in enormous quantities, which dehydrates the body. Edema becomes noticeable, and symptoms of severe shock appear. Intense pain is seldom a major factor. Symptoms of shock are low blood pressure, rapid pulse, pallor, and often considerable apprehension.

Intravenous Fluids. The primary concern is to replace body fluids that have been lost or immobilized at the burn areas. Because there is a distinct relationship between the extent of the surface area burned and the amount of fluid lost, the percentage of affected skin area as well as the classification of the burns must be estimated to determine the medical treatment (Fig. 13–13). The extent and depth of the burn and the expertise available within the hospital determine whether the child is treated at the general hospital or immediately transported to a burn unit.

An IV infusion site must be selected and fluids started; most often lactated Ringer's solution, isotonic saline, or plasma is used with a large-bore catheter to administer replacement fluids and maintain total parenteral nutrition (TPN). Intravenous fluids for maintenance and replacement of lost body fluids are estimated for the first 24 hours with half of this calculated requirement given during the first 8 hours. The patient's needs may change rapidly, however, necessitating a change in the rate of flow or the amount or type of fluid. The patient's urinary output, vital signs,

Depths of burns

Skin grafts

Superficial (1st degree)

Partial thickness (2nd degree)

Full thickness (3rd degree)

Epidermis

Dermis

Subcutaneous tissue

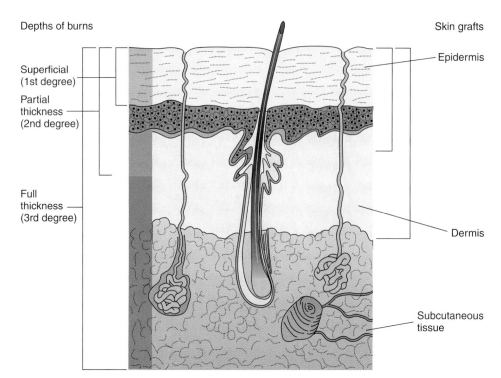

● *Figure 13.10* Cross section of the skin showing the relative depths of the types of burn injury.

and general appearance are all part of the information that the physician needs to determine the fluid requirements. With TPN, fluids can be administered to provide needed amino acids, glucose, fats, vitamins, and minerals so that large amounts of food do not need to be consumed orally. This nutrition is essential for tissue repair and healing.

Airway. The adequacy of the airway must be determined in case an endotracheal tube needs to be inserted or (rarely) a tracheostomy performed. Inhalation injury is a leading cause of complications in burns. If there are burns around the face and neck or if the burns occurred in a small enclosed space, inhalation injury should be suspected. In fires, toxic sub-

stances and the heat produced can cause damage to the respiratory tract. All these possibilities must be considered and the child should be observed for them.

Oral Fluids. The administration of oral fluids should be omitted or minimized for 1 or 2 days. Delayed gastric emptying causing acute gastric dilatation is a common complication of burns and can become a serious problem resulting in vomiting and anorexia. An NG tube on low suction prevents vomiting. IV fluids should relieve the child's thirst, which is usually severe, and sips of water may be allowed. Oral feedings can be started when bowel sounds are heard. Nasogastric feedings may be needed to supplement intake. The child's caloric and

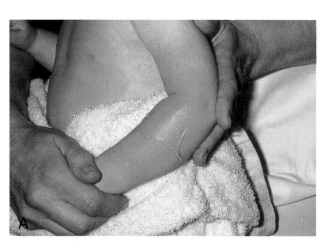

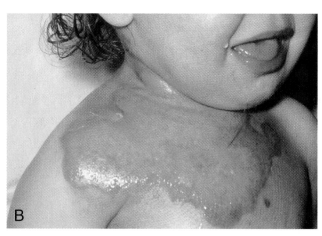

● *Figure 13.11* Partial-thickness burns. **(A)** Infant with first-degree burn on arm and chest caused by scalding. **(B)** Toddler with second-degree burn caused by scalding.

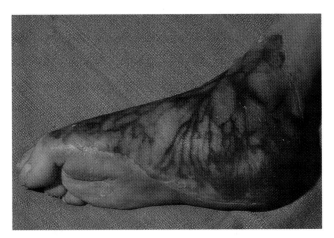

● *Figure 13.12* Full-thickness (third-degree) burn of the foot.

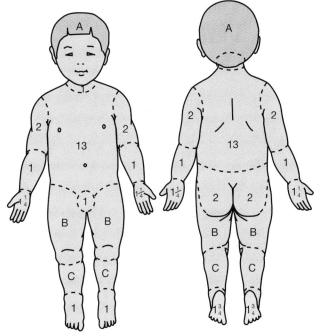

Relative Percentages of Areas Affected by Growth			
Area	Age 0	1	5
A = $\frac{1}{2}$ of head	$9\frac{1}{2}$	$8\frac{1}{2}$	$6\frac{1}{2}$
B = $\frac{1}{2}$ of one thigh	$2\frac{3}{4}$	$3\frac{1}{4}$	4
C = $\frac{1}{2}$ of one leg	$2\frac{1}{2}$	$2\frac{1}{2}$	$2\frac{3}{4}$

● *Figure 13.13* Determination of extent of burns in children.

nutritional requirements are two or three times those needed for normal growth; thus, nutritional supplements will most likely be needed.

Diuresis. Urinary output, which may be decreased because of the decrease in blood volume, must be monitored closely. Renal shutdown may be a threat. An output of 1 to 2 mL/kg/hr for children weighing 30 kg (66 lb) or less or 30 to 50 mL/hr for those over 30 kg is desirable. An indwelling catheter facilitates the accurate measurement of urine and specific gravity. After the first hour, the volume of urine should be relatively constant. Any change in volume or specific gravity should be reported.

After the initial fluid therapy has brought the burn shock under control and the extracellular fluid deficit has been compensated, the patient faces another hazard with the onset of the diuretic phase. This occurs within 24 to 96 hours after the accident. The plasma-like fluid is picked up and reabsorbed from the third space in the burn areas, and the patient may rapidly become **hypervolemic** (exhibit an abnormal increase in the blood volume in the circulatory system) even to the point of pulmonary edema. This is the principal reason for the extremely close check on all vital signs and for the close monitoring of IV fluids that must now be slowed or stopped entirely.

The nurse must notify the physician at once if any of the following signs of the onset of this phase occur:

- Rapid rise in urinary output; may increase to 250 mL/hr or higher
- Tachypnea followed by dyspnea
- Increase in pulse pressure; mean blood pressure also may increase. Central venous pressure, if measured, is elevated.

TABLE 13.4	**Classification of Burns**
Classification	Description
Minor	First-degree burn or second degree <10% of body surface or third degree <2% of body surface; no area of the face, feet, hand, or genitalia is burned
Moderate	Second-degree burn 10% to 20% body surface or on the face, hands, feet, or genitalia, or third-degree burn <10% body surface or if smoke inhalation has occurred
Severe	Second-degree burn >20% body surface or third-degree burn >10% body surface

Infection Control. The child has lost a portion of the integumentary system, which is a primary defense against infection. For this reason, measures must be taken to protect the child from infection. Antibiotics are not considered very effective in controlling infection of this type, most likely because the injured capillaries cannot carry the antibiotic to the site. If used, antibiotics are usually added to the IV fluids. Tetanus antitoxin or toxoid should be ordered according to the status of the child's previous immunization. If inoculations are up to date, a booster dose of tetanus toxoid is all that is required.

To protect the child from infection introduced into the burn, sterile equipment must be used in the child's care. Everyone who cares for the child must wear a gown, a mask, and a head cover. Visitors also are required to scrub, gown, and mask. Burn units are designed to be self-contained with treatment and operating areas, hydrotherapy units, and patient care areas. In hospitals where there is no specific burn unit, a private room with a door that can be closed should be set up as a burn unit. The strictest aseptic technique must be observed.

Wound Care. Two types of burn care are generally used: the open method and the closed method. The open method of burn care is most often used for superficial burns, burns of the face, and burns of the perineum. In open burn care, the wound is not covered but antimicrobial ointment is applied topically. This type of care requires strict aseptic precautions. In the closed burn method of burn care, nonadherent gauze is used to cover the burn. The child can be moved more easily, and the danger of added injury or pain is decreased. In the closed method though, dressing changes are very painful, and infection may occur under the dressings. Occlusive dressings help minimize pain because of the reduced exposure to air.

In both methods, daily **débridement** (removal of necrotic tissue) usually preceded by **hydrotherapy** (use of water in treatment) is performed. Débridement is extremely painful, and the child must have an analgesic administered before the therapy. The child is placed in the tub of water to soak the dressings; this helps to remove any sloughing tissue, **eschar** (hard crust or scab), exudate, and old medication. Often the tissue is trapped in the mesh gauze of the dressing, so soaking eases necrotic tissue removal. Loose tissue is trimmed before the burn is redressed. Hosing instead of tub soaking is used in some centers to reduce the risk of infection. Débridement is difficult emotionally for both the child and the nurse (Fig. 13–14). Diversionary activities may be used to help distract the child. Researchers also have found that children who are encouraged to participate actively in their burn care, even to help change dressings, experience healthy control over their situation and often suffer

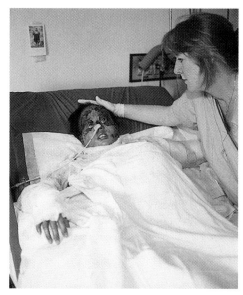

● *Figure 13.14* The nurse gives support to the child during debridement.

less anxiety than those who are completely dependent on the nurse. The child should never be scolded or reprimanded for uncooperative behavior. Praise for cooperation should be used generously.

Topical medications that may be used to reduce invading organisms are silver sulfadiazine (Silvadene), silver nitrate, mafenide acetate (Sulfamylon), Bacitracin, and povidone-iodine (Betadine). Each of these agents has advantages and disadvantages. The choice of agent is made by the physician and is determined, at least partially, by the organisms found in cultures of the burn area.

INTERNET EXERCISE 13.1

http://www.cooltheburn.com

Cool the Burn
Click on the logo, "Cool the Burn."
Click on "Learn about Burns."
Click on "The Burn Center" on the left side of the screen.
Click on "Bandages."

1. How could you use this site to help explain a dressing change to a child with a burn?

Click on "fun things."

2. Explain the activities available to use with a hospitalized child.

3. What is available on this site for caregivers of a child with a burn?

Grafting. Grafts may be **homografts, heterografts** (xenografts), or **autografts.** Homografts and heterografts are temporary grafts. A homograft consists of skin taken from another person, which is eventually rejected by the recipient tissue and sloughed off after 3 to 6 weeks. Skin from cadavers is often used in a procedure called an **allograft;** this skin can be stored and used up to several weeks, and permission for this use is seldom refused.

A heterograft is skin obtained from animals, usually pigs (porcine). Both homografts and heterografts provide a temporary dressing after débridement and have proved to be lifesaving measures for children with extensive burns.

An autograft, consisting of skin taken from the child's own body, is the only kind of skin accepted permanently by recipient tissues except for the skin from an identical twin. Obtaining enough healthy skin to cover a large area is usually impossible; therefore, homografts are of great value for immediate covering. If the donor site is kept free from infection and grafts of sufficient thinness are taken, the site should be ready for use again in 10 to 12 days.

After grafting, the donor and the graft sites are kept covered with sterile dressings.

Complications

Curling's ulcer (also called a stress ulcer) is a gastric or duodenal ulcer that often occurs after serious skin burns. It can easily be overlooked when the attention of nurses and physicians is directed toward the treatment of the burn area and the prevention of infection. Symptoms are those of any gastric ulcer but usually are vague, concerned with abdominal discomfort, are with or without localization, or are related to eating. Ulcers appear during the first 6 weeks. Blood in the stools combined with abdominal discomfort may be the basis for diagnosis. If desired, roentgenograms can confirm the diagnosis. Treatment consists of a bland diet and the use of antacids and antispasmodics.

The health care team must guard carefully against the complication of **contractures.** If the burn extends over a movable body part, fibrous scarring that forms in the healing process can cause serious deformities and limit movement. Joints must be positioned, possibly in overextension, so that maximal flexibility is maintained. Splinting, exercise, and pressure also are used to prevent contractures. In severe burns, pressure garments, which help decrease hypertrophy of scar tissue, may need to be worn for 12 to 18 months. The child must wear these garments continuously except when bathing.

Long-Term Care

The rehabilitative phase of care for the child is often long and difficult. Even after discharge from the health care facility, the child needs to return for further treatment or plastic surgery to release contrac-

tures and revise scar tissue. The emotional scars of the family and the child must be evaluated, and therapy must be initiated or continued. The impact of scarring and disfigurement may need to be resolved by both the child and members of the family. If the child is of school age, school work and social interaction must be considered. (See the Nursing Care Plan.)

● Nursing Process for the Child With a Burn

ASSESSMENT

Assessment of the child with a burn is complex and varies with the extent and depth of the burn, the stage of healing, and the age and general condition of the child. Initially the primary concerns are the cardiac and respiratory state, the assessment of shock, and an evaluation of the burns.

After the first phase (the first 24 to 48 hours), the healing of the child's burns must be evaluated and the child's nutrition, signs of infection, and pain level must be monitored. The emotional conditions of the child and the family also must be evaluated.

NURSING DIAGNOSES

Many nursing diagnoses may be identified over the child's extended hospitalization. The following are a few that may be appropriate:
- Risk for Infection related to the loss of protective layer (skin) secondary to burn injury
- Imbalanced Nutrition: Less Than Body Requirements related to increased caloric needs secondary to burns and anorexia
- Acute Pain related to tissue destruction and painful procedures
- Risk for Impaired Physical Mobility related to pain and scarring
- Anxiety related to changes in body image due to thermal injury
- Compromised Family Coping related to the impact of the injury on the child and family's life
- Deficient Caregiver Knowledge related to optimizing the child's healing process and to the long-term care required by the child

OUTCOME IDENTIFICATION AND PLANNING

During the first phase of care, the major goals relate to cardiopulmonary stabilization, fluid

NURSING CARE PLAN

for the Toddler With a Burn

Two-year-old JW was watching his mother fix dinner. She turned away from the stove where she had vegetables cooking. Jed climbed on his chair and grabbed the handle of the pan. Before his mother could react, the boiling liquid from the vegetables poured down over his right arm, the right side of his torso, and his right groin and leg. He is now in the pediatric unit for care of second- and third-degree burns of his right arm, right torso and groin, and right leg.

NURSING DIAGNOSIS
Risk for Infection related to the loss of a protective layer secondary to burn injury

GOAL: The child will be free from signs and symptoms of infection.

OUTCOME CRITERIA
- The child's burns show no signs of foul smelling drainage.
- The child's vital signs remain within normal limits: pulse ranging between 80–110, respirations 20–30, and temperature ranging between 98.6°–101°F (37°–38.4°C).

NURSING INTERVENTIONS	*RATIONALE*
Carry out conscientious handwashing and follow other infection control precautions including the use of sterile equipment and supplies. Wear sterile gown, mask and cap and use sterile gloves when giving direct care to the burned area.	Sterile technique decreases the introduction of microorganisms. Handwashing is the foundation of good medical asepsis. These procedures reduce the risk of infection.
Teach family and visitors sterile techniques especially handwashing.	Infection control procedures must include all who enter the child's room in order to be effective.
Screen visitors for signs of upper respiratory or skin infections.	The child with severe burns may be easily susceptible to upper respiratory and skin infections.
Note and document all drainage and any unusual odor; take regular cultures.	Early detection and prompt treatment of infection are essential as severe infection places an additional burden on the child's already stressed system.

NURSING DIAGNOSIS
Imbalanced Nutrition: Less than Body Requirements related to increased caloric needs secondary to burns and anorexia

GOAL
The child's caloric intake will be adequate to meet needs for tissue repair and growth.

OUTCOME CRITERIA
- The child will consume at least 80% of diet high in calories and protein.
- The child will maintains his preburn weight or will have weight gain appropriate for age.

NURSING INTERVENTIONS	*RATIONALE*
Offer a high-calorie, high-protein, bland diet.	Increased calories and high-protein are required to promote wound healing.
Plan appealing meals offering in small servings catering to the child's food likes and dislikes. Give choices when appropriate.	Small servings are more appealing to a child. Allowing Jed to make choices gives him some feeling of control and encourages his cooperation.
Weigh daily in the morning with only underwear on.	Daily or weekly weights provide information to determine nutritional status.

NURSING DIAGNOSIS
Acute Pain related to tissue destruction and painful procedures

GOAL: The child will show signs of being comfortable and pain will be kept at an acceptable level.

OUTCOME CRITERIA
- The child rests quietly with pulse between 80–110 bpm and respirations 20–30 and regular.
- The child uses the faces pain rating scale to indicate his pain level as appropriate for age (Chap. 4).
- Analgesics are administered before dressing changes and débridement procedures.

NURSING CARE PLAN continued

for the Toddler With a Burn

NURSING INTERVENTIONS	RATIONALE
Monitor every 2 to 4 hours to determine the child's comfort level, vital signs and if the child is restless.	Each individual reacts differently to pain and analgesics. Learning child's responses helps to effectively plan to reduce his pain.
Administer analgesics 20 to 30 minutes before dressing changes and débridement.	This gives the analgesics time to reach optimum effectiveness for pain relief during procedures.
Support and comfort during procedures. Plan a favorite activity after procedures to give child something pleasant to anticipate.	Acknowledging that the procedures are painful and his cooperation deserves a reward may help the child accept the inevitable.
Give opportunities to exercise some control when possible over timing, what gets done first, or other details.	A feeling of control over some aspects of his care and situation helps offset feelings of powerlessness.

NURSING DIAGNOSIS

Risk for Impaired Physical Mobility related to pain and scarring

GOAL: The child will have increased mobility and contractures will be minimal.

OUTCOME CRITERIA
- The child participates in range-of-motion activities and uses both arms and legs.
- The child's splints, pressure suit, and positions are maintained.
- The child has no evidence of contractures.
- The child participates in ambulatory activities.

NURSING INTERVENTIONS	RATIONALE
Position so that no two skin surfaces touch; give special attention to right armpit, right elbow, wrist and hand, right groin, and right knee.	When any two skin surfaces touch, scarring will occur that results in contractures and limited movement.
Maintain splints and pressure dressings to hyperextend joints.	Hyperextension limits the formation of contractures.
Plan self-care activities that give child some control and also will encourage movement of affected joints.	Encouraging child to do small activities to help himself promotes movement and decreases contractures.
Encourage active play and ambulation.	A child is more likely to cooperate in exercise and movement that is fun.

NURSING DIAGNOSIS

Deficient Caregiver Knowledge related to optimizing the child's healing process and to the long-term care required by the child

GOAL: The child's family caregivers will verbalize an understanding of the child's long-term home care.

OUTCOME CRITERIA
- Family caregivers demonstrate wound care and dressing changes.
- Family caregivers verbalize an understanding of the long-term management of child's care and needed treatment.
- The child's family secures the home care equipment needed for his care.
- The family caregivers plan for follow-up care and utilize social service assistance.

NURSING INTERVENTIONS	RATIONALE
Explain to mother and other family caregivers what you are doing and why as you give care and perform procedures for child.	Having a child with a burn is an overwhelming experience. Providing explanations as you give care helps the family to begin to grasp the care process.
Provide information to the child's mother and other family caregivers in small amounts, repeating information from one time to another. Allow ample opportunity for questions.	Family caregivers can absorb only so much information at a time. Repetition and patient, careful answering of questions helps the family to understand the long-term view.
Teach the child's family about the importance of diet, infection control, exercise, rest, activity, pressure suit, and all aspects of child's care.	The child's family needs to understand all aspects of care including how the pressure suit is worn, the care of the suit, and the need to change the suit as the child grows.

(nursing care plan continues on page 286)

NURSING CARE PLAN continued

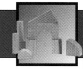

for the Toddler With a Burn

NURSING INTERVENTIONS	RATIONALE
Teach signs and symptoms that are important to note and what may need to be reported promptly.	Learning what to observe for and which signs or symptoms need to be reported promptly gives the family caregivers confidence in their ability and improves the level of home care that they give.
Provide family with information and contacts for social services, which will help in the care for the child.	Long-term care is improved and aided by contact and interaction with appropriate social services.

and electrolyte balance, and infection control. After the first 72 hours in the phase sometimes called the management or subacute phase, more long-term goals are developed. The child's goals are limited by his or her age and ability to communicate. Goals related to the child include preventing infection, maintaining adequate nutrition, reducing pain, increasing mobility, and relieving anxiety. The family caregiver goals include concerns about stress on the family related to the child's injury. Other goals relate to optimizing healing and decreasing complications to minimize permanent disability and gaining an understanding of the long-term implications of care.

IMPLEMENTATION

Preventing Infection. The immaturity of the child's immune system, the destruction of the skin layer, and the presence of necrotic tissue (an ideal medium for bacterial growth) contribute to a significant danger of infection. Conscientious handwashing is necessary by anyone who has contact with the child. Observe rigid infection control precautions and use only sterile equipment and supplies. Monitor vital signs including temperature on a 1-, 2-, or 4-hour schedule. Screen all people who have any contact with the child including visitors, family, or staff caretakers for any signs of upper respiratory or skin infection.

When caring for the burn, wear a sterile gown, mask, and cap. Wear sterile gloves or use a sterile tongue blade to apply ointment to the burn. Maintain the room temperature at around 80°F because water evaporates quickly through the denuded areas and even through

the leathery burn eschar with thermal loss resulting. Note and document all drainage. Report immediately and document any unusual odor. Cultures are done regularly usually several times a week. Avoid injury to the eschar and the donor site. Hair on the tissue adjacent to the burn area is usually shaved.

Ensuring Adequate Nutrition. The child who has received extensive burns requires special attention regarding nutritional needs. The nutritional problem is much more complex than simply getting a seriously ill child to eat. The child is in negative caloric balance from a number of causes, including
- Poor intake due to anorexia, ileus, Curling's ulcer, or diarrhea
- External loss due to exudative losses of protein through the burn wound
- Hypermetabolism due to fever, infection, and the state of toxicity

A bland diet high in protein (for healing and replacement) and calories is an essential component of therapy. Use every effort possible to interest the child in foods essential for tissue building and repair. Do not serve large servings because of anorexia as well as the child's physical condition. Foods are of no value if the child refuses to eat them. Try using colorful trays, foods with eye appeal, and any special touches to spur a child's appetite. Allow the child to have some control to encourage cooperation. Foods that may appeal are flavored milk shakes, ice cream shakes, high-protein drinks containing eggs and extra dried protein milk, ice cream, milk and egg desserts, and puréed meats and vegetables.

Even with the best efforts of nurses, dietitians, and the child, the burn patient seldom can eat enough food to meet the increased needs. Total parenteral nutrition (TPN) or tube feedings are often necessary as supplements to the oral intake. Commercial high-calorie formulas are available for tube feedings that meet the child's needs. Avoid using TPN or tube feedings as a threat to the child. Explain carefully to the child what is to be done and why and make sure the child understands. Try demonstrating the tube feeding process with a doll to help the child grasp the idea.

Weigh the child daily at the same time and with the same coverings. Carefully monitor intake and output.

Relieving Pain and Providing Comfort Measures. The pain of a thermal injury can be severe. As a result of the pain or the fear and anxiety that pain causes, the child may not sleep well, may suffer anorexia, and may be apprehensive and uncooperative during treatments and care. Analgesics must be administered to provide the most relief possible. Administer analgesics at least 20 to 30 minutes before dressing changes and débridement. Monitor the child's physiologic response to the pain and analgesics. Document the child's pupil reaction, heart and respiratory rates, and behavior in response to pain and analgesics. Schedule administration of pain medications so that the child is not too sedated at mealtimes.

Provide support and comfort during painful procedures. Use diversionary activities to help the child focus on something other than the pain. Promising a favorite activity after the dreaded procedure is acceptable. Television may be helpful, but be cautious not to overuse it. The younger child may enjoy learning new songs, playing age-appropriate games, or listening to someone reading stories. The older child may enjoy video or computer games, tape recordings, books, and board or card games. The child should never be admonished for crying or behaving "like a baby." Acknowledge the child's pain, give the child as much control as possible, and work with the child and the family to minimize the pain and to bring about the greatest rewards for all involved.

Preventing Contractures. Care must be taken to avoid contractures and scarring that limit movement. Never permit two burned body surfaces, such as fingers, to touch. If the neck is involved, the child may have to be kept with the neck hyperextended; the arms may need to be placed in a brace to prevent underarm contractures; joints of the knee or elbow must be extended to prevent scar formation from causing contractures that limit movement. Pressure dressings and pressure suits may be used for this purpose and may need to be worn for more than a year. Physical therapy may be needed, and splints may be used to position the body part to prevent contractures. All these measures can add to the child's discomfort.

Encourage range of motion, early ambulation, and self-help activities as additional means of preventing contractures. Use creativity to devise ways to involve the child in enjoyable activities that encourage movement of the affected part.

Reducing Anxiety About Changed Body Image. The child's age and level of understanding influence the amount of anxiety that he or she has about scarring and disability related to the burn. If the child is in a burn unit with other children, seeing others may cause unrealistic fears. Encourage the child to explore his or her feelings about changes in body image. Use therapeutic play with puppets or dolls if possible. Encourage both the family and the nursing staff to provide the child with continuous support.

Promoting Family Coping. The family may feel guilty about the injury; one member may feel especially responsible. These feelings affect the family's coping abilities. Give both the family and the child opportunities to discuss and express their feelings. Suggest counseling if necessary to help family members handle their feelings. Put the family in touch with support groups if available to help the family work through problems. Explain the child's care to family members and involve them in the care when possible. Avoid saying anything that might add to the guilt or anxiety that the family members are feeling.

Providing Family Teaching. Provide the family caregivers with explanations about the whole process of burns, the care, the healing process, and the long-term implications. Give information to the family as they are ready for it; do not thrust it on them all at once. To prepare for home care, teach the family about wound care, dressing changes, signs and symptoms to observe and report, and the importance of diet, rest, and activity. Help the family to find resources for any necessary supplies and equipment. Make a referral to social services to assist them in home care planning.

EVALUATION: GOALS AND OUTCOME CRITERIA

- *Goal:* The child will be free from signs or symptoms of infection.
  Criteria: The child's pulse and respirations are within normal limits for age; temperature is 98.6° to 101°F (37° to 38.4°C); there is no malodorous drainage.
- *Goal:* The child's caloric intake will be adequate to meet his needs for tissue repair and growth.
  Criteria: The child consumes at least 80% of diet high in calories and protein and maintains weight or has weight gain appropriate for age.
- *Goal:* The child will show signs of being comfortable.
  Criteria: The child rests quietly and does not cry or moan excessively; the pulse and respiratory rates are regular and normal for age.
- *Goal:* The child will have increased mobility and contractures will be minimal.
  Criteria: The child participates in range-of-motion activities; splints, pressure dressings and suits and positions are maintained; there is no evidence of contractures.
- *Goal:* The older child will express feelings related to body image changes.
  Criteria: The child expresses feelings and fears about body image and demonstrates a positive attitude of acceptance.
- *Goal:* The family caregivers will verbalize feelings related to the child's injury and take steps to develop coping skills.
  Criteria: The family caregivers verbalize fears, anxieties, and other feelings related to child's injury; discuss the impact of the injury on the child and family's life; cooperate with counseling; and become involved in support groups.
- *Goal:* The family caregivers will verbalize an understanding of the child's long-term home care management.
  Criteria: Family members demonstrate wound care and dressing changes, list signs and symptoms to observe for and report, secure needed home care equipment, and use social service assistance if appropriate.

Head Injuries

Head injuries are a significant cause of serious injury or death in children of all ages. The primary cause of a head injury varies with the child's age. Toddlers and young children may receive a head injury from a fall or child abuse; school-age children and adolescents usually experience such an injury as a result of a bicycling, in-line skating, or motor vehicle accident.

Toddlers seem to receive many head injuries. Fortunately most of them are not serious, but they are often frightening to the caregiver. If a scalp laceration is involved, the caregiver can be quite alarmed by the amount of bleeding due to the large blood supply to the head and scalp. The caregiver can apply an ice pack and pressure until the bleeding is controlled. Applying ice cubes in a zip-closure sandwich bag wrapped in a washcloth works well at home. An open wound should be cleaned with soap and water and a sterile dressing applied. For an injury without a break in the skin, the caregiver can apply ice for an hour or so to decrease the amount of swelling.

The caregiver should observe the child for at least 6 hours for vomiting or a change in the child's level of consciousness. If the child falls asleep, he or she should be awakened every 1 to 2 hours to determine that the level of consciousness has not changed. No analgesics or sedatives should be administered during this period of observation. The child's pupils are checked for reaction to light every 4 hours for 48 hours. The caregiver should notify the health care provider immediately if the child vomits more than three times, has pupillary changes, has double or blurred vision, has a change in level of consciousness, acts strange or confused, has trouble walking, or has a headache that becomes more severe or wakes him or her from sleep; these instructions should be provided in written form to the caregiver.

Family caregivers are wise to take the child to a health care facility to have the injury evaluated if they have any doubt about its seriousness. Complications of head injuries with or without skull fractures can include cerebral hemorrhage, cerebral edema, and increased intracranial pressure. These conditions require highly skilled intensive care, and victims are usually cared for in a pediatric neurologic or intensive care unit.

KEY POINTS

- Toddlerhood is a time of exploring and learning, when mobility and communication influence what happens to the child.
- Autism may become evident if the child does not

form relationships with parents and family.

▶ Respiratory infections may occur frequently in the toddler, causing anxiety for caregivers and possibly leading to respiratory emergencies.

▶ Hereditary diseases that affect nutrition include celiac syndrome and cystic fibrosis.

▶ Cystic fibrosis often causes respiratory involvement, which contributes to the severity of the disease.

▶ Toddlers need constant supervision because their inquiring minds have not developed judgment about things that are safe and those that are not. This trait sometimes results in accidents that can be life-threatening or cause permanent damage.

▶ Toddlers like to experience many things by tasting them. Thus toddlers may swallow poisons or objects that can cause serious systemic damage.

▶ Burns can cause lifelong damage.

BIBLIOGRAPHY

American Heart Association. (2001) *Basic life support for healthcare providers.* Dallas, TX.

Chisolm Jr. J J. (1999) Lead poisoning. In *Oski's pediatrics: Principles and practice* (3rd ed). Philadelphia: Lippincott Williams & Wilkins.

Cohen SM. (2001) Lead poisoning: A summary of treatment and prevention. *Pediatric Nursing,* 27(2), 125.

Corrarino J, Walsh P, Nadel E. (2001) Does teaching scald burn prevention to families of young children make a difference. *Journal of Pediatric Nursing,* 16(4), 256.

Davis PB. (2001) Cystic fibrosis. *Pediatrics in Review,* 22(8), 257.

Dudek, SG. (2000) *Nutrition essentials for nursing practice* (4th ed). Philadelphia: Lippincott Williams & Wilkins.

Hall-Long BA, Schell K, Corrigan V. (2001) Youth safety education and injury prevention program, *Pediatric Nursing,* 27(2), 141.

Herbst DD. (2001) Cystic fibrosis and lung transplantation: Ethical concerns. *Pediatric Nursing,* 27(1), 87.

Lifschitz CH. (1999) Celiac disease. In *Oski's pediatrics: Principles and practice* (3rd ed). Philadelphia: Lippincott Williams & Wilkins.

North American Nursing Diagnosis Association. (2001) *NANDA nursing diagnoses: Definitions and classification 2001–200.* Philadelphia: NANDA.

Pillitteri A. (2003) *Maternal and child health nursing* (4th ed). Philadelphia: Lippincott Williams & Wilkins.

Rosenstein BJ. (1999) Cystic fibrosis. In *Oski's pediatrics: Principles and practice* (3rd ed). Philadelphia: Lippincott Williams & Wilkins.

(2000) *Springhouse nurse's drug guide* (3rd ed). Springhouse, PA: Springhouse Corporation.

Sparks S, Taylor C. (2001) *Nursing diagnosis reference manual* (5th ed). Springhouse, PA: Springhouse Corporation.

Wiebelhaus P. (2001) Managing burn emergencies. *Nursing Management,* 32(7), 29–36.

Wong DL, Perry S, Hockenberry M. (2002) *Maternal child nursing care* (2nd ed). St. Louis: Mosby.

Wong DL, Hess C. (2000) *Wong and Whaley's clinical manual of pediatric nursing* (5th ed). St. Louis: Mosby.

Websites
Celiac Disease: *www.celiac.com*
www.NoMilk.com
www.familyvillage.wisc.edu/lib
www.cysticfibrosis.com
Cystic Fibrosis: *www.cff.org*
Burns: *www.ameriburn.org*

Workbook

NCLEX-STYLE REVIEW QUESTIONS

1. A toddler with a diagnosis of an upper respiratory disorder has a fever and a decreased urinary output. When planning care for this child which of the following goals would be MOST appropriate for this toddler? The child's

   a. anxiety will be reduced

   b. fluid intake will be increased

   c. caregivers will talk about their concerns

   d. caloric intake will be adequate for age

2. A child diagnosed with cystic fibrosis will have which of the following interventions included in the child's plan of care?

   a. Maintain a flat lying position when in bed.

   b. Provide low protein snacks between meals.

   c. Perform postural drainage in the morning and evening.

   d. Teach isolation procedures when hospitalized.

3. After discussing the disease with the caregiver of a child diagnosed with cystic fibrosis, the caregiver makes the following statements. Which of these statements indicates a need for further teaching?

   a. "It is good to know that my other children won't have the disease."

   b. "I will be sure to give my child the medication every time she eats."

   c. "It is important to let my child play with the other kids when she is at school."

   d. "When she exercises, I will feed her a salty snack."

4. The nurse is teaching a group of parents of toddlers about what to do in cases of poisoning. If a toddler has swallowed an unknown substance, which of the following should be the FIRST action of the caregiver? The caregiver should

   a. administer syrup of ipecac

   b. call the poison control center

   c. encourage the child to drink water

   d. place the child on a flat surface

5. In caring for a 3-½-year old child admitted after being severely burned, the nurse collects the following data. Which of following would be MOST important for the nurse to report immediately? The child's

   a. respiratory rate is 32 breaths a minute

   b. temperature is 38.4° celsius

   c. hourly urinary output is 150 ccs

   d. pain level is an 8 on the pain scale

STUDY ACTIVITIES

1. Draw a diagram to explain the heredity pattern of cystic fibrosis.

2. Research your community to find sources of help for families with children who have cystic fibrosis. What support groups and organizations are available that you might recommend to families of children with CF? Discuss with your peers what you found and make a list of resources to share.

3. Carmella has idiopathic celiac disease. Using the foods listed in the table below, identify the foods that would be recommended and those that would not be recommended in her meal plan. With the help of a nutrition text or by reading labels, state why each of those foods is either recommended or not recommended.

Food	Recommended	Not Recommended	Explanation of Why Food Would or Would Not Be Recommended
Ice cream Corn flakes Grits Rice pudding Whole-wheat bread Baked beans Hamburger Hot dog			

Food	Recommended	Not Recommended	Explanation of Why Food Would or Would Not Be Recommended
French fries			
Fresh vegetables			
Yogurt			
Oatmeal			
Rice Krispies			
Orange juice			
Graham crackers			
Corn chips			
Peanut butter			
Baked potato			
Tuna salad			
Pizza			

CRITICAL THINKING

1. Survey your house (or a house you select) and list the hazards for ingestion of poisonous substances, drowning, and burns. Include all types of burns. After the hazards are identified, formulate a plan to correct or lessen the hazards.

2. Your next-door neighbor has found their 18-month-old child with an empty bottle of children's acetaminophen. Describe the actions you should take. Using a drug reference, identify the specific antidote used in acetaminophen overdose.

3. Two-year-old Omar has partial- and total-thickness burns from a wood stove accident. Develop a teaching plan covering the importance of infection control for Omar during his convalescence.

4. *Dosage Calculation:* A toddler with a diagnosis of cystic fibrosis is being treated with the bronchodilator Theophylline. The child weighs 32 pounds. The usual dosage of this medication is 4 mg per kg per dose every 6 hours. Answer the following:
   a. How many kg does the child's weigh?
   b. How many mg per dose will be given?
   c. How many doses will the child receive in a day?
   d. How much Theophylline will be given in a 24-hour time period?

Growth and Development of the Preschool Child: 3 to 6 Years

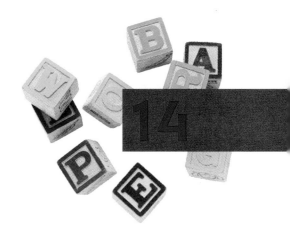

14

PHYSICAL DEVELOPMENT
Growth Rate
Dentition
Visual Development
Skeletal Growth
PSYCHOSOCIAL DEVELOPMENT
Language Development
Development of Imagination
Sexual Development
Social Development

NUTRITION
HEALTH PROMOTION AND MAINTENANCE
Routine Checkups
Family Teaching
Accident Prevention
Infection Prevention
THE HOSPITALIZED PRESCHOOLER

STUDENT OBJECTIVES

On completion of this chapter, the student will be able to

1. Briefly describe several social characteristics of the preschooler and state the ages included in this group.
2. Describe the growth rate of the preschooler.
3. State the age at which 20/20 vision usually is attained.
4. List four factors that may delay language development.
5. Discuss the role of magical thinking and imagination in the preschooler.
6. Describe the characteristics of dreams, nightmares, and imaginary playmates.
7. Discuss the nurse's role in helping parents understand their preschooler's sexual curiosity.
8. Discuss masturbation in the preschool age.
9. List six types of play in which preschoolers engage; define each type.
10. Discuss aggression in the preschooler: (a) verbal aggression, (b) physical aggression, (c) parents' tasks, (d) parents' example.
11. State the role of discipline for the preschooler: (a) caregiver behavior, (b) effect on child, (c) effect on caregiver.
12. Discuss the special needs of the disadvantaged preschooler.
13. Discuss the value of Head Start programs.
14. State preschool nutritional needs including (a) daily minimum needs, (b) appetite variations, (c) suggested snacks, (d) television commercials and other influences.
15. State the recommended health maintenance schedule for the preschooler.
16. List guidelines for accident prevention in the preschool-age population.
17. List nine health teachings for the preschooler concerning prevention of infection.
18. Identify the preschool social characteristic that increases the risk of infection.

KEY TERMS

associative play
cooperative play
dramatic play
magical thinking
noncommunicative language
onlooker play
parallel play
solitary independent play
unoccupied behavior

Preschoolers are fascinating creatures. As their social circles enlarge to include peers and adults outside the family, preschoolers' language, play patterns, and appearance change markedly. Their curiosity about the world around them grows, as does their ability to explore that world in greater detail and see new meanings in what they find (Fig. 14–1). Preschoolers can be said to soak up information "like a sponge." "Why?" and "how?" are favorite words. This curiosity also means that accidents are still a serious concern.

At 3 years of age, the child still has the chubby, baby-faced look of a toddler; by age 5, a leaner, taller, better-coordinated social being has emerged. The child works and plays tirelessly, "making things" and telling everyone about them. In children this age, exploring and learning go on continuously. They sometimes have problems separating fantasy from reality. According to Erikson, the developmental task of the preschool age is initiative versus guilt. Preschoolers often try to find ways to do things to help, but they may feel guilty if scolded when they fail because of inexperience or lack of skill.

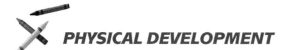

PHYSICAL DEVELOPMENT

Growth Rate

The preschool period is one of slow growth. The child gains about 3 to 5 lb each year (1.4 to 2.3 kg) and grows about 2.5 inches (6.3 cm). Because the increase in height is proportionately greater than the increase in weight, the 5-year-old child appears much thinner and less babyish than the 3-year-old does. Boys tend to be leaner than girls are during this time. Gross and fine motor skills continue to develop rapidly. Balance

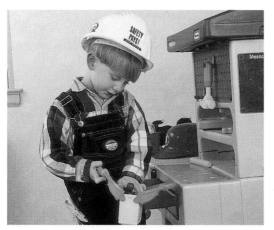

● *Figure 14.1* Preschoolers engage in meaningful play and are fascinated by what they find. They enjoy dressing up like the people they are playing.

improves and confidence emerges to try new activities. By age 5 the child generally can throw and catch a ball well, climb effectively, and ride a bicycle. Important milestones for growth and development are summarized in Table 14–1.

Dentition

By 6 years of age, the child's skull is 90% of its adult size. The deciduous teeth have completely emerged by the beginning of the preschool period. Toward the end of the preschool stage, these teeth begin to be replaced by permanent teeth. This is an event that most children anticipate as an indication that they are "growing up." Pictures of smiling 5- and 6-year-olds typically show missing front teeth (Fig. 14–2).

The age at which teeth erupt varies with individual children and with various ethnic and economic groups. Permanent teeth of African-American children erupt at least 6 months earlier than those of American children of European ancestry. The central incisors are usually the first to go, just as they were the first to erupt in infancy.

Visual Development

Although the preschooler's senses of taste and smell are acute, visual development is still immature at age 3. Eye-hand coordination is good, but judgment of distances generally is faulty, leading to many bumps and falls. During the preschool years, the child's vision should be checked to screen for amblyopia. Usually by age 6 the child has achieved 20/20 vision, but mature depth perception may not occur in some children until 8 to 10 years of age.

Skeletal Growth

Between the third and sixth birthdays, the greatest amount of skeletal growth occurs in the feet and legs. This contributes to the change from the wide-gaited, pot-bellied look of the toddler into the slim, taller figure of the 6-year-old. In addition, the carpals and tarsals mature in the hands and feet, which contributes to better hand and foot control.

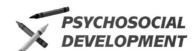

PSYCHOSOCIAL DEVELOPMENT

Language Development

Between the ages of 3 and 5 years, language development is generally rapid. Most 3-year-olds can construct simple sentences, but their speech has many

TABLE 14.1	Growth and Development: The Preschooler				
Age (yr)	Personal–Social	Fine Motor	Gross Motor	Language	Cognition
3	Begins Erikson's stage of "initiative vs. guilt." Conscience develops. Shy with strangers and inept with peers. Sufficiently independent to be interested in group experiences with age mates (e.g., nursery school)	Able to button clothes Copies ○ and + Uses pencils, crayons, paints Shows preference for right or left hand	Tends to watch motor activities before attempting them Can jump several feet Uses hands in broad movements Rides tricycle Negotiates stairs well	Vocabulary up to 1,000 words Articulates vowels accurately Talks a lot Sings and recites Asks many questions	Continues in preoperational state (2–7 years) characterized by: 1. *Centration,* or the inability to attend to more than one aspect of a situation 2. *Egocentricity,* or the inability to consider the perception of others 3. The static and irreversible quality of thought that makes the child unable to perceive the processes of change
4	Boisterous and inflammatory Aggressive physically and verbally but developing behaviors to become socially acceptable Becomes socially acceptable Accepts punishment for wrongdoing because it relieves guilt	Can use scissors; copies a square Adds three parts to stick figures	Has some hesitation but tends to try feats beyond ability Greater powers of balance and accuracy Hops on one foot; can control movements of hands	Vocabulary of about 1,500 words Constant questions Sentences of four or five words Uses profanity Reports fantasies as truth	Reality and fantasy are not always clear to the preschooler. Believes that words make things real—"magical thinking"
5	Initiates contacts with strangers and relates interesting little tales Interested in telling and comparing stories about self Peer relations are important ("best friends" abound) Responds to social values by assuming sex roles with rigidity	Ties shoelaces Copies a diamond and a triangle Prints a few letters or numbers May print first name Cuts food	Will not attempt feats beyond ability Throws and catches ball well Jumps rope Walks backward with heel to toe Skips and hops Adept on bicycle and climbing equipment	Vocabulary of 3,000 words Speech is intelligible Asks meanings of words Enjoys telling stories	Thinks feelings and thoughts can happen Intrusions into the body cause fear and anxiety (fear of mutilation and castration)

hesitations and repetitions as they search for the right word or try to make the right sound. Stuttering can develop during this period but usually disappears within 3 to 6 months. By the end of the fifth year, preschoolers use long, rather complex sentences; their vocabulary will have increased by more than 1,500 words since age 2.

Preschoolers' use of language changes during this period. Three-year-olds often talk to themselves or to their toys or pets without any apparent purpose other

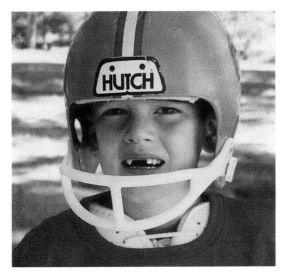

● *Figure 14.2* The smiling 6-year-old is often seen without his front teeth.

than the pleasure of using words. Piaget called this egocentric or **noncommunicative language.** By 4 years of age, children increase their use of communicative language, using words to transmit information other than their own needs and feelings.

Four- and 5-year-olds delight in using "naughty" words or swearing. Bathroom words become favorites, and taunts such as "you're a big doo-doo" bring heady excitement to them. Caregivers may become concerned by this turn of events, but the child simply may be trying words out to test their impact. A calm, matter-of-fact response that lets the child know that this is not language to use in the company of others may help defuse some of its power. Development of preschoolers' verbal abilities is summarized in Table 14–2.

One or more of the following may cause delays or other difficulties in language development:

- Hearing impairment or other physical problem
- Lack of stimulation
- Overprotection
- Lack of parental interest or rejection by parents.

Good language skills are developed as the child is engaged regularly in conversation with caregivers and others. The conversation should be on a level that the child can understand. Reading to the child is an excellent method of contributing to language development. Talking with the child about the pictures in storybooks can enhance this. Praise, approval, and encouragement are all part of supporting attempts at communication.

Family and cultural patterns also influence language development. Some children come from bilingual families and are trying to learn the rules of both languages. Others may come from geographic or social communities that have dialects different from the general population.

Development of Imagination

Preschoolers have learned to think about something without actually seeing it—to visualize or imagine. This normal development, sometimes called **magical thinking,** makes it difficult for them to separate fantasy from reality. Preschoolers believe that words or thoughts can make things real, and this belief can have either positive or negative results. For example in a moment of anger, a child may wish that a parent or a sibling would die; if that person later is hurt, the child feels responsible and suffers guilt. The child needs reassurance that this is not so.

TABLE 14.2	**Verbal Mastery by Preschoolers**	
Age (yr)	Characteristics of Language Usage	Vocabulary Size, Pattern, Comprehension, Rhythm
3–4	Loves to talk; talks a lot; makes up words; sings or recites own version of song; likes new words; asks many questions and wants answers. Not always logical in sentences and concepts. Uses four- or five-word phrases. Aggressive with words rather than actions.	Vocabulary of 900–1500 words; at 3 understands up to 3,600 words, up to 5,600 words by 4. By 4 years, speech understandable even with mispronunciations. May have hesitations, repetitions, and revisions while trying to imitate adult speech. Stuttering may occur but disappears within 3–6 months; may continue up to 2 years without being permanent.
4–5	Understands out-of-context words. Speech highly emotional. Difficulty finding right word; tells function rather than name of item. Changes subject rapidly. Boasts, brags, quarrels; loves "naughty" words. Relates fanciful tales.	Vocabulary of 3,000 words; understands up to 9,600 words by 5 years. Speech completely understandable.

Imagination makes preschoolers good audiences for storytelling, simple plays, and television as long as the characters and events are not too frightening or sad. When preschoolers see a television character die, they believe it is real and often cry. The child's television viewing should be supervised to avoid programs with negative impact or overstimulation.

During this stage, children often have imaginary playmates who are very real to them. This occurs particularly with only children for whom imaginary playmates fill times of loneliness. The imaginary friend often has the characteristics that the child might wish for. Sometimes the child blames the imaginary friend for breaking a toy or engaging in another act that the child does not want to take responsibility for. Caregivers need assurance that this is normal behavior.

The preschooler's active imagination often leads to a fear of the dark or nightmares. Consequently

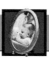

A PERSONAL GLIMPSE

We had just returned from a weekend visit to my parent's house. My two year old was sleeping quietly. I was in the laundry room doing the laundry from our weekend trip and my 5 year old (Kayla) was playing in the family room (or so I thought). Suddenly I heard a loud crashing sound that came from the kitchen. I asked, "What was that?" "Nothing Mom." I asked again, "What WAS that?" and headed toward the kitchen. When I got to the kitchen I discovered what the sound had been—the entire sugar canister was empty—the canister on its side, rolling on the floor with the contents all over the cabinet and kitchen floor. Clearly, SOMETHING had happened. I called to Kayla to come to the kitchen. This time I said, "Kayla, tell me how this happened." She told me, "I was playing Legos and Sandy (her imaginary friend) was making cookies just like at Grammas house and Sandy was getting the sugar and then it was all over the floor." As I looked at the mess she continued, "Like last time Sandy got the toothpaste all over the wall, only this time it was in the kitchen." As upset as I was at having to clean the mess, I thought it was creative of Kayla to use her "imaginary friend" as the mess maker.

Ann

▶ **LEARNING OPPORTUNITY:** What would you tell this mother regarding preschooler's and imaginary friends? What would you suggest this mother should say to respond to her child in this situation?

problems with sleep are common (see the discussion on sleep needs later in this chapter).

Sexual Development

The preschool period is the stage that Freud termed the *oedipal* or *phallic* (genital) *period*. During these years, children become acutely aware of their sexuality including sexual roles and organs. They generally develop a strong emotional attachment to the parent of the opposite sex. Children's curiosity about their own genitalia and those of peers and adults may make parents uncomfortable and evoke responses that indicate to the child that sex is dirty and something to be ashamed and guilty about.

Despite today's abundance of sexually oriented literature, many families find it difficult to deal with the young child's questions and actions. Nurses can help caregivers understand that the child's sexual curiosity is a normal, natural part of total curiosity about oneself and the surrounding world. The informed, understanding parent can help children develop positive attitudes toward sexuality and toward themselves as sexual human beings.

In addition to responsible teaching of sexual information, the caregiver also should teach the child about "good touch" and "bad touch." The child needs to understand that no one should touch the child's body in a way that is unpleasant.

Masturbation

Exploration of the genitalia is as natural for the preschooler as thumb-sucking is for the infant. It is one way the child learns to perceive the body as a possible source of pleasure and is the beginning of the acceptance of sex as natural and pleasurable.

Caregivers can be reassured that this is not uncommon behavior, and a calm, matter-of-fact response to the child found masturbating is the most effective approach. The child should be helped to understand that masturbation is not an activity that is appropriate in public. If the child seems to be masturbating excessively, counseling may be needed, especially if the child's life has been unsettled in other aspects.

Social Development

Preschoolers are outgoing, imaginative, social beings. They play vigorously and, in the process, learn about the world in which they live. As they gain control over their environment, preschoolers try to manipulate it, and this may lead to conflict with caregivers. Preschool children are delightful to watch as they go about the business of growing and learning.

Play

Play activities are one way that children learn. Normally by 3 years of age, children begin imitative play, pretending to be the mommy, the daddy, a policeman, a cowboy, an astronaut, or some well-known person or television character (Figs. 14–3 and 14–4). Caregivers can gain good insight into the way their child interprets family behavior by watching the child play. Listening to a preschooler scold a doll or stuffed animal for "bothering me while I'm busy talking on the phone" lets the adults hear how they sound to the child.

Dramatic play allows a child to act out troubling situations and to control the solution to the problem. This is important to remember when teaching children who are going to be hospitalized. Using dolls and puppets to explain procedures makes the experience less threatening.

Drawing is another form of play through which children learn to express themselves. During the preschool years as fine motor skills improve, children's drawings become much more complex and controlled and can be revealing about the child's self-concept and perception of the environment.

Preschoolers engage in various types of play: cooperative, associative, parallel, solitary independent, onlooker, and unoccupied behavior. In **cooperative play,** children play in an organized group with each

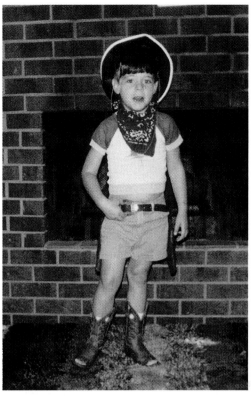

● *Figure 14.4* Imaginative play is common; this preschooler pretends to be a "cowboy."

other as in team sports. **Associative play** occurs when children play together and are engaged in a similar activity but without organization, rules, or a leader, and each child does what she or he wishes. In **parallel play,** children play alongside each other but independently. Although common among toddlers, parallel play exists in all age groups—for example, in a scout troop where each member is working on an individual project or craft. **Solitary independent play** means playing apart from others without making an effort to be part of the group or group activity. Watching television is one form of **onlooker play** in which there is observation without participation. In **unoccupied behavior,** the child may be daydreaming or fingering clothing or a toy without apparent purpose.

Children need all types of play to aid in their total development. Too much of one kind may signal a problem; for example, a youngster who spends most of the time unoccupied may be troubled, depressed, or not stimulated. Cooperative play helps to develop social interaction skills and often physical health.

Too much onlooker play, particularly television viewing, means that children are missing the benefits of other kinds of play and may be forming strong, highly inaccurate impressions of people and their behaviors. The amount of time that preschoolers spend watching television should be limited, and interactive play should be encouraged.

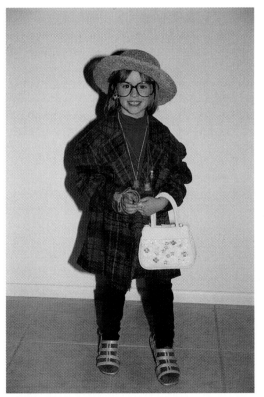

● *Figure 14.3* Preschoolers identify with adults. Dressing up like mommy is a favorite play activity.

Aggression

Temper tantrums are an early form of aggression. The preschooler with newly developed language skills uses words aggressively in name-calling and threats. Four-year-olds use physical aggression as well; they push, hit, and kick in an effort to manipulate the environment. The family caregivers' task during these years is to help the child understand that the anger and frustration that result in aggressive behavior are normal but need to be handled differently because aggressive behavior is not socially acceptable.

Children who come from unhappy home situations are likely to be more aggressive than children from a comfortable family situation. Their caregivers have served as role models, and their aggressive behavior toward each other has said to the child, "this is acceptable."

Discipline

Family caregivers need to remember that preschoolers are developing initiative and a sense of guilt. They want to be good and follow instructions, and they feel bad when they do not, even if they are not physically punished. Discipline during this time should strive to teach the child a sense of responsibility and inner control. All the child's caregivers must understand and agree to the limits and discipline measures for the child. If one caregiver says "no" and another one says "yes," the child soon learns to play one against the other, leading to confusion about limits. Spanking and other forms of physical punishment remove the responsibility from the child. Taking away a privilege from a child who has misbehaved until he or she can demonstrate that there has been an improvement in behavior is much more effective. Because the child's concept of time is not clear, the period should be comparatively brief (Fig. 14–5). Table 14–3 presents

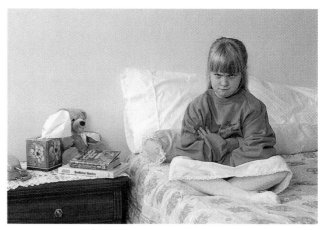

● **Figure 14.5** Although she may not like it, quiet solitude helps the preschooler develop inner control.

some examples of the effects of caregivers' positive and negative responses.

Nursery School or Day Care Experience

Group experiences with peers and adults outside the immediate family are important to a child's development. However, the transition to new experiences, new people, and new surroundings can be threatening to some preschoolers. Children vary in their willingness or ability to handle new situations; being introduced gradually according to individual readiness produces the most satisfactory adjustment. Some children spend only a few hours each week in a nursery school or other day care program; others must spend a great deal more time away from home and family because the adult family members work outside the home. The family should understand that this probably means that the child will demand more of their attention during the hours when they are together. As the child grows older and the attachment to peers becomes stronger, family caregivers sense a

TABLE 14.3	**Effects of Positive and Negative Caregiver Behavior**		
Behavior		Effect on Child	Effect on Adult
Attending only to desired behaviors Calm reasoning with expression of dislike of behavior Physical restraint with adult present Isolation of child for a period of time equal to 1 min per year of age Withholding of desired treats, outings, presents		Development of inner control	Feelings of adequacy as a parent
Yelling, screaming, and implying guilt and punishment Telling child that he or she is bad Physical punishment		Development of fears and compulsive behaviors	Feelings of guilt and inadequacy
Giving treats, presents, or food for lack of undesired behavior Physical punishment Threatening punishment from God or other authority figure		Development of control based on external forces	Feelings of being manipulated by child

decrease in the need for adult attention and a greater sense of independence in the child.

The Disadvantaged Child

Discussions of normal growth and development assume that children come from a secure, well-adjusted home in which there is ample opportunity for social, cultural, and intellectual enrichment. Many children, however, are deprived of such a background for many reasons. This population is the one most likely to have health problems and to need health services.

Children who have not been able to achieve a sense of security and trust, for whatever reason, need special understanding, warm acceptance, and intelligent guidance to grow into self-accepting people. Society is gradually awakening to the needs of these children and is trying to provide enriched nursery school and kindergarten experiences for those whose home life cannot do this for them, but much remains to be done. Further discussion of the problems of these children can be found in Unit IV: A Child in Crisis.

Head Start Programs

Recognition that environmental enrichment is often unavailable in families with limited social, cultural, and economic resources led to the establishment of Head Start programs. Head Start programs are funded by federal and local money and are free to the children enrolled. Children in such programs have an opportunity to broaden their horizons through varied experiences and to increase their understanding of the world in which they live. Family caregiver participation is a central component of the Head Start concept and often has a positive effect on other children in the household. In some programs, teachers go into the home to help the caregiver teach the young child motor, cognitive, self-help, and language skills. Counseling and referral services are also provided through Head Start programs. Children who have had a background of Head Start enrichment are better prepared to enter kindergarten or first grade and compete successfully with their peers.

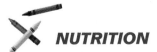

NUTRITION

The preschool period is not a time of rapid growth, so children do not need large quantities of food. Nevertheless, protein needs continue to remain high to provide for muscle growth. The preschooler's appetite is erratic; at one sitting the preschooler may devour everything on the plate and at the next meal he or she may be satisfied with just a few bites.

Portions are smaller than adult-sized portions, so the child may need to have meals supplemented with nutritious snacks (Box 14–1). Note that certain snacks are recommended only for the older child to avoid any danger of choking. The preschooler generally best accepts frequent, small meals with snacks in between.

Among the preschooler's favorites are soft foods, grain and dairy products, raw vegetables, and sweets. Television commercials for sugar-coated cereals, snacks, and fast foods of questionable nutritional value exert a powerful influence on the preschooler and can make supermarket shopping an emotional struggle between the caregiver and child. Caregivers should read labels carefully before making a purchase.

Preschoolers need guidance in choosing foods and are strongly influenced by the example of family members and peers. Food should never be used as a reward or bribe; otherwise, the child will continue to use food as a means to manipulate the environment and the behavior of others.

To meet the minimum daily requirements, the preschooler should have two or three glasses of milk each day and several small portions from each food group. Preschoolers have definite food preferences. They generally do not like highly spiced foods, often will eat raw vegetables but not cooked ones, and prefer plain foods rather than casseroles. New foods may be accepted but should be introduced one at a time to avoid overwhelming the child.

BOX 14.1	**Suggested Snacks for the Preschooler**

Raw vegetables: carrots,* cucumbers, celery,* green beans, green pepper, mushrooms, turnips, broccoli, cauliflower, tomatoes
Fresh fruits: apples, oranges, pears, peaches, grapes,* cherries,* melons
Unsalted whole-grain crackers
Whole-grain bread: cut to finger-sized sticks; plain, toasted, or with peanut butter
Small sandwiches: cut into quarters
Natural cheese: cut into cubes
Cooked meat: cut into small chunks or sliced thinly
*Nuts**
*Sunflower seeds**
Cookies: made with lightly sweetened whole grains
*Plain popcorn**
Yogurt: plain or with fresh fruit added

*Children younger than 2 years of age may choke on nuts, seeds, popcorn, celery strings, or carrot sticks. Avoid these until preschool years and then always cut into small, bite-sized pieces.

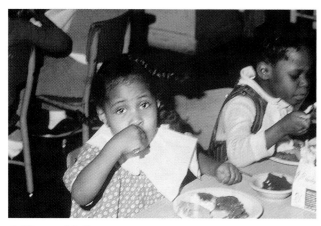

● *Figure 14.6* The preschooler may revert to using fingers when eating.

The preschooler shows growing independence and skill in eating. The 3-year-old tries to mimic adult behavior at the table but often reverts to eating with the fingers, spilling liquids, and squirming (Fig. 14–6). The 4-year-old is more skilled with the use of utensils, although an occasional misjudgment of abilities results in a mess. The 5-year-old uses utensils well, often can cut his or her own food, and can be taught to practice sophisticated table manners. Rituals such as using the same plate, cereal bowl, cup, or placemat may become important to the child's mealtime happiness.

HEALTH PROMOTION AND MAINTENANCE

Routine Checkups

Preschoolers with up-to-date immunizations need boosters of diphtheria-tetanus-pertussis, polio vaccine, and measles-mumps-rubella (MMR) vaccine between 4 and 6 years of age. These are required as preschool boosters for entrance into kindergarten.

An annual health examination is recommended to monitor the child's growth and development and to screen for potential health problems. Recommended screening procedures include urinalysis, hematocrit, lead level, tuberculin skin testing, and Denver Developmental Screening Test. The preschool child needs to be told in advance about the upcoming examination. Use simple explanations and provide an opportunity to ask questions and voice anxieties. A number of books available through public libraries are excellent for this purpose. Children who attend nursery school or a day care program are sometimes required to have an annual examination, but children who stay at home may not have this advantage. Particular attention should be paid to the child's vision

and hearing so that any problems can be treated before he or she enters school at age 5 or 6. A semiannual dental examination is also recommended.

Family Teaching

The nurse can use routine checkups and any other opportunities to teach caregivers about common aspects of everyday life with a preschooler. Preschoolers are busy learning and showing initiative as they are involved in their day-to-day life. Preschoolers are usually a pleasure to be around because they are so eager to learn anything new and are full of questions.

Bathing

Although preschoolers view themselves as "grownup," they still need continual supervision while bathing. The caregiver should run the bath water. The hot water heater should be turned down to 120°F (49°C) to avoid the danger of burns. Children should be taught to leave the faucets alone. Preschoolers can generally wash themselves with supervision. Ears, necks, and faces are spots that often need extra attention. Hands and fingernails often get soaked clean in the tub, but fingernails do need to be checked by the caregiver.

Preschoolers cannot wash their own hair, so this can be a time of tension between the child and caregiver. Shampooing in the tub with a nonirritating children's shampoo may work best. The child can lean the head back, look at the ceiling, and hold a washcloth on the forehead to keep water and soap from getting into the eyes. Shampoo protectors (clear plastic brims with no crowns) can be purchased if desired.

Bath time can be rather lengthy if the preschooler gets involved in playing with bath toys. This is something the caregiver can negotiate if limits need to be set. Some children this age are interested in taking a shower and may do so with adult supervision.

When washing their hands before meals or before or after going to the bathroom, preschoolers often wash only the fronts while totally ignoring their backs. If not supervised, the child may use only cold water and no soap. Again, the caregiver should turn the water on to a warm temperature to avoid burns.

Dental Care

The preschool child needs to be supervised in tooth brushing. Although the preschooler can brush well, the caregiver should check the cleanliness of the child's teeth. The caregiver should be responsible for flossing because the preschooler does not have the necessary motor skills. To help prevent tooth decay, the preschooler should be encouraged to eat healthy snacks such as fruits, raw vegetables, and natural cheeses rather than candy, cakes, or sugar-filled gum. Fluoridated water or fluoride supplements should be continued.

Dressing

The preschooler may have definite ideas about what he or she wants to wear. Giving the child the opportunity to choose what to wear each day is an excellent way to begin fostering a sense of control and to help the child learn to make decisions. Preschoolers do not have very good taste in what matches what, so some interesting outfits may result! Nevertheless, the child should be permitted to make these choices, and the caregivers (as well as older siblings and other adults) should accept the choices without negative comments. When it does matter—for the adults—how the child is dressed, the best plan is to give the child limited choices that will suit the occasion.

Toileting

By the preschool years, almost all children have succeeded in toilet training, although an occasional accident may occur. When the child does have an accident, treating it in a matter-of-fact way and providing the child with clean, dry clothing is best. The preschooler needs continual reminders to wash the hands before and after toileting. Little girls should be taught to wipe from front to back. Preschoolers may still need to be checked for careful wiping especially after a bowel movement.

Bedwetting is not uncommon for young preschoolers and is not a concern unless it continues past the age of 5 to 7 (see Chap. 17 for further discussion).

Sleep Needs

Preschoolers are often ready to give up their nap. This may depend partially on if they go to a preschool program that has a rest time. Often preschoolers will just curl up and fall asleep on a chair, a couch, or the floor. Bedtime can still be a challenge, but leading up to it with a period of quiet activities or stories encourages the child to wind down for the day.

Dreams and nightmares are common during the preschool period. Caregivers need to explain that "it was only a dream" and offer love and understanding until the fear has subsided. Fear of the dark is another common problem during these years. Children may be afraid to go to sleep in a dark bedroom. These are very real fears to the child. A small night-light may be reassuring to the child.

One mother solved this problem in an interesting fashion. The child was afraid of a monster in the closet or under the bed. The mother acknowledged the child's fears and purchased a spray can of room air freshener. At bedtime she ceremoniously sprayed around the room, in the closet, and under the bed. She assured the child that it was a special spray to kill monsters, just like bug spray kills bugs. The child was reassured and slept without fear.

Accident Prevention

Adults caring for preschoolers need to be just as attentive as they are with toddlers because a child's curiosity at this stage still exceeds his or her judgment. Burns, poisoning, and falls are common accidents. Preschoolers are often victims of motor vehicle accidents either because they dart into the street or driveway or fail to wear proper restraints. All states have laws that define safety seat and restraint requirements for children. Adults must teach and reinforce these rules. One primary responsibility of adults is always to wear seat belts themselves and to make certain that the child always is in a safety seat or has a seat belt on. A child can be calmly taught that the vehicle "won't go" unless the child is properly restrained.

By the age of 5 years, many preschoolers move from riding a tricycle to riding a bicycle. If the preschooler is not already wearing a bicycle helmet, it is important to educate caregivers that safety helmets are a necessary safety precaution. Lightweight, child-sized safety helmets that fit properly can be purchased, and the child should be taught that the helmet must be worn when riding a bike. Adults who wear helmets provide the best incentive to children. Safety rules for bicycle riding should be reinforced. The preschool child should be limited to protected areas for riding and should have adult supervision.

The preschool age is an excellent time to begin teaching safety rules. The rules for crossing the street and playing in an area near traffic are of vital

FAMILY TEACHING TIPS

Preschoolers Safety Teaching

1. Look both ways before crossing the street.
2. Cross the street only with an adult.
3. Watch for cars coming out of driveways.
4. Never play behind a car or truck.
5. Watch for cars or trucks backing up.
6. Wear a safety helmet when bike riding.
7. Learn your name, address, and phone number.
8. Stay away from strange dogs.
9. Stay away from any dog while it's eating.
10. Take only medicine that your caregiver gives you.
11. Don't play with matches or lighters.
12. Stay away from fires.
13. Don't run near a swimming pool.
14. Only swim when with an adult.
15. Don't go anywhere with someone you don't know.
16. Don't let anyone touch you in a way you don't like.

FAMILY TEACHING TIPS

Teaching to Prevent Infections

1. Cover your mouth when coughing or sneezing.
2. Throw away tissues used for nose blowing.
3. Wipe carefully after bowel movements (girls wipe front to back).
4. Wash hands after going to bathroom or blowing your nose.
5. Wash hands before eating.
6. Do not share food that you've partly eaten.
7. If food or an eating utensil falls on the floor, wash it right away.
8. Do not drink from another person's cup.
9. Do not share a toothbrush with someone else.

importance. Adults who care for preschool children should be careful to serve as good role models. These safety rules should extend into all aspects of the child's life. See Family Teaching Tips: Preschooler Safety Teaching.

Infection Prevention

Preschoolers who enjoy sound nutrition and adequate rest, exercise, and shelter usually are not seriously affected by simple childhood infections. Children who live in less than adequate economic circumstances, however, can be severely threatened by even a simple illness such as diarrhea or chickenpox. Immunizations are available for many childhood communicable diseases, but some caregivers do not have their children immunized until it is required for entrance to school. As a result, some children suffer unnecessary illnesses.

Preschoolers are just learning to share, and that can mean sharing infections with the entire family—and playmates as well. Teaching them basic precautions can help prevent the spread of infections. See Family Teaching Tips: Teaching to Prevent Infections.

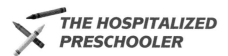

THE HOSPITALIZED PRESCHOOLER

The preschooler may view hospitalization as an exciting new adventure or as a frightening, dangerous experience depending on the preparation by caregivers and health professionals. As mentioned

earlier, play is an effective way to let children act out their anxieties and to learn what to expect from the hospital situation. Preschoolers are frightened about intrusive procedures; therefore, it is preferable to take the temperature with an oral or tympanic thermometer rather than with a rectal one. Children are less anxious about procedures if they are allowed to handle equipment beforehand and perhaps "use" it on a doll or another toy.

The hospitalized preschooler may revert to bedwetting but should not be scolded for it. The nurse should assure the family that this is normal. Explanations of where the bathrooms are and how to use the call light or bell to get help can help avoid problems with bedwetting. If a child is afraid of the dark, a night-light can be provided.

Hospital routines should follow home routines as closely as possible. The child should be allowed to participate in the care even though this may take longer. All procedures should be carefully explained

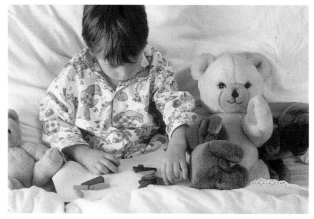

● **Figure 14.7** The hospitalized preschooler can enjoy age-appropriate activities, even when on bedrest.

to the child in words appropriate for the child's age; repeat the information as necessary.

If the child is ambulatory and not on infection-control precautions, the playroom can offer diversionary activities. If not, play materials can be provided for use in bed (Fig 14–7).

KEY POINTS

- During the preschool years, psychosocial growth is substantial but physical growth slows.
- Endless questions, boundless energy, and an ongoing struggle to separate fantasy from reality are characteristics of the preschooler.
- According to Erikson, the psychosocial developmental task for the preschool-age group is initiative versus guilt.
- Language develops rapidly during the preschool period, progressing from the ability to use simple sentences at age 3 to telling sometimes long and involved tales by age 5.
- Magical thinking and imagination contribute to fears and anxieties of the preschool child. The caregiver must acknowledge these concerns. Patient explanations and reassurance by the caregiver are important.
- The child needs to have limits set by caregivers within which he or she can be free to explore and learn and assert autonomy and initiative.
- Caregivers must serve as models of the kind of person they want the child to become, helping the child build confidence and self-esteem.
- Permitting preschoolers to decide what clothes they want to wear is a good way to begin helping them learn to make decisions.
- Safety promotion continues to be an important aspect of the care of the preschool child, because the child's curiosity still exceeds his or her judgment.
- During hospitalization, the child may regress to bedwetting, thumb sucking, and fussiness.

BIBLIOGRAPHY

Brazelton TB. (2001) *Touchpoints three to six: Your child's emotional and behavioral development.* Cambridge, MA: Perseus Publishing.

Brazelton TB, Greenspan S. (2001) *The irreducible needs of children: What every child must have to grow, learn, and flourish.* Cambridge, MA: Perseus Publishing.

Craven RF, Hirnle CJ. (1999) *Fundamentals of nursing* (3rd ed). Philadelphia: Lippincott Williams & Wilkins.

Dudek, SG. (2000) *Nutrition essentials for nursing practice* (4th ed). Philadelphia: Lippincott Williams & Wilkins.

Dworkin P. (2000) *Pediatrics* (4th ed). Philadelphia: Lippincott Williams & Wilkins.

Pillitteri A. (2003) *Maternal and child health nursing* (4th ed). Philadelphia: Lippincott Williams & Wilkins.

Spock B, et. al. (1998) *Dr. Spock's baby and child care.* New York: Pocket Books.

Wong DL. (1998) *Whaley and Wong's nursing care of infants and children* (6th ed). St. Louis: Mosby.

Wong DL, Perry S, Hockenberry M. (2002) *Maternal child nursing care* (2nd ed). St. Louis: Mosby.

Websites
Head Start Programs: *http://www2.acf.dhhs.gov/programs/hsb*
www.ecewebguide.com
www.earlychildhood.com

Workbook

NCLEX-STYLE REVIEW QUESTIONS

1. The nurse is assisting with a well child visit for a 5½-year-old. This child's records show that at the age of 3 years, this child weighed 32 pounds, was 35.5 inches tall, had 20 teeth, and slept 11 hours a day. If this child is following a normal pattern of growth and development, which of the following would the nurse expect to find in this visit? The child

   a. weighs 54 pounds

   b. measures 40 inches in height

   c. has 2 permanent teeth

   d. sleeps 2 hours for a morning nap

2. In working with a group of preschool children, which of the following activities would this age child MOST likely be doing?

   a. Pretending to be television characters

   b. Playing a game with large balls and blocks

   c. Participating in a group activity

   d. Collecting stamps or coins

3. The nurse is talking with a group of caregivers of preschool-age children. Which of the following statements made by a caregiver would require further data collection?

   a. "My child calls her sister bad names when she doesn't get her way."

   b. "She told me her imaginary friend broke my favorite picture frame."

   c. "My son always wants to eat cookies for lunch and for snacks."

   d. "Even when his friends are over to play, he wants to play by himself."

4. A caregiver of a preschool age child says to the nurse, "My 4-year-old touches her genitals sometimes when she is resting." Which of the following statements would be appropriate for the nurse to respond?

   a. "Masturbation is embarrassing to the parents; scolding the child will stop the behavior."

   b. "When children are angry or upset, they often masturbate."

   c. "When this age child masturbates, it can be unhealthy and dangerous."

   d. "Masturbation is a normal behavior, so providing another activity for the child would be appropriate."

5. In teaching caregivers of preschool children, the nurse would reinforce that which of the following would be MOST important for this age group? The preschool child should

   a. brush and floss teeth after snacks and meals

   b. cover mouth when coughing or sneezing

   c. be screened for amblyopia

   d. wear a seatbelt when riding in a vehicle

STUDY ACTIVITIES

1. List and compare the fine motor skills, gross motor skills, and language development in each of the following ages:

	3 Years	4 Years	5 Years
Fine motor skills			
Gross motor skills			
Language development			

2. Describe the guidelines you would give a family to help children develop good eating habits and encourage trying new foods. Write out a 1-day menu including snacks for a preschooler.

3. You are working with the staff in a day care facility to help them develop activities for their preschool program. Using your knowledge of preschool growth and development, make a list of behaviors you would teach the staff to look for in the preschooler. What activities would you suggest to encourage normal preschool growth and development?

CRITICAL THINKING

1. Four-year-olds are sometimes characterized as "the frustrating fours." After reviewing the preschool growth and development chart, identify the reasons you believe this may occur.

2. Clara has noticed her 4-year-old son Theo masturbating. She is upset and comes to you for help. Detail what you will tell her. Discuss with your peers the reactions and concerns that caregivers might express regarding masturbation in their preschool child.

3. Jackson reports that his 4-year-old son, Chad, wakes up screaming in the middle of the night. This is causing the family to lose sleep. Develop a plan of action for Jackson to use to ease the problem.

Health Problems of the Preschool Child

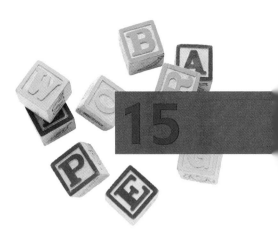

15

STUDENT OBJECTIVES

On completion of this chapter, the student will be able to

1. Differentiate between a child who is hard of hearing and one who is deaf.
2. Differentiate between rubella and rubeola: (a) length of illness, (b) signs and symptoms, (c) complications.
3. State the contagious period for chickenpox.
4. List two nursing measures to increase comfort and decrease scarring in chickenpox.
5. Describe cerebral palsy.
6. Discuss the causes of cerebral palsy: (a) prenatal, (b) perinatal, (c) postnatal.
7. Differentiate between spastic and athetoid cerebral palsy.
8. Identify the health care professionals involved in the care of the child with cerebral palsy.
9. List the causes of mental retardation: (a) prenatal, (b) perinatal, (c) postnatal.
10. Explain why Down's syndrome is also called trisomy 21.
11. List 10 signs and symptoms of Down's syndrome.
12. Name the most common complication of a tonsillectomy, and list the signs to observe for.
13. List four drugs commonly used in the treatment of acute lymphatic leukemia.
14. Name the most common type of hemophilia, and state how it is inherited.
15. Describe the symptoms of nephrotic syndrome.
16. Identify the cause of acute glomerulonephritis.
17. Name the most common presenting symptom of acute glomerulonephritis.
18. Compare nephrotic syndrome with acute glomerulonephritis.

KEY TERMS

adenoids
adenopathy
alopecia
ascites
astigmatism
ataxia
brachycephaly
clonus
dysarthria
granulocytes
hemarthrosis
hyperlipidemia
hyperopia
intercurrent infections
intrathecal administration
leukemia
leukopenia
lymphoblast
lymphocytes
monocytes
myopia
oliguria
petechiae
purpura
refraction
striae
tonsils

Today's preschoolers have a better opportunity for good health than ever before. Immunizations have dramatically reduced the threat of communicable childhood diseases. Antibiotics can minimize the dangers of infection. Early detection and proper nutrition can prevent certain kinds of mental retardation. Simpler, more effective screening techniques help to identify vision and hearing problems that need early treatment. Surgical advances have made possible the early repair of life-threatening heart problems. However, serious health problems do occur during the preschool period. These problems must be recognized and treated as soon as possible so that the child can be in optimum physical and emotional health when it is time to enter school, a landmark in the child's total development.

COMMUNICABLE DISEASES

Half a century ago, growing up meant being able to survive measles, mumps, whooping cough, diphtheria, and often poliomyelitis. These diseases were expected almost as routinely as the loss of the deciduous teeth. Immunization has changed that outcome so drastically that some caregivers have become less conscientious about having their children immunized until the immunization is required for entrance to school. Nevertheless, the incidence of childhood diseases has decreased with only an occasional outbreak in certain communities where many children are not immunized.

Understanding the various communicable diseases and their prevention, symptoms, and treatment (Table 15–1) requires knowledge of the terms in Box 15–1. Some communicable diseases require specific precautions to prevent spreading of the infection. Specific transmission precaution procedures can be found in the procedure manuals of individual institutions.

The nurse should explain to the child and the caregivers the reason for the transmission precautions; precautions are done to protect the child from the threat of infection or to protect others from the infection the child has. Otherwise, the child may feel that the precautions are a form of punishment. Families are more likely to follow the correct procedures if they understand the need for them. Transmission precautions may intensify the normal loneliness of being ill, so the child needs extra attention and stimulation during this time.

Prevention

The recommended schedule of infant immunization is found in Chapter 10. Caregivers of children whose

BOX 15.1	Common Terms in Communicable Disease Nursing

Antibody: a protective substance in the body produced in response to the introduction of an antigen
Antigen: a foreign protein that stimulates the formation of antibodies
Antitoxin: an antibody that unites with and neutralizes a specific toxin
Carrier: a person in apparently good health whose body harbors the specific organisms of a disease
Enanthem: an eruption on a mucous surface
Endemic: habitual presence of a disease within a given area
Epidemic: an outbreak in a community of a group of illnesses of similar nature in excess of the normal expectancy
Erythema: redness of the skin produced by congestion of the capillaries
Exanthem: an eruption appearing on the skin during an eruptive disease
Host: a human, animal, or plant that harbors or nourishes another organism
Immunity: Passive: immunity acquired by administration of an antibody. Active: immunity acquired by an individual as the result of his or her own reactions to pathogens. Natural: resistance of the normal animal to infection.
Incubation period: the time interval between the infection and the appearance of the first symptoms of the disease
Macule: a discolored skin spot not elevated above the surface
Pandemic: a worldwide epidemic
Papule: a small, circumscribed, solid elevation of the skin
Pustule: a small elevation of epidermis filled with pus
Toxin: a poisonous substance produced by certain organisms such as bacteria
Toxoid: a toxin that has been treated to destroy its toxicity but that retains its antigenic properties
Vaccine: a suspension of attenuated or killed microorganisms administered for the prevention of a specific infection

immunizations are incomplete must be urged to have the immunizations brought up to date. For families of limited means, free immunizations are available at clinics.

SENSORY DISORDERS

Hearing Impairment

Hearing loss is one of the most common disabilities in the United States with as many as 33 children a day born with a hearing impairment.[1] Depending on the degree of hearing loss and the age at detection, a child's development can be moderately to severely

text continued on page 311

TABLE 15.1   Infectious Diseases of Childhood

Disease/Causative Organism	Incubation	Communicable Period; When/How	Immunization/Immunity	Symptoms	Treatment/Nursing Implications	Type of Precautions	Complications
Rubeola (measles) Measles virus	10–21 days	Fifth incubation day until after first few days after rash erupts Direct or indirect contact with droplets	Attenuated live vaccine (part of MMR vaccine); disease gives lasting natural immunity	Occurs in winter or spring; high fever; coryza (runny nose); cough; enlarged lymph nodes (head and neck); Koplik spots (small red spots with blue-white centers on oral mucosa, specific to rubeola); conjunctivitis; photophobia; maculopapular rash starts at hairline and spreads to entire body	Soothing measures for rash include tepid baths, soothing lotion, maintaining dry skin; dimly lighted room for comfort; encourage fluids	Airborne	Otitis media, pneumonia, encephalitis, airway obstruction
Rubella (German measles) Rubella virus	14–21 days	5–7 days before until about 5 days after rash appears Direct or indirect contact with droplets	Attenuated live vaccine (part of MMR vaccine); disease gives lasting natural immunity	Low-grade fever; malaise; lymph glands of neck and head enlarged; pale small rash disappears in 3 days	Symptomatic relief	Droplet	Avoid contact with pregnant women; unborn fetus can suffer severe birth deformities if nonimmunized mother is exposed, especially in first trimester.
Parotitis (mumps) Paramyxovirus	14–21 days	Shortly before swelling appears until after it disappears Direct contact, droplet; indirect from contaminated articles	Attenuated live mumps vaccine (part of MMR vaccine); disease gives natural immunity Passive: mumps immune globulin	Parotid glands swollen, unilaterally or bilaterally; may have fever, headache, malaise, and complain of earache before	Chewing is painful, so liquids and soft foods are given; sour foods cause discomfort; analgesics for pain; antipyretics for fever; local compresses of	Droplet	In males past puberty, orchitis (inflammation of the testes); menigoen-cephalitis; may rarely cause severe hearing

Disease/Organism	Incubation; Period of Communicability	Immunity	Signs and Symptoms	Treatment	Transmission	Complications
						impairment
Varicella (chickenpox) Varicella zoster virus	10–21 days; 1 day before rash appears for about 6 days (until all vesicles crusted over); Direct or indirect contact with saliva or uncrusted vesicles	Lasting natural immunity; may reactivate in adult as herpes zoster; active artificial immunity available	Low-grade fever; malaise; successive crops of macules, papules, vesicles, and crusts, all present at the same time; itching is intense; scarring may occur when scabs are picked off before ready to fall off	Antihistamines to reduce itching; soothing baths and lotions may help; prevent scratching with short fingernails, mittens; acyclovir has been given to shorten the course of the disease. **Aspirin must not be given.** heat or cold may be soothing	Airborne, contact	Reye syndrome can occur if child has had aspirin during illness; super-infection of lesions if scratched; encephalitis
Pertussis (whooping cough) *Bordetella pertussis*	5–21 days; About 4–6 weeks; Direct contact, droplet; indirect from contaminated articles	Pertussis vaccine is part of the DTP vaccine; disease gives natural immunity	Begins with mild upper respiratory symptoms; in second week progresses to severe paroxysmal cough with inspiratory whoop, sometimes followed by vomiting; especially dangerous for young infants; may last 4–6 weeks	Bed rest; infants hospitalized; may need oxygen; observe for airway obstruction; provide high humidity; protect from secondary infections; encourage fluid intake; refeed child if vomiting occurs	Droplet	Pneumonia (can cause death of infant); otitis media; hemorrhage; convulsions

(table continues on page 310)

TABLE 15.1 (continued) | Infectious Diseases of Childhood

Disease/ Causative Organism	Incubation	Communicable Period; When/How	Immunization/ Immunity	Symptoms	Treatment/ Nursing Implications	Type of Precautions	Complications
Diphtheria Corynebacterium diphtheriae	2–5 days	As long as bacilli are present: 2–4 weeks or less with antibiotic therapy Direct contact with infected person, carrier, or contaminated article	Active immunity from diphtheria toxin in DTP vaccine; passive immunity with diphtheria antitoxin	Mucous membranes of nose and throat covered by gray membrane; purulent nasal discharge; brassy cough; toxin from organism passes through blood stream to heart and nervous system	Strict precautions maintained; intravenous antitoxin and antibiotics administered; bed rest; liquid to soft diet; analgesics for throat pain; nonimmunized contacts should be immunized	Contact, droplet	Neuritis; carditis; congestive heart failure; respiratory failure
Poliomyelitis (infantile paralysis) Poliovirus types 1, 2, 3	5–14 days	Variable: 1 week after symptoms for respiratory contact, up to 6 weeks for feces	Trivalent live oral polio vaccine; disease causes active immunity against specific strain	Fever, headache, nausea, vomiting, abdominal pain; stiff neck, pain and tenderness in lower extremities that proceed to paralysis	Bed rest; moist hot packs to extremities; range-of-motion exercises; supportive care; long-term ventilation if respiratory muscles involved	Standard	Permanent paralysis; respiratory arrest

impaired. Development of speech, human relationships, and understanding of the environment all depend on the ability to hear. Infants at high risk for hearing loss should be screened when they are between 3 and 6 months of age.

Hearing loss ranges from mild (hard of hearing) to profound (deaf) (Table 15–2). A child who is hard of hearing has a loss of hearing acuity but can learn speech and language by imitating sounds. A deaf child has no hearing ability.

Types of Hearing Impairment

There are four types of hearing loss: conductive, sensorineural, mixed, and central.

Conductive Hearing Loss. In this type of impairment, middle ear structures fail to carry sound waves to the inner ear. Conductive hearing loss is most often the result of chronic serous otitis media or other infection and can make hearing levels fluctuate. Chronic middle ear infection can destroy part of the eardrum or the ossicles, which leads to conductive deafness. This type of deafness is seldom complete and responds well to treatment.

Sensorineural (Perceptive) Hearing Loss. This type of hearing loss may be caused by damage to the nerve endings in the cochlea or to the nerve pathways leading to the brain. It is generally severe and unresponsive to medical treatment. Diseases such as meningitis and encephalitis, hereditary or congenital factors, and toxic reactions to certain drugs (such as streptomycin) may cause sensorineural hearing loss. Maternal rubella is believed to be the most common cause of sensorineural deafness in children.

Mixed Hearing Loss. Some children have both conductive and sensorineural hearing impairments. In these instances, the conduction level determines how well the child can hear.

Central Auditory Dysfunction. Although this child may have normal hearing, damage to or faulty development of the proper brain centers makes the child unable to use the auditory information received.

Clinical Manifestations

Mild to moderate hearing loss often remains undetected until the child moves outside the family circle into nursery school or kindergarten. The hearing loss may have been gradual, and the child may have become such a skilled lip reader that neither the child nor the family is aware of the partial deafness. Caregivers and teachers should be aware of the possibility of hearing loss in children who appear to be inattentive and noisy and who create disturbances in the classroom.

Certain reactions and mannerisms characterize a child with hearing loss. The child should be observed for an apparent inability to locate a sound and a turning of the head to one side when listening. The child who fails to comprehend when spoken to, who gives inappropriate answers to questions, who consistently turns up the volume on the television or radio, or who cannot whisper or talk softly may have hearing loss.

Diagnosis

Children who are profoundly deaf are more likely to be diagnosed before 1 year of age than are children with mild to moderate hearing losses. The child who is suspected of having a hearing loss should be referred for a complete audiologic assessment including pure-tone audiometric, speech reception, and speech discrimination tests. Children with

TABLE 15.2	Levels of Hearing Impairment
Decible Level	**Hearing Level Present**
Slight (<30 dB)	Unable to hear whispered word or faint speech No speech impairment present May not be aware of hearing difficulty Achieves well in school and home by compensating by leaning forward, speaking loudly
Mild (30–50 dB)	Beginning speech impairment may be present Difficulty hearing if not facing speaker; some difficulty with normal conversation
Moderate (55–70 dB)	Speech impairment present; may require speech therapy Difficulty with normal conversation
Severe (70–90 dB)	Difficulty with any but nearby loud voice Hears vowels easier than consonants Requires speech therapy for clear speech May still hear loud sounds such as jets or a train
Profound (>90 dB)	Hears almost no sound

From Pillitteri A. (2003). *Maternal and child health nursing* (4th ed). Philadelphia: Lippincott Williams & Wilkins.

sensorineural impairment generally have a greater loss of hearing acuity in the high-pitched tones. The loss may vary from slight to complete. Children with a conductive loss are more likely to have equal losses over a wide range of frequencies.

A child's hearing should be tested at all frequencies by a pure-tone audiometer in a soundproof room. Speech reception and speech discrimination tests measure the amount of hearing impairment for both speech and communication. Accurate measurements usually can be made in children as young as 3 years of age if the test is introduced as a game.

Infants and very young children must be tested in different ways. An infant with normal hearing should be able to locate a sound at 28 weeks, imitate sounds at 36 weeks, and associate sounds with people or objects at 1 year of age. A commonly used screening test for very young children uses noisemakers of varying intensity and pitch. The examiner stands beside or behind the child who has been given a toy. As the examiner produces sounds with a rattle, buzzer, bell, or other noisemaker, a hearing child is distracted and turns to the source of the new sound, whereas a deaf child does not react in a particular way.

Deafness, mental retardation, and autism are sometimes incorrectly diagnosed because the symptoms can be similar. Deaf children may fail to respond to sound or develop speech because they cannot hear. Mentally retarded or autistic children may show the same lack of response and development even though they do not have a hearing loss.

Treatment and Education

When the type and degree of hearing loss have been established, the child or even infant may be fitted with a hearing aid. Hearing aids are helpful only in conductive deafness not in sensorineural or central auditory dysfunction. These devices only amplify sound; they do not localize or clarify it. Many models are available including those in the ear, behind the ear, incorporated in glasses or on the body with a wire connection to the ear. FM receiver units also are available that can broadcast the speaker's voice from a greater distance and cut out the background noise. When the FM transmitter is turned off, this type of unit functions as an ordinary hearing aid.

It is believed that deaf children can best be taught to communicate by a combination of lip reading, sign language, and oral speech (Fig. 15–1). The family members are the child's first teachers; they must be aware of all phases of development—physical, emotional, social, intellectual, and language—and seek to aid this development.

A deaf child depends on sight to interpret the environment and to communicate. Thus it is

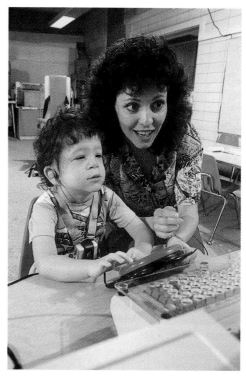

● **Figure 15.1** A young deaf girl learns to use the computer with the help of a speech therapist.

important to be sure that the child's vision is normal and if it is not, to correct that problem. The probability is twice as great that the child with a hearing loss also will have some vision impairment. Training in the use of all the other senses—sight, smell, taste, and touch—makes the deaf child better able to use any available hearing. Some researchers believe that most deaf children do have some hearing ability.

Preschool classes for deaf children exist in many large communities. These attempt to create an environment in which a deaf child can have the same experiences and activities that normal preschoolers have. Children are generally enrolled at age 2.5 years.

The John Tracy Clinic in Los Angeles founded in 1943 is dedicated to young children (birth through age 5) born with severe hearing loss or those who have lost hearing through illness before acquiring speech and language. The clinic's purpose is "to find, encourage, guide, and train the parents of deaf and hard-of-hearing children, first in order to reach and help the children, and second to help the parents themselves." With early diagnosis and intervention, hearing-impaired children can develop language and communication skills in the critical preschool period that enable many of them to speech-read and to speak. All services to parents and children are free. Full audiologic testing, parent-infant education, demonstration nursery school, parent education classes, and parent groups are offered. Many medical residents, nurses, and allied health care professionals come to observe the model programs at the clinic to see for themselves the benefits of early diagnosis.

The clinic also provides a correspondence course for parents. Three courses available in both English and Spanish are for deaf infants, deaf preschoolers, and deaf-blind children. These courses, which include written materials and videotapes, guide parents in encouraging their child to develop auditory awareness, speech-reading skills, and expressive language. Information about the clinic can be obtained by calling toll-free (800) 522-4582 or on the Internet at *http://www.johntracyclinic.org.*

Federal law requires free and appropriate education for all disabled children. Children with a hearing loss who cannot successfully function in regular classrooms are provided with supplementary services (speech therapist, speech interpreter, signer) in special classrooms or in a residential school.

Nursing Care for the Deaf Child

When the deaf child is in a health care facility, the child's primary caregiver should be present during the stay; caregiver presence is encouraged to help the child communicate needs and feelings, not as a convenience to the nursing staff.

The deaf child's anxiety about unfamiliar situations and procedures can be greater than that of the child with normal hearing. When speaking to the deaf child, stand or sit face to face on the child's level. Be certain that a deaf child can see you before you touch him or her. Demonstrate each procedure before it is performed, showing the child the equipment or pictures of the equipment to be used. Follow demonstrations with explanations to be sure the child understands. Keep a night-light in the child's room because sight is a critical sense to the deaf child. To understand the child's helpless feeling, imagine being in a soundless, dark room.

Hearing aids are expensive, so learning how to take care of and maintain them is wise. Put the aid in a safe place when the child is not wearing it. Check linens before putting them into the laundry so as not to discard a hearing aid along with the dirty linens.

Use family members as important resources to learn about the child's habits and communication patterns. In many communities signing classes are available for those working with hearing-impaired children and adults.

Vision Impairment

Like hearing, good vision is essential to a child's normal development. How well a child sees affects his or her learning process, social development, coordination, and safety. One in 1,000 children of school age has serious vision impairment. The sooner these impairments are corrected, the better a child's chances are for normal or near-normal development.

Children with vision impairments are classified as sighted with eye problems, partially sighted, or legally blind.

Types Of Vision Impairment

Eye Problems in Sighted Children. Among sighted children with eye problems, errors of **refraction** (the way light rays bend as they pass through the lens to the retina) are the most common. About 10% of school-age children have **myopia** (nearsightedness), which means that the child can see objects clearly at close range but not at a distance. When proper lenses are fitted, vision is corrected to normal. If uncorrected, this defect may cause a child to be labeled inattentive or retarded. Myopia tends to be familial and often progresses into adolescence then levels off.

Hyperopia (farsightedness) is a refractive condition in which the person can see objects better at a distance than close up. It is common in young children and often persists into the first grade or even later. The ocular specialist examining the child must decide whether or not corrective lenses are needed on an individual basis. Usually correction is not needed in a preschooler. Teachers and parents should be aware of the considerable eye fatigue that may result from efforts at accommodation for close work.

Astigmatism may occur with or without myopia or hyperopia and is caused by unequal curvatures in the cornea that bend the light rays in different directions; this produces a blurred image. Slight astigmatism often does not require correction; moderate degrees usually require glasses for reading and watching television and movies; severe astigmatism requires glasses at all times.

Partial Sight. Children with partial sight have a visual acuity between 20/20 and 20/200 in the better eye after all necessary medical or surgical correction. These children also have a high incidence of refractive errors particularly myopia. Eye injuries also cause loss of vision, as do conditions such as cataracts that can be improved by treatment but result in diminished sight.

Blindness. Blindness is legally defined as a corrected vision of 20/200 or less or peripheral vision of less than 20° in the better eye. Many causes of blindness have been reduced or eliminated such as retrolental fibroplasia (due to excessive oxygen concentrations in newborns) and trachoma, a viral infection. Maternal infections are still a common cause of blindness, although the incidence of maternal rubella has decreased because of immunization.

Between the ages of 5 and 7 years, children begin to form and retain visual images; they have memory with pictures. Children who become blind before 5 years of age are missing this crucial element in their development. Blindness can seriously hamper the child's ability to form human attachments; learn coordination, balance, and locomotion; distinguish fantasy from reality; and interpret the surrounding world. How well the blind child learns to cope depends on the family's ability to communicate, teach, and foster a sense of independence in the child.

Clinical Manifestations and Diagnosis

Squinting and frowning while trying to read a blackboard or other material at a distance, tearing, red-rimmed eyes, holding work too close to the eyes while reading or writing, and rubbing the eyes are all signs of possible vision impairment. Although blindness is likely to be detected in early infancy, partial sightedness or correctable vision problems may go unrecognized until a child enters school unless vision screening is part of routine health maintenance (Fig. 15–2).

A simple test kit for preschoolers is available for home use by family caregivers or visiting nurses (Fig. 15–3). This kit is an adaptation of the Snellen E chart used for testing children who have not learned to read. The child covers one eye and then points the fingers in the same direction as the "fingers" on each E, beginning with the largest. Some examiners refer to these as "legs on a table."

The Snellen Chart. This is the familiar test in which the letters on each line are smaller than those on the line above. If the child can read the 20-ft line standing 20 ft away from the chart, visual acuity is stated as 20/20. If the child can read only the line marked 100, acuity is stated as 20/100. The chart should be placed at eye level with good lighting and in a room free from distractions. One eye is tested at a time with the other eye covered. Normal preschool acuity is 20/30.

Picture charts for identification also are used but are not considered as accurate. An intelligent child can memorize the pictures and guess from the general shape without seeing distinctly.

Treatment and Education

Significant medical and surgical advances have occurred in the treatment of cataracts, strabismus, and amblyopia. The earlier the child is treated, the better the child's chances of adequate vision for normal development and function. Errors of refraction are usually correctable. Corrective lenses for minor vision impairments should be prescribed early and checked regularly to be sure they still provide adequate correction.

Children who are partially sighted or totally blind benefit from association with normally sighted children. In most communities, education for these special children is provided within the regular school or in special classes that offer the child more specialized equipment and instruction.

Special equipment includes printed material with large print, pencils with large leads for darker lines, tape recordings, magnifying glasses, and typewriters. For children with a serious impairment whose participation in regular activities is sharply curtailed, talking books, raised maps, and Braille equipment are needed as well. These devices prevent isolation of the visually impaired child and minimize any differences from the other children.

Nursing Care for the Visually Impaired Child

Children with a visual impairment have the same needs as other children, and these should not be overlooked. The child who is blind needs emotional comfort and sensory stimulation, much of which must be communicated by touch, sound, and smell. It is important for the nurse to explain sounds and other sensations that are new to the child and to let him or her touch the equipment that will be used in procedures. A tactile tour of the room helps orient the child to the location of furniture and other facilities. Awareness of safety hazards is particularly important when caring for the blind or partially sighted child.

Nurses and other personnel must identify themselves when they enter the room and must tell the child when they leave. Explanations of what is going to happen reduce the child's fear and anxiety and the possibility of being startled by an unexpected touch.

The child with a visual impairment should be involved with as many peers and their activities as possible. The child also should be encouraged to be as independent as possible. One step is to provide the child with finger foods and encourage self-feeding

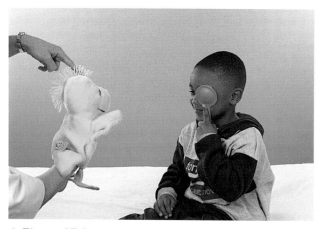

● *Figure 15.2* Vision screening on a preschool child as part of a routine exam.

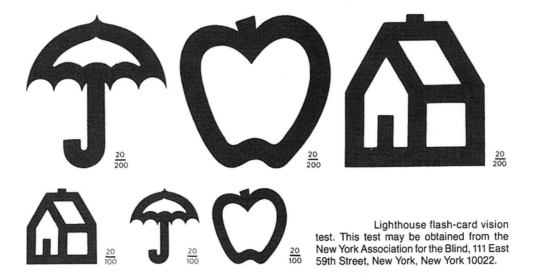

Lighthouse flash-card vision test. This test may be obtained from the New York Association for the Blind, 111 East 59th Street, New York, New York 10022.

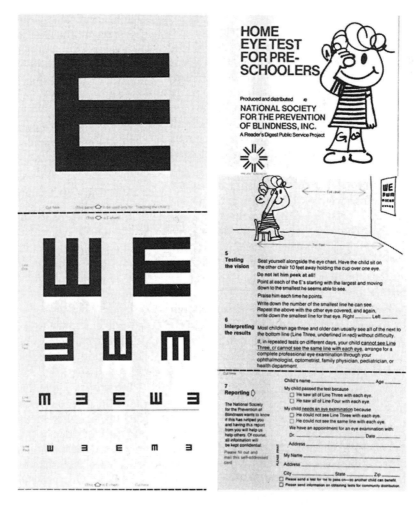

● *Figure 15.3* Home testing kit. This allows the very young preschooler to take the test in more familiar surroundings. The test may be obtained at www.preventblindness.org/children or by calling 1-800-331-2020.

after orienting the child to the plate. A small bowl, instead of a plate, is useful so that food can be scooped against the side to get it on the spoon. Eating is a time-consuming and messy affair, but it is essential to the growth of independence in all children.

INTERNET EXERCISE 15.1

http://www.preventblindness.org

On the left side of the screen, Click on "Children."
Click on "Eye Tests."
Click on "The Pointing Game."

1. What are the steps to following in administering this eye test to children?

Click on Back.
Click on "Distance Vision Test."

2. Print a copy of the Distance Vision Chart.

3. Following the instructions given, administer the distance vision test to a preschooler.

4. What did you discover about this child's vision?

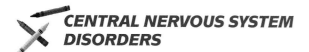

CENTRAL NERVOUS SYSTEM DISORDERS

Reye Syndrome

Reye syndrome (rhymes with "eye") is characterized by acute encephalopathy and fatty degeneration of the liver and other abdominal organs. It occurs in children of all ages but is seen more in young school-age children than in any other age group. Reye syndrome usually occurs after a viral illness, particularly after an upper respiratory infection or varicella (chickenpox). Administration of aspirin during the viral illness has been implicated as a contributing factor. As a result, the American Academy of Pedi-

atrics recommends that aspirin or aspirin compounds not be given to children with viral infections.

Clinical Manifestations

The symptoms appear within 3 to 5 days after the initial illness. The child is recuperating unremarkably when symptoms of severe vomiting, irritability, lethargy, and confusion occur. Immediate intervention is needed to prevent serious insult to the brain including respiratory arrest (Table 15–3).

Diagnosis

The history of a viral illness is an immediate clue. Liver function tests, including serum glutamic oxaloacetic transaminase (SGOT), serum glutamic pyruvic transaminase (SGPT), lactic dehydrogenase (LDH), and serum ammonia levels, are elevated because of poor liver function. The child is hypoglycemic and has delayed prothrombin time.

Treatment and Nursing Care

The child with Reye syndrome often is cared for in the intensive care unit because the disease may rapidly progress. Medical management focuses on supportive measures—improving respiratory function, reducing cerebral edema, and controlling hypoglycemia. The specific treatment is determined by the staging of the symptoms (refer to Table 15–3). The nurse carefully observes the child for overall physical status and any change in neurologic status. This is essential in evaluating the progression of the illness. Accurate intake and output determinations are necessary to determine when fluids need to be adjusted to control cerebral edema and prevent dehydration. Osmotic diuretics (e.g., mannitol) may be administered to reduce cerebral edema. The nurse monitors the blood glucose level and bleeding time. Low blood glucose levels can lead to seizures quickly in young children, and a prolonged bleeding time can indicate coagulation problems as a result of liver dysfunction.

TABLE 15.3	Staging of Reye Syndrome
Stage	**Symptoms Seen in Stage**
Stage I	Lethargic, vomiting, follows verbal commands, normal posture
Stage II	Combative or stuporous, inappropriate verbalizing, normal posture
Stage III	Comatose, decorticate posture and response to pain
Stage IV	Comatose, decerebrate posture and response to pain
Stage V	Comatose, flaccid, seizures, no papillary response, no response to pain

Adapted from the National Institutes of Health Staging System, Louis, PT. (1999). Reye syndrome. In *Oski's pediatrics: Principles and practice* (3rd ed). Philadelphia: Lippincott Williams & Wilkins.

This hospitalization period is a traumatic time for family members, so the nurse must give them opportunities to deal with their feelings. In addition, the family must be kept well informed about the child's care. Having a child in intensive care is a frightening experience, and every effort must be made to reassure the family with sincerity and honesty.

Since the American Academy of Pediatrics made its recommendation to avoid giving aspirin to children especially during viral illnesses, the number of cases of Reye syndrome has steadily decreased. The prognosis of children with Reye syndrome is greatly improved with early diagnosis and vigorous treatment. The nurse is responsible for teaching families with young children to avoid the use of aspirin.

Cerebral Palsy

Cerebral palsy (CP) is a group of disorders arising from a malfunction of motor centers and neural pathways in the brain. It is one of the most complex of the common permanent disabling conditions and often can be accompanied by seizures, mental retardation, sensory defects, and behavior disorders. Research in this area is directed at adapting biomedical technology to help people with cerebral palsy cope with the activities of daily living and achieve maximum function and independence.

Causes

Although the cause of CP cannot be identified in many cases, several causes are possible. It may be caused by damage to the parts of the brain that control movement; this damage generally occurs during the fetal or perinatal period particularly in premature infants.

Common *prenatal* causes are

- Any process that interferes with the oxygen supply to the brain such as separation of the placenta, compression of the cord, or bleeding
- Maternal infection (e.g., cytomegalovirus, toxoplasmosis, rubella)
- Nutritional deficiencies that may affect brain growth
- Kernicterus (brain damage caused by jaundice) resulting from Rh incompatibility
- Teratogenic factors such as drugs and radiation

Common *perinatal* causes are

- Anoxia immediately before, during, and after birth
- Intracranial bleeding
- Asphyxia or interference with respiratory function
- Maternal analgesia (e.g., morphine) that depresses the sensitive neonate's respiratory center

- Birth trauma
- Prematurity because immature blood vessels predispose the neonate to cerebral hemorrhage

About 10% to 20% of cases occur after birth. Common *postnatal* causes are

- Head trauma (e.g., due to a fall, motor vehicle accident)
- Infection (e.g., encephalitis, meningitis)
- Neoplasms
- Cerebrovascular accident

Prevention

Because brain damage in CP is irreversible, prevention is the most important aspect of care. Prevention of CP focuses on

- Prenatal care to improve nutrition, prevent infection, and decrease the incidence of prematurity
- Perinatal monitoring with appropriate interventions to decrease birth trauma
- Postnatal prevention of infection through breast-feeding, improved nutrition, and immunizations
- Protection from trauma of motor vehicle accidents, child abuse, and other childhood accidents

Clinical Manifestations and Types

Difficulty in controlling voluntary muscle movements is one manifestation of the central nervous system damage. Seizures, mental retardation, hearing and vision impairments, and behavior disorders often accompany the major problem. Delayed gross motor development, abnormal motor performance (e.g., poor sucking and feeding behaviors), abnormal postures, and persistence of primitive reflexes are other signs of CP. Diagnosis of CP seldom occurs before 2 months of age and may be delayed until the second or third year, when the toddler attempts to walk and caretakers notice an obvious lag in motor development. Diagnosis is based on observations of delayed growth and development through a process that rules out other diagnoses.

Several major types of CP occur; each has distinctive clinical manifestations.

Spastic Type. This is the most common type and is characterized by

- A hyperactive stretch reflex in associated muscle groups
- Increased activity of the deep tendon reflexes
- **Clonus** (rapid involuntary muscle contraction and relaxation)
- Contractures affecting the extensor muscles especially the heel cord
- Scissoring caused by severe hip adduction. When scissoring is present, the child's legs are crossed and the toes are pointed down (Fig 15–4). When

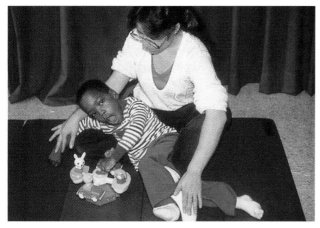

● *Figure 15.4* The physical therapist works with a child who has cerebral palsy. Note the scissoring of the legs.

standing, the child is on her or his toes. It is difficult for this child to walk on the heels or run.

Athetoid Type. Athetoid CP is marked by involuntary, uncoordinated motion with varying degrees of muscle tension. Children with this disorder are constantly in motion, and the whole body is in a state of slow, writhing muscle contractions whenever voluntary movement is attempted. Facial grimacing, poor swallowing, and tongue movements causing drooling and **dysarthria** (poor speech articulation) also are present. These children are likely to have average or above-average intelligence despite their abnormal appearance. Hearing loss is most common in this group.

Ataxia Type. Ataxia is essentially a lack of coordination caused by disturbances in the kinesthetic and balance senses. The least common type of CP, ataxia may not be diagnosed until the child starts to walk: the gait is awkward and wide-based.

Rigidity Type. This type is uncommon and is characterized by rigid postures and lack of active movement.

Mixed Type. Children with signs of more than one type of CP are usually severely disabled. The disorder may have been caused by postnatal injury.

Diagnosis

Children with CP may not be diagnosed with certainty until they have difficulties when attempting to walk. They may show signs of mental retardation, attention deficit disorder, or recurrent convulsions. Computed tomography, magnetic resonance imaging, and ultrasonography for infants before closure of skull sutures may be used to help determine the cause of CP.

Treatment and Special Aids

Treatment of CP focuses on helping the child to make the best use of residual abilities and achieve maxi-

mum satisfaction and enrichment in life. A team of health care professionals—physician, surgeon, physical therapist, occupational therapist, speech therapist, and perhaps a social worker—works with the family to set realistic goals. Dental care is important because enamel hypoplasia is common, and children whose seizure disorders are controlled with phenytoin (Dilantin) are likely to develop gingival hypertrophy. Medications such as baclofen, diazepam, and dantrolene may be used to help decrease spasticity.

Physical Therapy. Body control needed for purposeful physical activity is learned automatically by a normal child but must be consciously learned by a child who has problems with physical mobility (Fig. 15–5). Physical therapists attempt to teach activities of daily living that the child has been unable to accomplish. Methods must be suited to the needs of each child as well as to the general needs arising from the condition. These methods are based on principles of conditioning, relaxation, use of residual patterns, stimulation of contraction and relaxation of antagonistic muscles, and others. Various techniques are used. Because there are many variations in the disabilities caused by CP, each child must be considered individually and treated appropriately.

Orthopedic Management. Braces are used as supportive and control measures to facilitate muscle training, to reinforce weak or paralyzed muscles, or

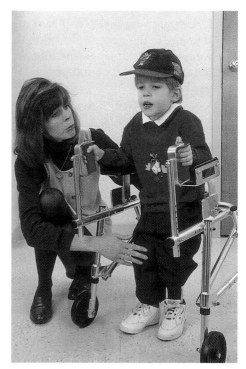

● *Figure 15.5* During a physical therapy session, this boy with CP works hard to take a step forward. His mom stays by his side to encourage him.

to counteract the pull of antagonistic muscles. Various types are available; each is designed for a specific purpose. Orthopedic surgery sometimes is used to improve function and to correct deformities such as the release of contractures and the lengthening of tight heel cords.

Technological Aids for Daily Living. Biomedical engineering, particularly in the field of electronics, has perfected a number of devices to help make the disabled person more functional and less dependent on others. The devices range from simple items, such as wheelchairs and specially constructed toilet seats, to completely electronic cottages furnished with a computer (even including a voice synthesizer), a tape recorder, a calculator, and other equipment that facilitates independence and useful study or work. Many of these devices can be controlled by a mouth stick, which is an extremely useful feature for people with poor hand coordination.

A child who has difficulty maintaining balance while sitting may need a high-backed chair with side pieces and a foot platform. Feeding may be a challenge, so caregivers may need help finding a method that works for feeding their child. Sometimes controlling and stabilizing the jaw will help with feeding (Fig 15–6). Feeding aids include spoons with enlarged handles for easy grasping or with bent handles that allow the spoon to be brought easily to the mouth. Plates with high rims and suction devices to prevent slipping enable a child to eat with little assistance. Covered cups set in holders with a hole in the lid to admit a straw help a child who does not

have hand control (Fig. 15–7). The severely disabled child may need a nasogastric or gastrostomy tube.

Manual skill can be aided by games that must be manipulated such as pegboards and cards. Keyboarding is an ego-boosting alternative for a child whose disability is too severe to permit legible writing. Computer programs have been designed to enable these children to communicate and improve their learning skills. Special keyboards, joysticks, and electronic devices help the child to have fun and gain a sense of achievement while learning. Computers also have expanded the opportunities for future employment for these children.

Nursing Care

The child with CP may be seen in the health care setting at any age level. Interview and observe the child and the family to determine the child's needs, the level of development, and the stage of family acceptance, and to set realistic long-range goals. The newly diagnosed child and family may have more potential nursing diagnoses than the child and family who have been successfully dealing with CP for a long time.

To ease the change of environment, the nurse needs to communicate with the family to learn as much as possible about the child's activities at home. The child should be encouraged to maintain current self-care activities and set goals for attaining new ones. Positioning to prevent contractures, providing modified feeding utensils, and suggesting appropriate educational play activities are all important

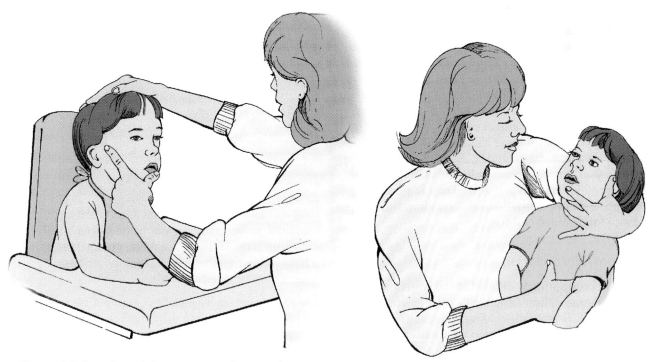

● **Figure 15.6** Feeding techniques to promote jaw control.

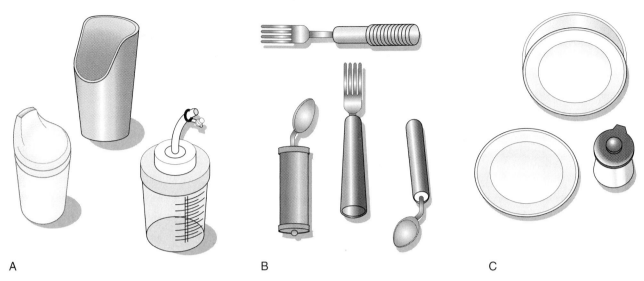

● **Figure 15.7** Feeding aids and devices: **(A)** cups; **(B)** utensils; **(C)** dishes.

aspects of the child's care. If the child has been admitted for surgery, the child and family need appropriate preoperative and postoperative teaching, emotional support, and assistance in setting realistic expectations. The family may need help to explore educational opportunities for the child.

Like any chronic condition, CP can become a devastating drain on the family's emotional and financial resources. The child's future depends on many variables: family attitudes; economic and therapeutic resources; the child's intelligence; and the availability of competent, understanding health care professionals. Some children, when given the emotional and physical support they need, can achieve a satisfactory degree of independence. Some have been able to attend college and find fulfilling work. Vocational training is also available to an increasing number of these young people. Some people with CP will always need a significant amount of nursing care with the possibility of institutionalized care when their families can no longer care for them.

The outlook for these children and their families is improving, but a great deal of work remains to be done. Working as a community member, the health care professional can play a vital role in promoting educational opportunities, rehabilitation, and acceptance for disabled children.

Mental Retardation

Mental retardation is defined in the American Psychiatric Association's *Diagnostic and Statistical Manual-TR Fourth Edition, Revised* using two criteria: significantly subaverage general intellectual functioning—an intelligence quotient (IQ) of 70 or lower—and concurrent deficits in adaptive functioning. *Adaptive functioning* refers to how well people can meet the standards of independence (activities of daily living) and social responsibility expected for their age and the cultural group to which they belong. Mental retardation often occurs in combination with other physical disorders.

Causes

Many factors can cause mental retardation. *Prenatal* causes include

- Inborn errors of metabolism such as phenylketonuria, galactosemia, or congenital hypothyroidism. Damage often can be prevented by early detection and treatment.
- Prenatal infection such as toxoplasmosis or cytomegalovirus. Microcephaly, hydrocephalus, cerebral palsy, and other brain damage can result from intrauterine infections.
- Teratogenic agents, such as drugs, radiation, and alcohol, can have devastating effects on the central nervous system of a developing fetus.
- Genetic factors—inborn variations of chromosomal patterns—result in a variety of deviations, the most common of which is Down's syndrome.

Perinatal causes of mental retardation include birth trauma, anoxia from various causes, prematurity, and difficult birth. In some instances, prenatal factors may have influenced the perinatal complications.

Postnatal causes include

- Poisoning such as lead poisoning. Children who develop encephalopathy from chronic lead poisoning usually have significant brain damage.
- Infections and trauma such as meningitis, convulsive disorders, and hydrocephalus.

A PERSONAL GLIMPSE

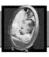

The mother of a developmentally delayed child knows her child has a problem before any doctor notices. Visually my son looked perfect. There were no outward signs of retardation. He was a beautiful baby but he was often ill—severe croup, pneumonia, bronchitis, grand mal seizures due to fever, hospital stays, EEGs, spinal taps, tests and more tests—but he always bounced back, much better than his parents recovered.

Slowly I started to notice that he was not the same as other kids his age. His vocabulary was Mom and DaDa where other 3 year olds were starting to put words together into little sentences. Everyone said he didn't talk because I spoiled him and got him everything he needed before he asked for it. I would try to believe people, including doctors, who would say, "Don't worry; you are just being an over-protective mother. Your son will be fine." You try to hide from the truth but slowly you realize you have to get others to see what you see. You have to get help for your child—someone has to listen to you.

Finally I forced my pediatrician to try some physical dexterity tests. My son failed these tests. I heard the doctor say the words that broke my heart: "I am sorry. I thought you were just another hysterical mother—but there is something wrong with your child. We must schedule him for more testing." Then I cried.

Patricia

> **LEARNING OPPORTUNITY:** What are some feelings parents of children diagnosed with mental retardation might have? What are some ways that the nurse can support the mother and the child in the above situation?

• Impoverished early environment such as inadequate nutrition and a lack of sensory stimulation. Emotional rejection in early life may do irreparable damage to a child's ability to respond to the environment.

The Mentally Retarded Child

About 3% of all children born in the United States have some level of cognitive impairment. About 20% of these are so severely retarded that diagnosis is made at birth or during the first year. Most of the other children are diagnosed as retarded when they begin school.

The most common classification of mental retardation is based on IQ. Although controversy exists about the validity of tests that measure intelligence, this system is still the most useful for grouping these children.

The child with an IQ of 70 to 50 is considered mildly mentally retarded. This child is a slow learner but can acquire basic skills. The child can learn to read, write, and do arithmetic to a fourth- or fifth-grade level but is slower than average in learning to walk, talk, and feed himself or herself. Retardation may not be obvious to casual acquaintances. With support and guidance, this child usually can develop social and vocational skills adequate for self-maintenance. About 80% of retarded children are classified in this category.

The moderately retarded child with an IQ of 55 to 35 has little, if any, ability to attain independence and academic skills and is referred to as *trainable*. Motor development and speech are noticeably delayed, but training in self-help activities is possible. This child may be able to learn repetitive skills in sheltered workshops. Some children may learn to travel alone, but few become capable of assuming complete self-maintenance. This category accounts for about 10% of retarded children.

The child considered severely retarded tests in the IQ range of 40 to 20. This child's development is markedly delayed during the first year of life. The child cannot learn academic skills but may be able to learn some self-care activities if sensorimotor stimulation is begun early. Eventually this child will probably learn to walk and develop some speech; however, a sheltered environment and careful supervision always will be required.

The profoundly retarded child has an IQ lower than 20. This child has minimal capacity for functioning and needs continuing care. Eventually the child may learn to walk and develop a primitive speech but will never be able to perform self-care activities. Only about 1% of retarded children are in this category.

Teaching and Education

Knowledge about teaching children with cognitive impairment has increased dramatically, and new teaching methods have been yielding encouraging results. Mildly and moderately retarded people are taught to perform tasks that enable them to achieve some degree of independence and usefulness. More and better services are being provided for all cognitively impaired children and adults.

The child with cognitive impairment may not be identified until well into the preschool stage, because slow development often can be excused in one way or another. The family may be the best judge of the child's development, and health care personnel must listen carefully to any concerns or questions that caregivers express.

When family members are faced with the fact that their child is retarded, they need to go through a grieving process, as do family members of any other child with a serious disorder. They need to mourn the loss of the normal child that was expected and resolve to give this child the best opportunities to develop his or her potential.

Early diagnosis and intervention are important tools to use in the care of the cognitively impaired child. Early infant tests are difficult to administer and the results are inaccurate, but they may provide the family with some idea about the child's potential. The family must be aware that these are only predictions based on unreliable test data.

The child is usually kept at home in the family environment. The current philosophy of care for such a child is to approach teaching in an aggressive manner by encouraging learning in a supportive home environment where the child can relate closely to a few people whose role is to stimulate and encourage maximum development. The individual attention, security, and sense of belonging to a family are important factors in every child's growth and development.

● Nursing Process for the Child With Cognitive Impairment

ASSESSMENT

The child who has a cognitive impairment is seen in the health care setting for diagnosis, treatment, and follow-up as well as the usual health maintenance visits. During these visits, health care personnel may be challenged to communicate with the child. A thorough interview with the child's caregiver can be helpful in learning about the child and family. Listen carefully to the caregiver, paying particular attention to any comments or concerns he or she has.

The interview and physical exam may be lengthy and detailed depending partially on the circumstances of the child's primary need for health care. Aside from the data collection needed as dictated by the current health care needs, the nurse also needs information about the child's habits, routines, and personal terminology (such as nicknames and toileting terms). Be careful to communicate at the child's level of understanding, and do not talk down to the child during the interview. Treat the child with respect. This approach helps gain cooperation from both the family and the child. Arrange the initial interview and physical exam so that they can be conducted in an unhurried atmosphere that avoids placing undue stress on the child or the family.

NURSING DIAGNOSES

The appropriate nursing diagnoses vary with the child's primary health care needs. Often the child with mental retardation also has physical disabilities that must be considered when a plan of care is being developed. Work with the child's caregiver to set realistic goals for the child. Some nursing diagnoses useful for the child with cognitive impairment are

- Self Care Deficit in Bathing/Hygiene, Dressing/Grooming, Feeding, and Toileting related to cognitive or neuromuscular impairment (or both)
- Impaired Verbal Communication related to impaired receptive or expressive skills
- Delayed Growth and Development related to physical and mental disability
- Risk for Injury related to physical or neurologic impairment (or both)
- Compromised Family Coping related to emotional stress or grief
- Risk for Social Isolation (family or child) related to fear of and embarrassment about the child's behavior or appearance

OUTCOME IDENTIFICATION AND PLANNING

The major goals for the cognitively impaired child depend entirely on the child's abilities determined during data collection and the interview. Common goals include learning self-care (within the child's ability), communicating with caregivers and nurses, reaching highest level of functioning (within the child's ability), and remaining free from injury. The goals for the family include learning new methods of working with the child, finding support and guidance, and learning about available resources.

IMPLEMENTATION

Promoting Self-Care. Teaching the mentally retarded child can be time-consuming, frustrating, challenging, and rewarding. When the child is first seen in a healthcare setting, a teaching program that reflects his or her developmental level must be designed. Be certain that all personnel who care for the child and any involved family members are aware of the program. Break each element of care to be taught into small segments and repeat those steps over and over. Patience is one of the most important aspects of teaching a mentally retarded child. Use praise generously, and give small material rewards as useful tools to aid in teaching. Challenge the child but make the immediate small goals realistic and attainable. Brushing teeth, brushing or combing the hair, bathing, washing the hands and face, feeding oneself, dressing independently, and basic safety are all self-care areas in which the child needs instruction and positive reinforcement.

Teaching the cognitively impaired child requires the same principles used in teaching any child: work at a level appropriate to the stage of the child's maturation, not the chronological age. If the child has physical disabilities in addition to retardation, the rate of physical development is also affected. One factor that makes the child with cognitive impairment different from the average child is the lack of ability to reason abstractly. This prevents transfer of learning or application of abstract principles to varied situations. Learning takes place by habit formation and emphasizing the "three Rs:" routine, repetition, and relaxation. Most cognitively impaired children increase in mental age although slowly and to a limited level. Therefore, each child needs to be watched for evidence of readiness for a new skill.

Environmental stimulation is essential for development in all children, but the cognitively impaired child needs much more environmental enrichment than the average child does. Suggested activities for providing this enrichment are summarized in Table 15–4.

TABLE 15.4	Examples of Developmental Stimulation and Sensorimotor Teaching for Retarded Infants and Young Children
Developmental Sequence	**Possible Activities to Encourage Development**
Sitting	
1. Sit with support in caretaker's lap	Hold child in sitting position on lap, supporting under armpits. Do several times a day, gradually lessening the support.
2. Sit independently when propped	Place child in sitting position against firm surface with pillow behind the back and on either side. Leave the child alone several times a day.
3. Sit with increasingly less support	Allow child to sit on equipment that provides increasingly less support such as baby swing, feeder, walker, high chair.
4. Sit in chair without assistance	Place child in a chair with arms. Provide balance support at first, then gradually withdraw. Leave for 10 minutes at a time.
5. Sit without support	Place child on floor. Gradually withdraw assistance.
Self-Feeding	
1. Sucking	Encourage child to suck by putting food on pacifier, putting a drop on tongue, and so forth.
2. Drink from a cup	Put small amount of fluid in a baby cup. Raise cup to mouth by placing hands under child.
3. Grasp piece of food and place in mouth	Place bit of favorite food in child's hand. Guide hand and food to mouth. Gradually reduce support.
4. Transfer food from spoon to mouth	Move spoon to child's mouth with hand supporting baby's. Gradually withdraw support.
5. Scoop up food and transfer to mouth	Have child hold spoon by handle, scoop up food, and transfer to mouth. Do not allow child to use fingers. Progress from bowl to flat plate.
Stimulation of Touch	
1. Body sensation	Hold, cuddle, rock child.
2. Explore environment through touch	Brush skin with objects of various textures (feathers, silk, sandpaper). Place objects of different textures near child. Move hand to object.
3. Explore environment through mouth	Give child objects that can be chewed. Guide hand to mouth at first.
4. Explore tactile sensations	Expose child to hard, soft, warm, and cold objects.
5. Explore with water	Place hands or feet in water.

Whether at home or in a health care facility, the child with cognitive impairment needs to know which behaviors are acceptable and which are unacceptable. Discipline is as important to this child as to any other. The limited ability of these children to adapt to varying circumstances makes consistent discipline essential with instructions given in simple, direct, concise language. Using a positive approach with many examples and demonstrations achieves better results than a constant stream of "don't touch" or "stop that."

Obedience is an important part of discipline especially for the child with faulty reasoning ability, but the objectives of discipline should be much broader than simply obedience. The child needs to know what to expect and finds security and support in routines and consistency. Use kindness, love, understanding, and physical comforting as a major part of discipline.

If discipline is needed, be certain it follows the misdeed immediately so that the cause-and-effect relationship is clear. Taking the child away from the group for a short time may help restore self-control. If the child is using misbehavior to get attention, praise and approval for good behavior may eliminate the need for wrongdoing.

Fostering Communication Skills. The child with cognitive impairment often has major problems with language skills. The child may have problems forming various speech sounds because of an enlarged tongue or other physical deviations, including hearing impairment. These problems can frustrate attempts at communication. In addition, the child may not be able to process the spoken word, which compounds communication problems. A speech therapist can evaluate the child and develop a program to help caregivers work with the child to improve both the child's understanding of what is said and the child's ability to use language.

Promoting Growth and Development. The child with cognitive impairment often has physical disabilities that affect growth and development. All but the most profoundly impaired children go through the sequence of normal development with delays at each stage; their abilities level off as the children reach the limits of their capabilities. A cognitively impaired child proceeds according to mental age rather than chronological age. Thus an impaired 6-year-old may be functioning on a mental level of 2 years, and the expected behavior must be essentially that of a 2-year-old. Teach the family caregivers about the important landmarks of normal growth and development to help them understand the progressive nature of maturation and to improve planning for the child.

Preventing Injury. The child with cognitive impairment has faulty reasoning ability and a short attention span. As a result, the caregivers must be responsible for protecting the child. The health care facility as well as the home must be made safe. Teach elementary safety rules and reinforce them continuously.

Promoting Family Coping. Before effective treatment can begin, the family must accept the reality of the child's problem and must want to cope with the difficult task of helping the child develop his or her full potential. Diagnosis made at birth or during the first year affords the greatest hope of early acceptance and beginning education and training.

The family's first reaction to learning that the child may have cognitive impairment is grief because this is not the perfect child of their dreams. A parent may feel shame, assuming that he or she cannot produce a perfect child. Some rejection of the child is almost inevitable at least in the initial stages, but this must be worked through for the family to cope. Some parents compensate for their early hostile feelings by overprotection or overconcern, making the child unnecessarily helpless and perhaps taking out their anger and frustration on the normal siblings. The family begins to function effectively only when the caregivers accept the child as another family member to be helped, loved, and disciplined.

Preventing Social Isolation. Family members need to know that their feelings are normal. Talking with other families of impaired children can offer some of the best support and guidance as caregivers seek information to help them deal with the problem. One group that includes both families and health care professionals is the National Association of Retarded Citizens, a volunteer organization with chapters in many communities (website *http://www.thearc.org*). The National Down Syndrome Society is another excellent resource for the family of a child with Down's syndrome (website *http://www.ndss.org*). Participating in the Special Olympics is a good way for children to begin to gain self-confidence.

EVALUATION: GOALS AND OUTCOME CRITERIA

- *Goal:* The child will develop skills to meet self-care needs within her or his ability.
  Criteria: The child practices basic hygiene habits as well as dressing/grooming, feeding, and toileting skills within his or her abilities with support and supervision.
- *Goal:* The child's communication skills will improve.
  Criteria: The child can communicate basic needs to staff and family.
- *Goal:* The child will attain the milestones of his or her stage of growth and development according to mental age and the family caregivers verbalize an understanding of the child's level of development.
  Criteria: The child attains the highest level of functioning for their mental age and the family caregivers identify the child's developmental level and set realistic goals.
- *Goal:* The child will be protected from injury by caregivers and will learn basic safety rules.
  Criteria: The child remains free from injury and cooperates with basic safety rules within his or her abilities.
- *Goal:* The family will effectively cope with the child's diagnosis.
  Criteria: The family verbalizes feelings, mourns the loss of the "perfect child," and provides appropriate care to help the child reach optimum functioning.
- *Goal:* The family will interact with social groups and support networks.
  Criteria: The family freely voices feelings and concerns about the child, makes contact with support systems, and establishes relationships with families of other cognitively impaired children.

Down's Syndrome

Down's syndrome is the most common chromosomal anomaly, occurring in about one in 700 to 800 births. Langdon Down first described the condition in 1866, but its cause was a mystery for many years. In 1932 it was suggested that a chromosomal anomaly might be the cause, but the anomaly was not demonstrated until 1959.

Down's syndrome has been observed in nearly all countries and races. The old term "mongolism" is

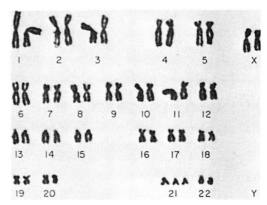

● *Figure 15.8* Karotype showing trisomy 21. Note three chromosomes in the 21 position.

inappropriate and no longer used. Most people with Down's syndrome have trisomy 21 (Fig. 15–8); a few have partial dislocation of chromosomes 15 and 21. A woman older than 35 years of age is at a greater risk of bearing a child with Down's syndrome than a younger woman, but children with Down's syndrome are born to women of all ages. Older women are more likely to choose to have an amniocentesis to determine if they are carrying a child with Down's syndrome, which may lead to a decision about abortion. The growing trend toward routine screening of all pregnant women for an elevated maternal serum alpha-fetoprotein level may reduce the number of children born with Down's syndrome because the parents will have the option to abort the pregnancy.

Clinical Manifestations

All forms of the condition show a variety of abnormal characteristics. Mental status is usually within the moderate to severe range of retardation with most children being moderately retarded. The most common anomalies include

- **Brachycephaly** (shortness of head)
- Retarded body growth
- Upward and outward slanted eyes (almond-shaped) with an epicanthic fold at the inner angle
- Short, flattened bridge of the nose
- Thick, fissured tongue
- Dry, cracked, fissured skin that may be mottled
- Dry and coarse hair
- Short hands with an incurved fifth finger
- A single horizontal palm crease (simian line)
- Wide space between the first and second toes
- Lax muscle tone (often referred to as "double jointed" by others)
- Heart and eye anomalies
- Greater susceptibility to leukemia than in the general population

Not all these physical signs are present in all people with Down's syndrome. Some may have only one or two characteristics; others may show nearly all the characteristics (Fig. 15–9).

Treatment and Care

The physical characteristics of the child with Down's syndrome determine the medical and nursing management. Lax muscles, congenital heart defects, and dry skin contribute to a large variety of problems. The child's relaxed muscle tone may contribute to respiratory complications as a result of decreased respiratory expansion. The relaxed skeletal muscles contribute to late motor development. Gastric motility is also decreased, leading to problems with constipation. Congenital heart defects and vision or hearing problems add to the complexities of the child's care.

In infancy, the child's large tongue and poor muscle tone may contribute to difficulty breast-feeding or ingesting formula and can cause great problems when the time comes to introduce solid foods. The family caregivers need support during these trying times. As the child gets older, concern about excessive weight gain becomes a primary consideration.

The family caregivers of the Down's syndrome child and other children who are cognitively impaired need strong support and guidance from the time the child is born. Early intervention programs have yielded some encouraging results, but the family must decide if they can manage the child at home. A cognitively impaired child who is undisciplined or improperly supervised may threaten the safety of others in the home and the neighborhood. Caring for the child may demand so much sacrifice from other family members that the family eventually disintegrates.

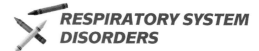

RESPIRATORY SYSTEM DISORDERS

Tonsillitis

Tonsillitis is a common illness in childhood resulting from pharyngitis. A brief description of the location and functions of the tonsils and adenoids serves as an introduction to the discussion of their infection and medical and surgical treatments.

A ring of lymphoid tissue encircles the pharynx, forming a protective barrier against upper respiratory infection. This ring consists of groups of lymphoid tonsils.

The faucial tonsils, the commonly known **tonsils,** are two oval masses attached to the side walls of the back of the mouth between the anterior and posterior pillars. The pharyngeal tonsils, known as the **adenoids,** are masses of lymphoid tissue in the nasal pharynx extending from the roof of the nasal pharynx to the free edge of the soft palate. The lingual tonsils are two masses of lymphoid tissue at the base of the tongue.

Lymphoid tissue normally enlarges progressively in childhood between the ages of 2 and 10 years and shrinks during preadolescence. If the tissue itself becomes a site of acute or chronic infection, it may become hypertrophied and can interfere with breathing, may cause partial deafness, or may become a source of infection in itself.

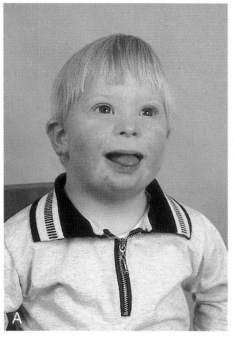
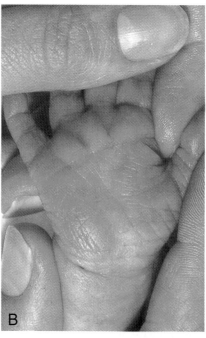

● **Figure 15.9** Typical features of a child with Down's syndrome: **(A)** facial features; **(B)** horizontal palm crease (simian line).

Clinical Manifestations and Diagnosis

The child with tonsillitis may have a fever of 101°F (38.4°C) or more, a sore throat, often with dysphagia (difficulty swallowing), hypertrophied tonsils, and erythema of the soft palate. Exudate may be visible on the tonsils. The symptoms vary somewhat with the causative organism. Throat cultures are performed to diagnose tonsillitis and the causative organism. Frequently the cause of tonsillitis is viral, although beta-hemolytic streptococcal infection also may be the cause.

Treatment

Medical treatment of tonsillitis consists of analgesics for pain, antipyretics for fever, and an antibiotic in the case of streptococcal infection. A standard 10-day course of antibiotics is recommended. Stress the importance of completing the full prescription of antibiotic to ensure that the streptococcal infection is eliminated. A soft or liquid diet is easier to swallow, and the child should be encouraged to maintain good fluid intake. A cool-mist vaporizer may be used to ease respirations.

Tonsillectomies and adenoidectomies are controversial. One can be performed independent of the other, but they are often done together. No conclusive evidence has been found that a tonsillectomy in itself improves a child's health by reducing the number of respiratory infections, increasing the appetite, or improving general well-being. Currently tonsillectomies generally are not performed unless other measures are ineffective or the tonsils are so hypertrophied that breathing and eating are difficult. Tonsillectomies are not performed while the tonsils are infected.

The adenoids are more susceptible to chronic infection. An indication for adenoidectomy is hypertrophy of the tissue to the extent of impairing hearing or interfering with breathing. Performing only an adenoidectomy if the tonsil tissue appears to be healthy is an increasingly common practice.

Tonsillectomy is postponed until after the age of 4 or 5 years except in the rare instance when it appears urgently needed. Often when a child has reached the acceptable age, the apparent need for the tonsillectomy has disappeared.

● Nursing Process for the Child Having a Tonsillectomy

ASSESSMENT

Much of the preoperative preparation, including complete blood count, bleeding and clotting time, and urinalysis, is done on a preadmission outpatient basis. In many facilities, the child is admitted on the day of surgery or the procedure is done in a day surgery setting. Psychological preparation is often accomplished through preadmission orientation. Acting out the forthcoming experience, particularly in a group, with the use of puppets, dolls, and play-doctor or play-nurse material helps the child develop security. The amount and the timing of preparation before admission depend on the child's age. The child may become frightened about losing a body part. Telling the child that the troublesome tonsils are going to be "fixed" is a much better choice than saying that they are going to be "taken out."

Include the child and the caregiver in the admission interview. Ask about any bleeding tendencies because postoperative bleeding is a concern. Carefully explain all procedures to the child, and be sensitive to the child's apprehension. Take and record vital signs to establish a baseline for postoperative monitoring. The temperature is an important part of the data collection to determine that the child has no upper respiratory infection. Observe the child for loose teeth that could cause a problem during administration of anesthesia; document findings.

NURSING DIAGNOSES

The information gathered during data collection is used to determine appropriate nursing diagnoses. Preoperative nursing diagnoses generally are those for any child undergoing a surgical procedure. Postoperative nursing diagnoses may include

- Risk for Aspiration postoperatively related to impaired swallowing and bleeding at the operative site
- Acute Pain related to surgical procedure
- Deficient Fluid Volume related to inadequate oral intake secondary to painful swallowing
- Deficient Knowledge related to caregivers understanding of post-discharge home care and signs and symptoms of complications

OUTCOME IDENTIFICATION AND PLANNING

The major postoperative goals for the child include preventing aspiration, relieving pain, and improving fluid intake especially while swallowing. The major goal for the family is to increase knowledge and understanding of post-discharge care and possible complications. Design the plan of care with these goals in mind.

IMPLEMENTATION

Preventing Aspiration Postoperatively. Immediately after a tonsillectomy, place the child in a partially prone position with head turned to one side until the child is completely awake. This position can be accomplished by turning the child partially over and by flexing the knee where the child is not resting to help maintain the position. Keeping the head slightly lower than the chest helps facilitate drainage of secretions. Avoid placing pillows under the chest and abdomen, which may hamper respiration. Encourage the child to expectorate all secretions, and place an ample supply of tissues and a waste container near him or her. Discourage the child from coughing. Check vital signs every 10 to 15 minutes until the child is fully awake, then check every 30 minutes to 1 hour. Note the child's preoperative baseline vital signs to interpret the vital signs correctly.

Hemorrhage is the most common complication of a tonsillectomy. Bleeding is most often a concern within the first 24 hours following surgery and the 5th to 7th day postoperatively. During the 24 hours after surgery, observe, document, and report any unusual restlessness or anxiety, frequent swallowing, or rapid pulse that may indicate bleeding. Vomiting dark, old blood may be expected, but bright, red-flecked emesis or oozing indicates fresh bleeding. Observe the pharynx with a flashlight each time vital signs are checked. Bleeding can occur when the clots dissolve between the 5th and 7th day postoperatively if new tissue is not yet present. Because the child is cared for at home by this time, the family should be given information concerning signs and symptoms to watch for (see Providing Family Teaching).

Providing Comfort and Relieving Pain. Apply an ice collar postoperatively; however, remove the collar if the child is uncomfortable with it. Administer pain medication as ordered. Liquid acetaminophen with codeine is often prescribed. Rectal or intravenous analgesics may be used. Encourage the caregiver to remain at the bedside to provide soothing reassurance. Crying irritates the raw throat and increases the child's discomfort; thus, it should be avoided if possible. Teach the caregiver what may be expected in drainage and signs that should be reported immediately to the nursing staff.

Encouraging Fluid Intake. When the child is fully awake from surgery, give small amounts of clear fluids or ice chips. Synthetic juices, carbonated beverages that are "flat," and juice popsicles are good choices. Avoid red liquids to eliminate confusion with bloody discharge. Also avoid irritating liquids such as orange juice and lemonade. Milk and ice cream products tend to cling to the surgical site and make swallowing more difficult; thus they are poor choices despite the old tradition of offering ice cream after a tonsillectomy. Continue administration of intravenous fluid and record intake and output until adequate oral intake is established.

Providing Family Teaching. The child is typically discharged on the day of or the day after surgery if no complications are present. Instruct the caregiver to keep the child relatively quiet for a few days after discharge. Recommend giving soft foods and nonirritating liquids for the first few days. Teach family members that if at any time following the surgery they note any signs of hemorrhage (bright red bleeding, frequent swallowing, restlessness), they should notify the care provider. Provide written instructions and phone numbers prior to discharge. Advise the caregivers that a mild earache may be expected about the third day.

EVALUATION: GOALS AND OUTCOME CRITERIA

- *Goal:* The child's airway will remain patent postoperatively.
  Criteria: The child's airway is open and clear and the child expectorates saliva and drainage with no aspiration.
- *Goal:* The child will show signs of being comfortable.
  Criteria: The child rests quietly and does not cry; pulse rate is regular and normal for age; child states that pain is lessened.
- *Goal:* The child's fluid intake will be adequate for age.
  Criteria: The child's skin turgor is good, mucous membranes are moist, and hourly urinary output is at least 20–30 mL. Parenteral fluids are maintained until the child's oral fluid intake is adequate.

- *Goal:* Family caregivers will verbalize an understanding of post-discharge care. *Criteria:* Family caregivers give appropriate responses when questioned about care at home, can state signs and symptoms of complications, and ask appropriate questions for clarification.

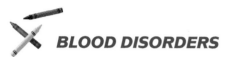

BLOOD DISORDERS

Several blood dyscrasias (abnormalities of the blood) may manifest themselves in the preschooler. Although leukemia, purpura, and hemophilia may be diagnosed at either an earlier or a later age, they are commonly associated with the preschool years. Children with these disorders are often chronically ill and require long-term care.

Acute Leukemia

Leukemia, the most common type of cancer in children, accounts for about 30% of all childhood cancers. *Acute lymphatic leukemia* (ALL) is responsible for about 70% to 75% of the childhood leukemias; *acute myeloid leukemia* (AML) for almost all the rest. Fortunately, ALL is also the most curable of all major forms of leukemia. The cure rate for AML is about 40%. The incidence of ALL is greatest between the ages of 2 and 6 years and is higher in boys; ALL is more common in white children than in African-American children. This discussion focuses on ALL.

Pathophysiology

Leukemia is the uncontrolled reproduction of deformed white blood cells. Despite intensive research, its cause is unknown. Mature leukocytes (white blood cells) are made up of three types of cells:

- **Monocytes** (5% to 10% of white blood cells) defend the body against infection.
- **Granulocytes** are divided into eosinophils, basophils, and neutrophils. Neutrophils (60% of the white blood cells) can pass through capillary walls to surround and destroy bacteria.
- **Lymphocytes** (30% of white blood cells) are divided into T cells that attack and destroy virus-infected cells, foreign tissue, and cancer cells, and B cells that produce antibodies (proteins that help destroy foreign matter).

An immature lymphocyte is called a **lymphoblast.** Leukemia occurs when lymphocytes reproduce so quickly that they are mostly in the blast, or immature, stage. This rapid increase in lymphocytes causes crowding, which in turn decreases the production of red blood cells and platelets. The decrease in red blood cells, platelets, and normal white blood cells causes the child to become easily fatigued and susceptible to infection and increased bleeding.

Clinical Manifestations

Clinical manifestations of leukemia appear with surprising abruptness in many affected children with few if any, warning signs. The symptoms result from the proliferation of lymphoblasts. Presenting manifestations are often fatigue, pallor, and low-grade fever caused by anemia. Other early or presenting symptoms are bone and joint pain caused by invasion of the periosteum by lymphocytes, widespread **petechiae** (pinpoint hemorrhages beneath the skin), and **purpura** (hemorrhages into the skin or mucous membranes) as a result of a low thrombocyte count. The lymph nodes often are enlarged.

Although they are seldom presenting signs, anorexia, nausea and vomiting, headache, diarrhea, and abdominal pain often occur during the course of the disease as a result of enlargement of the liver and spleen. Easy bruising is a constant problem. Ulceration of the gums and throat develops as a result of bacterial invasion and contributes to anorexia. Intracranial hemorrhages are not uncommon. Anemia becomes increasingly severe.

Diagnosis

In addition to the history, symptoms, and laboratory blood studies, a bone marrow aspiration must be done to confirm the diagnosis of leukemia. The preferred site for bone marrow aspiration in children is the iliac crest. Radiographs of the long bones demonstrate changes caused by the invasion of the lymphoblasts.

Treatment

The advances in the treatment of ALL have dramatically improved long-term survival. In children whose initial prognosis is good, about 90% have long-term survival. For children who have a relapse, survival rates are greatly reduced. Each succeeding relapse reduces the probability of survival.

Intensive chemotherapy is initially divided into three phases:

- *Induction*—geared to achieving a complete remission with no leukemia cells
- *Sanctuary*—preventing invasion of the central nervous system by leukemia cells (no sanctuary is given to the leukemia cells)
- *Maintenance*—maintaining the remission

A combination of drugs is used during the induction phase to bring about remission; among the drugs used are vincristine, prednisone, and asparaginase. During the sanctuary phase, **intrathecal administration** (drugs injected into the cerebrospinal fluid by lumbar puncture) of methotrexate is used to eradicate leukemia cells in the central nervous system. The maintenance phase may last 2 or 3 years and includes treatment with methotrexate, vincristine, prednisone, and 6-mercaptopurine. The drugs are often administered through a double-lumen catheter (Broviac) placed in the subclavian vein.

Two additional phases are instituted for children who suffer a relapse:

- *Reinduction*—administration of the drugs previously used plus additional drugs
- *Bone marrow transplant*—usually recommended after the second remission in children with ALL

● Nursing Process for the Child With Leukemia

ASSESSMENT

The process of collecting data on the child with leukemia varies according to the stage of the illness. Conduct the admission interview with both the family caregiver and the child. Do not allow the caregiver to monopolize the interview; give the child an opportunity to express feelings and fears and answer the questions.

The physical examination should include observing for **adenopathy** (enlarged lymph glands), abnormal vital signs (especially a low-grade fever), signs of bruising, petechiae, bleeding from or ulcerations of mucous membranes, abdominal pain or tenderness, and bone or joint pain. Observe the child for lethargic behavior, and question the caregiver about this. Note signs of local infection including edema, redness, and swelling, or any indication of systemic infection. The diagnosis of leukemia is devastating. Observe and note the child's and family's emotional states so that the nursing care plan can include helping them to discuss and resolve their feelings and fears.

NURSING DIAGNOSES

The data collected and the information gathered in the interview with both the child and the caregiver is used to develop nursing diagnoses. Some appropriate care diagnoses may be

- Risk for Infection related to increased susceptibility secondary to leukemic process and side effects of chemotherapy
- Risk for Injury related to bleeding tendencies
- Acute Pain related to the effects of chemotherapy and the disease process
- Fatigue related to disease; decreased energy and anxiety
- Delayed Growth and Development related to impaired ability to achieve developmental tasks secondary to limitations of disease and treatment
- Disturbed Body Image related to alopecia and weight loss
- Anticipatory Grieving by the family related to the prognosis

OUTCOME IDENTIFICATION AND PLANNING

Goals for the child with leukemia vary depending on individual circumstances. Preventing infection, preventing injury, relieving pain, and reducing fatigue are major goals. Other important goals for the child may be promoting normal growth and development and improving body image. The goal for the family may be to verbalize feelings and to increase coping abilities.

IMPLEMENTATION

Preventing Infection. The immune system is weakened by the uncontrolled growth of lymphoblasts that overpower the normal production of granulocytes (particularly neutrophils) and monocytes. In addition, the chemotherapy necessary to inhibit this proliferation of lymphoblasts causes immunosuppression. Thus these children are susceptible to infection especially during chemotherapy. Infections such as meningitis, septicemia, and pneumonia are the most common causes of death. The organism most often responsible is *Pseudomonas*. Other organisms that can be dangerous for the child are *Escherichia coli*, *Staphylococcus aureus*, *Klebsiella*, *Pneumocystis carinii*, *Candida albicans*, and *Histoplasmosis*. These infectious organisms can threaten the child's life.

To protect the child from infectious organisms, follow standard guidelines for protective isolation. Carefully screen staff, family, and visitors to eliminate any known infection. Enforce handwashing, gowning, and masking.

The social isolation that this imposes on the child can be difficult for the child to understand and tolerate, so spend additional time with the child beyond that necessary for direct care. Playing games, coloring, reading stories, and doing puzzles are all good activities that the child will enjoy. This also provides a much-needed break to the caregiver who may be staying with the child.

Preventing Bleeding and Injury. The mucous membranes bleed easily, so be gentle when doing oral hygiene. Use a soft, sponge-type brush or gauze strips wrapped around your finger. Mouthwash composed of one part hydrogen peroxide to four parts saline solution or normal saline solution may be used. Epistaxis (nosebleed) is a common problem that can usually be handled by applying external pressure to the nose. Apply pressure to sites of injections or venipunctures to prevent excessive bleeding. At least every 4 hours, monitor the child for other signs of bleeding such as petechiae, ecchymosis, hematemesis (bloody emesis), tarry stools, and swelling and tenderness of the joints. Protect the child from injury by external forces to prevent the possibility of hemorrhage from the injury. Take extra caution when the child's platelet count is especially low.

Reducing Pain. Pain from the invasion of lymphoblasts into the periosteum and bleeding into the joints can be excruciating. Use gentle handling: place sheepskin pads under bony prominences and position the child to help relieve discomfort and skin breakdown. Many times painful procedures must be done that add to the child's discomfort. Explain to the child that these procedures are necessary to help and are not in any way a form of punishment. Provide a pain scale to help the child rate the pain and communicate its intensity. The numeric and the faces pain rating scales are useful with children 3 years of age and older (see Fig. 4–4 in Chap. 4). Administer analgesics as ordered to achieve maximum comfort.

Promoting Energy Conservation and Relieving Anxiety. As a result of anemia, the child is fatigued. Pace procedures so that the child has as much uninterrupted rest as possible. Stress adds to the child's feelings of exhaustion; to decrease fatigue, help the child deal with the stress caused by the illness and treatments. To help relieve anxiety, encourage the child to talk about feelings and acknowledge the child's feelings as valid.

Promoting Normal Growth and Development. During treatment, the child frequently may be prevented from participating in normal activity. The social isolation that accompanies reverse isolation often interferes with normal development. Physical activities often are limited simply because of the child's lack of energy. Knowledge of normal growth and development expectations is important to consider when planning developmental activities. Stimulate growth and development within the child's physical capabilities. Stress positive developmental tasks, e.g., practicing or improving reading skills and learning or increasing computer skills. Encourage the family to help the child return to normal activities as much as possible during the treatment's maintenance phase when the child has been discharged from the hospital.

Promoting a Positive Body Image. The drugs administered in chemotherapy cause **alopecia** (loss of hair) (Fig. 15–10). Prepare the child and the family psychologically for this change in appearance. The child may want to wear a wig especially when returning to school. Encourage the family to choose the wig before chemotherapy is started so that it matches the child's hair and the child has time to get used to it. A cap or scarf often is appealing to a child, particularly if it carries a special meaning for him or her. Reassure the child and family that the hair will grow back in about 3 to 6 months. Wash the scalp regularly to avoid scaling.

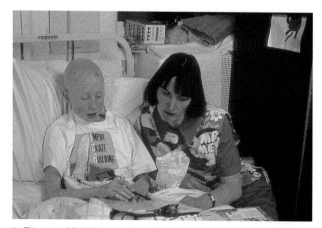

● *Figure 15.10* The child with alopecia needs support and encouragement.

Prednisone therapy may cause the child to have a moon-faced appearance, which may be upsetting to either the child or the family. Reassure them that this is temporary and will disappear when the drug is no longer needed.

The child may be hesitant for peers to see these changes. Encourage visits from peers before discharge, if possible, so that the child can be prepared to handle their reactions and questions. A schoolteacher can be invaluable in preparing classmates to welcome the child back with minimal reaction to the child's physical changes. Encourage the family to enlist the assistance of the child's teacher, school nurse, and pediatrician to ease the transition. Meeting other children who are undergoing chemotherapy and are in various stages of recovery often is helpful to the child and helps to relieve the feeling that no one else has ever looked like this. Provide the child and the family opportunities to express their feelings and apprehensions.

Promoting Family Coping. Family members often are devastated when they first learn that their child has leukemia. Provide support from the moment of the first diagnosis, through the hospitalization, and continuing through the maintenance phase. Family members live one day at a time, hoping that the remission will not end and that their child will be one who does not have a relapse and is finally considered cured. Provide opportunities for family members to freely express their feelings about the illness and treatment. The family will find comfort and stability in having one nurse caring for the child consistently. Involve the caregivers in the care of the child during hospitalization, and give them complete information about what to expect when caring for the child at home during the maintenance phase. Identify a contact person for the family to call to answer questions during this phase. Help the family work through feelings of overprotectiveness toward the child so that the child can lead as normal a life as possible.

Encourage the family to consider how siblings can fit into the child's return home. Siblings may have many questions about the seriousness of the illness and about the possible death of their brother or sister. Provide support for families to deal with these concerns. Most hospitals that provide care for pediatric oncology patients have caregiver support groups that meet regularly. Candlelighters is a national organization for parents

of young cancer patients (website *http://www.candlelighters.org*).

EVALUATION: GOALS AND OUTCOME CRITERIA

- *Goal:* The child will remain free of signs and symptoms of infection.
  Criteria: The child's temperature does not exceed 100°F (37.88C), there is no inflammation, discharge, or other signs of infection.
- *Goal:* The child will remain free from injury related to bleeding.
  Criteria: The child has no signs of petechiae, ecchymosis, hematemesis, tarry stools, and swelling and tenderness of the joints.
- *Goal:* The child will show signs of being comfortable.
  Criteria: The child rests quietly and uses a pain scale to indicate that the pain is at a tolerable level.
- *Goal:* The child's energy level will be maintained or will increase.
  Criteria: The child participates in activities and procedures paced so that the child has adequate rest periods. The child expresses anxieties.
- *Goal:* The child will accomplish appropriate growth and development milestones within the limits of the condition.
  Criteria: The child is involved in age-appropriate activities provided by staff and family.
- *Goal:* The child will accept changes in physical appearance.
  Criteria: The child shows pride and adjustment in changes in body image and shares feelings about body image changes.
- *Goal:* The family will verbalize feelings and develops coping mechanisms.
  Criteria: The family expresses feelings and fears about the child's prognosis and accepts counseling and support as needed.

Idiopathic Thrombocytopenic Purpura

Purpura is a blood disorder associated with a deficit of platelets in the circulatory system. The most common type of purpura is idiopathic thrombocytopenic purpura (ITP). Purpura is preceded by a viral infection in about half the diagnosed cases.

Clinical Manifestations and Diagnosis

The onset of ITP is often acute. Bruising and a generalized rash occur. In severe cases, hemorrhage may occur in the mucous membranes; hematuria or difficult-to-control epistaxis may be present. Rarely the serious complication of intracranial hemorrhage occurs. In most cases, symptoms disappear in a few weeks without serious hemorrhage. A few cases may continue in a chronic form of the disease.

In ITP, the platelet count may be 20,000/mm^3 (normal 150,000 to 300,000/mm^3) or lower. The bleeding time is prolonged, and the clot retraction time is abnormal. The white blood cell count remains normal, and anemia is not present unless excessive bleeding has occurred.

Treatment and Nursing Care

Corticosteroids are useful in reducing the severity and shortening the duration of the disease in some, but not all, cases of ITP. Intravenous gamma globulin has been used to increase the production of platelets until recovery occurs spontaneously. If the platelet count is higher than 20,000/mm^3, treatment may be delayed to see if a spontaneous remission will occur.

Nursing care consists of protecting the child from falls and trauma, observing for signs of external or internal bleeding, and providing a regular diet and general supportive care.

Hemophilia

Hemophilia is one of the oldest known hereditary diseases. Recent research has demonstrated that hemophilia is a syndrome of several distinct inborn errors of metabolism; all result in the delayed coagulation of blood. Defects in protein synthesis lead to deficiencies in any of the factors in the blood plasma needed for thromboplastic activity. The principal factors involved are factors VIII, IX, and XI.

Mechanism of Clot Formation

The mechanism of clot formation is complex. In a simplified form, it can best be described as occurring in three stages:

1. Prothrombin is formed through plasma-platelet interaction.
2. Prothrombin is converted to thrombin.
3. Fibrinogen is converted into fibrin by thrombin.

Fibrin forms a mesh that traps red and white blood cells and platelets into a clot, closing the defect in the injured vessel. A deficiency in one of the thromboplastin precursors may lead to hemophilia. This progression of events is shown in Figure 15–11. Refer to a specialized text on the circulatory system for a detailed discussion of the clot-forming mechanism.

Clinical Manifestations

Hemophilia is characterized by prolonged bleeding with frequent hemorrhages externally and into the skin, the joint spaces, and the intramuscular tissues. Bleeding from tooth extractions, brain hemorrhages, and crippling disabilities are serious complications. Death during infancy or early childhood is not unusual in severe hemophilia and results from a great loss of blood, intracranial bleeding, or respiratory obstruction caused by bleeding into the neck tissues.

An infant with hemophilia who is beginning to creep or walk bruises easily, and serious hemorrhages may result from minor lacerations. Bleeding often occurs from lip biting or from sharp objects put in the mouth. Tooth eruption seldom causes bleeding, but extractions require specialized handling and should be avoided by preventive care if possible. However, family caregivers must avoid overprotecting the child. The preschooler is active and plays hard, and injuries are practically unavoidable.

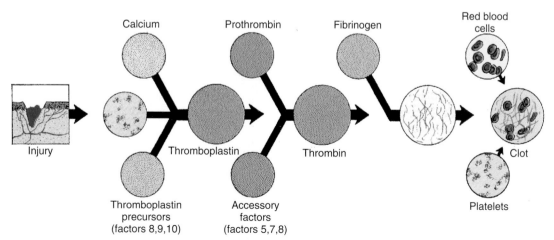

● **Figure 15.11** The mechanism of the formation of a blood clot is complex.

Clinical manifestations in any type of hemophilia are similar and are treated by administration of the deficient factor and by measures to prevent or treat complications. In severe bleeding, the quantities of fresh blood or frozen plasma needed may easily overload the circulatory system. Administration of factor VIII concentrate eliminates this problem.

Diagnosis

A careful examination of the family history and the type of bleeding present is conducted. Abnormal bleeding beginning in infancy when combined with a positive family history suggests hemophilia. A markedly prolonged clotting time is characteristic of severe factor VIII or IX deficiency, but mild conditions may have only a slightly prolonged clotting time. The partial prothrombin time is the test that most clearly demonstrates that factor VIII is low.

Common Types of Hemophilia

The two most common types of hemophilia are factor VIII deficiency and factor IX deficiency. These two types are briefly presented here.

Factor VIII Deficiency (Hemophilia A; Antihemophilic Globulin Deficiency; Classic Hemophilia). Classic hemophilia is inherited as a sex-linked recessive mendelian trait with transmission to affected males by carrier females. Hemophilia A (classic hemophilia), the most common type, occurs in about one in 10,000 people and is also the most severe. It is caused by a deficiency of antihemophilic globulin C, which is the factor VIII necessary for blood clotting.

Factor IX Deficiency (Hemophilia B; Plasma Thromboplastin Component Deficiency; Christmas Disease). Christmas disease was named after a 5-year-old boy who was one of the first patients diagnosed with a deficiency of factor IX. This deficiency constitutes about 15% of the hemophilias. It is a sex-linked recessive trait appearing in male offspring of carrier females and is caused by a deficiency of one of the necessary thromboplastin precursors, factor IX, the plasma thromboplastin component. Hemophilia B is indistinguishable from classic hemophilia in its clinical manifestations, particularly in its severe form. It also may exist in a mild form, probably more commonly than in hemophilia A.

In either hemophilia A or B, 25% or more of the affected people can trace no family history of the disease; it is assumed that spontaneous mutations have occurred in some cases.

Treatment

For many years, the only treatment for bleeding in hemophilia was the use of fresh blood or plasma. When fresh-frozen plasma came into use, it became the mainstay in hemophilia management. It has been particularly helpful in emergencies. Frozen plasma does, however, have several shortcomings. One major problem has been the large volumes needed to control bleeding. Another is the danger that injections of large amounts of plasma may lead to congestive heart failure. In addition, plasma must be given within 30 minutes because factor VIII loses its potency at room temperature.

Commercial preparations now are available that supply higher-potency factor VIII than previous preparations. These concentrates are supplied in dried form together with diluent for reconstitution. Directions for mixing and administration are included with the package. The preparations can be stored for a long time but have the disadvantage of exposing the recipient to a large number of donors. A synthetic preparation, DDAVP (1-deamino-8-D-arginine vasopressin), is used in mild factor VIII deficiencies and von Willebrand disease. Von Willebrand Disease (Vascular Hemophilia; Pseudohemophilia) is classified with the hemophilias. It is a mendelian dominant trait present in both sexes and is characterized by prolonged bleeding times.

One of the serious problems with using blood products of any kind has been the risk of exposure to hepatitis B and human immunodeficiency virus (HIV), the causative organism of acquired immunodeficiency syndrome (AIDS). Currently blood is screened thoroughly for viral contamination, which greatly diminishes the danger of HIV transmission. However, large numbers of hemophiliacs treated before the late 1980s were exposed to HIV and now test positive for HIV antibodies. Researchers continue to explore new ways to replace the missing factor while protecting the recipient from the threat of contracting an unknown illness.

● Nursing Process for the Child With Hemophilia

ASSESSMENT

Begin the nursing data collection by reviewing the child's history with the caregiver. Include previous episodes of bleeding, the usual treatment, medications the child takes, and the current episode of bleeding. Include the child in the interview if he or she is old enough to answer questions. Carefully observe the child for any signs of bleeding. Inspect the mucous membranes, examine the joints for tenderness and swelling, and check the skin for evidence of bruising. Question the child or caregiver about hematuria, hematemesis, headache, or black tarry stools.

NURSING DIAGNOSES

After data collection and the child's and family caregiver's interview, the information gathered is used to determine appropriate nursing diagnoses such as

- Acute Pain related to joint swelling and limitations secondary to hemarthrosis
- Impaired Physical Mobility related to pain and tenderness of joints
- Risk for Injury related to hemorrhage secondary to trauma
- Deficient Knowledge related to condition, treatments, and hazards
- Compromised Family Coping related to treatment and care of the child

OUTCOME IDENTIFICATION AND PLANNING

Use the information gathered to set goals with the cooperation and input of the caregiver and the child. The major goals for the child include stopping the bleeding, decreasing pain, increasing mobility, and preventing injury. The family goals include increasing knowledge about the child's condition and care and helping the family learn to cope with the disease condition.

IMPLEMENTATION

Relieving Pain. Bleeding into the joint cavities often occurs after some slight injury and seems nearly unavoidable if the child is allowed to lead a normal life. Extreme pain is caused by the pressure of the confined fluid in the narrow joint spaces and requires the use of sedatives or narcotics. Promptly immobilize the involved extremity to prevent contractures of soft tissues and the destruction of the bone and joint tissues. Immobilization helps to relieve pain and decrease bleeding. A bivalve plaster cast may be applied in the hospital to immobilize the affected part. Do not administer aspirin (or drugs containing aspirin) or other nonsteroidal anti-inflammatory drugs (NSAIDs), such as indomethacin, because of the danger of prolonging bleeding. Conversely ibuprofen, also an NSAID, has been proven safe for these children. Use of cold packs to stop bleeding is acceptable. The affected limb may be elevated above the level of the heart to slow blood flow. Use age-appropriate diversionary activities to help the child deal with the pain. Handle the affected joints carefully to prevent additional pain.

Preventing Joint Contractures. Passive range-of-motion exercises help prevent the development of joint contractures. Do not use them, however, after an acute episode because stretching of the joint capsule may cause bleeding. Encourage the child to do active range-of-motion exercises because he or she can recognize his or her own pain tolerance. Many patients who have had repeated episodes of **hemarthrosis** (bleeding into the joints) develop functional impairment of the joints despite careful treatment. Use splints and devices to position the limb in a functional position. Physical therapy is helpful after the bleeding episode is under control. Joint contractures are a serious risk, so make every effort to avoid them.

Preventing Injury. The child with hemophilia is continuously at risk for additional injury. Protect the child from trauma caused by necessary procedures. Limit invasive procedures as much as possible; if possible, collect blood samples by a finger stick. Avoid intramuscular injections. When an invasive procedure must be done, compress the site for 5 minutes or longer after the procedure, and apply cold compresses.

Remove any sharp objects from the child's environment. If the child is young, pad the crib sides to prevent bumping and bruising. Examine toys for sharp edges and hard surfaces. Soft toys are best for the young child. For mouth care, use a soft toothbrush or sponge-type brush to decrease the danger of bleeding gums. During daily hygiene, trim the nails to prevent scratching and give adequate skin care to prevent irritation.

Providing Family Teaching. Provide the family with a thorough explanation of hemophilia or reinforce information they already have. Review the family's knowledge about the disease and give additional information when needed. A child with hemophilia is healthy between bleeding episodes, but the fact that bleeding may occur as the result of slight trauma or often without any known injury causes considerable anxiety. For an unknown reason, bleeding episodes are more common in the spring and fall. Some evidence indicates that emotional stress can initiate bleeding episodes.

Topical fluoride applications to the teeth are particularly important in these children. Pay particular attention to proper oral hygiene, a well-balanced diet, and proper dental treatment, and teach the family about these considerations. Advise the family to select a dentist who understands the problems presented and who will set up an appropriate program of preventive dentistry.

Discuss safety measures for the home and the child's lifestyle. A young child may need a protective helmet and elbow and kneepads for everyday wear, especially when first becoming mobile. When possible, carpeting in the home helps to soften the falls of a toddler just learning to walk. An older child may need to wear the protective devices when playing outdoors. Playground areas can be treacherous for these children, but the child can participate in normal play activities within reason.

Instruct the family about medications, range-of-motion exercises, emergency measures to stop or limit bleeding, and all aspects of the child's care. Emergency splints should be kept in the home of every person with hemophilia. Ice packs also should be available for instant use. If possible, the bleeding area can be raised above the level of the heart. Before leaving for the health care facility, the caregiver should apply a splint and cold packs and give factor replacement according to the protocol established with the child's physician.

The family experiences continuous anxiety over how much activity to allow their child, how to keep from overprotecting him or her, and how to help the child achieve a healthy mental attitude, all the while preventing mishaps that may cause serious bleeding episodes. They must guide the child toward autonomy and independence within the framework of necessary limitations. At times, the emotional effects of social deprivation and restrained activity must be weighed against possible physical harm.

The financial strain on the family is considerable as it is with most families with a child who has a chronic condition. Children who have had several episodes of hemarthrosis may be disabled to the extent of needing crutches and braces or wheelchairs. Measures toward rehabilitation require hospitalization with possible surgery, casts, and other orthopedic appliances.

A hemophiliac child usually loses much school time. Any child who must frequently interrupt schooling for whatever reason experiences a considerable setback. Each child should be considered individually and provided with as normal an environment as possible.

Promoting Family Coping. Both the child and family must accept the limitations and yet realize the importance of having normal social experiences. School, health, and community agencies can offer the family counseling and encouragement and can help them raise the affected child in a healthy manner, both emotionally and physically. The National Hemophilia Foundation is a resource for services and publications (website *http://www.hemophilia.org*). Give the family information about other available support systems.

Review all these concerns with the family. Through discussion, questions, and demonstrations, confirm that the family understands the information provided. Counseling may be required for the family to learn to cope with the child's needs. Encourage family members to express their feelings about the impact the disease has on their lifestyle. The family may fear that the child will die from hemorrhaging. Guilt may play an important part in the family's reactions to the child. Recognizing and validating these feelings are important aspects of active listening. During hospitalization, involve the family in the child's care so they can learn how to help the child without causing additional pain.

EVALUATION: GOALS AND OUTCOME CRITERIA

- *Goal:* The child will experience diminished pain.
  Criteria: The child rests quietly with minimal pain as evidenced by the child using a pain scale to report decreased pain.
- *Goal:* The child will move freely with minimal pain.
  Criteria: There is no evidence of new joint contractures. The child maintains range of motion.
- *Goal:* The child will be protected from any new injuries.
  Criteria: The child is free from injuries or bleeding episodes caused as a result of procedures, treatments, or unsafe environment.

- *Goal:* The family caregivers will verbalize an understanding of the disease, injury prevention, and care of the child.
  Criteria: The family caregivers can list five safety measures to decrease the possibilities of injury to the child. The family can explain the disease and the child's home care and ask and answer appropriate questions.
- *Goal:* The family caregivers will develop appropriate coping mechanisms.
  Criteria: The family members express their feelings and demonstrate good coping mechanisms such as seeking help from appropriate support systems.

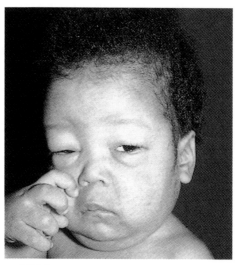

● *Figure 15.12* A child with nephrotic syndrome. Note the edema around the eyes.

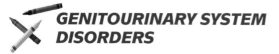

GENITOURINARY SYSTEM DISORDERS

Nephrotic Syndrome

Several different types of nephrosis have been identified in the nephrotic syndrome. The most common type in children is called *lipoid nephrosis, idiopathic nephrotic syndrome,* or *minimal change nephrotic syndrome* (MCNS). All forms of nephrosis have early characteristics of edema and proteinuria; therefore, definite clinical differentiation cannot be made early in the disease.

Nephrotic syndrome has a course of remissions and exacerbations that usually last for months. The recovery rate is generally good with the use of intensive steroid therapy and protection against infection.

The cause of MCNS is unknown. In rare cases, it is associated with other specific diseases. The nephrotic syndrome is present in as many as seven children per 100,000 population younger than 9 years of age. The average age of onset is 2.5 years with most cases occurring between the ages of 2 and 6 years.

Clinical Manifestations

Edema is usually the presenting symptom, appearing first around the eyes and ankles (Fig. 15–12). As the swelling advances, the edema becomes generalized with a pendulous abdomen full of fluid. Respiratory embarrassment may be severe, and edema of the scrotum on the male is characteristic. The edema shifts when the child changes position when lying quietly or walking about. Anorexia, irritability, and loss of appetite develop. Malnutrition may become severe. However, the generalized edema masks the loss of body tissue, causing the child to present a chubby appearance and to double his or her weight. After diuresis, the malnutrition becomes quite apparent. These children are usually susceptible to infection, and repeated acute respiratory conditions are the usual pattern. This is intensified by the immunosuppression caused by the administration of prednisone.

Diagnosis

Laboratory findings include marked proteinuria, especially albumin, with large numbers of hyaline and granular casts in the urine. Hematuria is not usually present, although a few red blood cells may appear in the urine. The blood serum protein level is reduced, and there is an increase in the level of cholesterol in the blood (**hyperlipidemia**).

Treatment

The management of nephrotic syndrome is a long process with remissions and recurrence of symptoms common. The use of corticosteroids has induced remissions in most cases and has reduced recurrences. Corticosteroid therapy usually produces diuresis in about 7 to 14 days, but the drug is continued until a remission occurs. Prednisone is the drug most commonly used. After the diuresis occurs, intermittent therapy is continued every other day or for 3 days a week. Daily urine testing for protein is continued whether the child is at home or in the hospital.

Diuretics may not be necessary when diuresis can be induced with steroids. Diuretics have not been effective in reducing the edema of nephrotic syndrome, although a loop diuretic (furosemide) may be administered if the edema causes respiratory embarrassment.

Immunosuppressant therapy may be used to reduce symptoms and prevent further relapses in children who do not respond adequately to corticosteroids. Cyclophosphamide (Cytoxan) is the drug most commonly used. Because cyclophosphamide has serious side effects, the family caregivers must be fully informed before therapy is started. **Leukopenia** (leukocyte count less than 5,000/mm^3) can be expected as well as the other common side effects of immunosuppressant therapy such as gastrointestinal symptoms, hematuria, and alopecia. The length of therapy is usually a brief period of 2 or 3 months.

A general diet is recommended that appeals to the child's poor appetite with frequent, small feedings if necessary. The addition of salt is discouraged. Family caregivers need encouragement and support for the long months ahead. Relapses usually become less frequent as the child gets older.

● Nursing Process for the Child With Nephrotic Syndrome

ASSESSMENT

Observe for edema when performing the physical examination of the child with nephrotic syndrome. Weigh the child and record the abdominal measurements to serve as a baseline. Obtain vital signs including blood pressure. Note any swelling about the eyes or the ankles and other dependent parts, and record the degree of pitting. Inspect the skin for pallor, irritation, or breakdown. Examine the scrotal area of the young boy for swelling, redness, and irritation. Question the caregiver about the onset of symptoms, the child's appetite, urine output, and signs of fatigue or irritability.

NURSING DIAGNOSES

After data collection and the child's and family caregiver's interview, the information gathered is used to determine appropriate nursing diagnoses to include the needs of the child and family. Among the nursing diagnoses that may be included are
- Excess Fluid Volume related to fluid accumulation in tissues and third spaces
- Risk for Imbalanced Nutrition: Less than Body Requirements related to anorexia
- Risk for Impaired Skin Integrity related to edema
- Fatigue related to edema and disease process

- Risk for Infection related to immunosuppression
- Deficient Caregiver Knowledge related to disease process, treatment and home care
- Compromised Family Coping related to care of a child with chronic illness

OUTCOME IDENTIFICATION AND PLANNING

The major goals for the child with nephrotic syndrome are relieving edema, improving nutritional status, maintaining skin integrity, conserving energy, and preventing infection. The family goals include learning about the disease and treatments as well as learning ways to cope with the child's long-term care. Design the nursing care plan to include all these goals.

Monitoring Fluid Intake and Output. Accurately monitor and document intake and output. Weigh the child at the same time every day on the same scale in the same clothing. Measure the child's abdomen daily at the level of the umbilicus, and make certain that all staff personnel measure at the same level. Note the desired location for measuring on the nursing care plan so that everyone follows the same practice. The abdomen may be greatly enlarged with **ascites** (edema in the peritoneal cavity). The abdomen can even become marked with **striae** (stretch marks). Test the urine regularly for albumin and specific gravity. Albumin can be tested with reagent strips dipped into the urine and read by comparison with a color chart on the container.

Improving Nutritional Intake. Although the child may look plump, underneath the edema is a thin, possibly malnourished child. The child's appetite is poor for several reasons:
- The ascites diminishes the appetite because of the full feeling in the abdomen.
- The child may be lethargic, apathetic, and simply not interested in eating.
- A no-added-salt diet may be unappealing to the child.
- Corticosteroid therapy may decrease the appetite.

Offer a visually appealing and nutritious diet. Consult the child and the family to learn which foods are appealing to the child. Cater to the child's wishes as much as possible to perk up a lagging appetite. A dietitian can help to plan appealing meals for the child. Serving six small meals may help increase the child's total intake better than the customary three meals a day.

Promoting Skin Integrity. The child's skin is stretched with edema and becomes thin and fragile. Inspect all skin surfaces regularly for breakdown. Because the child is lethargic, turn and position the child every 2 hours. Protect skin surfaces from pressure by means of pillows and padding. Protect overlapping skin surfaces from rubbing by careful placement of cotton gauze. Bathe the child regularly. Thoroughly wash the skin surfaces that touch each other with soap and water and dry them completely. A sheer dusting of cornstarch may be soothing. If the scrotum is edematous, use a soft cotton support to provide comfort.

Promoting Energy Conservation. Bed rest is common during the edema stage of the condition. The child rarely protests because of his or her fatigue. The sheer bulk of the edema makes movement difficult. When diuresis occurs several days after beginning prednisone, the child may be allowed more activity, but balance the activity with rest periods and encourage the child to rest when fatigued. Plan quiet, age-appropriate activities that interest the child. Most children love having someone read to them. Coloring books, dominoes, puzzles, and some kinds of computer and board games are quiet activities that many children enjoy. Involve the family in providing some of these activities. Avoid using television excessively as a diversion.

Preventing Infection. The child with nephrotic syndrome is especially at risk for respiratory infections because the edema and the corticosteroid therapy lower the body's defenses. Protect the child from anyone with an infection: staff, family, visitors, and other children. Handwashing and strict medical asepsis are essential. Monitor vital signs every 4 hours and observe for any early signs of infection.

Providing Family Teaching and Support. Children with nephrotic syndrome are usually hospitalized for diagnosis, thorough evaluation of their general health and specific condition, and institution of therapy. If the child has an infection, a course of antibiotic therapy may be given; unless unforeseen complications develop, the child is discharged with complete instructions for management. Provide a written plan to help family caregivers follow the program successfully. They must keep a careful record of home treatment for the health care provider to review at regular intervals.

Teach the family caregivers about reactions that may occur with the use of steroids and the adverse effects of abruptly discontinuing these drugs. If the family understands these aspects well, the incidence of forgetting to give the medication or of neglecting to refill the prescription may be reduced or eliminated. Encourage the family caregivers to report promptly any symptoms that they think are caused by the medication.

Teach the family that the necessary special care is important to keep the child in optimum health, and that **intercurrent infections** (those occurring during the course of an already existing disease) must be reported promptly. Also teach the family that exacerbations are common and that they need to understand these will probably occur. Stress the information that they should report including rapidly increasing weight, increased proteinuria, or signs of infections. Any of these may be a reason for altering the therapeutic regimen or changing the specific antibiotic agents used.

Provide the family caregivers with home care information appropriate for any chronically ill child. Bed rest is not indicated except during an intercurrent illness. Activity is restricted only by edema, which may slow the child down considerably; otherwise, normal activity is beneficial. Sufficient food intake may be a problem as in other types of chronic illness. Fortunately there are usually no food restrictions, and the appetite can be tempted by attractive, appealing foods.

As the name implies, MCNS causes few changes in the kidneys; these children have a good prognosis. Complications from kidney damage alter the course of treatment. Failure to achieve satisfactory diuresis or the need to discontinue steroids because of adverse reactions requires a reevaluation of treatment. The presence of gross hematuria suggests renal damage. In a few children, the persistence of abnormal urinary findings after diuresis presents a less hopeful outlook. A child who has frequent relapses lasting into adolescence or adulthood may develop renal failure and eventually be a candidate for a kidney transplant.

EVALUATION: GOALS AND OUTCOME CRITERIA

- *Goal:* The child's edema will be decreased.
  Criteria: The child has appropriate weight loss and decreased abdominal girth.
- *Goal:* The child will have an adequate nutritional intake to meet normal growth needs.
  Criteria: The child eats 80% or more of his or her meals.
- *Goal:* The child's skin integrity will be maintained.
  Criteria: The child's skin remains free of breakdown with no redness or irritation.
- *Goal:* The child's energy will be conserved.
  Criteria: The child rests as needed and engages in quiet diversional activities.
- *Goal:* The child will be free from signs and symptoms of infection.
  Criteria: The child has normal vital signs with no respiratory or gastrointestinal symptoms.
- *Goal:* The family caregivers will verbalize an understanding of the disease process, treatment and the child's home care needs.
  Criteria: The family can explain nephrotic syndrome and can describe aspects of medications given. They state signs and symptoms of infection, discuss home care, and ask and answer appropriate questions.

- *Goal:* The family caregivers will verbalize feelings and concerns.
  Criteria: The family verbalizes feelings and concerns related to caring for a child with a chronic illness; the family receives adequate support.

Acute Glomerulonephritis

Acute glomerulonephritis is a condition that appears to be an allergic reaction to a specific infection, most often group A beta-hemolytic streptococcal infection as in rheumatic fever. The antigen-antibody reaction causes a response that blocks the glomeruli, permitting red blood cells and protein to escape into the urine. Acute glomerulonephritis has a peak incidence in children 6 and 7 years of age and occurs twice as often in boys. The disease is discussed in this chapter so that it can be compared with nephrotic syndrome (Table 15–5). The prognosis is usually excellent, but a few children develop chronic nephritis.

Clinical Manifestations

Presenting symptoms appear 1 to 3 weeks after the onset of a streptococcal infection such as strep throat, otitis media, tonsillitis, or impetigo. Usually the presenting symptom is grossly bloody urine. The caregiver may describe the urine as smoky or bloody.

TABLE 15.5	**Comparison of Features of Acute Glomerulonephritis and Nephrotic Syndrome**	
Assessment Factor	**Acute Glomerulonephritis**	**Nephrotic Syndrome**
Cause	Immune reaction to group A β-hemolytic streptococcal infection	Idiopathic; possibly a hypersensitivity reaction
Onset	Abrupt	Insidious
Hematuria	Grossly bloody	Rare
Proteinuria	3+ or 4+ but not massive	Massive
Edema	Mild	Extreme
Hypertension	Marked	Mild
Hyperlipidemia	Rare or mild	Marked
Peak age frequency	5–10 y	2–3 y
Interventions	Limited activity; antihypertensives as needed; symptomatic therapy if congestive heart failure occurs	Bed rest during edema stage Corticosteroid administration Possible cyclophosphamide administration
Diet	Normal for age; no added salt if child is hypertensive	Nutritious for age; no added salt; small, frequent meals may be desirable
Prevention	Prevention through treatment of group A β-hemolytic streptococcal infections	None known
Course	Acute: up to 2–3 weeks	Chronic: may have relapses

Adapted from Pillitteri A. (2003) *Maternal and child health nursing* (4th ed.). Philadelphia: Lippincott Williams & Wilkins.

Periorbital edema may accompany or precede hematuria. Fever may be 103° to 104°F (39.4° to 40°C) at the onset but decreases in a few days to about 100°F (37.8°C). Slight headache and malaise are usual, and vomiting may occur. Hypertension appears in 60% to 70% of patients during the first 4 or 5 days. Both hematuria and hypertension disappear within 3 weeks.

Oliguria (production of a subnormal volume of urine) is usually present, and the urine has a high specific gravity and contains albumin, red and white blood cells, and casts. The blood urea nitrogen and serum creatinine levels and the sedimentation rates are elevated.

Cerebral symptoms consisting mainly of headache, drowsiness, convulsions, and vomiting occur in connection with hypertension in a few cases. When the blood pressure is reduced, these symptoms disappear. Cardiovascular disturbance may be revealed in electrocardiogram tracings, but few children have clinical signs. In most children, this condition is short-term; in some children, it progresses to congestive heart failure.

Treatment

Although the child usually feels well in a few days, activities should be limited until the clinical manifestations subside generally 2 to 4 weeks after the onset. Penicillin may be given during the acute stage to eradicate any existing infection; however, it does not affect the recovery from the disease because the condition is an immunologic response. The diet is generally not restricted, but additional salt may be limited if edema is excessive. Treatment of complications is symptomatic.

Nursing Care

Bed rest should be maintained until acute symptoms and gross hematuria have disappeared. The child must be protected from chilling and contact with people with infections. When the child is allowed out of bed, he or she must not become fatigued.

Urinary output should be monitored closely and recorded. The child must be weighed daily at the same time on the same scale in the same clothes. The amount of fluid the child is allowed may be based on output as well as on evidence of continued hypertension and oliguria. Fluid intake should be carefully recorded; special attention is needed to keep the intake within prescribed limits.

Blood pressure should be monitored regularly using the same arm and a properly fitting cuff. If hypertension develops, a diuretic may help reduce the blood pressure to normal levels. An antihypertensive drug may be added if the diastolic pressure is 90 mm Hg or higher. The urine must be tested regularly for protein and hematuria using dipstick tests.

Traces of protein in the urine may persist for months after the acute symptoms disappear, and an elevated Addis count indicating red blood cells in the urine persists as well. Family caregivers must learn to test for urinary protein routinely. If the urinary signs persist for more than 1 year, the disease has probably assumed a chronic form.

KEY POINTS

- The preschooler may view any illness as punishment for wrongdoing and must be reassured that this is not so.
- The preschooler can begin to understand simple explanations.
- Fear of bodily harm is common, so the child needs to be reassured about necessary procedures. Allowing the child to handle the equipment and act out procedures with dolls when possible can be helpful. Nurses must choose their words carefully so that the child does not misunderstand the explanation and perceive it as threatening.
- Magical thinking can cause anxieties and fears that are real to the child. Nurses must be alert for these perceptions so they can help the child acknowledge and deal with them.
- Encouraging and involving the child in bathing, dressing, feeding, and other activities of daily living can help preserve his or her developing independence.
- Many children are affected by hearing disabilities. The disability can range from mild to severe and can affect the child's speech development, social development, and learning.
- When working with a mentally retarded child, the nurse must be aware of the child's cognitive level and adjust the care plan accordingly.
- Illnesses that require isolation procedures either to protect the child (as in leukemia and nephrotic syndrome) or to prevent infection of other children (as in infectious diseases) cause feelings of rejection and separation. Thoughtful nursing care can decrease the trauma that children suffer when they are isolated for any reason.

REFERENCES

1. Ansel BM, Landa RM, Luethke LE. (1999) Development and disorders of speech, language and hearing. In *Oski's pediatrics: Principles and practice* (3rd ed). Philadelphia: Lippincott Williams & Wilkins.

BIBLIOGRAPHY

Accardo PJ, Capute AJ. (1999) Mental retardation. In *Oski's pediatrics: Principles and practice* (3rd ed). Philadelphia: Lippincott Williams & Wilkins.

American Psychiatric Association. (2000) *Diagnostic and statistical manual of mental disorders text revision* (4th ed). Washington, DC: APA.

Ecklund CR, Ross C. (2001) Over-the-counter medication use in preschool children. *Journal of Pediatric Health Care,* 15(4), 168.

Hagerman RJ. (1999) *Neurodevelopmental disorders: Diagnosis and treatment.* New York: Oxford University Press.

Naslund J. (2001) Modes of sensory stimulation. *Physiotherapy* 87(8), 13–23.

North American Nursing Diagnosis Association. (2001) *NANDA nursing diagnoses: Definitions and classification 2001–2002.* Philadelphia: NANDA.

Pillitteri A. (2003) *Maternal and child health nursing* (4th ed). Philadelphia: Lippincott Williams & Wilkins.

Sparks S, Taylor C. (2001) *Nursing diagnosis reference manual* (*5th ed*). Springhouse, PA: Springhouse Corporation.

(2000) *Springhouse nurse's drug guide* (3rd ed). Springhouse, PA: Springhouse Corporation.

Thomas D, Gaslin T. (2001) "Camping Up": Self-esteem in children with hemophilia. *Issues in Comprehensive Pediatric Nursing,* 24(4), 253.

VanRiper M, Cohen W. (2001) Caring for children with Down's syndrome and their families. *Journal of Pediatric Health Care,* 15(3), 123.

Wong DL. (1998) *Whaley and Wong's nursing care of infants and children* (6th ed). St. Louis: Mosby.

Wong DL, Perry S, Hockenberry M. (2002) *Maternal child nursing care* (2nd ed). St. Louis: Mosby.

Wong DL, Hess C. (2000) *Wong and Whaley's clinical manual of pediatric nursing* (5th ed). St. Louis: Mosby.

Websites

Reyes Syndrome: *http://www.reyessyndrome.org*
Mental Retardation: *www.aamr.org*
Hearing Loss: *www.johntracyclinic.org*
Hemophilia: *www.hemophilia.org*

Workbook

NCLEX-STYLE REVIEW QUESTIONS

1. A nurse admits a child with a diagnosis of possible leukemia. Of the following signs and symptoms, which would MOST likely be seen in the child with leukemia?

   a. Low grade fever, bone and joint pain

   b. High fever, sore throat

   c. Swelling around eyes, ankles, and abdomen

   d. Upward and outward slanted eyes

2. In planning care for a child diagnosed with leukemia, which of the following goals would be MOST important for this child? The child will

   a. remain free of signs and symptoms of infection

   b. participate in age-appropriate activities

   c. eat at least 60% of each meal

   d. share feelings about changes in body image

3. In caring for a child diagnosed with nephrotic syndrome, which of the following interventions will be included in the child's plan of care?

   a. Ambulate three to four times a day.

   b. Weigh on the same scale each day.

   c. Increase fluid intake by 50 cc an hour.

   d. Test the urine for glucose levels regularly.

4. A child diagnosed with acute glomerulonephritis will MOST likely have a history of which of the following?

   a. Sibling diagnosed with the same disease

   b. Recent illness such as strep throat

   c. Hemorrhage or history of bruising easily

   d. Hearing loss with impaired speech development

5. After discussing measures used to stop bleeding with the caregiver of a child diagnosed with hemophilia, the caregiver makes the following statements. Which of these statements indicates a need for further teaching?

   a. "I always have ice and cold packs in our freezer."

   b. "Keeping pressure on an injury usually helps stop the bleeding."

   c. "Whenever my child gets hurt, I have him sit up with his head elevated and his feet down."

   d. "I know how to keep his arm from moving by using splints."

STUDY ACTIVITIES

1. Using the table below, make a list of safety measures to help protect the child with hemophilia. Include measures to be taken at home, school, and in the hospital settings. Explain the reasons that these measures are important.

Safety Measure	Setting (Home, School, Hospital)	Reasons Measures Are Important

2. Four-year-old Todd is blind. You are helping with his care. Explain how you will orient him to the unit and prepare him for his hospital stay.

3. You are caring for 3½-year-old Missy, who has a mild hearing impairment. List the things you will do to adapt your nursing care to improve your communication with her.

CRITICAL THINKING

1. The family of Sean, a 3-year-old with hemophilia, is concerned that Sean might get AIDS from his treatments. What explanation will you give this family to reassure them? Discuss with your peers your thoughts and feelings about children who are HIV positive because of a transfusion they received.
2. Your friend asks you if cerebral palsy is inherited. Give a complete answer about the causes of cerebral palsy.

3. Jerome, a 6-year-old with Down's syndrome, has the mental age of a 3-year-old. Develop a plan to prepare him for a tonsillectomy.

4. *Dosage Calculation:* A preschool child with a diagnosis of nephrotic syndrome is being treated with Prednisolone. The child is being given a dose of 40 mg a day. The child weighs 44 pounds. Answer the following:

a. How many kg does the child's weigh?
b. How many mgs per kilogram is this child's dose?
c. If the dose is decreased to 30 mg a day, how many mgs per kilogram will this dose be?

_____

Growth and Development of the School-Age Child: 6 to 10 Years

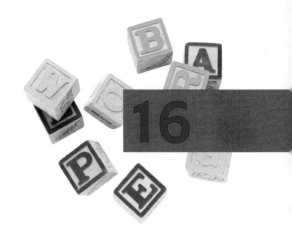

16

PHYSICAL DEVELOPMENT
  Growth
  Dentition
  Skeletal Growth
PSYCHOSOCIAL DEVELOPMENT
  The Child from Ages 6 to 7 Years
  The Child from Ages 7 to 10 Years
NUTRITION

HEALTH PROMOTION AND MAINTENANCE
  Routine Checkups
  Family Teaching
  Health Education
  Accident Prevention
THE SCHOOL-AGE CHILD IN THE HEALTH CARE FACILITY

STUDENT OBJECTIVES

On completion of this chapter, the student will be able to

1. State the major developmental task of the school-age group according to Erikson.
2. Discuss the physical growth patterns during the school-age years for (a) girls and (b) boys.
3. Describe dentition in this age group.
4. State factors that may deter successful completion of the developmental task of industry versus inferiority.
5. Describe the psychosocial characteristics of the 6- to 7-year-old child.
6. Discuss the importance of "gangs" to the 7- to 8-year-old child.
7. Briefly describe the progression in the 6- to 10-year-old child's concept of biology: (a) birth, (b) death, (c) human body, (d) health, (e) illness.
8. Identify nutritional influences on the school-age child, including (a) family attitudes, (b) mealtime atmosphere, (c) snacks, (d) school's role.
9. List three factors that contribute to obesity in the school-age child.
10. State two appropriate ways to help an obese child control weight.
11. State the usual amount of sleep the school-age child needs.
12. Describe practices that contribute to good dental hygiene for this age group.
13. Discuss the need for sex education in the school-age group: (a) family's role, (b) school's role, (c) others' role.
14. Identify common inhalant products that children may use as deliriants.
15. Discuss principles that a family caregiver can use to teach children about substance abuse.
16. Describe safety education appropriate for the school-age group.
17. State several factors that may influence the school-age child's hospital experience.

KEY TERMS

classification
conservation
decentration
deliriants
epiphyses
hierarchical arrangement
inhalants
reversibility
scoliosis

The first day of school marks a major milestone in a child's development, opening a new world of learning and growth. Between the ages of 6 and 10 years, dramatic changes occur in the child's thinking process, social skills, activities, attitudes, and use of language. The squirmy, boisterous 6-year-old child with a limited attention span bears little resemblance to the more reserved 10-year-old child who can become absorbed in a solitary craft activity for several hours.

Moving from the small circle of family into the school and community, children begin to see differences in their own lives and the lives of others. They constantly compare their families with other children's families and observe the way other children are disciplined, the foods they eat, the way they dress, and their homes. Every aspect of lifestyle is subject to comparison.

Most children reach school age with the necessary skills, abilities, and independence to function successfully in this new environment. They can feed and dress themselves, use the primary language of their culture to communicate their needs and feelings, and separate from their caregivers for extended periods. They show increasing interest in group activities and in making things. Children of this age work at many activities that involve motor, cognitive, and social skills. Success in these activities provides the child with self-confidence and a feeling of competence. Children who are unsuccessful during this stage, whether from physical, social, or cognitive disadvantages, develop a feeling of inferiority.

The health of the school-age child is no longer the exclusive concern of the family but of the community as well. Before admittance, most schools require that children have a physical examination and that immunizations meet state requirements. Generally this is a healthy period in the child's life, although minor respiratory disorders and other communicable diseases can spread quickly within a classroom. Few major diseases have their onset during this period. Accidents still pose a serious hazard; therefore, safety measures are an important part of learning.

PHYSICAL DEVELOPMENT

The physical development of the school-age child includes changes in weight and height as well as changes in dentition and the eruption of permanent teeth. The school age child's skeletal growth and changes are evident during this time period.

Growth

Between the ages of 6 and 10 years, growth is slow and steady. Average annual weight gain is about 5 to 6 lb (2 to 3 kg). By age 7, the child weighs about seven times as much as at birth. Annual height increase is about 2.5 inches (6 cm). This period ends in the preadolescent growth spurt in girls at about age 10 and in boys at about age 12.

Dentition

At about age 6, the child starts to lose the deciduous ("baby") teeth, usually beginning with the lower incisors. At about the same time, the first permanent teeth, the 6-year molars, appear directly behind the deciduous molars (Fig. 16–1). These 6-year molars are of the utmost importance: they are the key or pivot teeth that help to shape the jaw and affect the alignment of the permanent teeth. If these molars are allowed to decay so severely that they must be removed, the child will have dental problems later. (More information on care of the teeth is given later in this chapter.)

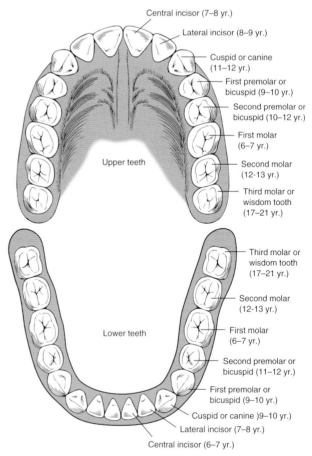

Central incisor (7–8 yr.)
Lateral incisor (8–9 yr.)
Cuspid or canine (11–12 yr.)
First premolar or bicuspid (9–10 yr.)
Second premolar or bicuspid (10–12 yr.)
First molar (6–7 yr.)
Upper teeth
Second molar (12-13 yr.)
Third molar or wisdom tooth (17–21 yr.)

Third molar or wisdom tooth (17–21 yr.)
Second molar (12-13 yr.)
First molar (6–7 yr.)
Lower teeth
Second premolar or bicuspid (11–12 yr.)
First premolar or bicuspid (9–10 yr.)
Cuspid or canine)9–10 yr.)
Lateral incisor (7–8 yr.)
Central incisor (6–7 yr.)

● **Figure 16.1** Chart showing the sequence of eruption of permanent teeth.

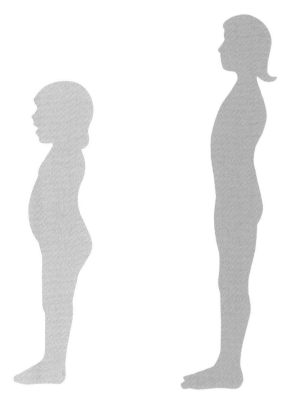

● *Figure 16.2* *(Left)* Profile of a 6-year-old showing protuberant abdomen. *(Right)* Profile of a 10-year-old showing flat abdomen and four curves of adult-like spine.

Skeletal Growth

The 6-year-old's silhouette is characterized by a protruding abdomen and lordosis ("swayback"). By the time the child has reached the age of 10 years, the spine is straighter, the abdomen flatter, and the body generally more slender and long-legged (Fig. 16–2).

Bone growth occurs mostly in the long bones and is gradual during the school years. Cartilage is being replaced by bone at the **epiphyses** (growth centers at the end of long bones and at the wrists). Skeletal maturation is more rapid in girls than in boys and in African-American children than in whites. Growth and development of the school-age child is summarized in Table 16–1.

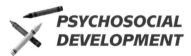

PSYCHOSOCIAL DEVELOPMENT

A sense of duty and accomplishment occupies the years from 6 to 12. This is the period Erikson calls *industry versus inferiority,* when the child is interested in engaging in meaningful projects and seeing them through to completion. The child applies the energies earlier put into play toward accomplishing tasks and often spends numerous sessions on one project. With

these attempts come the refinement of motor, cognitive, and social skills and development of a positive sense of self. Some school-age children, however, may not be ready for this stage because of environmental deprivation, a dysfunctional family, insecure attachment to parents, immaturity, or other reasons. Entering school at a disadvantage, these children may not be ready to be productive. Excessive or unrealistic goals set by a teacher or caregiver who is insensitive to this child's needs will defeat such a child and possibly lead to the child's feeling of inferiority rather than self-confidence.

When environmental support is adequate, several personality development tasks should be completed during these years. These tasks include developing coping mechanisms, a sense of right and wrong, a feeling of self-esteem, and an ability to care for oneself.

During the school-age years, the child's cognitive skills develop; at about the age of 7 years, the child enters the concrete operational stage identified by Piaget. The skills of **conservation** (the ability to recognize that a change in shape does not necessarily mean a change in amount or mass) are significant in this stage. This begins with the conservation of numbers, when the child understands that the number of cookies does not change even though they may be rearranged, along with the conservation of mass, when the child can see that an amount of cookie dough is the same whether in ball form or flattened for baking. This is followed by conservation of weight, in which the child recognizes that a pound is a pound regardless of whether plastic or bricks are weighed. Conservation of volume (for instance, a half-cup of water is the same amount regardless of the shape of the container) does not come until late in the concrete operational stage at about 11 or 12 years of age.

Each child is a product of personal heredity, environment, cognitive ability, and physical health. Every child needs love and acceptance, with understanding, support, and concern when mistakes are made. Children thrive on praise and recognition and will work to earn them (see Family Teaching Tips: Guiding Your School-Age Child).

The Child From Ages 6 to 7 Years

Children in the age group of 6 to 7 years are still characterized by magical thinking—believing in the tooth fairy, Santa Claus, the Easter bunny, and others. Keen imaginations contribute to fears, especially at night, about remote, fanciful, or imaginary events. Trouble distinguishing fantasy from reality can contribute to lying to escape punishment or to boost self-confidence.

TABLE 16.1	Developmental Milestones for the School-Age Child					
Age (yr)	Physical	Motor	Social	Language	Perceptual	Cognitive
6	Average height 45 inches (116 cm) Average weight 46 lb (21 kg) Loses first tooth (upper incisors) Six-year molars erupt Food "jags" Appetite increased	Tie shoes Can use scissors Runs, jumps, climbs, skips Can ride bicycle Can't sit for long periods Cuts, pastes, prints, draws with some detail	Increased need to socialize with same sex Egocentric—believes everyone thinks as they do Still in pre-operational stage until age 7	Uses every form of sentence structure Vocabulary of 2,500 words Sentence length about 5 words	Knows right from left May reverse letters Can discriminate vertical, horizontal, and oblique Perceives pictures in parts or whole but not both	Recognizes simple words Conservation of number Defines objects by use Can group according to an attribute to form subclasses
7	Weight is seven times birth weight Gains 4.4–6.6 lb/yr (2–3 kg) Grows 2–2.5 inches/yr (5–6 cm)	More cautious Swims Printing smaller than 6-year-old's Activity level lower than 6-year-old's	More cooperative Same-sex play group and friends Less egocentric	Can name day, month, season Produces all language sounds	b, p, d, q confusion resolved Can copy a diamond	Begins to use simple logic Can group in ascending order Grasps basic idea of addition and subtraction Conservation of substance Can tell time
8	Average height 49.5 inches (127 cm) Average weight 55 lb (25 kg)	Movements more graceful Writes in cursive Can throw and hit a baseball Has symmetric balance and can hop	Adheres to simple rules Hero worship begins Same-sex peer group	Gives precise definitions Articulation near adult level	Can catch a ball Visual acuity 20/20 Perceives pictures in parts and whole	Increasing memory span Interest in causal relation Conservation of length Seriation
9–10	Average height 51.5–53.5 inches (132–137 cm) Average weight 59.5–77 lb (27–35 kg)	Good coordination Can achieve the strength and speed needed for most sports	Enjoys team competition Moves from group to best friend Hero worship intensifies	Can use language to convey thoughts and look at other's point of view	Eye–hand coordination almost perfect	Classifies objects Understands explanations Conservation of area and weight Describes characteristics of objects Can group in descending order

Children who have attended a day care center, preschool, kindergarten, or Head Start program usually make the transition into first grade with pleasure, excitement, and little anxiety. Those without that experience may find it helpful to visit the school to experience separation from home and caregivers and to try getting along with other children on a trial basis. Most 6-year-old children can sit still for short periods of time and understand about taking turns. Those who have not matured sufficiently for this experience will find school unpleasant and may not do well.

Group activities are important to most 6-year-old children even if the groups include only two or three children. They delight in learning and show an intense interest in every experience. Judgment about acceptable and unacceptable behavior is not well developed and possibly results in name-calling and the use of vulgar words.

FAMILY TEACHING TIPS

Guiding Your School-Age Child

- Give your child consistent love and attention. Try to see the situation through your child's eyes. Do your best to avoid a hostile or angry reaction toward your child.
- Know where your child is at all times and who his or her friends are. Never leave your child home alone.
- Encourage your child to become involved in school and community activities. Become involved with your child's activities whenever possible. Encourage fair play and good sportsmanship.
- Show your children good examples by your behavior toward others.
- Never hit your children. Physical punishment shows them that it is all right to hit others and that they can solve problems in that way.
- Use positive nonphysical methods of discipline such as
  "Time out"—1 minute per year is an appropriate amount of time.
  "Grounding"—don't permit them to play with friends or take part in a special activity.
  Take away a special privilege.
- Set these limits for brief periods only. Consistency is extremely important in setting these restrictions.
- Be consistent. Make a reasonable rule, let your child know the rule, and then stick with it. You can involve your children in helping to set rules.
- Treat your child with love and respect. Always try to find the "positives" and praise the child for those behaviors. Don't treat your child in a manner that you would not use with an adult friend.
- Let the child know what you expect of him or her. Children who have responsibilities (age-appropriate) learn self-discipline and self-control.
- When you have a problem with your child, try to sit down and solve it together. Help him or her figure out ways to solve problems nonviolently.

Between the ages of 6 and 8 years, children begin to enjoy participating in real-life activities such as helping with gardening, housework, and other chores. They love making things such as drawings, paintings, and craft projects (Fig. 16–3).

The Child From Ages 7 to 10 Years

Between the seventh and eighth birthdays, children begin to shake off their acceptance of parental standards as the ultimate authority and become more impressed by the behavior of their peers. Interest in group play increases, and acceptance by the group or gang is tremendously important. These groups quickly become all-boy or all-girl groups and are often project-oriented, such as scout troops and athletic teams. Private clubs with homemade club-

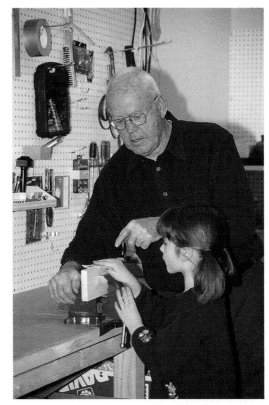

● **Figure 16.3** A 6-year-old works with her grandfather on a woodworking project.

houses, secret codes, and languages are popular. Individual friendships also are formed, and "best friends" are intensely loyal, if only for short periods. Table games, arts and crafts requiring skill and dexterity, computer games, school science projects, and science fairs are popular as are more active pursuits. This period includes the beginning of many neighborhood team sports including Little League, softball, football, and soccer (Fig. 16–4). Both boys and girls are actively involved in many of these sports.

Even though parents are no longer considered the ultimate authority, their standards have become part of the child's personality and conscience. Although the child may cheat, lie, or steal on occasion, he or she suffers considerable guilt if he or she learns that these are unacceptable behaviors.

Important changes occur in a child's thinking processes at about age 7 years, when there is movement from preoperational, egocentric thinking to concrete, operational, decentered thought. For the first time, children can see the world from someone else's point of view. **Decentration** means being able to see several aspects of a problem at the same time and to understand the relation of various parts to the whole situation. Cause-and-effect relations become clear; consequently, magical thinking begins to disappear.

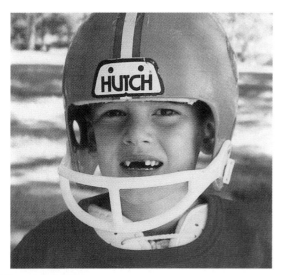

● **Figure 16.4** This boy enjoys being part of a team. (Note the dentition typical of an early school-age child!)

During the seventh or eighth year, children have an increased understanding of the conservation of continuous quantity. Understanding conservation depends on **reversibility,** the ability to think in either direction. Seven-year-olds can add and subtract, count forward and backward, and see how it is possible to put something back the way it was. A 7- or 8-year-old can understand that illness is probably only temporary, whereas a 6-year-old may think it is permanent.

Another important change in thinking during this period is **classification,** the ability to group objects into a **hierarchical arrangement** (grouping by some common system). Children in this age group love to collect sports cards, insects, rocks, stamps, coins, or anything else that strikes their fancy. These collections may be only a short-term interest, but some can develop into lifetime hobbies.

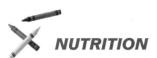

NUTRITION

As coordination improves, the child becomes increasingly active and requires more food to supply necessary energy. The nutritional needs of the school-age child should be met by choosing foods from all the food groups with the appropriate number of servings from each group in the child's daily diet (Table 16–2). Increased appetite and a tendency to go on food "jags" are typical of the 6-year-old child. This stage soon passes and is unimportant if the child generally gets the necessary nutrients. Allowing the child to express food dislikes and permitting refusal of the disliked food item are usually the best ways to handle this phase. As the child's tastes develop, once-disliked foods may become favorites unless earlier battles have been waged over the food. Children are more likely to learn to eat most foods if everyone else accepts them in a matter-of-fact way.

Children learn by the examples that caregivers and others set for them. They will accept more readily the importance of manners, calm voices, appropriate table conversation, and courtesy if they see them carried out consistently at home. To keep mealtime a positive and pleasant time, mealtime should never be used for nagging, finding fault, correcting manners, or discussing a poor report card. Hygiene should be taught in a cheerful but firm manner, even if the child must leave the table more than once to wash his or her hands adequately.

Most children prefer simple, plain foods and are good judges of their own needs if they are not coaxed, nagged, bribed, rewarded, or influenced by television commercials. Disease or strong emotions may cause loss of appetite. Forcing the child to eat is not helpful and can have harmful effects.

Caregivers must carefully supervise children's snacking habits to be sure that snacks are nutritious and not too frequent. Children should avoid junk food; continual nibbling can cause lack of interest at mealtime. They should be encouraged to eat a good breakfast to provide the energy and nutrients needed to perform well in school. Children need a clearly planned schedule that allows time for a good breakfast and tooth brushing before leaving for school.

Obesity can be a concern during this age. Some children may have a genetic tendency to obesity; environment and a sedentary lifestyle also play a part. In many families, children are urged to "clean your plate" or are encouraged to belong to the "clean plate club." In addition, many families now eat fast foods several times a week, which reinforces the problem because fast foods tend to have high fat and calorie content and contribute to obesity. Other children especially in the later elementary grades can be unkind to overweight children by teasing them, not choosing them in games, or avoiding them as friends. The child who becomes sensitive to being overweight is often miserable.

Encouraging physical activity and limiting dietary fat intake to 35% of total calories will help control the child's weight. Popular fad diets must be avoided because they do not supply adequate nutrients for the growing child. Caregivers must avoid nagging and creating feelings of inferiority or guilt, because the child may simply rebel. The child who is pressured too much to lose weight may become a food sneak, setting up patterns that will be

TABLE 16.2	Daily Nutritional Needs of the 6- to 10-year-old	
Food Group	**Number of Servings Daily**	**Examples of Serving Sizes**
Bread, cereal, rice and pasta group (especially whole grains)	9	1 slice bread ½ hamburger bun or English muffin a small roll, biscuit, muffin 3 or 4 small or 2 large crackers ½ cup cooked cereal, rice, pasta 1 oz ready-to-eat cereal
Vegetable group	4	½ cup cooked vegetables ½ cup chopped raw vegetables 1 cup leafy raw vegetables such as lettuce or spinach
Fruit group	3	1 apple, banana, orange ½ grapefruit a melon wedge ¾ cup juice ½ cup berries ½ cup cooked or canned fruit ¼ cup dried fruit
Milk, yogurt, cheese—milk group	2 or 3	1 cup milk 8 oz yogurt 1½ oz natural cheese 2 oz processed cheese

Meat, poultry, fish, dry beans, eggs, and nuts group	2 for a total of 6 oz	Total 6 oz a day—lean meat, poultry, fish
		Count as 1 oz
		  1 egg
		  ½ cup cooked beans
		  2 tablespoons peanut butter

Fats and sweets	Use sparingly, after recommended foods have been eaten	

Adapted from the U.S. Department of Agriculture, Home and Garden Bulletin, No. 232, 5th edition, 2000.

harmful later in life. In addition, anorexia nervosa (see Chap. 19) has become a problem for some girls in the older school-age group.

Health teaching at school should reinforce the importance of a proper diet. Family and cultural food patterns are strong, however, and tend to persist despite nutrition education. Some families are making a positive effort to reduce fat and cholesterol when preparing meals. Most schools have subsidized lunch programs for eligible children, and some have breakfast programs. These provide well-balanced meals, but often children eat only part of what they are offered. Some families post the school lunch menu on the refrigerator or kitchen bulletin board so that children can decide whether to eat the school's lunch or pack their own on any particular day. This way the child can avoid lunches he or she dislikes or simply refuses to eat. School-age children are old enough to be at least partially responsible for preparing their own lunch.

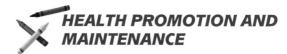

HEALTH PROMOTION AND MAINTENANCE

The school years are generally healthy years for most children. However, routine health care and health education, including health habits, safety, sex education, and substance abuse, are very important aspects of well-planned health promotion and maintenance programs for school-age children.

Routine Checkups

The school-age child should have a physical examination by a physician or other health care provider every year. Additional visits are commonly made throughout the year for minor illness. The school-age child should visit the dentist at least twice a year for a cleaning and application of fluoride.

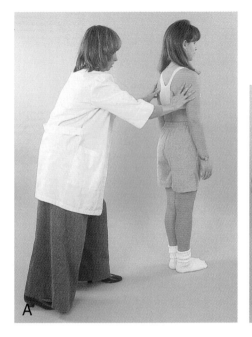
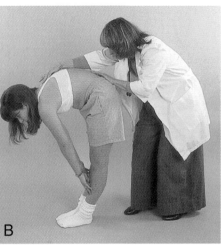

● *Figure 16.5* Scoliosis checkup. **(A)** Viewing from the back, the examiner checks the symmetry of the girl's shoulders. She will also look for a prominent shoulder blade, an unequal distance between the girl's arms and waist, a higher or more prominent hip, and curvature of the spinal column. **(B)** With the child bending over and touching her toes, the examiner checks for a curvature of the spinal column. She will also look for a rib hump.

Most states have immunization requirements that must be met when the child enters school. A booster of tetanus-diphtheria vaccine is recommended every 10 years lifelong. In addition, physical and dental examinations may be required at specific intervals during the elementary school years. During a physical examination at about the age of 10 to 11 years, the child is initially examined for signs of **scoliosis** (lateral curvature of the spine). The child is monitored on an ongoing basis and reexamined during adolescence (Fig. 16–5; refer to Chap. 17). Vision and hearing screening should be performed before entrance to school and on a periodic basis (annual or biannual) thereafter. The school nurse often conducts these examinations.

Elementary school children generally are healthy with only minor illnesses that are usually respiratory or gastrointestinal in nature. The leading cause of death in this age group continues to be accidents.

Family Teaching

The school-age child generally incorporates healthy habits into his or her daily routine, but reinforcement by caregivers is still needed. Education for the care of the teeth with particular attention to the 6-year molars is important. Proper dental hygiene includes a routine inspection and conscientious brushing after meals. A well-balanced diet with plenty of calcium and phosphorus and minimal sugar is important to healthy teeth. Foods containing sugar should be eaten only at mealtimes and should be followed immediately by proper brushing (Fig. 16–6).

Exercise and sufficient rest also are important during this period. Caregivers need to help school-age children to balance their rest needs and their extracurricular activities. Extracurricular activities help the child remain fit, bond with peers, and establish positive, lifelong attitudes toward exercise. The school-age child needs 10 to 12 hours of sleep per night. The 6-year-old needs 12 hours of sleep and

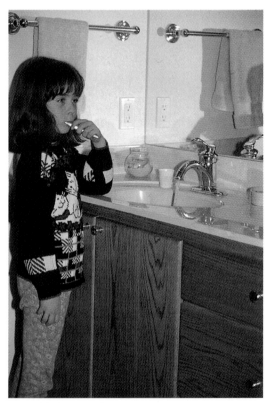

● *Figure 16.6* The school-age child needs encouragement to brush after meals and at bedtime as part of a good dental hygiene program.

should be provided with a quiet time after school to recharge after a busy day in the classroom. The nurse should take an opportunity to highlight these important aspects of daily health care to both the caregivers and child.

Health Education

Health teaching in the home and at school is essential. Caregivers have a responsibility to teach the child about basic hygiene, sexual functioning, substance abuse, and accident prevention. Schools must include these topics in the curriculum because many families are not well informed enough to cover them adequately. Some schools offer health classes taught by a health educator at each grade level. In other schools, health and sex education are integrated into the curriculum and taught by each classroom teacher. Nurses should become active in their community to ensure that these kinds of programs are available to children.

Sex Education

Children learn about femininity and masculinity from the time they are born. Behaviors, attitudes, and actions of the men and women in the child's life, especially their actions toward the child and toward each other, form impressions in the child that last a lifetime. The proper time and place for formal sex education have been very controversial. Part of the problem seems to be that many people automatically think that sex education means just adult sexuality and reproduction. However, sex education includes helping children develop positive attitudes toward their own bodies, their own sex, and their own sexual role to achieve optimum satisfaction in being a boy or a girl.

In some schools, sex education is limited to one class, usually in the fifth grade, in which children are shown films about menstruation and their developing bodies. Often these are taught in separate classes for boys and girls. Some health educators strongly recommend that sex education should be started in kindergarten and developed gradually over the successive grades. Learning about reproduction of plants and animals, about birth and nurturing in other animals, and about the roles of the male and the female in family units can lead to the natural introduction of human reproduction, male and female roles, families, and nurturing. If all children grew up in secure, loving, ideal families, much of this could be learned at home. However, many children do not have this type of home, so they need healthy, positive information to help them develop healthy attitudes about their own sexuality. Feelings of self-worth woven into these lessons help children feel good about themselves and who they are.

Caregivers who feel uncomfortable discussing sex with their children may find it helpful to use books or pamphlets available for various age groups. Generally a female caregiver finds it easier to discuss sex with a girl, and a male caregiver feels more comfortable with a boy. This can pose special problems for the single caregiver with a child of the opposite sex. Again, printed materials may be helpful. Nurses may be called on to help a caregiver provide information and must be comfortable with their own sexuality to handle these discussions well.

At a young age, children are exposed to a large amount of sexually provocative information through the media. Children who do not get accurate information at home or at school will learn what they want to know from their peers; this information is often inaccurate, which makes sex education even more urgent. In addition, the U.S. Centers for Disease Control currently recommends that elementary school children be taught about acquired immunodeficiency syndrome (AIDS) and how it is spread. Many school districts are working hard to integrate this information into the health curriculum at all grade levels in a sensitive, age-appropriate manner.

Substance Abuse

In addition to nutrition, health practices, safety, and sex education, school-age children also need substance abuse education. Programs that teach children to "just say no" are one way that children can learn that they are in control of the choices they make regarding substance abuse. Teaching children the unhealthy aspects of tobacco and alcohol use and drug abuse should be started in elementary school as

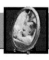

A PERSONAL GLIMPSE

When we had the program on drugs at school, I learned some things. Like when you take drugs, you can get sick or even die. In one part of the lesson, we watched a video where a kid took drugs and almost died and during the other part the school nurse showed us samples of drugs. Even though I leaned about drugs from the program, I think that all children should be taught this subject by their parent or guardian.

Stephen, age 11

▶ **LEARNING OPPORTUNITY:** What do you think is the most effective way to teach school-age children about the dangers of substance abuse? List some ways you can help to reduce substance abuse among school-age children.

a good foundation for more advanced information in adolescence.

Age, race, and socioeconomic status are not limiting factors in this problem, despite the stereotype that children who abuse substances are children of the ghetto. The use of alcohol and other substances to provide mind-altering excitement occurs in children as young as 8 or 9 years of age. Many children, even those as young as elementary school age, from every level of society smoke cigarettes. The risk for starting to smoke is greatest in the sixth and seventh grades. Forty percent of children try cigarettes before they enter high school; the total reaches 70% before the end of high school. Twelve percent of boys have chewed tobacco or snuff, which is just as addictive and harmful as smoking.

Children may experiment with **inhalants** (substances whose volatile vapors can be abused) because they are readily available and may seem no more threatening than an innocent prank. Inhalants classified as **deliriants** contain chemicals that give off fumes that can produce symptoms of confusion, disorientation, excitement, and hallucinations. Many inhalants are commonly found in the home (Box 16–1). The fumes are mind-altering when inhaled. The child initially may experience a temporary high, giddiness, nausea, coughing, nosebleed, fatigue, lack of coordination, or loss of appetite. Overdose can cause loss of consciousness and possible death from suffocation by replacing oxygen in the lungs or depressing the central nervous system, thereby causing respiratory arrest. Permanent damage to the lungs, the nervous system, or the liver can result. Children who experiment with inhalants may

FAMILY TEACHING TIPS

Guidelines to Prevent Substance Abuse

1. Openly communicate values by talking about the importance of honesty, responsibility, and self-reliance. Encourage decision-making. Help children see how each decision builds on previous decisions.
2. Provide a good role model for the child to copy. Children tend to copy parent's habits of smoking and drinking alcohol and attitudes about drug use, whether they are over-the-counter, prescription, or illicit drugs.
3. Avoid conflicts between what you say and what you do. For example, don't ask the child to lie that you are not home when you are or encourage the child to lie about age when trying to get a lower admission price at amusement centers.
4. Talk about values during family times. Give the child "what if" examples, and discuss the best responses when faced with a difficult situation. For example, "What would you do if you found money that someone dropped?"
5. Set strong rules about using alcohol and other drugs. Make specific rules with specific punishments. Discuss these rules and the reasons for them.
6. Be consistent in applying the rules that you set.
7. Be reasonable; don't make wild threats. Respond calmly and carry out the expected punishment.
8. Get the facts about alcohol and other drugs, and provide children with current, correct information. This helps you in discussions with children and also helps you to recognize symptoms if a child has been using them.

(From *The parent's guide to drug prevention: Growing up drug free.* Washington, DC: U.S. Department of Education, 1998.)

BOX 16.1	Common Products Inhaled as Deliriants

Model glue
Rubber cement
Cleaning fluids
Kerosene vapors
Gasoline vapors
Butane lighter fluid
Paint sprays
Paint thinner
Varnish
Shellac
Hair spray
Nail polish remover
Liquid typing correction fluid
Propellant in whipped-cream spray cans
Aerosol paint cans
Upholstery-fabric-protection spray cans
Solvents

proceed to abuse other drugs in an attempt to get similar effects. Addiction occurs in younger children more rapidly than in adults.

Family caregivers must work to develop a strong, loving relationship with the children in the family, teach the children the family's values and the difference between right and wrong, set and enforce rules for acceptable behavior of family members, learn facts about drugs and alcohol, and actively listen to the children in the family (see Family Teaching Tips: Guidelines to Prevent Substance Abuse). An excellent reference for family caregivers is *The Parents Guide to Drug Prevention: Growing Up Drug Free*, which is published by the United States Department of Education and can be ordered free by calling the Department of Education's toll-free number, (800) 624-0100, or via the Internet at *http://www.ed.gov/offices/OESE/SDFS/*.

Accident Prevention

As stated earlier, accidents continue to be a leading cause of death during this period. Even though school-age children do not require constant supervision, they must be taught certain safety rules and practice them until they are routine (Fig. 16–7). They should understand the function of traffic lights. Family members should obey traffic lights as a matter of course, because example is the best teacher for any child. Every child should know her or his full name, the caregivers' names, and his or her own home address and telephone number. Children should be taught the appropriate way to call for emergency help in their community (911 in a community that has such a system). Many communities have safe-home programs that designate homes where children can go if they have a problem on the way home from school. These homes are clearly marked in a way that children are taught to recognize. In many communities, local police officers or firefighters are interested in coming into the classroom to help teach safety. Children benefit from meeting police officers and understanding that the officer's duty is to help children, not to punish them. Safety rules should be stressed at home and at school. The Family Teaching Tips box summarizes important safety considerations for school-age children.

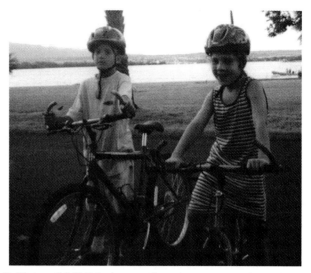

● **Figure 16.7** Helmets are an important aspect of bike safety.

Nurses who care for school-age children should understand how concepts about birth, death, the body, health, and illness change between the ages of 6 and 10 years (Table 16–3). All procedures must be

INTERNET EXERCISE 16.1

http://arizonachildcare.org/childproof/bicyclesfty.html

Read the section entitled "General Tips of Bicycle Safety."

1. List seven things that you would check when following this bike safety checklist.

2. Describe how a bicycle helmet works.

3. After reading this site, if the parent of a school age child asks, "Does my child really need a bicycle helmet?" how would you answer that question?

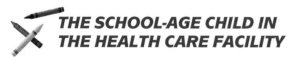

THE SCHOOL-AGE CHILD IN THE HEALTH CARE FACILITY

Increased understanding of their bodies, continuing curiosity about how things work, and development of concrete thinking all contribute to helping school-age children understand and accept a health care experience better than younger children do. They can communicate better with health care providers, understand cause and effect, and tolerate longer separations from their family.

FAMILY TEACHING TIPS

Safety Topics for Elementary School–Age Children

1. Traffic signals and safe pedestrian practices
2. Safety belt use for car passengers
3. Bicycle safety
   a. Wear a helmet.
   b. Use hand signals.
   c. Ride with traffic.
   d. Be sure others see you.
4. Skateboard and skating safety
   a. Wear a helmet.
   b. Wear elbow and knee pads.
   c. Skate only in safe skating areas.
5. Swimming safety
   a. Learn to swim.
   b. Never swim alone.
   c. Always know the water depth.
   d. Don't dive head first.
   e. No running or horseplay at a pool.
6. Danger of projectile toys
7. Danger of all-terrain vehicles
8. Use of life jacket when boating
9. Stranger safety
   a. Who is a stranger?
   b. Never accept a ride from someone you don't know.
   c. If offered a ride, check the vehicle license number and try to remember it.
   d. Never accept food or gifts from someone you don't know.
10. Good touch and bad touch

TABLE 16.3	Children's Concept of Biology		
Concept	6 to 8 Years	8 to 10 Years	Implications for Nursing
Birth	Gradually see babies as the result of three factors: social and sexual intercourse and biogenetic fusion Tend to see baby as emerging from female only; many still see baby as manufactured by outside force—created whole Boys less knowledgeable about baby formation than girls	Begin to put three components together; recognize that sperm and egg come together but may not be sure why Fewer discrepancies in knowledge based on sex differences	Cultural and educational factors play a part in development of where babies come from. Nurse should assess children's ideas about birth and if they can understand where babies come from and how before teaching. Explanations about roles of both parents can begin, but the idea of sperm and egg union may not be understood until 8 or 9 years of age.
Death	May be viewed as reversible Animism (attribution of life) may be seen in some children; death is viewed as result of outside force. Experiences with death facilitate concept development.	Considered irreversible Ideas about what happens after death unclear; related to concreteness of thinking and socio-religious upbringing	Change from vague view of death as reversible and caused by external forces to awareness of irreversibility and bodily causes Fears about death more common at 8; adults should be alert to this Explanations about death, the fact that their thoughts will not cause a death, and they will not die (if illness is not fatal) are needed.
Human body	Know body holds everything inside Use outside world to explain Aware of major organs Interested in visible functions of body	Can understand physiology; use general principles to explain body functions; interested in invisible functions of body	Cultural factors may play a part in ability and willingness to discuss bodily functions. Educational programs can be very effective because of natural interest. Assess knowledge of body by using diagrams before teaching.
Health	See health as doing desired activities List concrete practices as components of health Many do not see sickness as related to health; may not consider cause and effect	See health as doing desired activities Understand cause and effect Believe it is possible to be part healthy and part not at the same time; can reverse from health to sickness and back to health	Need assistance in seeing cause and effect Capitalize on positiveness of concept; health lets you do what you really want to do. Young children who are sick may feel they will never get well again.
Illness	Sick children may see illness as punishment; evidence suggests that healthy children do not see illness as punishment. Highly anxious children more likely to view illness as disruptive. Sickness is a diffuse state; rely on others to tell them when they are ill	Same as 6–8 years of age; can identify illness states, report bodily discomfort, recognize that illness is caused by specific factors	Social factors play a part in illness concept. Recognize that some see illness as punishment. Encourage self-care and self-help behavior, especially in older children.

explained to children and their families; showing the equipment and materials to be used (or pictures of them) and outlining realistic expectations of procedures and treatments are helpful. Children's questions including those about pain should be answered truthfully. Children of this age have

anxieties about looking different from other children. An opportunity to verbalize these anxieties will help a child deal with them. School-age children need privacy more than younger children do and may not want to have physical contact with adults; this wish should be respected. Boys may be uncomfortable

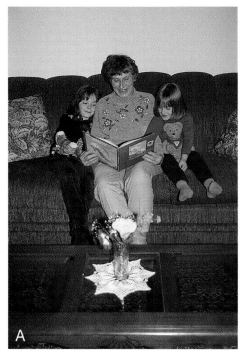
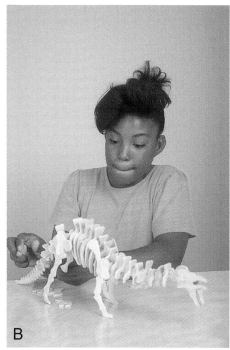

A

B

● **Figure 16.8 (A)** School-age children still like to listen to stories, in either the hospital or the home setting, **(B)** Hospitalized school-age children enjoy projects and crafts.

having a female nurse bathe them, and girls may feel uncomfortable with a male nurse. These attitudes should be recognized and handled in a way that ensures as much privacy as possible.

Family caregivers may feel guilty about the child's need for hospitalization and, as a result, may overindulge the child. The child may regress in response to this, but this regression should not be encouraged. Sometimes the family needs as much reassurance as the child does.

Discipline and rules have a place on a pediatric unit. Families and children must be informed about the rules as part of the admission routine. Opportunities for interaction with peers, learning situations, and doing crafts and projects can help make the child's experience more tolerable (Fig. 16–8).

KEY POINTS

▶ Growth and development during the school-age years is steady at all levels—emotional, social, intellectual, and physical.

▶ According to Erikson, the developmental task of school-age children is industry versus inferiority. The child engages in many activities using motor, cognitive, and social skills. Success in these activities is necessary for the child to develop a sense of competency.

▶ A child's successes or failures during this period

can have a lifelong impact on attitudes and performance.

▶ The school-age child gains a real sense of self with individualized moral standards and conscience.

▶ The family is still the major sustaining force, even though much time is spent with peers in activities outside the home.

▶ Substance abuse is an ever-increasing concern during this age. Family caregivers must make every effort to be alert to children's use of inhalants, deliriants, alcohol, or tobacco.

▶ School-age children need privacy, and this must be respected when planning their care.

▶ Children's interest in science creates a fascination with their bodies and how they work.

▶ The changes in a school-age child's understanding of biology influence the child's view of his or her own health care. The nurse needs to understand these concepts to plan nursing care for the school-age child.

BIBLIOGRAPHY

Berger KS. (2001) *The developing person through the life span* (5th ed). New York: Worth Publishers.

Brazelton TB, Greenspan S. (2001) *The irreducible needs of children: What every child must have to grow, learn, and flourish.* Cambridge, MA: Perseus Publishing.

Brown RL, et. al. (2002) All-terrain vehicle and bicycle crashes in children: Epidemiology and comparison of injury severity. *Journal of Pediatric Surgery*, 37(3), 375–80.

Craven RF, Hirnle CJ. (1999) *Fundamentals of nursing* (3rd ed). Philadelphia: Lippincott Williams & Wilkins.

Dudek, SG. (2000) *Nutrition essentials for nursing practice* (4th ed). Philadelphia: Lippincott Williams & Wilkins.

(2001) Counseling about bicycle safety. *Pediatrics in Review*, 22 (9), 321–322.

McClowry SG. (2002) The temperament profiles of school-age children. *Journal of Pediatric Nursing*, 17(1), 3–10.

Pillitteri A. (2003) *Maternal and child health nursing* (4th ed). Philadelphia: Lippincott Williams & Wilkins.

Sanford CC. (2001) Delivering health care to children on their turf: An elementary school school-based wellness center. *Journal of Pediatric Health Care*, 15(3), 132.

Schmidt CK. (2001) Development of children's body knowledge, Using knowledge of the lungs as an exemplar. *Issues in Comprehensive Pediatric Nursing*, 24(3), 177–91.

Spock B, et. al. (1998) *Dr. Spock's baby and child care*. New York: Pocket Books.

Wong DL. (1998) *Whaley and Wong's nursing care of infants and children* (6th ed). St. Louis: Mosby.

Wong DL, Perry S, Hockenberry M. (2002) *Maternal child nursing care* (2nd ed). St. Louis: Mosby.

Websites

Substance Abuse: *www.toughlove.org*

Family Support Groups:
http://home.earthlink.net/famanon/index.html
www.keepkidshealthy.com/schoolage

Workbook

NCLEX-STYLE REVIEW QUESTIONS

1. The nurse is assisting with a well child visit for a 7 year old. This child's records show that at birth this child weighed 7 pounds and 8 ounces. At the age of 6 years, this child was 45 inches tall. If this child is following a normal pattern of growth and development, which of the following would the nurse expect to find in this visit? The child

   a. weighs 54 pounds

   b. measures 50 inches in height

   c. has 4 molars in the lower jaw

   d. has an apical pulse of 60 beats a minute

2. In working with a group of school-age children, which of the following activities would this age child MOST likely be doing?

   a. Pretending to be television characters

   b. Playing a game with large balls and blocks

   c. Participating in a group activity

   d. Telling stories about themselves

3. During the school-age years according to Erikson, the child is in the stage of growth and development known as industry versus inferiority. If the caregivers of a group of children made the following statements, which statement reflects that the child is developing industry?

   a. "When my child falls down, he tries so hard to just get up and not cry."

   b. "My child was so excited when she finished her science project all by herself."

   c. "Every night my child follows the same routine at bedtime."

   e. "My child loves to make up stories about tall, big buildings."

4. In teaching caregivers of school-age children, the nurse would reinforce that which of the following would be MOST important for this age group? The school-age child should be

   a. encouraged to brush teeth

   b. taught basic sex education

   c. screened for scoliosis

   d. required to wear a bicycle helmet

5. The nurse is teaching a group of caregivers of school-age children about the importance of setting a consistent bedtime for the school-age child. Which of the following statements made by a caregiver indicates an understanding of the sleep patterns and needs of the school-age child?

   a. "My child sleeps between 11 and 12 hours a night."

   b. "She stays up late when she takes a nap after school."

   c. "My son doesn't even know when he is tired."

   d. "My teenage child doesn't sleep as much as my 9-year-old does."

STUDY ACTIVITIES

1. List and compare the motor skills, social skills, and cognitive development in each of the following ages:

	6 Years	7 Years	8 Years	9–10 Years
Motor skills				
Social skills				
Cognitive development				

2. Make a safety poster or teaching aid to use in an elementary school classroom. Perhaps you can make this a class project and donate the posters to your pediatric unit or nearby school.

3. Survey your home and make a list of all the products available that a child could use as an inhalant for a deliriant effect.

CRITICAL THINKING

1. Delsey, the mother of 6-year-old Jasmine, is upset because Jasmine is a picky eater and often does not want to eat what Delsey has prepared. Discuss the information would you share with her to advise and reassure her.

2. Steve, the primary family caregiver of 8-year-old Carolyn, feels that he should offer her sex education and asks for your advice. Describe what you would say to Steve in response. Explain the reasons for your answer.

3. Substance abuse education including alcohol and tobacco should be included in the school health program. Discuss effective methods that you believe should be used to present these programs to children.

Health Problems of the School-Age Child

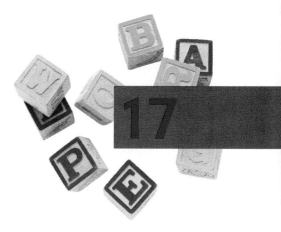

17

BEHAVIORAL PROBLEMS
School Phobia
CENTRAL NERVOUS SYSTEM DISORDERS
Attention Deficit Hyperactivity Disorder
Seizure Disorders
ALLERGIC REACTIONS
Allergic Rhinitis (Hay Fever)
Asthma
Nursing Process for the Child With Asthma
GASTROINTESTINAL SYSTEM DISORDERS
Appendicitis
Nursing Process for the Child With Appendicitis
Intestinal Parasites

DISORDERS OF ELIMINATION
Enuresis
Encopresis
CARDIOVASCULAR SYSTEM DISORDERS
Rheumatic Fever
Nursing Process for the Child With Rheumatic Fever
ENDOCRINE SYSTEM DISORDERS
Type 1 Diabetes Mellitus
Nursing Process for the Child With Type 1 Diabetes Mellitus
MUSCULOSKELETAL SYSTEM DISORDERS
Scoliosis
Nursing Process for the Child With Scoliosis

Legg-Calvé-Perthes Disease (Coxa Plana)
Osteomyelitis
Muscular Dystrophy
Juvenile Rheumatoid Arthritis
Fractures
SKIN DISORDERS
Fungal Infections
Parasitic Infections
Skin Allergies
Bites

STUDENT OBJECTIVES

On completion of this chapter, the student will be able to

1. Identify 10 characteristics that may be seen in a child with attention deficit hyperactivity disorder.
2. Describe (a) simple partial motor seizures, (b) simple partial sensory seizures and (c) complex partial (psychomotor) seizures.
3. Describe (a) tonic-clonic seizures, (b) absence seizures, (c) atonic or akinetic seizures, (d) myoclonic seizures, and (e) infantile spasms.
4. List factors that can trigger an asthmatic attack.
5. Describe the physiologic response that occurs in the respiratory tract in an asthmatic attack.
6. List the symptoms of appendicitis; differentiate symptoms of the older and the younger child.
7. Identify three intestinal parasites common to children, and state the route of entry for each.
8. Name the bacterium usually responsible for the infection that leads to a child developing rheumatic fever.
9. List the major manifestations of rheumatic fever.
10. Describe what would be included in a teaching plan for an 8-year-old child with Type 1 diabetes mellitus.
11. Discuss the importance of good skin care, correct insulin administration, and exercise in the diabetic child.
12. Describe scoliosis and identify three methods of correction.
13. Identify the most common form of muscular dystrophy; describe its characteristics.
14. Name the drugs of choice in the treatment of juvenile rheumatoid arthritis, and state the primary purpose of these drugs.
15. Describe the purpose of doing neurovascular checks in a child with a musculoskeletal disorder.
16. List and define the five Ps to observe, record, and report when caring for a child in a cast.
17. Describe the treatment for pediculosis of the scalp, and state the protection the nurse must use when treating a child with this condition in the hospital.

KEY TERMS

absence
akinetic
allergen
ankylosis
anthelmintic
arthralgia
atonic
aura
carditis
chorea
diabetic ketoacidosis
encopresis
enuresis
halo traction
hirsutism
hyposensitization
infantile spasms
insulin reaction
Kussmaul breathing
kyphosis
lordosis
metered-dose inhaler
myoclonic
nebulizer
partial
polyarthritis
polydipsia
polyphagia
polyuria
school phobia
seizure
skeletal traction
skin traction
synovitis
tinea
tonic-clonic
traction
wheezing

Entering school is a stressful time for every child, but especially so for the child with a chronic health problem. Imitation of peers is important during this time; sometimes this is impossible for the child with a learning disorder, severe allergies, or problems that limit physical mobility or make the child feel different from peers. These children must cope with all the normal developmental stresses of their age group and the additional stress that the health problem causes.

Given enough information and guidance, school-age children can learn to understand, cope with, and manage health problems such as diabetes and asthma. Nurses and caregivers who care for these children should foster maximum independence and a life as normal as possible.

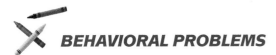

BEHAVIORAL PROBLEMS

A number of behavioral problems are common in the school-age group. These problems can interfere with the child's socialization, education, and development. Some of these have definite organic causes; for others, the causes are not clearly defined.

School Phobia

School absenteeism is a national problem. Children are absent from school for a variety of reasons, one of which may be **school phobia.** Children who develop school phobia may be good students; more girls than boys are affected. Teachers and nurses can help detect school phobia by paying close attention to absence patterns. School-phobic children may have a strong attachment to one parent, usually the mother, and they fear separation from that parent perhaps because of anxiety about losing her or him while away from home. School phobia may be the child's unconscious reaction to a seemingly overwhelming problem at school. The parent can unwittingly reinforce school phobia by permitting the child to stay home. The symptoms—vomiting, diarrhea, abdominal or other pain, and even a low-grade fever—are genuine and are caused by anxiety that may approach panic. They disappear with relief of the immediate anxiety after the child has been given permission to stay home.

Treatment includes a complete medical examination to rule out any organic cause for the symptoms and school-family conferences to help the child return to school. Those working with these children must recognize that they really do want to go to school but for whatever reason cannot make themselves go;

these children are not delinquents. The school nurse and teacher along with other professionals, such as a social worker, psychologist, or psychiatrist, all may contribute to resolving the problem. If the child fears a specific factor at school, such as an overly critical teacher, the child may need to be moved to another class or school.

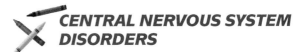

CENTRAL NERVOUS SYSTEM DISORDERS

Although the health problems discussed in this section—attention deficit hyperactivity disorder and seizure disorders—may not be classified simply as central nervous system disorders, the central nervous system plays an important part in each of them. Both conditions have a great impact on a child's success in school and throughout life. Continuing research will help identify the causes and improve treatment. The future holds great promise for children with these conditions.

Attention Deficit Hyperactivity Disorder

Attention deficit hyperactivity disorder (ADHD), or attention deficit disorder, is a syndrome characterized by degrees of inattention, impulsive behavior, and hyperactivity. About 3% to 5% of all American school-age children have ADHD; boys are more commonly affected than girls are. The cause of the disorder is unclear: developmental lag, biochemical disorder, and food sensitivities are all theories under consideration. The disorder affects every part of the child's life. The child with ADHD may have these characteristics:

- Impulsive
- Easily distracted
- Often fidgets or squirms
- Has difficulty sitting still
- Has problems following through on instructions despite being able to understand them
- Inattentive when spoken to
- Often loses things
- Goes from one uncompleted activity to another
- Has difficulty taking turns
- Often talks excessively
- Often engages in dangerous activities without considering the consequences

These children also often demonstrate signs of clumsiness or poor coordination, such as the inability to use a pencil or scissors well, that are inappropriate for their age group. No one child has all these symptoms. Although it was believed that these symptoms are resolved by late adolescence, it is now apparent that they continue into adulthood at least for some people.

Although these children may have poor success in the classroom because of their inability to pay attention, they are not intellectually impaired. The child's poor impulse control also contributes to disciplinary problems in the classroom. Some children with ADHD may have learning disorders such as dyslexia and perceptual deficits. The child's self-confidence can suffer from feeling inferior to the other children in the class. Special arrangements can be made to provide an educational atmosphere that is supportive for the child without the need for the child to leave the classroom.

Diagnosis

Diagnosis can be made after the child is 3 years old but often is not made until the child reaches school age and has trouble settling into the routine of being in the classroom setting. Diagnosis can be difficult and also may be controversial because many of the symptoms are subjective and rely on the assessment of caregivers and teachers. Some authorities have expressed concern that teachers incorrectly label children as hyperactive. The symptoms may be a result of environmental factors that can include broken homes, stress, and nonsupportive caregivers.

The multidisciplinary approach is most effective for diagnosis, i.e., one involving pediatric and education specialists, a psychologist, the classroom teacher, family caregivers, and others. A careful, detailed history including school and social functioning, psychological testing, and physical and neurologic examinations can help make the diagnosis.

Treatment and Nursing Care

Treatment is also multidisciplinary. Learning situations should be structured so that the child has minimal distractions and a supportive teacher. Home support is necessary and requires structured, consistent guidance from the caregivers. Medication is used for some children. Stimulant medications, such as methylphenidate (Ritalin) and dextroamphetamine (Dexedrine), have often been used. When given in large amounts, these medications may suppress the appetite and affect the child's growth. Pemoline (Cylert) has been used but generally with less success than methylphenidate and dextroamphetamine. Using stimulants for a hyperactive child seems paradoxical, but these drugs apparently stimulate the area of the child's brain that aids in concentration, thus enabling the child to have better control.

In the health care setting, the nurse should maintain a calm, patient attitude toward the child with ADHD. The child should be given only one simple instruction at a time. Limiting distractions, using consistency, and offering praise for accomplishments are invaluable methods of working with these children. The families of children with ADHD need a great deal of support. Primary family caregivers in particular can become frustrated and upset by the constant challenge of dealing with a child with ADHD. Building the child's self-esteem, confidence, and academic success must be the primary goal of all who work with these children.

INTERNET EXERCISE 17.1

http://www.add.org

Under the Information section, Click on "Kids Area."

1. List seven areas available on this site that you could share with a child who is diagnosed with ADD.

Click on "School and me with ADD."

2. What suggestions could you offer to a child who has ADD to help them be more successful in school?

Click on the back arrow.
Click on "Medicine, Me, and ADD."

3. Share this story with a school age child who is diagnosed with ADD. What was this child's reaction?

A PERSONAL GLIMPSE

I don't really mind it. When I don't take my meds, I go crazy or bonkers (sometimes). I'm on my pills cause of my behavor [sic] and anger. And also to control my anger and ways I talk (like so I won't say bad words or other bad langnage [sic]). I was taught about to control your anger, don't let your anger control you.

Eddie, a 9-year-old who takes medication for behavior problems.

▶ **LEARNING OPPORTUNITY:** What feelings do you think this child experiences in those times when he is not able to control his anger? What would you say to this child to encourage him to talk about his disorder and his feelings?

Seizure Disorders

Seizure disorders, also referred to as convulsive disorders, are not uncommon in children and may result from a variety of causes. A common form of seizures is the acute febrile seizure that occurs with fevers and acute infections (see Chap. 11). Epilepsy, on the other hand, is a recurrent and chronic seizure disorder. Epilepsy can be classified as primary (idiopathic) with no known cause or secondary resulting from infection, head trauma, hemorrhage, tumor, or other organic or degenerative factor. Primary epilepsy is the most common; its onset generally is between ages 4 and 8 years.

Clinical Manifestations

Seizures are the characteristic clinical manifestation of both types of epilepsy and may be either **partial** (focal) or generalized. Partial seizures are limited to a particular area of the brain; generalized seizures involve both hemispheres of the brain.

Partial Seizures. Manifestations of partial seizures vary depending on the area of the brain from which they arise. Loss of consciousness or awareness may not occur. Partial seizures are classified as simple partial motor, simple partial sensory, or complex partial (psychomotor).

Simple Partial Motor Seizures. These cause a localized motor activity such as shaking of an arm, leg, or other part of the body. These may be limited to one side of the body or may spread to other parts.

Simple partial sensory seizures may include sensory symptoms called an **aura** (a sensation that signals an impending attack) involving sight, sound, taste, smell, touch, or emotions (a feeling of fear, for example). The child may also have numbness, tingling, paresthesia, or pain.

Complex Partial (Psychomotor) Seizures. These also begin in a small area of the brain and change or alter consciousness. They cause memory loss and staring. Nonpurposeful movements such as hand rubbing, lip smacking, arm dropping, and swallowing may occur. Following the seizure the child may sleep or be confused for a few minutes. The child is often unaware of the seizure. These can be the most difficult seizures to control.

Generalized Seizures. Types of generalized seizures include tonic-clonic (formerly called grand mal), absence (formerly called petit mal), atonic or akinetic (formerly called "drop attacks"), myoclonic, and infantile spasms.

Tonic-Clonic Seizures. These consist of four stages: the prodromal period, which can be days or hours; the aura, which is a warning, immediately before the seizure; the tonic-clonic movements; and the postictal stage. Not all these stages occur with every seizure: the seizure may just begin with a sudden loss of consciousness. During the prodromal period the child might be drowsy, dizzy, or have a lack of coordination. If the seizure is preceded by an aura, it is identified as a generalized seizure secondary to a partial seizure. The aura may reflect in which part of the brain the seizure originates. Young children may have difficulty describing an aura, but may cry out in response to it. In the tonic phase the child's muscles contract, the child may fall, and the child's extremities may stiffen. The contraction of respiratory muscles during the tonic phase may cause the child to become cyanotic and appear briefly to have respiratory arrest. The eyes roll upward and the child might utter a guttural cry. The initial rigidity of the tonic phase changes rapidly to generalized jerking muscle movements in the clonic phase. The child may bite the tongue or lose control of bladder and bowel functions. The jerking movements gradually diminish then disappear, and the child relaxes. The seizure can be brief, lasting less than 1 minute, or it can last 30 minutes or longer. The period after the tonic-clonic phase is called the postictal period. The child may sleep soundly for several hours during this stage or return rapidly to an alert state. Many have a period of confusion, and others experience a prolonged period of stupor.

Absence Seizures. These rarely last longer than 20 seconds. The child loses awareness and stares straight ahead but does not fall. The child may have blinking or twitching of the mouth or an extremity along with the staring. Immediately after the seizure, the child is alert and continues conversation but does not know what was said or done during the episode. Absence seizures can recur frequently, sometimes as often as 50 to 100 a day. If seizures are not fully controlled, the caregiver needs to be especially aware of dangerous situations that might occur in the child's day such as crossing a street on the way to school. These seizures often decrease significantly or stop entirely at adolescence.

Atonic or Akinetic Seizures. These cause a sudden momentary loss of consciousness, muscle tone, and postural control and can cause the child to fall. They can result in serious facial, head, or shoulder injuries. They may recur frequently, particularly in the morning. Following the seizure the child can stand and walk as normal.

Myoclonic Seizures. These are characterized by a sudden jerking of a muscle or group of muscles, often in the arms or legs without loss of consciousness. Myoclonus occurs during the early stages of falling asleep in people who do not have epilepsy.

Infantile Spasms. These occur between 3 and 12 months of age, almost always indicate a cerebral defect, and have a poor prognosis despite treatment. These seizures occur twice as often in boys as in girls and are preceded or followed by a cry. Muscle contractions are sudden, brief, symmetric, and accompanied by rolling eyes. Loss of consciousness does not always occur.

Status Epilepticus. Status epilepticus is the term used to describe a seizure that lasts longer than 30 minutes or a series of seizures where the child does not return to a normal level of consciousness. This emergency situation requires immediate treatment to decrease the likelihood of permanent brain injury, respiratory failure, or even death.

Diagnosis

The types of seizures can be differentiated through the use of EEG (electroencephalography), video and ambulatory EEG, skull radiography, CT (computed tomography), MRI (magnetic resonance imaging), a brain scan, and physical and neurologic assessments. The child's seizure history is an important part of determining the diagnosis.

Treatment

The main goal of treatment, complete control of seizures, can be achieved for most people through the use of anticonvulsant drug therapy. A number of anticonvulsant drugs are available (Table 17–1). The choice of drug is made based on its effectiveness in controlling seizures and side effects and on its degree of toxicity. Chewable or tablet forms of the medications are often used because suspensions separate and sometimes are not shaken well, causing the possibility of inaccurate dosage. The oldest and most popular drug is phenytoin (Dilantin). It can cause hypertrophy of the gums (gingival hyperplasia) after prolonged use.

A few children may be candidates for surgical intervention when the focal point of the seizures is in an area of the brain that is accessible surgically and is not an area critical to functioning. If the cause of the seizures is a tumor or other lesion, surgical removal is sometimes possible.

Ketogenic diets (high in fat and low in carbohydrates and protein) cause the child to have high levels of ketones, which helps to reduce seizure activity. These diets are prescribed, but long-term maintenance is difficult because the diets are difficult to follow and are unappealing to the child.

Nursing Care

In the hospital or home setting, keeping the child safe during a seizure is the highest priority. The caregiver of a child who has a seizure disorder needs to be taught how to prevent injury if the child has a seizure (see Family Teaching Tips: Precautions Before and During Seizures). In the hospital setting, the siderails are padded; objects that could cause harm are kept away from the bed; oxygen and suction are kept at the bedside; and the siderails are in the raised position and the bed lowered when the child is sleeping or resting.

If the child begins having a seizure, the child is placed on her or his side with the head turned toward one side. The nurse stays calm and removes any objects from around the child, protects the child's head, and loosens tight clothing. During the seizure, the nurse notes

- Time the seizure started
- What the child was doing when the seizure began
- Any factor present just before the seizure (bright light, noise)
- Part of the body where seizure activity began
- Movement and parts of the body involved
- Any cyanosis
- Eye position and movement
- Incontinence of urine or stool
- Time seizure ended
- Child's activity following the seizure

When the seizure is over, the nurse should monitor the child, closely paying attention to his or her level of consciousness, motor functions, and behavior. The nurse documents the information noted during the seizure activity. The child may be able to describe the aura or sensation that occurred just prior to the seizure. This information is important to document.

Education and counseling of the child and the family caregivers are important parts of nursing care. They need complete, accurate information about the disorder and the results that can be realistically expected from treatment. Epilepsy does not lead inevitably to mental retardation, but continued and uncontrolled seizures do increase its possibility. Thus, early diagnosis and control of seizures are very important.

Although the outlook for a normal, well-adjusted life is favorable, the nurse should inform the child and family about restrictions that may be encountered. Children with epilepsy should be encouraged to participate in physical activities but should not participate in sports in which a fall could cause serious injury. In many states a person with uncontrolled epilepsy is legally forbidden to drive a motor vehicle; this could limit choice of vocation and lifestyle. Despite attempts to educate the general public about epilepsy, many people remain prejudiced about this disorder, and this can limit the epileptic person's social and vocational acceptance.

TABLE 17.1	Antiepileptic-Anticonvulsive Therapeutic Agents		
Drug	Indication	Side Effects	Nursing Implications
Carbamazepine (Tegretol)	Generalized tonic-clonic, simple partial, complex partial	Drowsiness, dry mouth, vomiting, double vision, leukopenia, GI upset, thrombocytopenia	There may be dizziness and drowsiness with initial doses. This should subside within 3–14 days.
Clonazepam (Klonopin)	Absence seizures, generalized tonic-clonic, myoclonic, simple partial, complex partial	Double vision, drowsiness, increased salivation, changes in behavior, bone marrow depression	Obtain periodic liver function tests and complete blood count. Monitor for drowsiness, lethargy.
Ethosuximide (Zarontin)	Absence seizures, myoclonic	Dry mouth, anorexia, dizziness, headache, nausea, vomiting, GI upset, lethargy, bone marrow depression	Use with caution in hepatic or renal disease.
Phenobarbital (Luminol)	Generalized tonic-clonic, myoclonic, simple partial, complex partial	Drowsiness, alteration in sleep patterns, irritability, respiratory and cardiac depression, restlessness, headache	Alcohol can enhance the effects of phenobarbital. Monitor blood levels of drug. Liver function studies are necessary with prolonged use.
Phenytoin (Dilantin)	Generalized tonic-clonic, simple partial, complex partial	Double vision, blurred vision, slurred speech, nystagmus, ataxia, gingival hyperplasia, hirsutism, cardiac arrhythmias, bone marrow depression	Alcohol, antacids, and folic acid decrease the effect of phenytoin. Instruct the child or caregiver to notify the dentist that he or she is taking phenytoin to monitor hyperplasia of the gums. Inform the child or caregiver that the drug may color the urine pink to red-brown.
Primidone (Mysoline)	Generalized tonic-clonic, simple partial, complex partial	Behavior changes, drowsiness, hyperactivity, ataxia, bone marrow depression	Adverse effects are the same as for phenobarbital. Sedation and dizziness may be severe during initial therapy; dosage may need to be adjusted by the physician.
Valproic acid (Depakene)	Absence, generalized tonic-clonic, myoclonic, simple partial, complex partial	Nausea, vomiting, or increased appetite, tremors, elevated liver enzymes, constipation, headaches, depression, lymphocytosis, leukopenia, increased prothrombin time	Physical dependency may result when used for prolonged period. Tablets and capsules should be taken whole. Elixir should be taken alone, not mixed with carbonated beverages. Increased toxicity may occur with administration of salicylates (aspirin).

General Nursing Considerations With Anticonvulsant Therapy
General nursing considerations with anticonvulsant therapy that apply to all or most of drugs given to children include:
1. Warn the patient and family that patients should avoid activities that require alertness and complex psychomotor coordination (e.g., climbing).
2. Medication can be given with meals to minimize gastric irritation.
3. The anticonvulsant medications should not be discontinued abruptly as this can precipitate status epilepticus.
4. Anticonvulsant medications generally have a cumulative effect, both therapeutically and adversely.
5. Alcohol ingestion increases the effects of anticonvulsant drugs, exaggerating central nervous system depression.
6. Many of the drugs can cause bone marrow depression (leukopenia, thrombocytopenia, neutropenia, megaloblastic anemia). Regular complete blood cell counts, including WBCs, RBCs, and platelets, are necessary to evaluate bone marrow production.
7. The child should receive periodic blood tests to monitor therapeutic levels as opposed to toxic levels.

FAMILY TEACHING TIPS

Precautions Before and During Seizures

BEFORE
• Have child swim with a companion.
• Have child use protective helmet and padding for bicycle riding, skate boarding.
• Supervise when using power equipment.
• Carry or wear medical ID bracelet.
• Discuss the child's condition with teachers and school nurse.
• Know factors that trigger seizure activity.

DURING
• Stay calm.
• Move furniture or objects that could cause injury.
• Turn child on side with head turned to one side.
• Remove glasses.
• Protect child's head.
• Don't restrain.
• Don't try to put anything between child's teeth.
• Keep people from crowding around child.
• After seizure, notify care provider for follow-up.
• If seizures continue without stopping, call for emergency help.

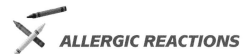

ALLERGIC REACTIONS

Millions of Americans suffer from allergic diseases, most of which begin in childhood. Children with allergies are hampered because of poor appetites, poor sleep, and restricted physical activity in play and at school, all of which often result in altered physical and personality development. Children whose parents or grandparents have allergies are more likely to become allergic than other children are.

An allergic condition is caused by sensitivity to a substance called an **allergen** (an antigen that causes an allergy). Thousands of allergens exist. Some of the most common are

• Pollen
• Mold
• Dust
• Animal dander
• Insect bites
• Tobacco smoke
• Nuts
• Chocolate
• Milk
• Fish
• Shellfish

Drugs, particularly aspirin and penicillin, can be allergens as well. Some plants and chemicals cause allergic reactions on the skin. These are discussed later in this chapter.

Allergens may enter the body through various routes, the most common being the nose, throat, eyes, skin, digestive tract , and bronchial tissues in the lungs. The first time the child comes in contact with an allergen, no reaction may be evident but an immune response is stimulated—helper lymphocytes stimulate B lymphocytes to make immunoglobulin E (IgE) antibody. The IgE antibody attaches to mast cells and macrophages. When contacted again, the allergen attaches to the IgE receptor sites and a response occurs in which certain substances, such as histamine, are released; these substances produce the symptoms known as allergy.

Diagnosis of an allergy requires a careful history and physical examination and possibly skin and blood tests including a complete blood count, serum protein electrophoresis, and immunoelectrophoresis. Skin testing is generally done when removal of obvious allergens is impossible or has not brought relief. If a food allergy is suspected, an elimination diet may help identify the allergen. Eliminating the food suspected is sometimes difficult because there are often "hidden" ingredients in food products. For instance, when the caregivers of a child allergic to peanuts begins reading labels of food products they find many unsuspecting products contain peanuts or peanut oil. When specific allergens have been identified, patients can either avoid them or, if this is impossible, undergo immunization therapy by injection. This process is called **hyposensitization** or immunotherapy.

Hyposensitization is performed for the allergens that produce a positive reaction on skin testing. The allergist sets up a schedule for injections in gradually increasing doses until a maintenance dose is reached. The patient should remain in the physician's office for 20 to 30 minutes after the injection in case any reaction occurs. Reactions are treated with epinephrine. Severe reactions in children are uncommon, and hyposensitization is considered a safe procedure with considerable benefit for some children.

Symptomatic relief in allergic reactions can be gained through antihistamine or steroid therapy, but the best treatment is prevention.

Allergic Rhinitis (Hay Fever)

Allergic rhinitis in children is most often due to sensitization to animal dander, house dust, pollens, and molds. Pollen allergy seldom appears before 4 or 5 years of age.

Clinical Manifestations

A watery nasal discharge, postnasal drip, sneezing, and allergic conjunctivitis are the usual symptoms of allergic rhinitis. Continued sniffing, itching of the nose and palate, and the "allergic salute" in which the child pushes his or her nose upward and backward to relieve itching and open the air passages in the nose are common complaints. Because of congestion in the nose, there is back pressure to the blood circulation around the eyes and dark circles are visible under the eyes (Fig. 17–1).

Treatment

When possible, offending allergens are avoided or removed from the environment. Antihistamine-decongestant preparations, such as Dimetapp, Actifed, and others, can be helpful for some patients. Hyposensitization can be implemented, particularly if antihistamines are not helpful or are needed chronically.

Asthma

Asthma is a spasm of the bronchial tubes due to hypersensitivity of the airways in the bronchial system and inflammation that leads to mucosal edema and mucus hypersecretion. Asthma is also sometimes referred to as reactive airway disease. This reversible obstructive airway disease affects millions of people in the United States, including 5% to 10% of all U.S. children.

Asthma attacks are often triggered by a hypersensitive response to allergens. In young children, asthma may be a response to certain foods. Asthma is often triggered by exercise, exposure to cold weather, irritants such as wood-burning stoves, cigarette smoke, dust, pet dander, and foods such as chocolate, milk, eggs, nuts, and grains. Infections, such as bronchitis and upper respiratory infection, can provoke asthma attacks. In children with asthmatic tendencies, emotional stress or anxiety can trigger an attack. Some children with asthma may have no evidence of an immunologic cause for the symptoms.

Asthma can be either intermittent with extended periods when the child has no symptoms and does not need medication or chronic with the need for frequent or continuous therapy. Chronic asthma affects the child's school performance and general activities and may contribute to poor self-confidence and dependency. Asthma is the most common single cause of school absence.[1]

Pathophysiology

Spasms of the smooth muscles cause the lumina of the bronchi and bronchioles to narrow. Edema of the mucous membranes lining these bronchial branches and increased production of thick mucus within them combine with the spasm to cause respiratory obstruction (Fig. 17–2).

Clinical Manifestations

The onset of an attack may be very abrupt or it may progress over several days as evidenced by a dry,

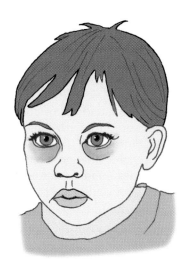

● **Figure 17.1** Back pressure to blood circulation around the eyes leads to dark areas under the eyes in the child with allergic rhinitis.

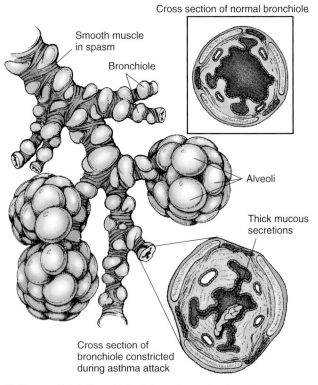

Cross section of normal bronchiole

Smooth muscle in spasm

Bronchiole

Alveoli

Thick mucous secretions

Cross section of bronchiole constricted during asthma attack

● **Figure 17.2** Bronchiole airflow obstruction in asthma.

hacking cough; **wheezing** (the sound of expired air being pushed through obstructed bronchioles); and difficulty breathing. Asthma attacks often occur at night and awaken the child from sleep. The child must sit up and is totally preoccupied with efforts to breathe. Attacks may last for only a short time or may continue for several days. Thick, tenacious mucus may be coughed up or vomited after a coughing episode. In some asthmatic patients, coughing is the major symptom and wheezing occurs rarely if at all. Many children no longer have symptoms after puberty, but this is not predictable. Other allergies may develop in adulthood.

Diagnosis

The history and physical examination are of primary importance in diagnosing asthma. When listening to the child's breathing (auscultation), the examiner hears dyspnea and wheezing, which are usually generalized over all lung fields. Mucus production may be profuse. Pulmonary function tests are valuable diagnostic tools and indicate the amount of obstruction in the bronchial airways especially in the smallest airways of the lungs. A definitive diagnosis of asthma is made when the obstruction in the airways is reversed with bronchodilators.

Treatment

Prevention is the most important aspect in the treatment of asthma. Children and their families must be taught to recognize the symptoms that lead to an acute attack so that they can be treated as early as possible. These symptoms include respiratory retractions and wheezing and an increased amount of coughing at night, in the early morning, or with activity. Use of a peak flow meter is an objective way to measure airway obstruction, and children as young as 4 or 5 years of age can be taught to use one (see Family Teaching Tips: How to Use a Peak Flow Meter) (Fig. 17–3). A peak flow diary should be maintained and also can include symptoms, exacerbations, actions taken, and outcomes. Families must make every effort to eliminate any possible allergens from the home. The goals of asthma treatment include preventing symptoms, maintaining near normal lung function and activity levels, preventing recurring exacerbations and hospitalizations, and providing the best medication treatment with the fewest adverse effects. Depending on the frequency and severity of symptoms and exacerbations, a stepwise approach to the treatment of asthma is used to manage the disease. The steps are used to determine combinations of medications to be used (Table 17–2).

Medications used to treat asthma are divided into two categories: quick-relief medications for

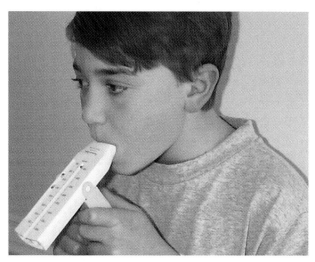

● *Figure 17.3* The child with asthma uses a peak flow meter and keeps track of readings on a daily basis.

immediate treatment of symptoms and exacerbations and long-term control medications to achieve and maintain control of the symptoms. The classifications of drugs used to treat asthma include bronchodilators (sympathomimetics and xanthine derivatives) as well as other antiasthmatic drugs (corticosteroids, leukotriene inhibitors and mast cell stabilizers). See Table 17–3 for a list of some of the other medications used to treat asthma. Many of these drugs can be given either by a **nebulizer** (tube attached to a wall unit or cylinder that delivers moist air via a face mask) or a MDI **metered-dose inhaler** (hand-held plastic device that delivers a premeasured dose). The MDI may have a spacer unit attached that makes it easier for the young child to use (Fig. 17–4).

Bronchodilators. Bronchodilators are used for quick relief of acute exacerbations of asthma symptoms. They are short-acting and available in pill, liquid, or inhalant form. These drugs are administered every 6 to 8 hours or every 4 to 6 hours by inhalation, if breathing difficulty continues. In severe attacks, epinephrine by subcutaneous injection often affords quick relief of symptoms. Some bronchodilators such as salmeterol (Serevent) are used in long-term control.

Theophylline preparations have long been used in the treatment of asthma. The drug is available in short-acting and long-acting forms. The short-acting forms are given about every 6 hours. Because they enter the bloodstream quickly, they are most effective when used only as needed for intermittent episodes of asthma. Long-acting preparations of theophylline are given every 8 to 12 hours. Some of these preparations come in sustained release forms. These are helpful in patients who continually need medication,

TABLE 17.2	Stepwise Approach to Treating Asthma
Steps	**Symptoms**
Step One	
Mild intermittent	Symptoms occur less than 2 times a week No symptoms between exacerbations Exacerbations brief Nighttime symptoms less than 2 times a month
Step Two	
Mild persistent	Symptoms occur more than 2 times a week but less than one time a day Exacerbations may affect activity Nighttime symptoms greater than 2 times a month
Step Three	
Moderate persistent	Daily symptoms Daily use of inhaled short-acting beta-2 agonist Exacerbations affect activity Exacerbations more than 2 times a week, may last days Nighttime symptoms more than 1 time a week
Step Four	
Severe persistent	Continual symptoms Limited physical activity Frequent exacerbations Frequent nighttime symptoms

because these drugs sustain more consistent theophylline levels in the blood than short-acting forms do. Patients hospitalized for status asthmaticus may receive theophylline intravenously (IV).

Corticosteroids. Corticosteroids are anti-inflammatory drugs used to control severe or chronic cases of asthma. Steroids may be given in inhaled form to decrease the systemic effects that accompany oral steroid administration.

Leukotriene Inhibitors. These are given by mouth along with other asthma medications for long-term control and prevention of mild, persistent asthma. Leukotrienes are bronchoconstrictive substances, which are released in the body during the inflammatory process. These drugs inhibit leukotriene production, which helps with bronchodilation and decreases airway edema.

Mast Cell Stabilizers. These help to stabilize the cell membrane by preventing mast cells from releasing the chemical mediators that cause bronchospasm and mucous membrane inflammation They are used to help decrease wheezing and exercise-induced asthma attacks. These are nonsteroidal anti-inflammatory drugs (NSAID) and have relatively few side effects. A bronchodilator often is given to open up the airways just before the mast cell stabilizer is used. Children dislike the taste of the medication, but

receiving sips of water following the administration minimizes the distaste.

Chest Physiotherapy. Because asthma has multiple causes, treatment and continued management of the disease require more than medication. Chest physiotherapy includes breathing exercises, physical training, and inhalation therapy. Studies have shown that breathing exercises to improve respiratory function and help control asthma attacks can be an important adjunct to using medications for treatment. These exercises teach children how to help control their own symptoms and thereby build self-confidence, which is sometimes lacking in asthmatic children. If the exercises can be taught as part of play activities, children are more likely to find them fun and to practice them more often.

● Nursing Process for the Child With Asthma

ASSESSMENT

Obtain information from the caregiver about the asthma history, the medications the child takes,

FAMILY TEACHING TIPS

How to Use a Peak Flow Meter

INTRODUCTION

Your child cannot feel early changes in the airway. By the time the child feels tightness in the chest or starts to wheeze, he or she is already far into an asthma episode. The most reliable early sign of an asthma episode is a drop in the child's peak expiratory flow rate, or the ability to breathe out quickly, which can be measured by a peak flow meter. Almost every asthmatic child over the age of 4 years can and should learn to use a peak flow meter (Figs. *A* and *B*.)

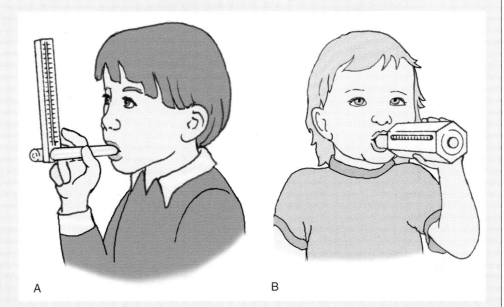

(A) The Assess peak flow meter. **(B)** The Mini-Wright peak flow meter.

A   B

STEPS TO ACCURATE MEASUREMENTS

1. Remove gum or food from the mouth.
2. Move the pointer on the meter to zero.
3. Stand up and hold the meter horizontally with fingers away from the vent holes and marker.
4. With mouth wide open, slowly breathe in as much air as possible.
5. Put the mouthpiece on the tongue and place lips around it.
6. Blow out as hard and fast as you can. Give a short, sharp blast, not a slow blow. The meter measures the fastest puff, not the longest.
7. Repeat steps 1–6 three times. Wait at least 10 seconds between puffs. Move the pointer to zero after each puff.
8. Record the best reading.

GUIDELINES FOR TREATMENT

Each child has a unique pattern of asthma episodes. Most episodes begin gradually, and a drop in peak flow can alert you to start medications before the actual symptoms appear. This early treatment can prevent a flare-up from getting out of hand. One way to look at peak flow scores is to match the scores with three colors:

Green	Yellow	Red
80%–100% personal best	50%–80% personal best	Below 50% personal best
No symptoms	Mild to moderate symptoms	Serious distress
Full breathing reserve	Diminished reserve	Pulmonary function is significantly impaired
Mild trigger may not cause symptoms	A minor trigger produces noticeable symptoms	Any trigger may lead to severe distress
Continue current management	Augment present treatment regimen	Contact physician

Remember, treatment should be adjusted to fit the individual's needs. Your physician will develop a home management plan with you. When in doubt, consult your physician.

TABLE 17.3	Medications Used in the Treatment of Asthma			
Generic Name	Trade Name	Dose Form	Uses	Adverse Reactions/Side Effects
Bronchodilators				
Sympathomimetics (Beta-2-receptor Agonists)				
albuterol sulfate	Proventil, Ventolin	MDI PO Nebulizer	Quick relief	Restlessness, anxiety, fear, palpitations, insomnia, tremors
metaproterenol hydrochloride	Alupent, Metaprel	MDI PO Nebulizer	Quick relief Short-term control	Tremors, anxiety, insomnia, dizziness, tachycardia
terbutaline sulfate	Brethine	MDI PO	MDI—Quick relief PO—Long-term control	Tremors, anxiety, insomnia, dizziness, tachycardia
salmeterol	Serevent	MDI	Long-term control	Headache, tremors, tachycardia
Xanthine Derivative				
Theophylline	Slo-Phyllin, Elixophyllin Theo-Dur	PO Timed-release	Long-term control	Nausea, vomiting, headache, nervousness, irritability, insomnia
Antiasthma Drugs				
Corticosteroids				
beclomethasone	Beclovent	MDI	Long-term control	Throat irritation, cough, nausea, dizziness
triamcinolone	Azamacort	MDI	Long-term control	Throat irritation, cough, nausea, dizziness
Leukotriene Inhibitors				
Montelukast	Singulair	PO	Long-term control	Headache, nausea, abdominal pain, diarrhea
Mast Cell Stabilizers				
Cromolyn	Intal	Intranasal nebulizer	Long-term control	Nasal irritation, unpleasant taste, headache, nausea, dry throat

MDI = metered-dose inhaler.

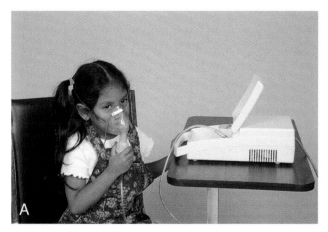
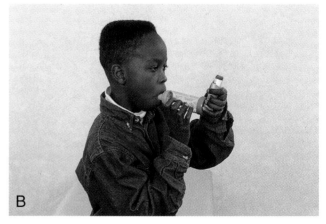

● *Figure 17.4* (**A**) Girl using a nebulizer with a mask. (**B**) Boy using a metered-dose inhaler with spacer.

and the medications taken within the last 24 hours. Ask if the child has vomited, because vomiting would prevent absorption of oral medications. Ask about any history of respiratory infections; possible allergens in the household such as pets; type of furniture and toys; if there is a damp basement (which would contain mold spores); and a history of breathing problems after exercise. In the physical examination, include vital signs, observation for diaphoresis and cyanosis, position, type of breathing, alertness, chest movement, intercostal retractions, and breath sounds. Note any wheezing.

If the child is old enough and alert enough to cooperate, involve him or her in gathering the history, and encourage the child to add information. Ask questions that can be answered "yes" or "no" to minimize tiring the distressed child.

NURSING DIAGNOSES

The information gathered during data collection is used to determine appropriate nursing diagnoses. The nurse works with the child and the child's caregiver to develop a plan of care for the child. Consider the apprehensions of both the child and the family. Nursing diagnoses may include
- Ineffective Airway Clearance related to bronchospasm and increased pulmonary secretions
- Risk for Deficient Fluid Volume related to water loss from tachypnea and diaphoresis and reduced oral intake
- Fatigue related to dyspnea
- Anxiety related to sudden attacks of breathlessness
- Deficient Caregiver Knowledge related to disease process, treatment, home care and control of disease

OUTCOME IDENTIFICATION AND PLANNING

The initial major goals for the child include maintaining a clear airway and an adequate fluid intake as well as relieving fatigue and anxiety. The family's goals include learning how to manage the child's life with asthma. Base the nursing plan of care on these goals.

IMPLEMENTATION

Monitoring Respiratory Function. Continuously monitor the child while he or she is in acute distress from an asthma attack using pulse oximetry and a cardiopulmonary monitor. If this equipment is unavailable, take the child's respirations every 15 minutes during an acute attack and every 1 or 2 hours after the crisis is over. Listening to lung sounds should be done to further monitor the respiratory function. Observe for nasal flaring and chest retractions; observe the skin for color and diaphoresis. Elevate the child's head. An older child may be more comfortable resting forward on a pillow placed on an overbed table. Monitor the child for response to medications and their side effects such as restlessness, gastrointestinal (GI) upset, and seizures. Use humidified oxygen and suction as needed during periods of acute distress.

Monitoring and Improving Fluid Intake. During an acute attack, the child may lose a great quantity of fluid through the respiratory tract and may have a poor oral intake because of coughing and vomiting. Theophylline administration also has a diuretic effect, which compounds the problem. Monitor intake and output. Encourage oral fluids that the child likes. IV fluids are administered as ordered. IV fluid intake is monitored and all precautions for parenteral administration are followed. Note the skin turgor and observe the mucous membranes at least every 8 hours. Weigh the child daily to help determine fluid losses.

Promoting Energy Conservation. The child may become extremely tired from the exertion of trying to breathe. Activities and patient care should be spaced to provide maximum periods of uninterrupted rest. Provide quiet activities when the child needs diversion. Keep visitors to a minimum and maintain a quiet environment.

Reducing Child and Parent Anxiety. The sudden onset of an asthma attack can be frightening to the child and the family caregivers. Respond quickly when the child has an attack. Reassure the child and the family during an episode of dyspnea. The child's fear of attacks can be increased by the caregiver's behavior. Teach the child and the caregiver the symptoms of an impending attack and the immediate response needed to decrease the threat of an attack. This knowledge will help them to cope with impending attacks and plan how to handle the attacks. When they are prepared with information, the child and family may be less fearful. Give the child examples of sports figures, entertainers, actors and actresses, and political leaders who have or have had asthma, for example, Olympic track and field athlete Jackie Joyner Kersee and President John F. Kennedy.

Providing Family Teaching. Child and family caregiver teaching is of primary importance in the care of asthmatic children. Family caregivers may overprotect the child because of the fear that an attack will occur when the child is with a babysitter, at school, or anywhere away from the caregiver. Asthma attacks can be prevented or decreased by prompt and adequate intervention. Teach the caregiver and child within the scope of the child's ability to understand about the disease process, recognition of symptoms of an impending attack, environmental control, avoidance of infection, exercise, drug therapy, and chest physiotherapy.

Teach the caregiver and the child how to use metered-dose inhaler medications and have them demonstrate correct usage (see Family Teaching Tips: How to Use a Metered-Dose Inhaler). Give instructions on home use of a peak flow meter. Urge them to maintain a diary to record the peak flow as well as asthma symptoms, onset of attacks, action taken, and results. Include instructions about administering premedication before the child is exposed to situations in which an attack may occur.

Inform caregivers of allergens that may be in the child's environment, and encourage them to eliminate or control the allergens as needed. Stress the importance of quick response when the child has a respiratory infection. Give instructions for exercise and chest physiotherapy.

Stress to the caregivers the importance of informing the child's classroom teacher, physical education teacher, school nurse, babysitter, and others who are responsible for the child about the child's condition. With a physician's order including directions for use, the child should be permitted to bring medications to school and keep them so they can be used when needed.

FAMILY TEACHING TIPS

How to Use a Metered-Dose Inhaler

1. When ready to use, shake the inhaler well with the cap still on. The child should stand, if possible.
2. Remove the cap.
3. Hold the inhaler with the mouthpiece down, facing the child.
4. Be sure the child's mouth is empty.
5. Hold the mouthpiece about 1 to 1½ inches from the lips.*
6. Breathe out normally. Open mouth wide and begin to breathe in.
7. Press top of medication canister firmly while inhaling deeply. Hold breath as long as possible (at least 10 seconds—teach child to count slowly to 10).
8. Breathe out *slowly* through nose or pursed lips.
9. Relax 2 to 5 minutes and repeat as directed by physician.

*The mouthpiece can also be put between the lips with the lips forming an airtight seal, or a spacer can be attached to the inhaler and the mouthpiece held between the lips.

Provide information on support groups available in the area. The American Lung Association has many materials available to families and can provide information about support groups, camps, and workshops (web site: *http://www.lungusa.org*). The Asthma and Allergy Foundation of America (web site: *http://www.aafa.org*) and the National Heart, Lung, Blood Institute (website *http://www.nhlbl.nih.gov*) are also resources.

EVALUATION: GOALS AND OUTCOME CRITERIA

- *Goal:* The child's airway will remain open.
  Criteria: The child's breath sounds are clear with no wheezing, retractions, or nasal flaring; the skin color is good; and the pulse rate is within normal limits.
- *Goal:* The child's fluid intake will be adequate.
  Criteria: The child's hourly urine output is 30–40 ml; mucous membranes are moist; skin turgor is good; weight remains stable.
- *Goal:* The child will have less fatigue.
  Criteria: The child has extended periods of rest; activities are well spaced to avoid tiring the child.

- *Goal:* The child's and caregivers' anxiety and fear related to impending attacks will be minimized.
  Criteria: The child and the caregiver list the symptoms of an impending attack, describe appropriate responses and display confidence in their ability to handle an attack.
- *Goal:* The child and the caregiver will gain knowledge of how to live with asthma.
  Criteria: The child and the caregiver verbalize an understanding of the disease process, treatment, and control. They interact with health care personnel and ask and answer relevant questions. The caregiver obtains information and makes contact with support groups.

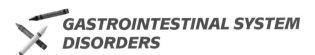

GASTROINTESTINAL SYSTEM DISORDERS

The school-age child may have periodic complaints about a stomach ache or abdominal pain. Usually these aches and pains are minor, benign, and self-limiting. However, the child's complaints should not be dismissed without being assessed, especially if they seem to be acute, have a regular pattern, or are accompanied by other symptoms.

Appendicitis

Most cases of appendicitis (inflammation of the appendix) in childhood occur in the school-age child. In young children, the symptoms may be difficult to evaluate.

The appendix is a blind pouch located in the cecum near the ileocecal junction. Obstruction of the lumen of the appendix is the primary cause of appendicitis. The obstruction usually is caused by hardened fecal matter or a foreign body. This obstruction causes circulation to be slowed or interrupted resulting in pain and necrosis of the appendix. The necrotic area can rupture causing escape of fecal matter and bacteria into the peritoneal cavity and resulting in the complication of peritonitis.

Clinical Manifestations

Symptoms in the older child may be the same as in an adult: pain and tenderness in the right lower quadrant of the abdomen, nausea and vomiting, fever, and constipation. These symptoms are uncommon in young children, however, because many children already have a ruptured appendix when first seen by the physician. The young child has difficulty localizing the pain, may act restless and irritable, and may have a slight fever, a flushed face, and a rapid pulse. Usually the white blood cell count is slightly elevated. It may take several hours to rule out other conditions and make a positive diagnosis. When appendicitis is suspected, laxatives and enemas are contraindicated because they increase peristalsis, which increases the possibility of rupturing an inflamed appendix.

Treatment

Surgical removal of the appendix is necessary and should be performed as soon as possible after diagnosis. If the appendix has not ruptured before surgery, the operative risk is nearly negligible. Even after perforation has occurred, the mortality rate is less than 1%.

Food and fluids by mouth are withheld before surgery. If the child is dehydrated, IV fluids are ordered. If fever is present, the temperature should be reduced to below 102°F (38.9°C).

Recovery is rapid and usually uneventful. The child is ambulated early and can leave the hospital a few days after surgery. If peritonitis or a localized abscess occurs, gastric suction, parenteral fluids, and antibiotics may be ordered.

● Nursing Process for the Child With Appendicitis

ASSESSMENT

When a child is admitted with a diagnosis of possible appendicitis, an emergency situation exists. The family caregiver who brings the child to the hospital is often upset and anxious. The admission exam and assessment must be performed quickly and skillfully. Obtain information about the child's condition for the last several days to formulate a picture of how the condition has developed. Emphasize GI complaints, appetite, bowel movements for the last few days, and general activity level. During the physical exam, include vital signs especially noting any elevation of temperature, presence of bowel sounds, abdominal guarding, and nausea or vomiting. Report immediately diminished or absent bowel sounds. Provide the child and caregiver with careful explanations about all procedures to be performed. Use special empathy and understanding to alleviate the child's and family's anxieties.

NURSING DIAGNOSES

As soon as the medical diagnosis of appendicitis has been confirmed, the child is prepared for surgery. Some nursing diagnoses might include
- Fear of child and family caregiver related to emergency surgery
- Acute Pain related to necrosis of appendix and surgical procedure
- Risk for Deficient Fluid Volume related to decreased intake
- Deficient Caregiver Knowledge related to post op and home care needs

OUTCOME IDENTIFICATION AND PLANNING

Because of the urgent nature of the child's admission and preparation for surgery, great efforts must be taken to provide calm, reassuring care both to the child and the caregivers. A major goal for both the child and the caregivers is relieving fear. Additional goals for the child are relieving pain and maintaining fluid intake. Another goal for the family is increasing knowledge of the postoperative and home care needs of the child.

Reducing Fear. Although procedures must be performed quickly, consider both the child's and the family's fear. The child may be extremely frightened by the sudden change of events and also may be in considerable pain. The family caregiver may be apprehensive about impending surgery. Introduce various health care team members by name and title as they come into the child's room to perform procedures. Explain to the child and the family what is happening and why. Explain the postanesthesia care unit (recovery room) to the child and the family. Encourage the family and child to verbalize fears, and try to allay these fears as much as possible. Let family members know where to wait during surgery, how long the surgery will last, where dining facilities are located, and where the surgeon will expect to find them after surgery. If possible, demonstrate deep breathing, coughing, and abdominal splinting to the child and have her or him practice it. Throughout the preoperative care, be

sensitive to verbalized or nonverbalized fears and provide understanding care.

Reducing Pain. Preoperatively, analgesics are not given because they may conceal signs of tenderness that are important for diagnosis. Provide comfort through positioning and gentle care while performing preoperative procedures. Heat to the abdomen is contraindicated because of the danger of rupture of the appendix. Postoperatively, observe the child hourly for indications of pain and administer analgesics as ordered. Provide quiet activities to help divert the child's attention from the pain. The child may fear ambulation postoperatively because of pain. Many children (and adults too) are worried that the stitches will pull out. Reassure the child that this worry is understood but that the sutures (or staples) are intended to withstand the strain of walking and moving. Activity is essential to the child's recovery but should be as pain-free as possible. Help the child understand that as activity increases, the pain will decrease. The child whose appendix ruptured before surgery may also have pain related to the nasogastric tube, abdominal distention, or constipation.

Monitoring Fluid Intake. Dehydration can be a concern, especially if the child has had nausea and vomiting preoperatively. On admission to the hospital, the child is maintained NPO until after surgery. Accurately measure and record intake and output. IV fluids are administered as ordered. Postoperatively, check dressings to detect evidence of excessive drainage or bleeding that indicate loss of fluids. Clear oral fluids are usually ordered soon after surgery. After the child takes and retains fluids successfully, a progressive diet is ordered. Monitor, record, and report bowel sounds at least every 4 hours because the physician may use this as a gauge to determine when the child can have solid food.

Providing Family Teaching. The child who has had an uncomplicated appendectomy usually convalesces quickly and can return to school within 1 or 2 weeks. Teach the caregiver to keep the incision clean and dry. Activities are limited according to the physician's recommendations. The child whose appendix ruptured may be hospitalized for up to a week and is more limited in activities postoperatively. Instruct the family to observe for signs and symptoms of complications postoperatively including fever, abdominal distention, and pain. Emphasize the need for making and keeping follow-up appointments.

EVALUATION: GOALS AND OUTCOME CRITERIA

- *Goal:* The child and family caregivers will have reduced or alleviated fear.
  Criteria: The child and family verbalize fears and ask questions preoperatively; the child cooperates with health care personnel.
- *Goal:* The child's pain will be controlled.
  Criteria: The child's pain is at an acceptable level, as evidenced by the child's verbalization of pain according to a pain scale (see Chap. 4).
- *Goal:* The child will have adequate fluid intake.
  Criteria: The child's skin turgor is good, vital signs are within normal limits, and hourly urine output is at least 30–40 mL.
- *Goal:* The family caregivers will verbalize an understanding of post op and home care needs of the child.
  Criteria: The family caregivers discuss recovery expectations, demonstrate wound care as needed, and list signs and symptoms to report.

Intestinal Parasites

A few intestinal parasites are common in the United States especially in young and school-age children. Hand-to-mouth practices contribute to infestations.

Enterobiasis (Pinworm Infection)

The pinworm (*Enterobius vermicularis*) is a white, threadlike worm that invades the cecum and may enter the appendix. Articles contaminated with pinworm eggs spread pinworms from person to person. The infestation is common in children and occurs when the pinworm eggs are swallowed. The eggs hatch in the intestinal tract and grow to maturity in the cecum. The female worm, when ready to lay her eggs, crawls out of the anus and lays the eggs on the perineum.

Itching around the anus causes the child to scratch and trap new eggs under the fingernails, which often causes reinfection when the child's fingers go into the mouth. Clothing, bedding, food, toilet seats, and other articles become infected, and the infestation spreads to other members of the family. Pinworm eggs also can float in the air and be inhaled.

The life cycle of these worms is 6 to 8 weeks after which reinfestation commonly occurs without treatment. The incidence is highest in school-age children and next highest in preschoolers. All members of the family are susceptible.

Clinical Manifestation and Diagnosis. Intense perianal itching is the primary symptom of pinworms. Young children who cannot clearly verbalize their feelings may be restless, sleep poorly, or have episodes of bedwetting.

The usual method of diagnosis is to use cellophane tape to capture the eggs from around the anus and to examine them under a microscope. Adult worms also may be seen as they emerge from the anus when the child is lying quietly or sleeping. The cellophane tape test for identifying worms is performed in the early morning just before or as soon as the child wakens:

1. Wind clear cellophane tape around the end of a tongue blade, sticky side outward.
2. Spread the child's buttocks and press the tape against the anus, rolling from side to side.
3. Transfer the tape to a microscope slide and cover with a clean slide to send to the laboratory. The tongue blade can be placed in a plastic bag if the caregiver does not have slides or a commercially prepared kit.
4. The tape is examined microscopically for eggs in the laboratory.

Treatment and Nursing Care. Treatment consists of the use of an **anthelmintic** (or vermifugal, a medication that expels intestinal worms). Mebendazole (Vermox) is the most commonly used product. The medication should be repeated in 2 or 3 weeks to eliminate any parasites that hatch after the initial treatment. Because pinworms are easily transmitted, the nurse should encourage all family members to be treated as well.

It is often disturbing to children and caregivers for the child to be found to have pinworms. They may need reassurance from the nurse that pinworm infestation is as common as an infection or a cold. This support is important when caring for a child with any type of intestinal parasite.

As a preventive measure, the nurse should teach the child to wash the hands after bowel movements and before eating. The child should also be encouraged to observe other hygiene measures such as regular bathing and daily change of underclothing. The nurse must teach caregivers to keep the child's fingernails short and clean. Caregivers also need to know that bedding should be changed frequently to avoid reinfestation. All bedding and clothing, especially underclothing, should be washed in hot water.

Roundworms

Ascaris lumbricoides is a large intestinal worm found only in humans. Infestation is from the feces of infested people. It is usually found in areas where sanitary facilities are lacking and human excreta are deposited on the ground.

The adult worm is pink and 9 inches to 12 inches long. The eggs hatch in the intestinal tract, and the larvae migrate to the liver and lungs. The larvae reaching the lungs ascend up through the bronchi, are swallowed, and reach the intestine where they grow to maturity and mate. Eggs are then discharged into the feces. Full development requires about 2 months. In tropical countries where infestation may be heavy, bowel obstructions may present serious problems. Generally, however, no symptoms are present in ordinary infestations. Identification is made by means of microscopic examination of feces for eggs. Pyrantel pamoate (Antiminth) is the medication commonly used. The nurse must teach caregivers that improved hygiene practices with sanitary disposal of feces including diapers are necessary to prevent infestation.

Hookworms

The hookworm lives in the human intestinal tract, where it attaches itself to the wall of the small intestine. Eggs are discharged in the feces of the host. These parasites are prevalent in areas where infected human excreta is deposited on the ground and where the soil, moisture, and temperature are favorable for the development of infective larvae of the worm. In the southeastern United States and tropical West Africa, the prevailing species is *Necator americanus.*

Clinical Manifestation and Diagnosis. After feces containing eggs are deposited on the ground, larvae hatch. They can survive there as long as 6 weeks and usually penetrate the skin of barefoot people. They produce an itching dermatitis on the feet (ground itch). The larvae pass through the bloodstream to the lungs and into the pharynx, where they are swallowed and reach the small intestine. In the small intestine, they attach themselves to the intestinal wall, where they feed on blood. Heavy infestation may cause anemia through loss of blood. Chronic infestation produces listlessness, fatigue, and malnutrition. Identification is made by examination of the stool under the microscope.

Treatment and Nursing Care. Pyrantel pamoate or mebendazole may be used in the treatment of hookworms. The nurse must stress the need for the affected child to receive a well-balanced diet with additional protein and iron. Transfusions are rarely necessary. To prevent hookworm infestation, the nurse should instruct caregivers to keep children from running barefoot where there is any possibility of ground contamination with feces.

Giardiasis

Giardiasis is not caused by a worm but by a protozoan parasite, *Giardia lamblia.* It is a common cause of diarrhea in world travelers and is also prevalent in children who attend day care centers and other types of residential facilities; it may be found in contaminated mountain streams or pools frequented by diapered infants. The child ingests the cyst containing the protozoa. The cyst is activated by stomach acid and passes into the duodenum, where it matures and causes diarrhea, weight loss, and abdominal cramps. Identification and diagnosis are made through examination of stool under the microscope.

Metronidazole (Flagyl) or quinacrine (Atabrine) is effective in treating the infestation. The nurse should alert the caregiver that quinacrine causes a yellow discoloration of the skin. To prevent infestations, the nurse should stress to caregivers the importance of careful handling of soiled diapers especially in a child care facility. Handwashing, avoiding pools and streams used by diapered infants, and avoiding contact with infected persons are also important.

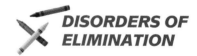

DISORDERS OF ELIMINATION

Although difficulties with diarrhea or constipation are common in school-age children, the most common cause for stress in the child and the caregiver is incontinence. Enuresis or encopresis can cause many days of frustration and discouragement for both the child and the caregiver.

Enuresis

Enuresis, or bedwetting, is involuntary urination beyond the age when control of urination commonly is acquired. Many children do not acquire complete nighttime control before 5 to 7 years of age, and occasional bedwetting may be seen in children as late as 9 or 10 years of age. Boys have more difficulty than girls do, and in some instances enuresis may persist into the adult years.

Enuresis may have a physiologic or psychological cause and may indicate a need for further exploration and treatment. Physiologic causes may include a small bladder capacity, urinary tract infection, and lack of awareness of the signal to empty the bladder because of sleeping too soundly. Persistent bedwetting in a 5- or 6-year-old child may be a result of rigorous toilet training before the child was physically or psychologically ready. Enuresis in the older child may express resentment toward family caregivers or a desire to regress to an earlier level of development to receive more care and attention. Emotional stress can be a precipitating factor. The health care team also needs to consider the possibility that enuresis can be a symptom of sexual abuse.

If a physiologic cause has been ruled out, efforts should be made to discover possible causes including emotional stress. If the child is interested in achieving control—for instance, to go to camp or visit friends overnight—waking the child during the night to go to the toilet or limiting fluids before retiring may be helpful. However, these measures should not be used as a replacement for searching for the cause. Help from a pediatric mental health professional may be needed.

The family caregiver may become extremely frustrated about having to deal with smelly, wet bedding every morning. The child may go to great efforts to hide the fact that the bed is wet. Health care personnel must take a supportive, understanding attitude toward the problems of the caregiver and the child, allowing each of them to ventilate feelings and providing a place where emotions can be freely expressed.

Encopresis

Encopresis is chronic involuntary fecal soiling beyond the age when control is expected (about 3 years of age). Speech and learning disabilities may accompany this problem. If no organic causes (e.g., worms, megacolon) exist, encopresis indicates a serious emotional problem and a need for counseling for the child and the family caregivers. Some experts believe that overcontrol or undercontrol by a caregiver can cause encopresis. Recommendations for treatment differ; the most important goal, however, is recognition of the problem and referral for treatment and counseling.

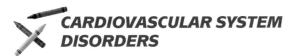

CARDIOVASCULAR SYSTEM DISORDERS

The child's cardiovascular system experiences a period of slow growth with few problems through the school-age years. The primary threat to the cardiovascular system during this age is rheumatic heart disease as a complication of rheumatic fever.

Rheumatic Fever

Rheumatic fever is a chronic disease of childhood, affecting the connective tissue of the heart, joints, lungs, and brain. An autoimmune reaction to group A beta-hemolytic streptococcal infections, rheumatic fever occurs throughout the world particularly in the temperate zones. It has become less common in developed countries, but there have been recent indications of increased occurrences in some areas of the United States.

Rheumatic fever is precipitated by a streptococcal infection such as strep throat, tonsillitis, scarlet fever, or pharyngitis, which may be undiagnosed or untreated. The resultant rheumatic fever manifestation may be the first indication of trouble. An elevation of antistreptococcal antibodies that indicates recent streptococcal infection, however, can be demonstrated in about 95% of the rheumatic fever patients tested within the first 2 months of onset. An antistreptolysin-O titer (ASO titer) measures these antibodies.

Clinical Manifestations

A latent period of 1 to 5 weeks follows the initial infection. The onset is often slow and subtle. The child may be listless, anorectic, and pale. He or she may lose weight and complain of vague muscle, joint, or abdominal pains. Often there is a low-grade late afternoon fever. None of these is diagnostic by itself but if such signs persist, the child should have a medical examination.

Major manifestations of rheumatic fever are **carditis** (inflammation of the heart), **polyarthritis** (migratory arthritis), and **chorea** (disorder characterized by emotional instability, purposeless movements, and muscular weakness). The onset may be acute rather than insidious with severe carditis or arthritis as the presenting symptom. Chorea generally has an insidious onset.

Carditis. Carditis is the major cause of permanent heart damage and disability among children with rheumatic fever. Carditis may occur alone or as a complication of either arthritis or chorea. Presenting symptoms may be vague enough to be missed. The child may have a poor appetite, pallor, a low-grade fever, listlessness, or moderate anemia. Careful observation may reveal slight dyspnea on exertion. Physical examination shows a soft systolic murmur over the apex of the heart. Unfortunately such a child may have been in poor physical health for some time before the murmur is discovered.

Acute carditis may be the presenting symptom particularly in young children. An abrupt onset of high fever (perhaps as high as 104°F (40°C)), tachycardia, pallor, poor pulse quality, and a rapid decrease in hemoglobin are characteristic. Weakness, prostration, cyanosis, and intense precordial pain are common. Cardiac dilatation usually occurs. The pericardium, myocardium, or endocardium may be affected.

Polyarthritis. Polyarthritis moves from one major joint to another (ankles, knees, hips, wrists, elbows, shoulders). The joint becomes painful to either touch or movement (**arthralgia**) and hot and swollen. Body temperature is moderately elevated; the erythrocyte sedimentation rate (ESR) is increased. Although extremely painful, this type of arthritis does not lead to the disabling deformities that occur in rheumatoid arthritis.

Chorea. The onset of chorea is gradual with increasing incoordination, facial grimaces, and repetitive involuntary movements. Movements may be mild and remain so, or they may become increasingly severe. Active arthritis is rarely present when chorea is the major manifestation. Carditis occurs, although less commonly than when polyarthritis is the major condition. Attacks tend to be recurrent and prolonged but are rare after puberty. It is seldom possible to demonstrate an increase in the antistreptococcal antibody level because of the generally prolonged latency period.

Corticosteroids and salicylates are of little value in the treatment of uncomplicated chorea. The child may be sedated with phenobarbital, chlorpromazine (Thorazine), haloperidol (Haldol), or diazepam (Valium). Bed rest is necessary with protection such as padding the bedsides if the movements are severe.

Diagnosis

Rheumatic fever is difficult to diagnose and sometimes impossible to differentiate from other diseases. The possible serious effect of the disease demands early and conscientious medical treatment. However, avoid causing apprehension and disruption of the child's life because the condition could prove to be something less serious. The nurse should not attempt a diagnosis but should understand the criteria on which a presumptive diagnosis is based.

The modified Jones criteria (Fig. 17–5) are generally accepted as a useful rule for guidance when deciding whether or not to treat the patient for rheumatic fever. The criteria are divided into major and minor categories. The presence of two major or one major and two minor criteria indicates a high probability of rheumatic fever if supported by evidence of a preceding streptococcal infection. This system is not infallible, however, because no one criterion is specific to the disease; additional manifestations can help confirm the diagnosis.

Treatment

The chief concern in caring for a child with rheumatic fever is the prevention of residual heart disease. As long as the rheumatic process is active,

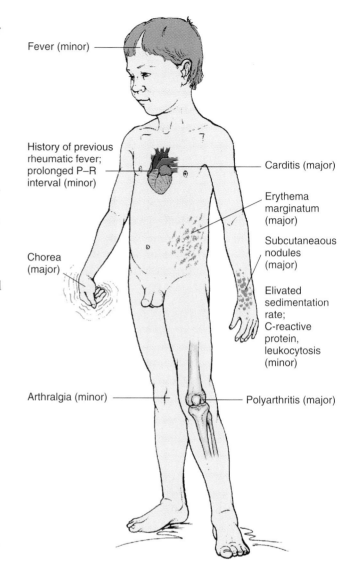

Fever (minor)

History of previous rheumatic fever; prolonged P–R interval (minor)

Carditis (major)

Erythema marginatum (major)

Subcutaneaous nodules (major)

Chorea (major)

Elivated sedimentation rate; C-reactive protein, leukocytosis (minor)

Arthralgia (minor)

Polyarthritis (major)

● **Figure 17.5** Major and minor manifestations of rheumatic fever.

progressive heart damage is possible. Bed rest, therefore, is essential to reduce the heart's workload. The length bed rest is determined by the degree of carditis present. This may be from 2 weeks to several weeks, depending on how long heart failure is present.

Residual heart disease is treated in accordance with its severity and its type with digitalis, restricted activities, diuretics, and a low-sodium diet as indicated.

Laboratory tests, although nonspecific, provide an evaluation of the disease activity to guide treatment. Two commonly used indicators are the ESR and the presence of C-reactive protein. The ESR is elevated in the presence of an inflammatory process and is nearly always increased in the polyarthritis or carditis manifestation of rheumatic fever. It remains elevated until clinical manifestations have ceased and any subclinical activity has subsided. It seldom increases in uncomplicated chorea. Therefore, ESR elevation in a choreic patient may indicate cardiac involvement.

C-reactive protein is not normally present in the blood of healthy people, but it appears in the serum of acutely ill people including people ill with rheumatic fever. As the patient improves, C-reactive protein disappears.

Leukocytosis is also an indication of an inflammatory process. Until the leukocyte count returns to a normal level, the disease probably is still active.

Drug Therapy. Medications used in the treatment of rheumatic fever include penicillin, salicylates, and corticosteroids. Penicillin is administered to eliminate the hemolytic streptococci. If the child is allergic to penicillin, erythromycin is used. Penicillin administration continues after the acute phase of the illness to prevent the recurrence of rheumatic fever.

Salicylates are given in the form of acetylsalicylic acid (aspirin) to children with the daily dosage calculated according to the child's weight. Aspirin relieves pain and reduces the inflammation of polyarthritis. It is also used for its antipyretic effect. The continued administration of a relatively large dosage may cause toxic effects; individual tolerance differs greatly.

For mild or severe carditis, corticosteroids appear to be the drug of choice because of their prompt, dramatic action.

Administration of salicylates or corticosteroids is not expected to alter the course of the disease, but the control of the toxic manifestations enhances the child's comfort and sense of well-being and helps reduce the burden on the heart. This is of particular importance in acute carditis with congestive heart failure. Diuretics may be administered when needed in severe carditis.

Prevention

Because the peak of onset of rheumatic fever occurs in school-age children, health services for this age group take on added importance. The overall approach is to promote continuous health supervision for all children including the school-age child. The use of well-child conferences or clinics needs to increase to provide continuity of care for school-age children. The nurse who has contact in any way with school-age children must be aware of the importance of teaching the public about the need to have upper respiratory infections evaluated for group A beta-hemolytic streptococcus and the need for treatment with penicillin. The nurse also should stress that the child must take the complete prescription of penicillin (usually 10 days' supply) even though the symptoms disappear and the child feels well.

● Nursing Process for the Child With Rheumatic Fever

ASSESSMENT

Conduct a thorough exam of the child. Begin with a careful review of all systems and note the child's physical condition. Observe for any signs that may be classified as major or minor manifestations. In the physical exam, include observation for elevated temperature and pulse and careful examination for erythema marginatum, subcutaneous nodules, swollen or painful joints, or signs of chorea. A throat culture determines if there is an active infection. Obtain a complete, up-to-date history from the child and the caregiver. Ask about a recent sore throat or upper respiratory infection. Find out when the symptoms began, the extent of the illness, and what if any treatment was obtained. Include the school-age child in the nursing interview to help contribute to the history.

NURSING DIAGNOSES

The nursing diagnoses vary depending on the manifestations displayed. The data collected in the physical exam and review of systems is used to determine appropriate diagnoses such as

- Acute Pain related to joint pain when extremities are touched or moved
- Deficient Diversional Activity related to prescribed bed rest
- Activity Intolerance related to carditis or arthralgia
- Risk for Injury related to chorea
- Risk for Noncompliance with prophylactic drug therapy related to financial or emotional burden of lifelong therapy
- Deficient Caregiver Knowledge related to the condition, need for long-term therapy, and risk factors

OUTCOME IDENTIFICATION AND PLANNING

The goals are determined in cooperation with the child and the caregiver. Goals for the child include reducing pain, providing diversional activities and sensory stimulation, conserving energy, and preventing injury. Goals for the caregiver include complying with drug therapy and increasing knowledge about the long-term care of the child. Throughout planning and implementation, bear in mind the child's developmental stage.

IMPLEMENTATION

Providing Comfort Measures and Reducing Pain. Position the child to relieve joint pain. Large joints, including the knees, ankles, wrists, and elbows, usually are involved. Carefully handle the joints when moving the child to help minimize pain. Even the weight of blankets may cause pain; be alert to this possibility and improvise covering as needed. Warm baths and gentle range-of-motion exercises will help to alleviate some joint discomfort. Use pain indicator scales with children so they are able to express the level of their pain (see Fig. 4–4 in Chap. 4).

Salicylates are administered in the form of aspirin to reduce fever and relieve joint inflammation and pain. Because of the risks of long-term administration of salicylates, note any signs of toxicity and record and report them promptly. Tinnitus, nausea, vomiting, and headache are all important signs of toxicity. Administer aspirin after meals or with a glass of milk to lessen GI irritation. Enteric-coated aspirin is also available for patients who are sensitive to its effects. Large doses may alter the prothrombin time and thus interfere with the clotting mechanism. Salicylate therapy is usually continued until all laboratory findings are normal.

The child whose pain is not controlled with salicylates may be administered corticosteroids. Side effects such as **hirsutism** (abnormal hair growth) and "moon face" may be upsetting to the child and family. Toxic reactions such as euphoria, insomnia, gastric irritation, and growth suppression must be watched for and reported. Because premature withdrawal of a steroid drug is likely to cause a relapse, it is important to discontinue the drug gradually by decreasing dosages.

Providing Diversional Activities and Sensory Stimulation. Children vary greatly in how ill they feel during the acute phase of rheumatic fever. For those who do not feel very ill, bed rest can cause distress or resentment. Be creative in finding diversional activities that allow bed rest but prevent restlessness and boredom. This may be a good time to choose a book that involves the child's imagination and that has enough excitement to create ongoing

interest. Do not use the television as an all-day babysitter. Quiet games can provide some entertainment. Use of a computer can be beneficial because both entertaining and educational games are available, and most children enjoy working with a computer. Simple needlework and model building are other useful diversional activities. During the school year, make efforts (or encourage the caregiver) to provide the child with a tutor and work from school; this helps relieve boredom and also maintains contact with peers. Plan all activities with the child's developmental age in mind. The pain of arthralgia may be so great that the child will not want to be involved in any kind of activity. Administer analgesics as ordered to help decrease the inflammation of the joints and decrease the pain, so the child will feel like participating in age appropriate activities.

Promoting Energy Conservation. Provide rest periods between activities to help pace the child's energies and provide for maximum comfort. During times of increased cardiac involvement or exacerbations of joint pain, the child may want to rest and perhaps have someone read a story. Peers may be encouraged to visit, but these visits must be monitored so that the child is not overly tired. The child's classroom could be encouraged to write to the child to provide contact with everyday school activities and keep the child in touch. If the child has chorea, inform visitors that the child cannot control these movements, which are as upsetting to the child as they are to others.

Preventing Injury. The child with chorea may be frustrated with his or her inability to control the movements. Provide an opportunity for the child to express feelings. Protect the child from injury by keeping the side rails up and padding them. Do not leave a child with chorea unattended in a wheelchair. Use all appropriate safety measures.

Promoting Compliance with Drug Therapy. A child does not become immune from future attacks of rheumatic fever after the first illness. Rheumatic fever can recur whenever the child has a group A beta-hemolytic streptococcal infection if the child is not properly treated. For this reason, the child who has had rheumatic fever must be maintained on prophylactic doses of penicillin for 5 years or longer. Whenever the child is to have oral surgery, including dental work, extra prophylactic precautions should be taken even into adulthood. Because of this long-term therapy, noncompliance can become a problem for both financial and emotional reasons. Oral penicillin is usually prescribed, but if compliance is poor, monthly injections of Bicillin can be substituted. Encourage the family to contact the local chapter of the American Heart Association for help finding economical sources of penicillin (web site: *www.americanheart.org*). Become informed about other resources that may be available in your community. Emphasize to the child and the family the need to prevent recurrence of the disease because of the danger of heart damage. Follow-up care must be ongoing even into adulthood.

Providing Family Teaching. Inform the family and child about the importance of having all upper respiratory infections checked by a health care provider to prevent another bout of a streptococcal infection. Be certain that they understand that the child can have recurrences and that a future recurrence could have much more serious effects. If the child has had carditis and heart damage has occurred, instruct the caregiver that the child must be regularly followed to evaluate the damage. The child may need to be maintained on cardiac medications. Instruct the family about these medications. Mitral valve dysfunction is a common aftereffect of severe carditis. A girl who has had mitral valve damage from cardiac involvement may have problems in adulthood during pregnancy. Inform the caregiver that heart failure for such a girl is a possibility during pregnancy and that she should be followed closely to determine heart problems in the event that a mitral valve replacement is needed.

Teaching time is an excellent opportunity to stress the importance of preventing rheumatic fever. Other children in the family may benefit if caregivers are given this information.

EVALUATION: GOALS AND OUTCOME CRITERIA

- *Goal:* The child's joint pain will be minimal.
  Criteria: The child verbalizes or indicates that the pain level is decreased by using a pain scale to express degree of pain.
- *Goal:* The child will become engaged in activities while on bed rest.

  Criteria: The child displays interest and is actively involved in age-appropriate activities.
- *Goal:* The child will learn when and how to conserve energy.
  Criteria: The child rests quietly during rest periods, identifies when he or she needs rest, and engages in quiet diversional activities.
- *Goal:* The child remains free of injury from chorea movements and a safe environment is maintained.
  Criteria: The child has no evidence of injury and safety measures are followed.
- *Goal:* The family caregivers will comply with follow-up drug therapy and the child will take prophylactic medications.
  Criteria: The child and family caregivers verbalize an understanding of the importance of prophylactic medication and identify means for obtaining it.
- *Goal:* The family caregivers will verbalize an understanding of the child's condition, need for long-term therapy, and risk factors.
  Criteria: The caregivers discuss the child's condition, need for follow-up care for the child, and indicate how they will obtain it.

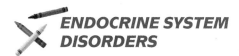

ENDOCRINE SYSTEM DISORDERS

Type 1 diabetes mellitus is the most significant endocrine disorder that affects children of school age. Other conditions that may affect schoolchildren are disorders of the pituitary gland that alter growth and diabetes insipidus. The incidence of these latter conditions is low.

Type 1 Diabetes Mellitus

At least 15 million Americans have been diagnosed with diabetes. A significant number of them are children: Type 1 diabetes mellitus is estimated to affect about one in 600 children between the ages of 5 and 15 years. The incidence of this condition continues to increase.

Diabetes is often considered an adult disease, but at least 5% of cases begin in childhood, usually at about 6 years of age or around the time of puberty. Management of diabetes in children is different from that in adults and requires conscientious care geared to the child's developmental stage.

Diabetes is classified into two major types: Type 1 diabetes that formerly was called insulin-dependent diabetes mellitus (IDDM) or juvenile diabetes and Type 2 diabetes that formerly was called non-insulin-dependent diabetes mellitus. As noted in Table 17–4, diabetes in children is Type 1.

Pathogenesis

The exact pathophysiology of diabetes is not completely understood; however, it is known to result from dysfunction of the beta (insulin-secreting) cells of the islets of Langerhans in the pancreas. Some researchers believe that the presence of an acute infection during childhood may trigger a mechanism in genetically susceptible children, activating beta-cell dysfunction and disrupting insulin secretion. Other conditions that may contribute to Type 1 diabetes are pancreatic tumors, pancreatitis, and long-term corticosteroid use. Normally the sugar derived from digestion and assimilation of foods is burned to provide energy for the body's activities. Excess sugar is converted into fat or glycogen and stored in the body tissues. Insulin, a hormone secreted by the pancreas, is responsible for the burning and storage of sugar. In diabetes, the secretion of insulin is inadequate or nonexistent, allowing sugar to accumulate in the bloodstream and spill over into the urine. In children, diabetes causes an abrupt, pronounced decrease in insulin production, resulting in decreased ability to derive energy from the food eaten. Large amounts of protein and fat are used to supply the child's energy needs, causing loss of weight and slowed growth. This combination of failure to gain weight and lack of energy may be the initial reason the child is brought to the health care provider's attention. However, a health care provider may not see the child until symptoms of ketoacidosis are evident.

Clinical Manifestations

Classic symptoms of Type 1 diabetes mellitus are **polyuria** (dramatic increase in urinary output probably with enuresis), **polydipsia** (increased thirst), and **polyphagia** (increased hunger and food consumption). These symptoms are usually accompanied by weight loss or failure to gain weight and lack of energy, even though the child has increased food consumption. Symptoms of diabetes in children often have an abrupt onset.

If the child's symptoms are not noted and referred for diagnosis, the disorder is likely to progress to **diabetic ketoacidosis.** Because of inadequate insulin production, carbohydrates are not converted into fuel for energy production. Fats are then mobilized for energy but are incompletely oxidized in the absence of glucose. Ketone bodies (acetone, diacetic acid, and oxybutyric acid) accumulate. They are readily excreted in the urine, but the acid-base balance of body fluids excreted is upset and results in acidosis. Diabetic ketoacidosis is characterized by drowsiness, dry skin, flushed cheeks and cherry-red lips, acetone breath with a fruity smell, and **Kussmaul breathing** (abnormal increase in the depth and rate of the respiratory movements). Nausea and vomiting may occur. If untreated, the child lapses into coma and exhibits dehydration, elec-

TABLE 17.4	Comparison of Type 1 and Type 2 Diabetes	
Assessment	Type 1 Diabetes	Type 2 Diabetes
Age of onset	5–7 y or at puberty	40–65 y
Type of onset	Abrupt	Gradual
Weight changes	Marked weight loss is often initial sign	Associated with obesity
Other symptoms	Polydipsia	Polydipsia
	Polyuria (often begins as bed-wetting)	Polyuria
	Fatigue (marks fall in school)	Fatigue
	Blurred vision (marks fall in school)	Blurred vision
	Glycosuria	Glycosuria
	Polyphagia	Pruritus
	Pruritus	Mood changes
	Mood changes (may cause behavior problems in school)	
Therapy	Hypoglycemic agents never effective; insulin needed	Managed by diet, oral hypoglycemic agents, or insulin
	Diet only moderately restricted; no dietary foods used	Diet tends to be strict
	Common-sense foot care for growing children	Good skin and foot care necessary
Period of remission	Period of remission for 1–12 mo generally follows initial diagnosis	Not demonstrable

Adapted from Pillitteri A. (2003). *Maternal and child health nursing* (4th ed). Philadelphia: Lippincott Williams & Wilkins.

trolyte imbalance, rapid pulse, and subnormal temperature and blood pressure.

Treatment for ketoacidosis requires skilled nursing care, and the child may be admitted to a pediatric intensive care unit. Fluid depletion is corrected; blood and urine glucose levels and other blood studies are monitored closely to evaluate the degree of ketoacidosis and electrolyte imbalance. If the child cannot urinate, a catheter is inserted. Regular insulin is given IV along with IV electrolyte fluids.

Diagnosis

Early detection and control are critical in postponing or minimizing later complications of diabetes. The nurse should observe carefully for any signs or symptoms in all members of a family with a history of diabetes. The family also should be taught to observe the children for frequent thirst, urination, and weight loss. All relatives of diabetics are considered a high-risk group and should have periodic testing.

At each visit to a health care provider, children who have a family history of diabetes should be monitored for glycosuria using a finger stick glucose test or urine dipstick testing. If the blood glucose level is elevated or glycosuria is present, a fasting blood sugar (FBS) is performed. A FBS of 200 mg/dL or higher almost certainly is diagnostic for diabetes when other signs such as polyuria and weight loss despite polyphagia are present.

Although glucose tolerance tests are performed in adults to confirm diabetes, they are not commonly used in children. The traditional oral glucose tolerance test is often unsuccessful in children because they may vomit the concentrated glucose that must be swallowed.

Treatment

Management of diabetes in children includes insulin therapy and a meal and exercise plan. Treatment of the diabetic child involves the family and child and a number of health team members such as the nurse,

the pediatrician, the nutritionist, and the diabetic nurse educator. After diabetes is diagnosed, the child may be hospitalized for a period of time. This allows the condition to be stabilized under supervision. This is a trying time, and the nurse must plan care with an understanding of the emotional impact of the diagnosis. The child's teacher, the school nurse, and others who supervise the child during daily activities must be informed of the diagnosis.

Insulin. Insulin therapy is an essential part of the treatment of diabetes in children. The dosage of insulin is adjusted according to blood glucose levels so that the levels are maintained near normal. Two kinds of insulin are often combined for the best results. Insulin can be grouped into rapid-acting, short-acting, intermediate-acting, and long-acting (Table 17–5). The introduction of the rapid acting insulin Lispro or Humalog has greatly changed insulin administration in children.[2] This insulin can be administered immediately after the child has eaten so the amount of food eaten can be taken into consideration when determining the dosage. The onset of action of Lispro is less than 15 minutes. An intermediate-acting and a short-acting insulin often are given together. Some preparations come in a premixed proportion of 70% intermediate-acting and 30% short-acting insulin, eliminating the need for mixing. Many children are controlled on an insulin regimen in which a dose containing a short-acting insulin and an intermediate-acting insulin are given at two times during the day: once before breakfast and the second before the evening meal. Children's insulin doses have to be individually regulated to keep their blood glucose levels as close to normal as possible.

Insulin reaction (insulin shock, hypoglycemia) is caused by insulin overload, resulting in too rapid metabolism of the body's glucose. This may be due to a change in the body's requirement, carelessness in diet (such as failure to eat proper amounts of food), an error in insulin measurement, or excessive exercise. Because diabetes in children is very labile (unstable, fluctuating), the child is subject to insulin

TABLE 17.5	Types of Insulin: Onset, Peak, and Duration			
Action	Preparation	Onset (hrs)	Peak (hrs)	Duration (hrs)
Rapid-acting	Lispro Humalog	0.25	0.5–1	3–4
Short-acting	Regular	0.5–1	2–4	5–7
Intermediate-acting	NPH	1.5–2	6–12	18–24
	Lente	1.5–2	6–12	18–24
Long-acting	Ultralente	4–6	18–24	36–48

*References may vary slightly on these figures.

reactions. Some symptoms of impending insulin shock in children are any type of odd, unusual, or antisocial behavior; weakness; nervousness; lethargy; headache; blurred vision and dizziness; and undue fatigue or hunger. Other symptoms might include pallor, sweating, convulsions, and coma. Children often have hypoglycemic reactions in the early morning. The nurse must observe the child at least every 2 hours during the night. Note tossed bedding, which would indicate restlessness, and any excessive perspiration. If necessary, try to arouse the child. As the child becomes regulated and observes a careful diet at home, parents need not watch so closely but should have a thorough understanding of all aspects of this condition. Blood glucose monitoring often is scheduled for this early morning time in an effort to detect abnormal glucose levels.

Treatment of an insulin reaction should be *immediate*. Give the child sugar, candy, orange juice, or one of the commercial products designed for this emergency. Repeated or impending reactions require consultation with the physician.

If the child cannot take a sugar source orally, glucagon should be administered subcutaneously to bring about a prompt increase in the blood glucose level. Every adult responsible for a diabetic child should clearly understand the procedure for administering this drug and should have easy access to it. Glucagon is a hormone produced by alpha cells of the pancreatic islets. An elevation in the blood glucose level results in insulin release in a normal person, but a decrease in the blood glucose level stimulates glucagon release. The released glucagon in the bloodstream acts on the liver to promote glycogen breakdown and glucose release. Glucagon is available as a pharmaceutical product and is packaged in prefilled syringes for immediate use. It is administered in the same manner as insulin.

Glucagon acts within minutes to restore consciousness, after which the child can take candy or sugar. This treatment prevents the long delay while waiting for a physician to administer glucose IV or for an ambulance to reach the child. It is, however, not a substitute for proper medical supervision.

Insulin Regimen. Most newly diagnosed diabetic children show a decreased need for insulin during the first weeks or months after control is established. This is often referred to as the "honeymoon period," and it should be explained to the family in advance to avoid false hope. As the child grows, the need for insulin increases and continues to do so until the child reaches full growth. Again, family caregivers need to know that this is normal and that the child's condition is not getting worse.

Methods of Giving Insulin. The child may not be able to take over management of the insulin dose as early as blood glucose monitoring, but he or she can watch the preparation of the syringe and learn the technique for drawing up the dosage. It may be helpful to encourage the child to watch the process until it becomes routine. By 8 or 9 years of age, the child should be encouraged to talk with the caregiver about the dose and to practice working with the syringe. The child also may draw up the dose and prepare for self-administration. The age at which this is possible varies. No two children mature at the same rate; some may be able to do this much earlier than others. Automatic injection devices can help the child self-administer insulin at a younger age. The child should be encouraged to take over the management of the therapy when ready. If included in decision-making, the child can learn the importance of the routine and accept the restrictions the disease imposes.

Insulin Pumps. An insulin pump is a method of continuous insulin administration useful for some diabetics. The pump is about the size of a transistor radio and can be worn strapped to the waist or on a shoulder strap. It delivers a steady low dose of insulin through a syringe housed in the pump and connected by polyethylene tubing to a small-gauge subcutaneous needle implanted in the abdomen. Extra insulin is released at mealtimes and other times when needed by pressing a button. The pump does not sense the blood glucose level; therefore, careful blood glucose monitoring at least four times a day is necessary to adjust the dosage as needed. The pump must be removed to bathe, swim, or shower. The child may want to wear loose clothing that will hide the pump. The needle site must be regularly observed for redness and irritation. The site is changed every 24 to 48 hours using aseptic technique.

Unique Needs of the Adolescent. Adolescence is an extremely trying period for many diabetics, as it is for other young people. Diabetics, like normal adolescents, must work from dependence to independence. Even when an adolescent has accepted responsibility for self-care, it is not unusual for him or her to rebel against the control that this condition demands, become impatient, and appear to ignore future health. The adolescent may skip meals, drop diet controls, or neglect glucose monitoring. Going barefoot and neglecting proper foot care also can cause problems for the diabetic adolescent. It can be a difficult time for both the family and the adolescent. The caregivers naturally become concerned and are apt to give the adolescent more controls to rebel against. Special care should be taken by the family, teachers, nurses, and physicians to see that these young people find enough maturing satisfaction in other areas and do not need to rebel in this vital area.

The adolescent who completely understands all aspects of the condition (especially if allowed to assume control of treatment previously) should be allowed to continue managing her or his own treatment. Should the adolescent run into difficulty, an adolescent clinic can be of great value. Here the adolescent can discuss problems with understanding people who respond with care and provide dignity and attentive listening.

● Nursing Process for the Child With Type 1 Diabetes Mellitus

ASSESSMENT

When collecting data, ask the caregiver about the child's symptoms leading up to the present illness. Ask about the child's appetite, weight loss or gain, evidence of polyuria or enuresis in a previously toilet-trained child, polydipsia, dehydration (which may include constipation), irritability, and fatigue. Include the child in the interview and encourage him or her to contribute information. Observe for evidence of the child's developmental stage to help to determine appropriate nursing diagnoses and planning effective care (Table 17–6). If the child is first seen in diabetic coma, adjust the initial nursing interview accordingly.

In the physical exam, measure the height and weight and examine the skin for evidence of dryness or slowly healing sores. Note signs of hyperglycemia, record vital signs, and collect a urine specimen. Perform a blood glucose level determination using a bedside glucose monitor (Fig. 17–6).

NURSING DIAGNOSES

The nursing diagnoses are selected based on the data collected with adjustments for the child's developmental stage. The understanding the child and family have regarding the disease and treatment are important aspects for the healthcare team to consider when nursing diagnoses are being chosen. Nursing diagnoses might include

- Altered Nutrition: Less than Body Requirements related to insufficient caloric intake to meet growth and development needs and the inability of the body to use nutrients
- Risk for Impaired Skin Integrity related to slow healing process and decreased circulation
- Risk for Infection related to elevated glucose levels

- Effective Therapeutic Regimen Management related to blood glucose levels
- Deficient Knowledge related to complications of hypoglycemia and hyperglycemia
- Deficient Knowledge related to insulin administration
- Deficient Knowledge related to appropriate exercise and activity
- Compromised Family Coping related to the impact of the disease on the child and family's life
- Risk for Impaired Adjustment related to long term management of chronic disease

OUTCOME IDENTIFICATION AND PLANNING

The major goals for the child include maintaining adequate nutrition and skin integrity, preventing infection, regulating glucose levels, and learning to adjust to having a chronic disease. Goals for the child and family include learning about and managing hypoglycemia and hyperglycemia, insulin administration, and exercise needs for the child. An additional goal is for family members to express their concerns about coping with the child's illness.

IMPLEMENTATION

Ensuring Adequate and Appropriate Nutrition. The child with diabetes needs a sound nutritional program that provides adequate nutrition for normal growth while it maintains the blood glucose at near-normal levels. The food plan should be well balanced with foods that take into consideration the child's food preferences, cultural customs, and lifestyle (see Family Teaching Tips: Child's Diabetic Food Plan). Help the child and caregiver to understand the importance of eating regularly scheduled meals. Special occasions can be planned so that the child does not feel left out of celebrations. If a particular meal is going to be late, the child should have a complex carbohydrate and protein snack. Children should be included in meal planning when possible so that they learn what is permissible and what is not. In this way they will be able to handle eating when they are on their own in school and in social situations.

Preventing Skin Breakdown. Skin breakdowns, such as blisters and minor cuts, can become

TABLE 17.6	Developmental Guidelines for Diabetic Child Responsibilities*					
Issue	Age (yr)					
	Under 4	4–5	6–7	8–10	11–13	14+
Food	Teaching focuses on parents	Knows likes and dislikes	Can begin to tell sugar content of food and know foods he or she should *not* have	Has more ability to select foods according to criteria like exchange lists	Knows if foods fit own diet plan	Helps plan meals and snacks
Insulin	Parents take responsibility for care	Can tell where injection should be Can pinch the skin	Can begin to help with aspects of injections	Gives own injections with supervision	Can learn to measure insulin	Can mix two insulins
Testing		Can choose finger for finger stick Can wash finger with soap and water Collects urine; should watch caregiver do testing; helps with recording	Can do own finger stick using automatic puncture device. Can help with some aspects of blood test. Can do own urine test and record results.	Can do blood tests with supervision	Can see test results forming a pattern	Can begin to use test results to adjust insulin
Psychological		Identifies with being "bad" or "good"; these words should be avoided. A child this age may think he or she is bad if the test is said to be "bad."	Needs many reminders and supervision	Needs reminders and supervision Understands only immediate consequences, not long-term consequences, of diabetes control. "Scientific" mind developing; intrigued by tests	May be somewhat rebellious Concerned with being "different"	Understands long-term consequences of actions including diabetes control Independence and self-image are important. Rebellion continues and some supervision and continued support are still needed.

These are only guidelines. Each child is an individual. Talk to your health care provider about any concerns you may have.

major problems for the diabetic child. Teach the caregiver and child to inspect the skin daily and promptly treat even small breaks in the skin. Encourage daily bathing. Teach the child and caregiver to dry the skin well after bathing, and give careful attention to any area where skin touches skin such as the groin, axilla, or other skin folds. Emphasize good foot care. This includes wearing well-fitting shoes, inspecting between toes for cracks, trimming nails straight across, wearing clean socks, and not going barefoot. Establishing these habits early will help the child prepare for lifelong care of diabetes.

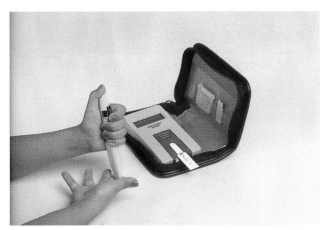

● *Figure 17.6* Child uses an automatic lancet to get blood sample (*left*) and blood glucose monitor to determine blood glucose level (*right*).

Preventing Infection. Diabetic children may be more susceptible to urinary tract and upper respiratory infections. Teach the child and caregiver to be alert for signs of urinary tract infection such as itching and burning on

urination. Instruct them to report signs of urinary tract or upper respiratory infections to the care provider promptly.

Many children are subject to minor infections and illnesses during the school years with little long-term effect. However, the diabetic child is more susceptible to long-term complications. When the diabetic child has an infection and fever, the temperature and metabolic rate increase and the body needs more sugar and, therefore, more insulin to make the sugar available to the body. Although the child may not be eating due to vomiting or anorexia, the body still needs insulin. Insulin should never be skipped during illness. Blood glucose levels should be checked every 2 to 4 hours during this time. Fluids need to be increased. Instruct the caregivers to contact the care provider when the child becomes ill, especially if the child is vomiting, cannot eat, or has diarrhea, so that close supervision can be maintained. Give the caregiver guidelines for care of an ill child with the initial diabetic instructions.

It is extremely important for the child to wear a Medic Alert identification medal or a bracelet with information about diabetic status. Identification cards, such as those carried by many adult diabetics, are seldom practical for a child.

Regulating Glucose Levels. The child who is seen in the health care facility with diabetes may be newly diagnosed or may be experiencing an unstable episode as a result of illness or changing needs. The child's blood glucose level must be monitored to maintain it within normal limits. Determine the blood glucose level at least twice a day, before breakfast and before the evening meal, by means of bedside glucose monitoring (see Fig. 17–6).

On initial diagnosis of diabetes, the blood glucose level should be checked as often as every 4 hours until some stability is achieved. Because regular monitoring of the blood glucose level is necessary, teach the child and the caregiver how to perform monitoring. Because this procedure involves a finger stick, the child may object and resist it. Offer encouragement and support, helping the child to express fears and acknowledging that the finger stick does hurt and it is acceptable to dislike it. Consider the child's developmental stage when performing the testing. School-age children can be involved in much of the process. Encourage the child to choose the finger to be used and clean it

---

FAMILY TEACHING TIPS

Child's Diabetic Food Plan

1. Plan well-balanced meals that are appealing to child.
2. Be positive with child when talking about foods that he or she can eat; downplay the negatives.
3. Space three meals and three snacks throughout the day. Daily caloric intake is divided to provide 20% at breakfast, 20% at lunch, 30% at dinner, and 10% at each of the snacks.
4. Calories should be made up of 50% to 60% carbohydrates, 15% to 20% protein, and no more than 30% fat.
5. Avoid concentrated sweets such as jelly, syrup, pie, candy bars, and soda pop.
6. Artificial sweeteners may be used.
7. Child must not skip meals. Make every effort to plan meals with foods that the child likes.
8. Include foods that contain dietary fiber such as whole grains, cereals, fruits and vegetables, nuts, seeds, and legumes. Fiber helps prevent hyperglycemia.
9. Dietetic food is expensive and unnecessary.
10. Keep complex carbohydrates available to be eaten before exercise and sports activities to provide sustained carbohydrate energy sources.
11. Teach child day by day about the food plan to encourage independence in food selections when at school or away from home.

with soap and water. Automatic-release instruments make it easier for the child to do the finger stick. Teach the child to read the results and learn the desired level. School-age children are in the stage of industry versus inferiority and usually are interested in learning new information. Appeal to this developmental characteristic to gain the child's cooperation.

Providing Child and Family Teaching in the Management of Hypoglycemia and Hyperglycemia. The child is monitored closely for signs of hypoglycemia or hyperglycemia. If the blood glucose level is higher than 240 mg/dL, the urine may be tested for ketones. Be aware of the most likely times for an increase or decrease in the blood glucose level in relation to the insulin the child is receiving. Teach the child and family the signs of both hypoglycemia and hyperglycemia (see Family Teaching Tips: Signs of Hypoglycemia and Hyperglycemia) and how to be prepared to take the appropriate action if necessary. They must be alert to signs of hypoglycemia especially when insulin is at peak action (see Table 17–5). Teach them to treat blood glucose levels lower than 60 mg/dL with juice, sugar, or nondiet soda. If the blood glucose level cannot be checked promptly, the child should still consume a simple carbohydrate if there are any signs of hypoglycemia.

If the child cannot swallow, glucagon or dextrose should be administered following the physician's orders. Glucagon is commercially available and can be administered intramuscularly or subcutaneously. Teach the caregiver how to mix and administer it.

Instruct the child to get help immediately when signs of hypoglycemia occur and to carry and take sugar cubes, Lifesavers, gumdrops, or a small tube of cake frosting. The reaction should be followed with a snack of a complex carbohydrate such as crackers and a protein such as cheese, peanut butter, or half of a meat sandwich. The snack is needed to maintain the increase in blood glucose level created by the simple carbohydrates and to prevent another hypoglycemic reaction.

Reassure the caregiver and the child that hypoglycemia is much more likely to occur than hyperglycemia. If there is any doubt as to whether the child is having a hypoglycemic or a hyperglycemic reaction, treat it like hypoglycemia. Instruct caregivers to keep a record of the hypoglycemic reactions to determine if there

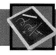

FAMILY TEACHING TIPS

Signs of Hypoglycemia and Hyperglycemia

HYPOGLYCEMIA
- Shaking
- Irritability
- Hunger
- Diaphoresis
- Dizziness
- Drowsiness
- Pallor
- Changed level of consciousness
- Feeling "strange"

HYPERGLYCEMIA
- Polyphagia (excessive hunger)
- Polyuria (excessive urination)
- Dry mucous membranes
- Poor skin turgor
- Lethargy
- Change in level of consciousness

is a pattern and if the insulin schedule or food plan needs adjustment.

Providing Child and Family Teaching on Insulin Administration. Teach the family caregiver and the child the correct way to give insulin. Disposable syringes make caring for equipment relatively easy. A doll may be used to practice the actual administration until the caregiver (and child, if old enough) is comfortable and confident. Provide direct supervision until proficiency is demonstrated.

This part of the treatment is probably the most threatening aspect of the illness. Remember your feelings when you gave your first injection in nursing school. The child and family need a great deal of empathy and warm support. Increasing their confidence and skills of insulin administration will reduce their fear.

Give clear instructions concerning the importance of rotating injection sites (Fig. 17–7). If used too frequently, a site is apt to become indurated and eventually fibrosed, which hinders proper insulin absorption. The atrophic hollows in the skin, or the lumps of hypertrophied tissue, are unsightly as well. Some people appear to have greater skin sensitivity than others do. Areas on the upper arms, upper thighs, abdomen, and buttocks can be used. Use of a careful plan allows several weeks to elapse before a site is used again. Usually 4 to 6 injec-

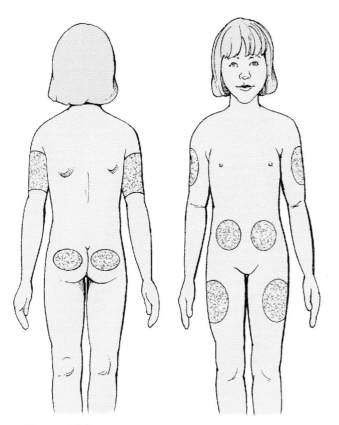

● **Figure 17.7** Subcutaneous injection sites.

tions are given in one area before going on to the next area. Starting from the inner, upper corner of the area, each injection is given ½ inches below the preceding one, going down in a vertical line. The next series of injections in this area would start ½ inches outward at the upper level. If there is any sign of induration, the local site should be avoided for a few weeks after all signs of irritation have disappeared. A chart recording the sites used and the rotation schedule is recommended.

Providing Child and Family Teaching About Exercise and Activity. Exercise decreases the blood glucose level because carbohydrates are being burned for energy. The therapeutic program should be adjusted to allow for this increase in energy requirements to avoid hypoglycemia. Adjustments also may be needed in the child's school schedule. For instance, physical education should never be scheduled right before lunch for a diabetic child. Also, the diabetic child should not be scheduled for a late lunch period.

Promoting Family Coping. When the diagnosis of diabetes is confirmed, the family

caregiver may feel devastated. A young child will not understand the implications, but the school-age or adolescent child will experience a great amount of fear and anxiety. The caregiver may have feelings of guilt, resentment, or denial. Other family members also may experience strong feelings about the illness. All these feelings and concerns must be recognized and resolved to work successfully with the diabetic child. Encourage the family to express these feelings and fears. To help him or her deal with feelings, involve the caregiver in the child's caring during hospitalization. Carefully listen to questions and answer them completely and honestly. Many written materials are available to give to the caregiver, but be sure the caregiver can read and understand them. Videos are also available that are helpful in educating the diabetic and the family. Recommend available community support groups. Cover home care in detail. Provide the family caregiver with a support person to contact when questions arise after discharge.

Because so much information must be absorbed in a brief time, the caregivers may seem forgetful or confused. Careful, patient repetition of all aspects of diabetes and the child's care is necessary. When anxiety levels are high, information is often heard but not digested. Provide written material in an understandable form. Have caregivers repeat information, and question them to confirm that they understand. Demonstrate warmth and caring throughout the teaching to increase the family's comfort; this also will develop their confidence in nursing responses that they can expect to their questions and apprehensions.

Promoting Self-Care and Positive Self-Esteem. The school-age or older child may experience some strong feelings of inadequacy or being "sick." These feelings must be expressed and handled. To help allay fear, teach the child as much as is appropriate for his or her age. Tell the child about athletes and other famous people who are diabetic. When possible, another child who is diabetic may visit so that the child does not feel so alone. Encourage the child to become active in helping with self-care. Answer questions about how diabetes will affect the child's activities. Summer camps for children with diabetes are available in many areas and can help develop the child's self-assurance.

The diabetic child can participate in normal activities. However, at least one friend should be told about the diabetic condition, and the child should not go swimming or hiking without a responsible person nearby who knows what to look for and what to do if the child should have a reaction.

Some older children are sensitive about their condition and fear that they seem different from their friends. Even with the best instruction and preparation, they may feel this way and wish to keep their condition secret. They must understand that a teacher or some other adult in their environment must be acquainted with their condition. Classroom teachers need to know which of their students have such a condition and should understand the signs of an impending reaction.

Diabetic children under good control need not be kept from such activities as campouts, overnight trips with the school band, or other similar activities away from home. Of course, these children must first be capable of measuring their insulin and giving their own injections. Some young people may find that a desire to participate in such an activity can be the factor that helps them overcome reluctance to measure and administer their own insulin.

EVALUATION: GOALS AND OUTCOME CRITERIA

- *Goal:* The child's caloric intake will be adequate to meet nutritional needs and to maintain appropriate growth.
  Criteria: The child eats food at meals and snack times, maintains normal weight for age and height, and the child and caregiver demonstrate understanding of meal planning by making appropriate menu selections.
- *Goal:* The child's skin integrity will be maintained.
  Criteria: The child's skin is intact with no signs of breakdown; the child and caregiver describe skin inspection and care.
- *Goal:* The child will be free from signs and symptoms of infection.
  Criteria: The child shows no signs of infection; temperature is within normal range; the child and caregiver discuss the importance of promptly reporting infections.
- *Goal:* The child will maintain normal glucose levels.

Criteria: The child's blood glucose level is 60 to 100 mg/dL; the urine is negative for acetone; there are no signs of hypoglycemia or hyperglycemia.
- *Goal:* The child and caregiver will verbalize an understanding of the signs, symptoms, and management of hypoglycemia and hyperglycemia.
  Criteria: The child and caregiver list the signs of hypoglycemia and hyperglycemia and discuss how to handle each; they ask questions to clarify information.
- *Goal:* The child and caregiver will verbalize an understanding of insulin administration.
  Criteria: The child and caregiver demonstrate insulin injection, describe various types of insulin and their reaction and peak times, and develop a site rotation schedule.
- *Goal:* The child and caregiver will verbalize an understanding of exercise and activity for a diabetic child.
  Criteria: The child and caregiver describe the effects of exercise on the blood glucose levels.
- *Goal:* The child and caregiver will express their concerns about coping with the child's illness.
  Criteria: As appropriate for age, the child discusses necessary adjustments to the daily schedule and activities and names several people to inform about the diabetic condition. The caregiver demonstrates support of the child in managing daily and long-term care of diabetes.
- *Goal:* The child will show adjustment and have a positive attitude about the condition.
  Criteria: The child expresses feelings about having diabetes and participates in age appropriate activities and realistic goal planning.

MUSCULOSKELETAL SYSTEM DISORDERS

The long bones of the extremities grow rapidly during the school-age period. "Growing pains" are a frequent complaint but rarely indicate serious disease. School age is a time of increasing physical activity including team sports. Peer approval and group or team participation at school and in after-school activities are important to the school-age child. Minor skeletal injuries, such as sprains and minor fractures, may make the child a temporary celebrity.

However, a serious skeletal defect or injury may influence the child's ability to cope with peer relationships and create social adjustment problems.

Scoliosis

Scoliosis, a lateral curvature of the spine, occurs in two forms: structural and functional (postural). The latter is more common. Rotated and malformed vertebrae cause structural scoliosis. Functional scoliosis can have several causes: poor posture, muscle spasm due to trauma, or unequal length of legs. When the primary problem is corrected, elimination of the functional scoliosis begins.

Most cases of structural scoliosis are idiopathic (no cause is known); a few are caused by congenital deformities or infection. Idiopathic scoliosis is seen in older school-age children at 10 years of age and older. Although mild curves occur as often in boys as in girls, idiopathic scoliosis requiring treatment occurs eight times more frequently in girls than in boys.[3]

Diagnosis

Nurses play an important role in screening for scoliosis. School nurses and others who work in health care settings with children aged 10 years and older should conduct or assist with screening programs. Many states require regular examination of students for scoliosis, beginning in the fifth or sixth grade. Scoliosis screening should last through at least eighth grade. A school nurse often does the initial screening. Nurses in other health care settings are responsible for further screening of these children during regular well-child visits.

During examination, observe the undressed child from the back and note any lateral curvature of the spinal column, asymmetry of the shoulders, shoulder blades, or hips, and an unequal distance between the arms and waist (Fig. 17–8). The examiner then asks the child to bend at the hips (touch the toes) and observes for prominence of the scapula on one side and curvature of the spinal column.

Treatment

Treatment depends on many factors and is either nonsurgical or surgical. Electrical stimulation may be used for mild curvatures, but its effectiveness is unclear. Other nonsurgical treatment includes the use of braces or traction. Surgical treatment includes the use of rods, screws, hooks, and spinal fusion. Curvatures of less than 25 degrees are observed closely but not treated. Curvatures between 25 degrees and 40 degrees are corrected with a brace. The Milwaukee brace was the first used for treatment and is still used to treat some spinal curvatures such as kyphosis, but is not used as frequently now. The Boston brace or TLSO braces are commonly used. Curvatures of more than 40 degrees are usually corrected surgically. Treatment is long term and often lasts through the rest of the child's growth cycle.

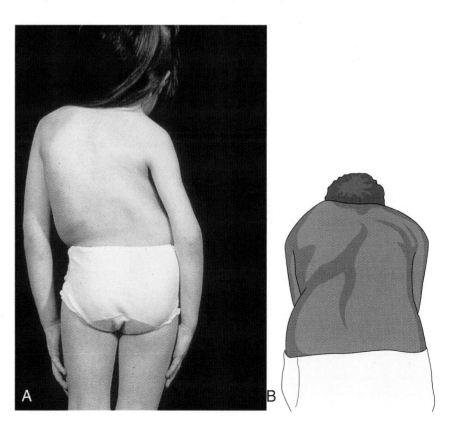

● *Figure 17.8* **(A)** Posterior view of child's back with lateral curvature. **(B)** View of child bending over with prominence of scapular area and asymmetry of flank demonstrated.

Electrical Stimulation. Electrical stimulation may be used as an alternative to bracing for the child with a mild to moderate curvature. Electrodes are applied to the skin or surgically implanted. Treatment occurs at night while the child is asleep. The leads are placed to stimulate muscles on the convex side of the curvature to contract as impulses are transmitted. This causes the spine to straighten. If external electrodes are used, the skin under the leads must be checked regularly for irritation. This treatment is the least disruptive to the child's life, but there is some controversy about its effectiveness.

Braces. The Milwaukee brace was the first type of brace used for scoliosis but is now more commonly used to treat **kyphosis,** an abnormal rounded out curvature of the spine that is also called humpback. The Boston brace or the TLSO (thoracic-lumbar-sacral orthotic) brace is used to treat scoliosis (Fig. 17–9). The Boston brace and the TLSO brace are made of plastic and are customized to fit the child.

The brace should be worn constantly except during bathing or swimming to achieve the greatest benefit. It is worn over a T-shirt or undershirt to protect the skin. The fit of the device is monitored closely and the child and caregiver should be taught to notify the healthcare provider if there is any rubbing. During the first couple weeks of wearing the brace, the child can be given a mild analgesic for discomfort and aching. The child's provider may also prescribe certain exercises to be done several times a day. These are taught before the brace is applied but are done while the brace is in place.

Wearing a brace creates a distinct change in body image, especially in the older school-age child or in adolescence at a time when body consciousness is at an all-time high. Clothing choices are a challenge when wearing a brace, but wearing clothing similar to what peers are wearing helps the child to feel more

accepted. The need to wear the brace and deal with the limitations it involves may cause anger; the change in body image can cause a grief reaction. Handling these feelings successfully requires understanding support from the nurse, family, and peers. It is important for the child to have an opportunity to talk about his or her feelings. Sometimes it is helpful for the patient in a brace to talk with other scoliosis patients and learn how they have coped. Understanding the disorder itself and the important benefits of treatment also can ease the adjustment.

Traction. When a child has a severe spinal curvature or cervical instability, a form of traction known as **halo traction** (Fig. 17–10) may be used to reduce spinal curves and straighten the spine. Halo traction is achieved by using stainless steel pins inserted into the skull while countertraction is applied by using pins inserted into the femur. Weights are increased gradually to promote correction. When the curvature has been corrected, spinal fusion is performed. In some cases, halo traction might be used following surgery if there is cervical instability.

The strange appearance of the halo traction apparatus magnifies the problems of body image; in addition, the head may need to be shaved. The child needs a thorough explanation of what will occur during the procedure and should be given the opportunity to talk about his or her feelings. Frequent shampooing, cleansing of the pin sites, and observation for signs of complications are critical in the care of children in halo traction.

Surgical Treatment. Various types of instruments such as rods, screws, and hooks may be placed along the spinal column to realign the spine, then spinal fusion is performed to maintain the corrected position. This procedure, which is done in cases of severe curvatures, is frightening to the child and

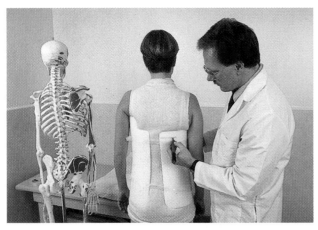

● *Figure 17.9* A girl with scoliosis being fitted with a TLSO brace for treatment.

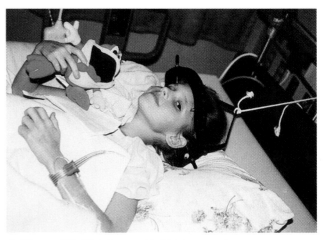

● *Figure 17.10* A 9-year-old girl in halo traction.

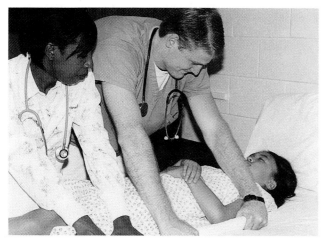

● *Figure 17.11* Two nurses use a draw-sheet to log roll the child to a side-lying position.

family. It is major surgery, and the child and family must be well prepared for it. Because this is an elective procedure, thorough preoperative teaching can be carried out for the child and the family. The child can expect to have postoperative pain and will have to endure days of remaining flat in bed, being turned only in a log-rolling fashion (Fig. 17–11). Postoperatively the neurovascular status of the extremities is monitored closely. The child may be given a patient-controlled analgesia pump to control pain. A Foley catheter is usually inserted because of the need to remain flat. The rods remain in place permanently. In some cases the child may be placed in a body cast for a period of time to ensure fusion of the spine. About 6 months after surgery, the child will be able to take part in most activities except contact sports (such as tackle football, gymnastics, and wrestling). Because the bones are fused and rods are implanted, this procedure arrests the child's growth in height, which contributes to the emotional adjustment that the child and family must make.

● Nursing Process for the Child With Scoliosis

ASSESSMENT

The child with scoliosis must be reassessed every 4 to 6 months. Document the degree of curvature and related impairments. This is a sensitive age for children, when privacy and the importance of being like everyone else are top priorities. Keep this in mind when interviewing and during examination of the child. Provide privacy and protect the child's modesty.

The child who is admitted to a health care facility for application of a brace or other instrumentation may be carrying a lot of unseen emotional baggage. Be sensitive to this emotional state. The family caregivers also may be upset but trying to hide it for the child's sake. In addition to routine observations, look for clues to the emotional state of both the child and family caregivers.

NURSING DIAGNOSES

When collecting data, pay attention to evidence of the emotional states of the child and caregiver. The types of treatment involved as well as the emotional state of the child and caregiver help in determining appropriate nursing diagnoses. Some diagnoses for application of a brace might include
- Impaired Physical Mobility related to restricted movement
- Risk for Injury related to decreased mobility
- Risk for Impaired Skin Integrity related to irritation of brace
- Risk for Disturbed Body Image related to wearing a brace continuously
- Risk for Noncompliance related to long-term treatment

OUTCOME IDENTIFICATION AND PLANNING

Consult the child and caregiver when establishing nursing goals. Be especially sensitive to the child's needs. Goals for the child may include minimizing the disruption of activities, preventing injury, and maintaining skin integrity and self-image. Goals for the child and caregiver include complying with long-term care.

IMPLEMENTATION

Promoting Mobility. Prescribed exercises must be practiced and performed as directed. Encourage and support the child during these exercises. The child may need to be in traction for 1 or 2 weeks before the brace is applied. This can be emotionally traumatic.

Preventing Injury. Evaluate the child's environment after the brace has been applied and take precautions to prevent injury. Help the child practice moving about safely: going up and down stairs; getting in and out of vehicles, chairs, and desks; and getting out of bed. Teach the child to avoid hazardous surfaces. Listen carefully to the child and the family caregiver to determine any other hazards in the home or school environment. Advise the family caregiver to contact school personnel to ensure that the child has comfortable, supportive seating at school and that adjustments are made in the physical education program.

Preventing Skin Irritation. When the brace is first applied, check the child regularly to confirm proper fit. Observe for any areas of rubbing, discomfort, or skin irritation and adjust the brace as necessary. Teach the child how to inspect all areas under the brace daily. Instruct the child and caregiver that reddened areas should be reported to the care provider so that adjustments can be made. Skin under the pads should be massaged daily. Daily bathing is essential, and clean cotton underwear or a T-shirt should be worn under the brace to provide protection.

Promoting Positive Body Image. The child should be involved in all aspects of care planning. Self-image and the need to be like others are very important at this age. Learning to be confident enough to handle the comments of peers can be difficult for the child. Give the child frequent opportunities to ventilate feelings about being different. Help the child select clothing that blends with current styles but is loose enough to hide the brace. Encourage the child to find extracurricular activities with which the brace will not interfere. Active sports are not permitted, but many other activities are available. Help the child focus and enhance a positive attribute about characteristics such as hair or complexion. Encourage the child and caregiver to discuss accommodations with school personnel together.

Promoting Compliance with Therapy. The child must wear the brace for years until the spinal growth is completed and needs to be weaned from it gradually for another 1 or 2 years by wearing it only at night. During this period, the caregivers and the child need emotional support from healthcare personnel. Be certain that the child and caregivers have a complete understanding of the importance of wearing the brace continually. To encourage compliance, teach them about the complications that may occur if correction is unsuccessful. Inform the caregiver about the need to monitor the child for

compliance. Help the caregiver understand the importance of being empathetic to the child's need to be like others during this period of development. Offer ways in which the caregiver can help the child deal with adjustment to the therapy.

EVALUATION: GOALS AND OUTCOME CRITERIA

- *Goal:* The child will move effectively within the limits of the brace.
  Criteria: The child ambulates and participates in daily activities.
- *Goal:* The child will remain free from injury while in brace.
  Criteria: The child demonstrates safe practices related to everyday activities at home and in the school environment.
- *Goal:* The child's skin will remain intact.
  Criteria: The child uses methods to reduce skin irritation and bathes regularly. Skin remains free from irritation and breakdown.
- *Goal:* The child will exhibit positive coping behaviors.
  Criteria: The child is self-confident, has an attractive, well-groomed appearance, and verbalizes feelings about the need to wear the brace.
- *Goal:* The child will comply with therapy.
  Criteria: The child wears the brace as directed. Caregivers report compliance, and the child's condition shows evidence of compliance.

Legg-Calvé-Perthes Disease (Coxa Plana)

Legg-Calvé-Perthes disease is an aseptic necrosis of the head of the femur. It occurs four to five times more often in boys than in girls and 10 times more often in whites than in other ethnic groups. It can be caused by trauma to the hip, but generally the cause is unknown. Symptoms first noticed are pain in the hip or groin and a limp accompanied by muscle spasms and limitation of motion. These symptoms mimic **synovitis** (inflammation of a joint, which is most commonly the hip in children), which makes immediate diagnosis difficult. Radiographic examination may need to be repeated several weeks after the initial visit to demonstrate vascular necrosis for a definitive diagnosis.

There are three stages of the disease; each lasts 9 months to 1 year. In the first stage, radiographic studies show opacity of the epiphysis. In the second stage, the epiphysis becomes mottled and fragmented; during the third stage, reossification occurs.

In the past, immobilization of the hip through the use of braces and crutches and bed rest with traction or casting was considered essential for recovery without deformity. However, restricting a child's activity for 2 years or more was extremely difficult. Current treatment focuses on containing the femoral head within the acetabulum during the revascularization process so that the new femoral head will form to make a smoothly functioning joint. The method of containment varies with the portion of the head affected. Use of a brace that holds the necrotic portions of the head in place during healing is considered an effective method of containment. Reconstructive surgery is now possible, enabling the child to return to normal activities within 3 to 4 months.

The prognosis for complete recovery without difficulty later in life depends on the child's age at the time of onset, the amount of involvement, and the cooperation of the child and the family caregivers. Nursing care focuses on helping the child and caregivers to manage the corrective device and the importance of compliance to promote healing and avoid long-term disability.

Osteomyelitis

Osteomyelitis is an infection of the bone usually caused by *Staphylococcus aureus*. Acute osteomyelitis is twice as common in boys and results from a primary infection such as a staphylococcal skin infection (impetigo), burns, a furuncle (boil), a penetrating wound, or a fracture. The bacteria enter the bloodstream and are carried to the metaphysis of a bone, where an abscess forms, ruptures, and spreads the infection along the bone under the periosteum.

Symptoms usually begin abruptly with fever, malaise, as well as pain and localized tenderness over the metaphysis of the affected bone. Joint motion is limited. Diagnosis is based on laboratory findings of leukocytosis (15,000–25,000 cells or more), an increased ESR, and positive blood cultures. Radiographic examination does not reveal the process until 5 to 10 days after the onset.

Treatment for acute osteomyelitis must be immediate. Intravenous antibiotic therapy is started at once and is continued for at least 6 weeks. Depending on the physician and the compliance of the child and family, a short course of IV antibiotics may be followed by administration of oral antibiotics to complete treatment. Surgical drainage of the involved metaphysis may be performed. If the abscess has ruptured into the subperiosteal space, chronic osteomyelitis follows.

If prompt, specific antibiotic treatment is vigorously employed, acute osteomyelitis may be brought under control rapidly and extensive bone destruction of chronic osteomyelitis is prevented. If extensive destruction of bone has occurred before treatment, surgical removal of necrotic bone becomes necessary.

During the acute stage, nursing care includes reducing pain by positioning the affected limb, minimizing movement of the limb, and administering medication. Transmission-based precautions may be required if the wound is open and draining. Follow the usual procedure for IV antibiotic therapy including careful observance of the venipuncture site and monitoring the rate, dosage, and time of antibiotic. An intermittent infusion device or peripherally inserted central catheter may be used for long-term IV therapy.

Monitor oral nutrition and fluids because the child's appetite may be poor during the acute phase and may improve in later stages. Weight-bearing on the affected limb must be avoided until healing has occurred because pathologic fractures occur very easily in the weakened stage. Physical therapy helps restore limb function.

Muscular Dystrophy

Muscular dystrophy is a hereditary, progressive, degenerative disease of the muscles. The most common form of muscular dystrophy is Duchenne (pseudohypertrophic) muscular dystrophy. Duchenne muscular dystrophy, an X-linked recessive hereditary disease, occurs almost exclusively in males and is carried by females. When muscular dystrophy has been diagnosed in a child, the mother and the siblings should be tested to see if they have the disease or are carriers.

The first signs are noted in infancy or childhood when the child finds it difficult to stand or walk, which is usually at about 3 years of age; later, trunk muscle weakness develops. Mild mental retardation often accompanies this disease. The child cannot rise easily to an upright position from a sitting position on the floor; instead he or she rises by climbing up the lower extremities with the hands (Fig. 17–12). Weakness of leg, arm, and shoulder muscles progresses gradually. Increasing abnormalities in gait and posture appear by school age with **lordosis** (forward curvature of the lumbar spine, or swayback), pelvic waddling, and frequent falling (Fig. 17–13). The child becomes progressively weaker usually becoming wheelchair-bound by 10 to 12 years of age (middle school or junior high school age). The disease continues into adolescence and young adulthood, when the patient usually succumbs to respiratory or heart failure.

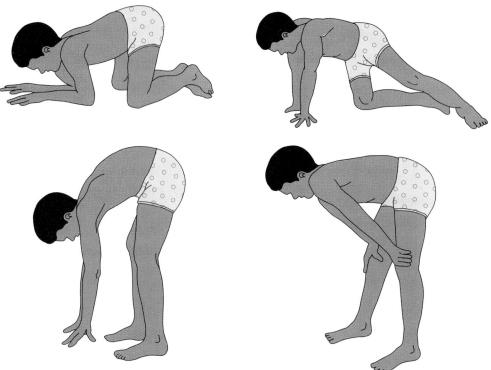

● **Figure 17.12** Child "climbing up" lower extremities.

In addition to symptoms in the first 2 years of life, highly increased serum creatinine phosphokinase levels as well as a decrease in muscle fibers seen in a muscle biopsy can confirm the diagnosis.

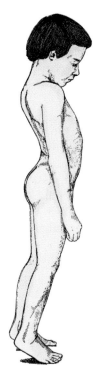

● **Figure 17.13** Characteristic posture of a child with Duchenne muscular dystrophy. Along with the typical toe gait, the child develops a lordotic posture as Duchenne dystrophy causes further deterioration.

No effective treatment for the disease has been found, but research is rapidly closing in on genetic identification, which promises exciting changes in treatment in the future. The child is encouraged to be as active as possible to delay muscle atrophy and contractures. To help keep the child active, physiotherapy, diet to avoid obesity, and parental encouragement are important.

When a child becomes wheelchair-bound, kyphosis (hunchback) develops and causes a decrease in respiratory function and an increase in the incidence of infections. Breathing exercises are a daily necessity for these children.

The nurse should advise the family to keep the child's life as normal as possible, which may be difficult. This disease can drain the emotional and financial reserves of the entire family. The nurse might suggest assistance through the Muscular Dystrophy Association–USA (National Headquarters, 3300 E. Sunrise Drive Tucson, AZ 85718, 800-572-1717, website: *http://www.mdausa.org*), through local chapters of this organization, and by talking with other parents who face the same problem.

Juvenile Rheumatoid Arthritis

Juvenile rheumatoid arthritis (JRA) is the most common connective tissue disease of childhood. Connective tissues are those that provide a supportive framework and protective covering for the body such as the musculoskeletal system and skin and mucous membranes. Joint inflammation occurs first; if

TABLE 17.7	Characteristics of Different Types of Juvenile Rheumatoid Arthritis		
Sign/Symptom of Onset	Polyarthritis	Oligoarthritis (Pauciarticular)	Systemic
Frequency of cases	30%–40%	50%–60%	10%–15%
Number of joints involved	5 or more	4 or fewer	Variable
Sex ratio (F:M)	3:1	5:1	1:1
Systemic involvement	Moderate	Not present	Prominent
Uveitis*	5%	20%	Rare
Sensitivity			
Rheumatoid factors	10%	Rare	Rare
Antinuclear bodies	40%–50%	75%–85%	10%
Course	Systemic disease is generally mild; articular involvement may be unremitting	Systemic disease is absent; major cause of morbidity is uveitis	Systemic disease is often self-limited; arthritis is chronic and destructive in 50%
Prognosis	Guarded to moderately good	Excellent except for eyesight	Moderate to poor

*Uveitis—an inflammation of the middle (vascular) tunic of the eye; includes the iris, ciliary body, and choroid.

Adapted from Cassidy JT. (1999) Rheumatic disease of childhood. In *Oski's pediatrics: Principles and practice* (3rd ed). Philadelphia: Lippincott Williams & Wilkins.

untreated, inflammation leads to irreversible changes in joint cartilage, ligaments, and menisci (the crescent-shaped fibrocartilage in the knee joints) eventually causing complete immobility. The occurrence of JRA appears to peak at two age levels: 1 to 3 years and 8 to 12 years. It can be subdivided into three different types: systemic; polyarticular, involving five or more joints; and oligoarthritis (pauciarticular), involving four or fewer joints that are most often the knees and the ankles (Table 17–7). This disease has a long duration, but 85% of children with JRA reach adulthood without serious disability.[4]

The treatment goal is to maintain mobility and preserve joint function. Treatment can include drugs, physical therapy, and surgery. Early diagnosis and drug therapy to control inflammation and other systemic changes can reduce the need for other types of treatment.

Enteric-coated aspirin has long been the drug of choice for JRA but because of the concern of aspirin therapy and Reye syndrome (see Chap. 15), NSAIDs (nonsteroidal anti-inflammatory drugs) are being used frequently to replace aspirin in treatment of JRA. Aspirin may still be used because it is an effective anti-inflammatory drug, is inexpensive, is easily administered, and has few side effects when carefully regulated. Both aspirin and NSAID drugs such as Naproxen and Ibuprofen may cause GI irritation and bleeding. To decrease these side effects, the drugs should be administered with food or milk. Acetaminophen is not an appropriate substitute because it lacks anti-inflammatory properties. Teach family caregivers the importance of regular administration of the medications even when the child is not experiencing pain. The primary purpose of aspirin or NSAIDs is not to relieve pain but to decrease joint inflammation.

When aspirin or NSAIDs are no longer effective, gold preparations, steroids, D-penicillamine, or immunosuppressives may be used. All these are toxic and must be closely monitored.

Physical therapy includes exercise, application of splints, and heat. Implementing this program at home requires the cooperation of the nurse, physical therapist, and care provider. Joints must be immobilized by splinting during active disease, but gentle daily exercise is necessary to prevent **ankylosis** (immobility of a joint). Stress to the caregivers the importance of encouraging the child to perform independent activities of daily living to maintain function and independence. The family caregiver must be patient, allowing the child time to accomplish necessary tasks.

Depending on the degree of disease, activity, range-of-motion exercises, isometric exercises, swimming, and riding a tricycle or bicycle may be part of the treatment plan. Inform caregivers that these exercises should not increase pain; if exercise does trigger increased pain, the amount of exercise should be decreased.

Fractures

A fracture is a break in a bone that is usually accompanied by vascular and soft-tissue damage and is characterized by pain, swelling, and tenderness. Children's fractures differ from those of adults in that generally they are less complicated, heal more

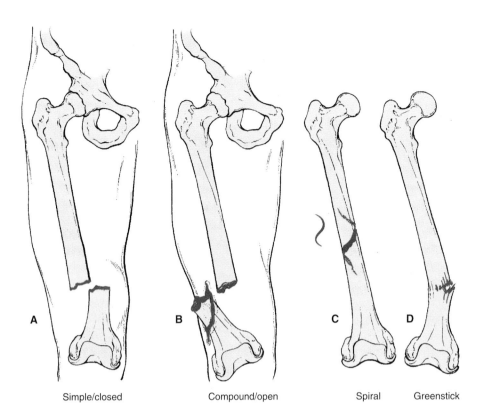

Simple/closed   Compound/open   Spiral   Greenstick

● *Figure 17.14* Types of fractures. All are examples of complete fractures except *D*, which is an incomplete fracture.

quickly, and usually occur from different causes. The child has an urge to explore the environment but lacks the experience and judgment to recognize possible hazards. In some instances, caregivers may be negligent in their supervision, but often the child uses immature judgment or is simply too fast for them.

The bones most commonly fractured in childhood are the clavicle, femur, tibia, humerus, wrist, and fingers. The classification of a fracture reflects the kind of bone injury sustained (Fig. 17–14). If the fragments of fractured bone are separated, the fracture is said to be complete. If fragments remain partially joined, the fracture is termed incomplete. Greenstick fractures are one kind of incomplete fracture common in children due to incomplete ossification. When a broken bone penetrates the skin, the fracture is called compound, or open. A simple, or closed, fracture is a single break in the bone without penetration of the skin. Spiral fractures, which twist around the bone, are frequently associated with child abuse and are caused by a wrenching force. Fractures in the area of the epiphyseal plate (growth plate) can cause permanent damage and severely impair growth (Fig. 17–15).

Treatment

Most childhood fractures are treated by realignment and immobilization using either traction or closed manipulation and casting. A few patients with severe fractures or additional injuries, such as burns and other soft-tissue damage, may require surgical

reduction, internal or external fixation, or both. Internal fixation devices include rods, pins, screws, and plates made of inert materials that will not trigger an immune reaction. They allow early mobilization of the child to a wheelchair, crutches, or a walker.

External fixation devices are used primarily in complex fractures often with other injuries or compli-

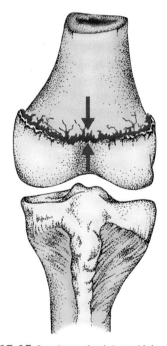

● *Figure 17.15* One form of epiphyseal injury; a crushing injury (as might occur in a fall from a height) can destroy the layer of germinal cells of the epiphysis, resulting in disturbance of growth.

COMMUNICATIONS BOX 17.1

Seven-year-old Jimmy is in skeletal traction for a severely fractured elbow. As the nurse enters his room, he turns his head away from the door.

LESS EFFECTIVE COMMUNICATION	*MORE EFFECTIVE COMMUNICATION*
Nurse: Hey, Jimmy. What's the trouble?	*Nurse:* Hi, Jimmy. You look like you are having some pain. Tell me where it hurts.
Jimmy: Nothin'.	*Jimmy:* (Points to elbow)
Nurse: What do you mean, "nothin?"	*Nurse:* Can you tell me how it feels?
Jimmy: (Just shrugs)	*Jimmy:* It feels kind of burny.
Nurse: What's the matter . . . Cat got your tongue?	*Nurse:* Kind of burny? Show me exactly where the burny feeling is.
Jimmy: (Shrugs again)	*Jimmy:* Right here (pointing). And it kind of feels jabby.
Nurse: Jimmy, I can't help you if you won't talk to me.	*Nurse:* OK, Jimmy. You did a good job of showing me exactly how it feels. I'll get some medicine to make it feel better. After I give you the medicine, I'll read a story to you if you like.
Jimmy: (Turns away from the nurse)	
Nurse: OK, Sport. When you decide to talk, let me know. (Leaves the room)	

▶ *The nurse treats Jimmy as "pal" but isn't skilled at using open-ended questions. The response "cat got your tongue?" is almost a sure turn-off to a youngster. The nurse ends up leaving the room without finding out what Jimmy's problem was. He will continue to have pain until it builds to a point where he can't stand it any more, and then it will take longer for the pain medication to bring comfort.*

▶ *The nurse recognized Jimmy had some kind of problem. Pain was the most likely choice. If it had not been pain, Jimmy would have most likely responded verbally to set her straight. By asking open-ended questions that couldn't be answered with just "yes" or "no," the nurse got more definite responses from Jimmy. After telling Jimmy that he/she would get him medicine for the pain, the nurse offered the special treat of a story.*

cations. These devices are applied under sterile conditions in the operating room and may be augmented by soft dressings and elevated by means of an overhead traction rope. External fixation devices rarely are used on young children.

Casts. The kind of cast used is determined by the age of the child, the severity of the fracture, the type of bone involved, and the amount of weight-bearing that the child will be allowed to have on the extremity. Most casts are formed from gauze strips impregnated with plaster of Paris or other synthetic material such as fiberglass or polyurethane resin, which is pliable when wet but hardens when dry. Synthetic materials are lighter in weight and present a cleaner appearance because they can be sponged with water when soiled; they are even available in colors. Synthetic casts dry more rapidly than plaster of Paris. The lightweight casts tend to be used as arm casts and hip spica casts that are used to treat infants with congenital hip conditions (Fig. 17–16). The hip spica cast covers the lower part of the body usually

from the waist down and either one or both legs while leaving the feet open. The cast maintains the legs in a frog like position. Usually there is a bar placed between the legs to help support the cast.

The child and the family should be taught what to expect after the cast is applied and how to care for the casted area. A stockinette is applied over the area to be casted, and the bony prominences are padded before the wet plaster rolls are applied. Although the wet plaster of Paris feels cool on the skin when applied, evaporation soon causes a temporary sensation of warmth. The cast will feel heavy and cumbersome.

A wet cast should be handled only with open palms because fingertips can cause indentations and result in pressure points. If the cast has no protective edge, it should be petaled (see Fig. 9–22 in Chap. 9) with adhesive tape strips. If the cast is near the genital area, plastic should be taped around the edge to prevent wetting and soiling of the cast.

After the fracture has been immobilized, any complaints of pain signal possible complications such

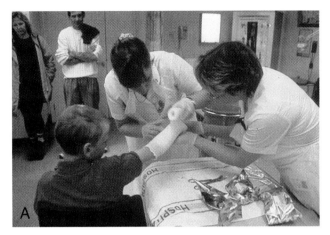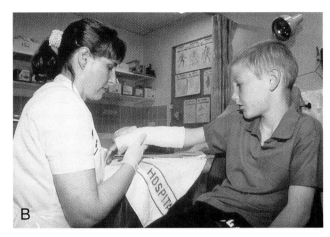

● ***Figure 17.16*** **(A)** Fiberglass cast is being applied. **(B)** Following cast application, a nurse checks the circulation in the hand.

as compartment syndrome and should be recorded and reported immediately. Compartment syndrome is a serious neurovascular concern that occurs when increasing pressure within the muscle compartment causes decreased circulation. It is important for the nurse to monitor the child's neurovascular status frequently because of the risk of tissue and nerve damage. Monitoring the neurovascular status is sometimes referred to as CMS (circulation, movement, sensation) checks and includes observing, documenting, and reporting the five Ps:

- *Pain:* Any sign of pain should be noted and the exact area determined.
- *Pulse:* If an upper extremity is involved, brachial, radial, ulnar, and digital pulses should be checked. If a lower extremity is involved, femoral, popliteal, posterior tibial, and dorsalis pedis pulses should be monitored.
- *Paresthesia:* Check for any diminished or absent sensation or for numbness or tingling.
- *Paralysis:* Check hand function by having the child try to hyperextend the thumb or wrist, oppose the thumb and little finger, and adduct all fingers. Check function of the foot by having the child try to dorsiflex and plantarflex the ankles and flex and extend the toes.
- *Pallor:* Check the extremity and the nail beds distal to the site of the fracture for color. Pallor, discoloration, and coldness indicate circulatory impairment.

In addition to the five Ps, any foul odor or drainage on or under the cast, "hot spots" on the cast (areas warm to touch), looseness or tightness, or any elevation of temperature must be noted, documented, and reported. Family caregivers should be instructed to watch carefully for these same danger signals.

Children and caregivers should be cautioned not to put anything inside the cast, no matter how much

the casted area itches. Small toys and sticks or sticklike objects should be kept out of reach until the cast has been removed. Blowing cool air through the cast with a hair dryer set on a cool temperature or using a fan may help to relieve the discomfort.

When the fracture has healed, the cast is removed with a cast cutter. This can be frightening for the child unless the person using the cast cutter explains and demonstrates that the device will not cut flesh but only the hard surface of the cast. The child should be told that there will be vibration from the cast cutter, but it will not burn.

After cast removal, the casted area should be soaked in warm water to help remove the crusty layer of accumulated skin. Application of oil or lotion may prove comforting. Family caregivers and the child must be cautioned against scrubbing or scraping this area because the tender layer of new skin underneath the crust may bleed.

Traction. Traction is a pulling force applied to an extremity or other part of the body. A body part is pulled in one direction against a counterpull or countertraction exerted in the opposite direction. A system of weights, ropes, and pulleys is used to realign and immobilize fractures, reduce or eliminate muscle spasm, and prevent fracture deformity and joint contractures.

Two basic types of traction are used: skin traction and skeletal traction. **Skin traction** pulls on tape, rubber, or a plastic material attached to the skin, which indirectly exerts pull on the musculoskeletal system. Examples of skin traction are Bryant's traction, Buck extension traction, and Russell traction. **Skeletal traction** exerts pull directly on skeletal structures by means of a pin, wire, tongs, or other device surgically inserted through a bone. Examples of skeletal traction are 90-degree traction and balanced suspension traction. Dunlop's traction, sometimes used for fractures of the humerus or the elbow, can be

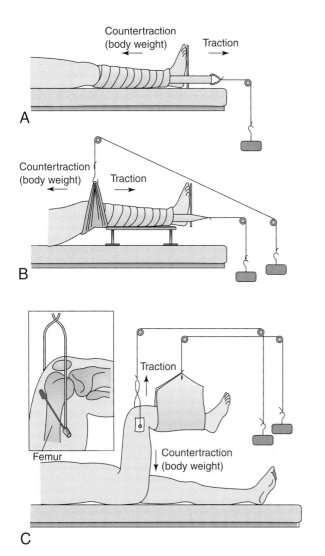

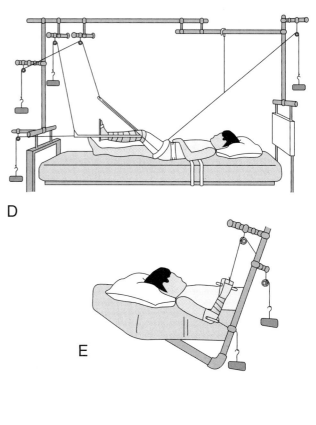

● *Figure 17.17* Types of traction. **(A)** Buck extension, skin traction. **(B)** Russell traction, skin traction. Two lines of traction (one horizontal and one vertical) allow for good bone alignment for healing. **(C)** 90°–90° (skeletal) traction; a wire pin is inserted into the distal femur. **(D)** Balanced suspension traction. **(E)** Dunlop's traction (skeletal).

either skin or skeletal traction if a pin is inserted into the bone to immobilize the extremity (Fig. 17–17).

Bryant's traction (Fig. 17–18) is often used for the treatment of a fractured femur in children younger

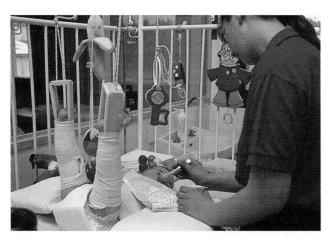

● *Figure 17.18* An infant in Bryant's traction is being fed.

than 2 years of age. These fractures are often transverse (crosswise to the long axis of the bone) or spiral fractures. The use of Bryant's traction entails some risk of compromised circulation and may result in contractures of the foot and lower leg particularly in an older child. The child's legs are wrapped with elastic bandages that should be removed at least daily to observe the skin then rewrapped. Skin temperature and the color of the legs and feet must be checked frequently to detect any circulatory impairment. Severe pain may indicate circulatory difficulty and should be reported immediately. When a child is in Bryant's traction, the hips should not rest on the bed; the nurse should be able to pass a hand between the child's buttocks and the sheet.

Buck extension traction, in which the child's body provides the countertraction to the weights, is used for short-term immobilization. It is used to correct contractures and bone deformities such as Legg-Calvé-Perthes disease. Russell traction seems to be more effective for older children. A child in either type of traction, however, tends to slide down until the weights rest on the bed or the floor. The child should be pulled up to keep the weights free, the ropes must be in alignment with the pulleys, and the alignment should be checked frequently. An older child may try to coax a roommate to remove the weights or the sandbags used as weights.

Children in any kind of traction must be carefully monitored to detect any signs of neurovascular complications. Skin temperature and color, presence or absence of edema, peripheral pulse, sensation, and motion must be monitored every hour for the first 24 hours after traction has been applied and every 4 hours after the first 24 hours unless ordered otherwise. Skin care must be meticulous. Skin preparation (Skin-Prep) should be used to toughen the skin rather than lotions or oils that soften the skin and contribute to tissue breakdown.

Children in skeletal traction require special attention to pin sites. Pin care should be performed every 8 hours. The provider may order that povidone-iodine or a hydrogen peroxide solution be used to clean the pin sites. Standard precautions and aseptic technique reduce the risk for infection. Any sign of infection (odor, local inflammation, or elevated temperature) must be recorded and reported at once. (See the Nursing Care Plan.)

External Fixation Devices. In children who have severe fractures or conditions such as having one extremity shorter than the other, external fixation devices are used to correct the condition (Fig. 17–19). When an external fixation device is used, special skin care at the pin sites is also necessary. The sites are left open to the air and should be inspected and cleansed every 8 hours. The appearance of the pins puncturing the skin and the unusual appearance of the device can be upsetting to the child, so be sensitive to any anxiety the child expresses.

As early as possible, the child (if old enough) or family caregivers should be taught to care for the pin sites. External fixation devices are sometimes left in place for as long as 1 year; therefore, it is important that the child accepts this temporary change in body image and learns to care for the affected site. Children with these devices will probably work with a physical therapist during the rehabilitation period and will have specific exercises to perform. Before discharge from the hospital, the child should feel comfortable moving about and should be able to recognize the signs of pin infection.

Crutches. Children with fractures of the lower extremities and other lower leg injuries often must learn to use crutches to avoid weight-bearing on the injured area. Several types of crutches are available. The most common are axillary crutches, which are principally used for temporary situations. Forearm,

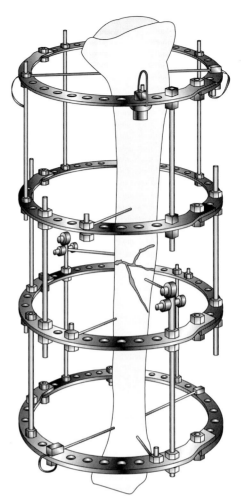

● *Figure 17.19* External fixation device.

or Canadian, crutches usually are recommended for children who need crutches permanently such as paraplegic children with braces. Trough, or platform, crutches are more suitable for children with limited strength or function in the arms and hands.

The use of crutches is generally taught by a physical therapist, but it can be the responsibility of nurses. The type of crutch gait taught is determined by the amount of weight-bearing permitted, the child's degree of stability, whether or not the knees can be flexed, and the specific treatment goal.

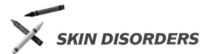

SKIN DISORDERS

School-age children often have minor bruises, abrasions, or rashes that generally cause few problems. Some common fungal and parasitic disorders, however, can become serious if not controlled and cured. Allergic skin reactions are not uncommon. Because a large part of the school-age

NURSING CARE PLAN

for the Child in Traction

TD is a 9-year-old boy who has been hospitalized following a serious bicycle accident in which he was struck by a motor vehicle. In the accident he sustained a fractured right femur and several cuts and abrasions. He has been placed in balanced suspension traction and will be in traction for several weeks before the extremity can be cast. He is in the fourth grade at school and plays soccer and basketball.

NURSING DIAGNOSIS
Risk for Peripheral Neurovascular Dysfunction related to fracture or effects of traction

GOAL: The child will maintain circulation and normal neurovascular status in extremities.

OUTCOME CRITERIA
- The child's pulse rate is within a normal range with adequate pulses and capillary refill in all extremities.
- The child has good skin color and temperature, appropriate movement and sensation in all extremities.

NURSING INTERVENTIONS	*RATIONALE*
Maintain proper body alignment with traction weights and pulleys hanging free of bed and off the floor.	Body alignment must be maintained to prevent permanent injury or disalignment and decreased range of motion in effected extremity.
Monitor pulses in right leg and compare to pulses in other extremity.	Comparison helps to determine if circulation is adequate in affected extremity.
Monitor skin in extremities for color, temperature, sensation, and movement.	Any change in neurovascular status could indicate impaired nerve function.
Record and report any change in neurovascular status.	Immediate reporting leads to rapid treatment and decreases likelihood of long-term damage.

NURSING DIAGNOSIS
Impaired Skin Integrity related to abrasions
High Risk for Impaired Skin Integrity related to immobility

GOAL: The child will exhibit healed skin abrasions and no further skin breakdown.

OUTCOME CRITERIA
- The child's skin abrasions heal without signs or symptoms of infection.
- The child's skin remains intact without redness or irritation.

NURSING INTERVENTIONS	*RATIONALE*
Wash and thoroughly dry skin every day.	Stimulates circulation and keeps skin clean
Inspect skin at least every 4 hours for evidence of redness or broken skin.	Early detection and treatment of skin breakdown can prevent long-term complications.
Change position every 2 hours within restraints of traction.	Relieves pressure and decreases likelihood of skin breakdown and decreased circulation.
Clean pin sites as ordered following standard precautions.	Decreases risk of infection
Observe for redness, drainage at pin sites, and elevated temperature.	Signs and symptoms of possible infection

NURSING DIAGNOSIS
Activity Intolerance related to skeletal traction and bedrest

GOAL: The child will maintain adequate range of motion.

OUTCOME CRITERIA
- The child performs range of motion within limits of traction.
- The child does own self-care activities.
- The child participates in age appropriate activities within restrictions of traction.

(nursing care plan continues on page 406)

NURSING CARE PLAN continued

for the Child in Traction

NURSING INTERVENTIONS	RATIONALE
Teach child active and passive range-of-motion exercises. Encourage child to become active in self-care.	Maintains joint function and increases circulation. Provides a feeling of control over hospitalization; increases use of parts of body not immobilized to allow normal muscle function.

NURSING DIAGNOSIS
Deficient Diversional Activity related to lengthy hospitalization

GOAL: The child will achieve developmental tasks appropriate for age.

OUTCOME CRITERIA
• The child selects and participates in age-appropriate activities and play.
• The child shows enjoyment in participating in activities.
• The child communicates and interacts with peers.

NURSING INTERVENTIONS	RATIONALE
Provide age-appropriate games, supplies, and activities that the child can do while in traction such as books, puzzles, computer games.	Access to age appropriate activities helps the child to develop and achieve milestones of growth and development.
Encourage child to communicate with peers by telephone, letter, computer.	Allows for normal growth and development opportunities
Move child's bed to hallway or playroom to enable participation in activities.	Increases interaction with other children; decreases boredom

child's time is spent away from home, the child is exposed to poisonous plants that cause allergic reactions or to bites from insects, animals, or snakes; these need attention.

Fungal Infections

Fungal infections of the skin are superficial infections caused by fungi that live in the outer (dead) layers of the skin, the hair, and nails. **Tinea** (ringworm) is the term commonly applied to these infections, which are further differentiated by the part of the body infected.

Tinea Capitis (Ringworm of the Scalp)

Ringworm of the scalp is called *tinea capitis* or *tinea tonsurans.* The most common cause is *Microsporum audouinii,* which is transmitted from person to person through combs, towels, hats, barber scissors, or direct contact. A less common type, *Microsporum canis,* is transmitted from animal to child. Tinea capitis begins as a small papule on the scalp and spreads, leaving scaly patches of baldness. The hairs become brittle and break off easily. Griseofulvin, an oral antifungal

antibiotic, is the medication of choice. Because treatment may be prolonged (3 months or more), compliance must be reinforced. Children who are being properly treated may attend school. Hair loss is not permanent.

Tinea Corporis (Ringworm of the Body)

Tinea corporis is ringworm of the body that affects the epidermal skin layer. The lesions appear as a scaly ring with clearing in the center and may occur on any part of the body. They resemble the lesions of scalp ringworm. The child usually contracts tinea corporis from contact with an infected dog or cat. Topical antifungal agents, such as clotrimazole, econazole nitrate, tolnaftate, and miconazole, are effective. Griseofulvin also is used in this condition.

Tinea Pedis (Ringworm of the Feet; Athlete's Foot)

Tinea pedis (athlete's foot) is the scaling or cracking of the skin between the toes. Examination under a microscope of scrapings from the lesions is necessary for definite diagnosis. Transmission is by direct or indirect contact with skin lesions from infected people. Contaminated sidewalks, floors, pool decks, and shower stalls spread the condition to those who walk barefoot. Tinea pedis, usually found in adolescents and adults, is becoming more prevalent among school-age children due to the popularity of plastic shoes.

Care includes washing the feet with soap and water, then gently removing scabs and crusts and applying a topical agent such as tolnaftate. Griseofulvin by mouth is also useful. During the chronic phase, the use of ointment, scrupulous foot hygiene, frequent changing of white cotton socks, and avoidance of plastic footwear are helpful. Continuing application of a topical agent for up to 6 weeks is recommended.

Tinea Cruris (Ringworm of the Inner Thighs and Inguinal Area)

Tinea cruris (jock itch) is caused by the same organisms that cause tinea corporis. It is more common in athletes and is uncommon in preadolescent children. Tinea cruris is pruritic and localized to the area. Treatment is the same as for tinea corporis. Sitz baths also may be soothing.

Parasitic Infections

Parasites are organisms that live on or within another living organism from which they obtain their food supply. Lice and the scabies mite live by sucking the blood of the host.

Pediculosis

Pediculosis (lice infestation) may be caused by *Pediculus humanus capitis* (head lice), *Pediculus humanus corporis* (body lice), or *Phthirus pubis* (pubic lice). Head lice are the most common infestation in children. Animal lice are not transferred to humans.

Head lice are passed from child to child by direct contact or indirectly by contact with combs, headgear, or bed linen. Lice, which are rarely seen, lay their eggs called nits on the head where they attach to hair strands. The nits can be seen as tiny pearly white flecks attached to the hair shafts. They look much like dandruff, but dandruff flakes can be flicked off easily, whereas the nits are tightly attached and not easily removed. The nits hatch in about 1 week, and the lice become sexually mature in about 2 weeks. Severe itching of the scalp is the most obvious symptom.

Use of lindane (Kwell) shampoo, which is prescribed by a physician, gives the most satisfactory results. After wetting the hair with warm water, the Kwell is applied like any ordinary shampoo; about 1 oz is used. The head should be lathered for 4

minutes, then rinsed thoroughly and dried. After the hair is dry, it should be combed with a fine-toothed comb dipped in warm white vinegar to remove remaining nits and nit shells. Shampooing may be repeated in 2 weeks to remove any lice that may have been missed as nits and since hatched. Avoid getting Kwell into the eyes or on mucous membranes. When treating a child in the hospital for pediculosis, wear a disposable gown, gloves, and head cover for protection.

Family caregivers are often embarrassed when the school nurse sends word that the child has head lice. They can be reassured that lice infestation is common and can happen to any child; it is not a reflection on the caregiver's housekeeping. All family members should be inspected and treated as needed. See Family Teaching Tips: Eliminating Pediculi Infestations for other useful information.

Scabies

Scabies is a skin infestation caused by the scabies mite, *Sarcoptes scabiei*. The female mite burrows in areas between the fingers and toes and in warm folds of the body, such as the axilla and groin, to lay eggs. Burrows are visible as dark lines, and the mite is seen as a black dot at the end of the burrow. Severe itching occurs, causing scratching with resulting secondary infection.

The areas are treated with lindane lotion or crotamiton (Eurax). The body is first scrubbed with soap and water, then the lotion is applied on all areas of the body except the face. With lindane, a second coat can be applied, then all washed off in 24 hours. For crotamiton, a second coat is applied in 24

FAMILY TEACHING TIPS

Eliminating Pediculi Infestations

1. Wash all child's bedding and clothing in hot water and dry in hot dryer.
2. Vacuum carpets, car seats, mattresses, and upholstered furniture very thoroughly. Discard vacuum dust bag.
3. Wash pillows, stuffed animals, and other washable items the same way clothing is washed.
4. Dry-clean non-washable items.
5. If items cannot be washed or dry-cleaned, seal in plastic bag for 2 weeks to break reproductive cycle of lice.
6. Wash combs, brushes, and other hair items (rollers, curlers, barrettes, etc.) in shampoo and soak for 1 hour.
7. If you discover the infestation, report to child's school or day care.
8. Schools should disinfect headphones.

hours; the patient waits an additional 48 hours to wash it off. Caregivers should follow the tips recommended for pediculosis. All who had close contact with the child within a 30- to 60-day period should be treated. The rash and itch may continue for several weeks even though the mites have been successfully eliminated.

Skin Allergies

One of the most common allergic skin reactions is eczema (atopic dermatitis), which is discussed in Chapter 11. Other skin disorders of allergic origin include hives (urticaria) and giant swellings (angioedema) and rashes caused by poison ivy, poison oak, and other plants or drug reactions. Skin rashes are common in school-age children. Infectious diseases cause some and allergies cause others. Whatever the cause, rashes are usually treated with topical preparations such as lotions, ointments, and greases, plus cool soaks. The itching must be relieved as much as possible because scratching can introduce additional pathogens to the affected area.

Hives (Urticaria) and Giant Swellings (Angioedema)

Hives appear in different sizes on many different parts of the body and are usually caused by foods or drugs. They are bright red and itchy and can occur on the eyelids, tongue, mouth, hands, feet or in the brain or stomach. When affecting the mouth or tongue, hives can cause difficulty in breathing; in the stomach, the swelling can produce pain, nausea, and vomiting. Swelling in brain tissue causes headache and other neurologic symptoms.

Foods such as chocolate, nuts, shellfish, berries or other raw fruit, fish, and highly seasoned foods are likely to cause hives. Possible drug allergens include aspirin and related drugs, laxatives, anti-inflammatory drugs, tranquilizers, and antibiotics (penicillin is the most common allergen of this group). Sometimes it is impossible to identify the cause.

Treatment is aimed at reducing the swelling and relieving the itching. If the allergen can be identified, it can be removed from the child's environment and hyposensitization can be performed. If the allergen is a certain food, that food must be eliminated from the child's diet. Antihistamines (topical or systemic) are used to relieve itching and reduce swelling. Cool soaks also help to relieve itching. Fingernails should be kept short and clean. In severe cases, corticosteroids may be necessary.

Plant Allergies

Poison ivy, oak, and sumac are common causes of contact dermatitis. Of these, poison ivy is the worst offender, particularly during the summer (Fig. 17–20). The cause of the allergy is the extremely potent oil, urushiol, which is present in all parts of these plants. Its effects vary from slight inflammation and itching to severe, extensive swelling that can virtually immobilize the child. This disorder causes intense itching (pruritus) and forms tiny blisters that weep and continue to spread the inflammation.

Antihistamines or oral steroids help to relieve itching and prevent scratching. Cool soaks, Aveeno baths, calamine lotion, or topical steroids help minimize discomfort. The child should be taught to recognize and avoid the poisonous plants. The plants also should be removed from the environment when possible.

Bites

Because school-age children are active, inquisitive, and not completely inhibited in their actions, they commonly suffer animal and human bites as well as insect stings and bites. Many of these are minor particularly if the skin is not broken. Some, however, can have life-threatening implications if proper care is not given.

Animal Bites

Children enjoy pets, but often they are not alert to possibly dangerous encounters with pets or wild animals. Dog bites are common. Fortunately because of rabies vaccination programs for dogs, few dog bites cause rabies; in fact, cats are the domestic animal most likely to carry rabies. Any pet that bites should be held until it can be determined if the animal has been vaccinated against rabies. If not, the child must undergo a series of injections to prevent this potentially fatal disease. The series consists of both active and passive immunizations. Active immunity is established with five injections of human diploid cell vaccine beginning on the day of the bite and on days

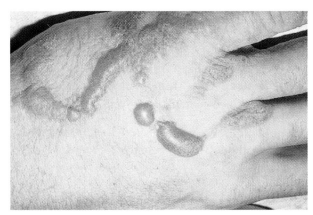

● *Figure 17.20* Poison ivy on a child's hand.

3, 7, 14, and 28. Human rabies immune globulin is given on the first day along with the diploid cell vaccine.

All animal and human bites should be thoroughly washed with soap and water. An antiseptic such as 70% alcohol or povidone-iodine should be applied after the wound has been thoroughly rinsed. The wound must be observed for signs of infection until well healed. Animal bites should be promptly reported to the proper authorities.

Children should be taught at an early age about the danger of animal bites, particularly of strange or wild animals such as skunks, raccoons, bats, and squirrels.

Spider Bites

Spider bites can cause serious illness if untreated. Bites of black widow spiders, brown recluse spiders, and scorpions demand medical attention. Applying ice to the affected area until medical care is obtained can slow absorption of the poison.

Tick Bites

Wood ticks carried by chipmunks, ground squirrels, weasels, and wood rats can cause Rocky Mountain spotted fever. Most cases are found in the South Atlantic, South Central, and Southeastern United States. Dogs are often the carriers to humans. People living in areas where ticks are common can be immunized against this disease.

Deer ticks, carried by white-footed mice and white-tailed deer found in the Northeast, Midwest, and West, can carry the organism that causes Lyme disease. The first stage of the disease begins with a lesion at the site of the bite. The lesion appears as a macule with a clear center. The second stage occurs several weeks to months later if the patient is not treated. The symptoms of this stage may affect the central nervous system and the heart. If untreated, the third stage may occur months to years later, causing arthritis, neurologic disorders, and bone and joint disease.

Children and adults should wear long pants, long-sleeved shirts, and insect repellent when walking in the woods. Pant legs should be tucked into socks. If a tick is found on the body, alcohol may be applied and the tick carefully removed with tweezers. To prevent the release of pathogenic organisms, care should be taken not to crush the tick. A health care provider must be consulted if there is any suspicion that a deer tick has bitten a child or an adult.

Snake Bites

Snake bites demand immediate medical intervention. The wound should be washed, ice applied, and the involved body part immobilized. Prompt transport to the nearest medical facility is essential.

Insect Stings or Bites

Insect stings or bites can prove fatal to children who are sensitized. Swelling may be localized or may include an entire extremity. Circulatory collapse, airway obstruction, and anaphylactic shock can cause death within 30 minutes if the child is untreated. Immediate treatment is necessary and may include injection of epinephrine, antihistamines, or steroids. These children should wear a Medic Alert bracelet and carry an anaphylaxis kit that includes a plastic syringe of epinephrine and an antihistamine. The teacher, school nurse, and anyone who cares for the child should be alerted to the child's allergy and should know where the anaphylaxis kit is and how to use it when necessary.

KEY POINTS

▶ Most illnesses during the school-age years are short-term and minor, but for some children this is a time of visits to a health care facility and many trips to the health care provider.

▶ Children with long-term or chronic diseases such as scoliosis, asthma, rheumatic fever, or diabetes may be self-conscious about being different from their classmates.

▶ Children need to have positive self-esteem. Illness may threaten the child's self-confidence and can contribute to self-doubt.

▶ School-age children can be involved in their health care by learning how the illness affects their bodies, how to help care for themselves, and what the future may hold for them.

▶ An important aspect of teaching the asthmatic child and family is helping them learn to anticipate an impending episode and respond appropriately. Exercise and activity are an essential part of therapy for the child with asthma.

▶ The diabetes of childhood is Type 1 insulin-dependent diabetes mellitus, which is managed by insulin replacement, diet, and exercise.

▶ The diabetic child and family members must be included when teaching about all aspects of caring for the child's diabetes.

▶ Nurses who care for school-age children have a responsibility to be observant for scoliosis.

▶ Goals in caring for a child with juvenile rheumatoid arthritis include preserving joint function and preventing physical deformities.

▶ The adventurous school-age child often explores

new horizons and because of immature judgment may be exposed to the dangers of fractures, poison ivy, and animal bites particularly when in hazardous or wooded areas.

REFERENCES

1. Eggleston PA. (1999) Asthma. In *Oski's pediatrics: Principles and practice* (3rd ed). Philadelphia: Lippincott Williams & Wilkins.
2. Kelekman J, et al. (1999) Diabetes update in the pediatric population. *Pediatric Nursing*, 25(6), 666.
3. Sponseller PD. (1999) Bone, joint, and muscle problems. In *Oski's pediatrics: Principles and practice* (3rd ed). Philadelphia: Lippincott Williams & Wilkins.
4. Cassidy JT. (1999) Rheumatic diseases of childhood. In *Oski's pediatrics: Principles and practice* (3rd ed). Philadelphia: Lippincott Williams & Wilkins.

BIBLIOGRAPHY

Azar R, Solomon CR. (2001) Coping strategies of parents facing child diabetes mellitus. *Journal of Pediatric Nursing*, 16(6), 418.

Cassidy JT. (1999) Rheumatic diseases of childhood. In *Oski's pediatrics: Principles and practice* (3rd ed). Philadelphia: Lippincott Williams & Wilkins.

Chin K R, et. al. (2001) A guide to early detection of scoliosis. *Contemporary Pediatrics*, 18(9) 77.

El-Said GM. (1999) Rheumatic fever. In *Oski's Pediatrics: Principles and practice* (3rd ed). Philadelphia: Lippincott Williams & Wilkins.

England AC, Dalheim Rydstrom I, Astrid N. (2001) Being the parent of a child with asthma. *Pediatric Nursing*, 27(4), 365.

Guevara J, et. al. (2001) Health care costs for children with attention deficit disorder,. *Pediatrics*. 108(1), 71.

Katz DR. (2001) Adolescent idiopathic scoliosis: The effect of brace treatment on the incidence of surgery. *Physical Therapy*, 81(9), 1591.

Kelekman J, et. al. (1999) Diabetes update in the pediatric population. *Pediatric Nursing*, 25(6), 666.

Lawless MR, McElderry DH. (2001) Nocturnal enuresis: Current concepts. *Pediatrics in Review*, 22(12), 399–407.

Maniatis A K, et al. (2001) Continuous subcutaneous insulin infusion therapy for children and adolescents: An option for routine diabetes care. *Pediatrics*, 107(2), 351.

Meaux JB. (2000) Stop, look, listen: The challenge for children with ADHD. *Issues in Comprehensive Pediatric Nursing*, 23(1), 1–13.

North American Nursing Diagnosis Association. (2001) *NANDA nursing diagnoses: Definitions and classification 2001–2002*. Philadelphia: NANDA.

Palmer EA. (2001) Family caregiver experiences with asthma in school age children. *Pediatric Nursing*, 27(1), 75.

Pillitteri A. (2003). *Maternal and child health nursing* (4th ed). Philadelphia: Lippincott Williams & Wilkins.

Powell ET, Austin A. (1998) Developing a pediatric diabetes critical pathway. *Pediatric Nursing*, 24(6), 558.

(2001) *Questions and answers about scoliosis in children and adolescents*. National Institute of Arthritis and Musculoskeletal and Skin Diseases, National Institutes of Health, *www.niams.nih.gov/hi/index.htm*.

Skoner DP. (2002) Balancing safety and efficacy in pediatric asthma management. *Pediatrics*, 109(2), 381.

Smeltzer SC, Bare BG. (2000) *Textbook of medical-surgical nursing* (9th ed). Philadelphia: Lippincott Williams & Wilkins.

Sparks S, Taylor C. (2001) *Nursing diagnosis reference manual* (5th ed). Springhouse, PA: Springhouse Corporation.

Splete H. (2001) Catch curves like scoliosis in time for bracing. *Pediatric News*, 35(11), 42.

(2000) *Springhouse nurse's drug guide* (3rd ed). Springhouse, PA: Springhouse Corporation.

Stadtler AC, et al. (2001) The Touchpoints pediatric asthma program. *Pediatric Nursing*, 27(5), 459.

Wong DL. (1998) *Whaley and Wong's nursing care of infants and children* (6th ed). St. Louis: Mosby.

Wong DL, Perry S, Hockenberry M . (2002) *Maternal child nursing care* (2nd ed). St. Louis: Mosby.

Wong DL, Hess C. (2000) *Wong and Whaley's clinical manual of pediatric nursing* (5th ed). St. Louis: Mosby.

Websites
Scoliosis: *www.scoliosis-assoc.org*
Diabetes: *www.jdf.org*
Diabetes: *www.childrenwithdiabetes.com*
Epilepsy: *www.efa.org*
Asthma: *www.aaaai.org*
Asthma: *www.aafa.org*

Workbook

NCLEX-STYLE REVIEW QUESTIONS

1. The nurse is teaching a group of caregivers of children who have asthma. The caregivers made the following statements. Which of these statements indicates a need for further teaching?

   a. "We need to identify the things that trigger our child's attacks."

   b. "I always have him use his bronchodilator before he uses his steroid inhaler."

   c. "We will be sure our child does not exercise to prevent attacks."

   d. "She drinks lots of water which I know helps to thin her secretions."

2. A nurse admits a child with a diagnosis of possible appendicitis. Of the following signs and symptoms which would MOST likely be seen in the child with appendicitis?

   a. Sore throat, bone and joint pain

   b. Itching, swelling around eyes and ankles

   c. Convulsions, weight gain or loss

   d. Fever, nausea and vomiting

3. The nurse is doing patient teaching with a child who has been placed in a brace to treat scoliosis. Which of the following statements made by the child indicates an understanding of the treatment?

   a. "I am so glad I can take this brace off for the school dance."

   b. "At least when I take a shower I have a few minutes out of this brace."

   c. "Wearing this brace only during the night won't be so embarrassing."

   d. "When I start feeling tired, I can just take my brace off for a few minutes."

4. The nurse is working with a 12-year-old child diagnosed with Type 1 diabetes mellitus. The child asks the nurse why she can't take pills instead of shots like her grandmother does. Which of the following would be the BEST response by the nurse?

   a. "The pills correct another type of diabetes than you have."

   b. "When your blood glucose levels are better controlled, you can take the pills too."

   c. "Your body does not make its own insulin so the insulin injections help replace it."

   d. "The pills only work for adults who have diabetes. Maybe when you are older, you can take the pills."

5. A child diagnosed with rheumatic fever will MOST likely have a history of which of the following?

   a. A sibling diagnosed with the disease

   b. A recent strep throat infection

   c. Bruising easily

   d. Increased urinary output

STUDY ACTIVITIES

1. Using the table below, list the areas that must be checked and monitored when doing a neurovascular status check (CMS check) on a child with a fracture. Include the area to be monitored, the definition or explanation, observations, and documentation.

2. Develop a teaching aid or poster to use in teaching diabetic children how to administer their own insulin injections. Include how you will help this child make an insulin site rotation chart. Present your project to your peers.

Area to Be Monitored (the 5 Ps)	Definition or Explanation	Observations (What Signs to Look for)	Documentation

3. A coworker says to you, "That Jeff in room 204 is bouncing off the walls." You are assigned to this child, who has a diagnosis of attention deficit hyperactive disorder (ADHD). Make a list of behavior techniques to use with the child who has ADHD. Develop a plan of care you could use to care for Jeff.

CRITICAL THINKING

1. You are in the grocery store and see a child having a seizure. No other adult is around. Explain step by step what you will do.

2. Five-year-old Malcolm has been sent home from kindergarten with a note advising of an outbreak of pinworms. There are five children between 2 and 8 years of age in the household where he lives, including cousins. Explain to his aunt, who cares for the children, what she should do to handle the problem.

3. Twelve-year-old Carrie has scoliosis and must wear a TLSO brace. She says she thinks it's really ugly. Describe the feelings Carrie might be going through in this situation. How will you respond to Carrie? Write out a therapeutic conversation you might have with this child.

4. *Dosage Calculation:* A school-age child with a diagnosis of a seizure disorder is being treated with Dilantin. The child weighs 58 pounds. The child is being given a dose of 6 mg/kg a day in 3 divided doses. Answer the following:
   a. How many kg does the child's weigh?
   b. How many mgs of Dilantin will the child receive in a 24-hour period of time?
   c. How many mgs of Dilantin will the child receive in each dose?
   d. If the dose is increased by 20 mg a dose, how many milligrams will then be in each dose?
   e. How many milligrams will the child receive in a 24-hour period after the dose has been increased?

Growth and Development of the Adolescent: 11 to 18 Years

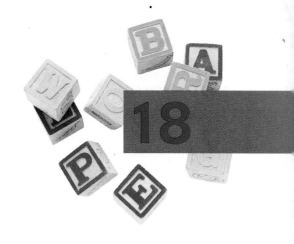

18

PREADOLESCENT DEVELOPMENT
  Physical Development
  Preparation for Adolescence
ADOLESCENT DEVELOPMENT
  Physical Development
  Psychosocial Development
  Personality Development
  Body Image
NUTRITION
  Ethnic and Cultural Influences

HEALTH PROMOTION AND MAINTENANCE
  Routine Checkups
  Family Teaching
  Health Education and Counseling
  Accident Prevention
THE ADOLESCENT IN THE HEALTH CARE FACILITY

STUDENT OBJECTIVES

On completion of this chapter, the student will be able to

1. Define key terms.
2. State the age of (a) the preadolescent and (b) the adolescent.
3. Describe the psychosocial development of the preadolescent.
4. Name the physical changes that make the child appear uncoordinated in early adolescence.
5. List the secondary sexual characteristics that appear (a) in adolescent boys and (b) in adolescent girls.
6. State (a) the major cognitive task of the adolescent according to Piaget and (b) the psychosocial task according to Erikson.
7. Explain some problems that adolescents face when making career choices today.
8. Discuss the necessity for orderly psychosocial development of identity and trust before adolescents are ready for intimate relationships.
9. Discuss the adolescent's need to conform to peers.
10. Discuss the influence of peer pressure on psychosocial development.
11. Discuss adolescent body image and associated problems.
12. Name the nutrients commonly deficient in the diets of adolescents.
13. Discuss the aspects of sexual maturity that impact the needs for health education in the adolescent.
14. Discuss the issues that the adolescent faces in making decisions related to sexual responsibility and substance use.

KEY TERMS

early adolescence
heterosexual
homosexual
malocclusion
menarche
nocturnal emissions
orthodontia
puberty

"**A**dolescence" comes from the Latin word meaning "to come to maturity," a fitting description of this stage of life. The adolescent is maturing physically and emotionally, growing from childhood toward adulthood, and seeking to understand what it means to be grown up.

Early adolescence (preadolescence, pubescence) begins at about age 10 in girls and about age 12 in boys with a dramatic growth spurt that signals the advent of **puberty** (reproductive maturity). During this stage, the child's body begins to take on adult-like contours, the primary sex organs enlarge, secondary sexual characteristics appear, and hormonal activity increases. This early period ends with the onset of menstruation in the female and the production of sperm in the male. The bone growth that began during intrauterine life continues through adolescence and is usually completed by the end of this period.

Adolescents are fascinated and sometimes fearful and confused by the changes occurring in their bodies and their thinking processes. They begin to look grown up, but they do not have the judgment or independence to participate in society as an adult. These young people are strongly influenced by their peer group and often resent parental authority. Roller-coaster emotions characterize this age group, as does intense interest in romantic relationships (Fig. 18–1).

The adolescent years can be a time of turmoil and uncertainty that creates conflict between family caregivers and children. If these conflicts are resolved, normal development can continue. Unresolved conflicts can foster delays in development and prevent the young person from maturing into a fully functioning adult.

Body image is critical to adolescents. Health problems that threaten body image, such as acne, obesity, dental or vision problems, and trauma, can seriously interfere with development.

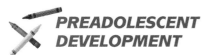

PREADOLESCENT DEVELOPMENT

During the period between 10 and 12 years of age, the rate of growth varies greatly in boys and girls. This variability in growth and maturation can be a concern to the child who develops rapidly or the one who develops more slowly than his or her peers. Children of this age do not want to be different from their friends. The developmental characteristics of the preadolescent child in late school age stage overlap with those of early adolescence; nevertheless there are unique characteristics to set this stage apart (Table 18–1).

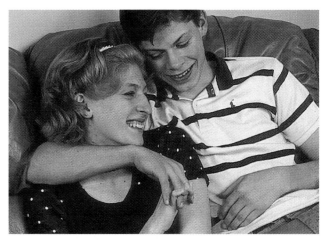

● *Figure 18.1* Intense interest in the opposite sex characterizes adolescence.

Physical Development

Preadolescence begins in the female between the ages of 9 and 11 years and is marked by a growth spurt that lasts for about 18 months. Girls grow about 3 inches each year until **menarche** (the beginning of menstruation), after which growth slows considerably. Early in adolescence, girls begin to develop a figure, the pelvis broadens, and axillary and pubic hair begins to appear along with many changes in hormone levels. The variation between girls is great and often is a cause for much concern by the "early bloomer" or the "late bloomer." Young girls who begin to develop physically as early as 9 years of age are often embarrassed by these physical changes. In girls, the onset of menarche marks the end of the preadolescent period.

Boys enter preadolescence a little later usually between 11 and 13 years of age and grow generally at a slower, steadier rate than do girls. During this time, the scrotum and testes begin to enlarge, the skin of the scrotum begins to change in coloring and texture, and sparse hair begins to show at the base of the penis. Boys who start their growth spurt later often are concerned about being shorter than their peers. In boys, the appearance of **nocturnal emissions** ("wet dreams") is often used as the indication that the preadolescent period has ended.

Preparation for Adolescence

Preadolescents need information about their changing bodies and feelings. Sex education that includes information about the hormonal changes that are occurring or will be occurring is necessary to help them through this developmental stage.

Girls need information that will help them handle their early menstrual periods with minimal apprehension. Most girls have irregular periods for the first year or so; they need to know that this is not a cause for worry. They have many questions about protec-

TABLE 18.1	Growth and Development of the Preadolescent: 10–13 Years				
Physical	**Motor**	**Personal-Social**	**Language**	**Perceptual**	**Cognitive**
Average height 56¾ inches–59 inches (144–150 cm) Average weight 77–88 lb (35–40 kg) Pubescence may begin Girls may surpass boys in height Remaining permanent teeth erupt	Refines gross and fine motor skills May have difficulty with some fine motor coordination due to growth of large muscles before that of small muscle growth; hands and feet are first structures to increase in size; thus, actions may appear uncoordinated during early preadolescence Can do crafts Uses tools increasingly well	Attends school primarily for peer association Peer relationships of greatest importance Intolerant of violation of group norms Can follow rules of group and adapt to another point of view Can use stored knowledge to make independent judgments	Fluent in spoken language Vocabulary 50,000 words for reading; oral vocabulary of 7,200 words Uses slang words and terms, vulgarities, jeers, jokes, and sayings	Can catch or intercept ball thrown from a distance Possible growth spurts may cause myopia	Begins abstract thinking Conservation of volume Understands relation among time, speed, and distance Ability to sympathize, love, and reason are all evolving. Right and wrong become logically clear

tion during the menstrual period and the advisability of using sanitary pads or tampons. They may fear that "everybody will know" when they have their first period and must be allowed to express this fear and be reassured.

Boys also need information about their bodies. Erections and nocturnal emissions are topics they need to discuss, as well as the development of other male secondary sex characteristics.

Both boys and girls need information about changes in the opposite sex, including discussions that address their questions. This kind of information helps them increase their understanding of human sexuality. School programs may provide a good foundation for sex education, but each preadolescent needs an adult to turn to with particular questions. Even a well-planned program does not address all the needs of the preadolescent. The best school program begins early and builds from year to year as the child's needs progress (see Chap. 16).

Preadolescence is an appropriate time for discussions that will help the young teen resist pressures to become sexually active too early. Family caregivers may turn to a nurse acquaintance for guidance in preparing their child. Perhaps the most important aspect of discussions about sexuality is that honest, straightforward answers must be given in an atmosphere of caring concern. Children whose need for information is not met through family, school, or community programs will get their information—often inaccurate—from peers, movies, television, or other media.

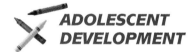

ADOLESCENT DEVELOPMENT

Adolescence spans the ages of about 13 to 18 years. Some males do not complete adolescence until they are 20 years old. The rate of development during adolescence varies greatly from one teen to another. It is a time of many physical, emotional, and social changes. During this period, the adolescent is engaged in a struggle to master the developmental tasks that lead to successful completion of this stage of development (Table 18–2). Completion of the developmental tasks of earlier developmental stages is a prerequisite for the completion of these tasks.

Physical Development

Rapid growth occurs during adolescence. Girls begin growing during the preadolescent period and achieve 98% of their adult height by the age of 16. Boys start growing around 13 years of age and may continue to grow until 20 years of age. The skeletal system's rapid

TABLE 18.2	Developmental Tasks of Adolescence
Basic Task	**Associated Tasks**
Appreciate own uniqueness*	Identify interests, skills, and talents
	Identify differences from peers
	Accept strengths and limitations
	Challenge own skill levels
Develop independent internal identity*	Value self as a person
	Separate physical self from psychological self
	Differentiate personal worth from cultural stereotypes
	Separate internal value from societal feedback
Determine own value system*	Identify options
	Establish priorities
	Commit self to decisions made
	Translate values into behaviors
	Resist peer and cultural pressures to conform to their value system
	Find comfortable balance between own and peer/cultural standards, behaviors, and needs
Develop self-evaluation skills*	Develop basis for self-evaluation and monitoring
	Evaluate quality of products
	Assess approach to tasks and responsibilities
	Develop sensitivity to intrapersonal relationships
	Evaluate dynamics of interpersonal relationships
Assume increasing responsibility for own behavior*	Quality of work, chores
	Emotional tone
	Money management
	Time management
	Decision making
	Personal habits
	Social behaviors
Find meaning in life	Accept and integrate meaning of death
	Develop philosophy of life
	Begin to identify life or career goals
Acquire skills essential for adult living	Acquire skills essential to independent living
	Develop social and emotional abilities and temperament
	Refine sociocultural amenities
	Identify and experiment with alternatives for facing life
	Acquire employment skills
	Seek growth-inducing activities
Seek affiliations outside of family	Seek companionship with compatible peers
	Affiliate with organizations that support uniqueness
	Actively seek models or mentors
	Identify potential emotional support systems
	Differentiate between acquaintances and friends
	Identify ways to express sexuality
Adapt to adult body functioning	Adapt to somatic (body) changes
	Refine balance and coordination
	Develop physical strength
	Consider sexuality and reproduction issues

*Tasks deemed crucial to continued maturation

growth, which outpaces muscular system growth, causes the long and lanky appearance of many teens and contributes to the clumsiness often seen during this age.

During the first menstrual cycles, ovulation does not usually occur because increased estrogen levels are needed to produce an ovum mature enough to be released. However, at 13 to 15 years of age, the cycle becomes ovulatory, and pregnancy is possible. The girl's breasts take on an adult appearance by age 16, and pubic hair is curly and abundant.

By the age of 16 years, the penis, testes, and scrotum are adult in size and shape, and mature spermatozoa are produced. Male pubic hair also is adult in appearance and amount. After age 13, muscle strength and coordination develop rapidly. The larynx and vocal cords enlarge, and the voice deepens. The "change of voice" makes the teenage male's voice vary unexpectedly, which occasionally causes embarrassment for the teen.

Psychosocial Development

Adolescence is a time of transition from childhood to adulthood. Between the ages of 10 and 18 years, adolescents move from Freud's latency stage to the genital stage, from Erikson's industry versus inferiority to identity versus role confusion, and from Piaget's concrete operational thinking to formal operational thought. They develop a sense of moral judgment and a system of values and beliefs that will affect their entire lives. The foundation provided by family, religious groups, school, and community experiences is still a strong influence, but the peer group exerts tremendous power. Trends and fads among adolescents dictate clothing choices, hairstyles, music, and other recreational choices (Fig. 18–2). The adolescent whose family caregivers make it difficult to conform are adding another stress to an already emotion-laden period. Peer pressure to experiment with potentially dangerous practices such as drugs, alcohol, and reckless driving also can be strong; adolescents may need careful guidance and understanding support to help resist this peer influence.

Personality Development

Erikson considered the central task of adolescence to be the establishment of identity. Adolescents spend a

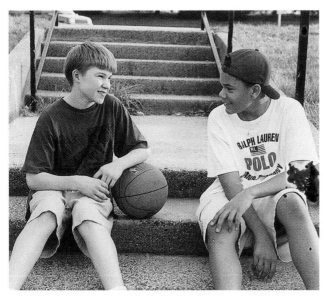

● *Figure 18.2* For many teens, hanging out with friends is an important way to share common interests and gain a sense of belonging.

lot of time asking themselves, "Who am I as a person? What will I do with my life? Marry? Have children? Will I go to college? If so, where? If not, why not? What kind of career should I choose?"

Adolescents are confronted with a greater variety of choices than ever before. Sex role stereotypes have been shattered in most careers and professions. More women are becoming lawyers, physicians, plumbers, and carpenters; more men are entering nursing or choosing to become house-husbands while their wives earn the primary family income. Transportation has made greater geographic mobility possible, so that many youngsters can spend summers or a full school year in a foreign country, plan to attend college thousands of miles from home, and begin a career in an even more remote location. Making decisions and choices is never simple. With such a tremendous variety of options, it is understandable that adolescents often are preoccupied with their own concerns.

When identity has been established generally between the ages of 16 and 18 years, adolescents seek intimate relationships usually with members of the opposite sex. *Intimacy*, which is mutual sharing of one's deepest feelings with another person, is impossible unless both persons have established a sense of trust and a sense of identity. Intimate relationships are a preparation for long-term relationships, and people who fail to achieve intimacy may develop feelings of isolation and experience chronic difficulty in communicating with others.

Most intimate relationships during adolescence are **heterosexual,** or between members of the opposite sex. Sometimes, however, young people form intimate attachments with members of the same sex, or **homosexual** relationships. Because our culture is predominately heterosexual and is still struggling with trying to understand homosexual relationships, these relationships can cause great anxiety for family caregivers and children. Although some parts of American society are beginning to accept homosexual relationships as no more than another lifestyle, prejudice still exists. So great a stigma has been attached to homosexuality that many adolescents fear they are homosexual if they are uncomfortable about heterosexual intimacy. However, this discomfort is normal as adolescents move from same-sex peer group activities to dating peers of the opposite sex.

Body Image

Body image is closely related to self-esteem. Seeing one's body as attractive and functional contributes to a positive sense of self-esteem. During adolescence, the desire not to be different can extend to feelings about one's body and can cause adolescents to feel that their bodies are inadequate even though they are actually healthy and attractive.

American culture tends to equate a slender figure with feminine beauty and acceptability and a lean, tall, muscular figure with masculine virility and strength. Adolescents, particularly males, who feel that they are underdeveloped suffer great anxiety. Adolescent girls have even undergone plastic surgery to augment their breasts to relieve this anxiety. Girls in this age group often feel that they are too fat and try strange, nutritionally unsound diets to reduce their weight. Some literally starve themselves. Even after their bodies have become emaciated, they truly believe that they are still fat and, therefore, unattractive. This condition is called *anorexia nervosa* and is discussed further in Chapter 19.

Adolescents need to establish a positive body image by the end of their developmental stage. Because bone growth is completed during adolescence, a person's height will remain basically the same throughout adult life even though weight can fluctuate greatly. Tall girls who long to be petite and boys who would like to be 6 feet tall may need guidance and support to bring their expectations in line with reality and learn to have positive feelings about their bodies and accept them the way they are.

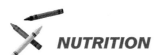

NUTRITION

Nutritional requirements are greatly increased during periods of rapid growth in adolescence. Adolescent boys need more calories than do girls throughout the growth period. Appetites increase, and most teens eat frequently. Families with teenage boys often jokingly say that they cannot keep the refrigerator filled. Nutritional needs are related to growth and sexual maturity rather than age.

Even though adolescents understand something about nutrition, they may not relate this understanding to their dietary habits. Their accelerated growth rate and increased physical activities for some mean that they need more food to meet their energy requirements. Because adolescents are seeking to establish their independence, their food choices are sometimes not wise and tend to be influenced by peer preference rather than parental advice. Teens frequently skip meals especially breakfast, snack on foods that provide empty calories, and eat a lot of fast foods. The era of fast-food meals has given adolescents easy access to high-calorie, nutritionally unbalanced meals. Too many fast-food meals and nutritionally empty snacks can result in nutritional deficiencies (Fig. 18–3).

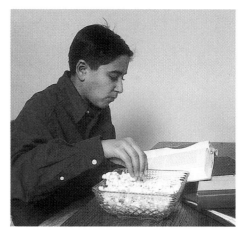

● **Figure 18.3** Teens are always hungry, but often choose convenient junk foods, which lack nutritional value.

When good nutritional habits have been established in early childhood, adolescent nutrition is likely to be better balanced than when nutritional teaching has been insufficient. Being part of a family that practices sound nutrition helps ensure that occasional lapses into sweets, fast foods, and other peer group food preferences will not create serious deficiencies. Nutrients that are often deficient in the teen's diet include calcium, iron, zinc, vitamins A, D, B_6, and folic acid. Calcium needs increase during skeletal growth. Girls need additional iron because of losses during menstruation. Boys also need additional iron during this growth period (Table 18–3).

In their quest for identity and independence, some adolescents experiment with food fads and diets. Adolescent girls, worried about being fat, fall prey to a variety of fad diets. Athletes also may follow fad diets that may include supplements in the belief that these diets enhance bodybuilding. These diets often include increased amounts of protein and amino acids that cause diuresis and calcium loss. Carbohydrate loading, which some practice during the week before an athletic event, increases the muscle glycogen level to two to three times normal and may hinder heart function. A meal that is low in fat and high in complex carbohydrates eaten 3 to 4 hours before an event is much more appropriate for the teen athlete.

Adolescents need a balanced diet consisting of three servings from the milk-dairy group, two or three servings (6 to 7 oz total) from the meat group, three or four servings from the fruit group, four or five servings from the vegetable group, and 9 to 11 servings from the grain group (Fig. 18–4). Adolescents often resist pressure from family members to eat balanced meals; all family caregivers can do is to provide nutritious meals and snacks and regular mealtimes. A good example may be the best teacher at this point. A refrigerator stocked with ready-to-eat

TABLE 18.3	Food Sources of Nutrients Commonly Deficient in Preadolescent and Adolescent Diets

Common Nutrient Deficiencies	Food Sources
Vitamin A	Liver, whole milk, butter, cheese; sources of carotene such as yellow vegetables, green leafy vegetables, tomatoes, yellow fruits
Vitamin D	Fortified milk, egg yolk, butter
Vitamin B_6 (pyridoxine)	Chicken, fish, peanuts, bananas, pork, egg yolks, whole-grain cereals
Folate (folic acid)	Green leafy vegetables, enriched cereals, liver, dried peas and beans, whole grains
Calcium	Milk, hard cheese, yogurt, ice cream, small fish eaten with bones (e.g., sardines), dark-green vegetables, tofu, soybeans, calcium-enriched orange juice
Iron	Lean meats, liver, legumes, dried fruits, green leafy vegetables, whole-grain and fortified cereals
Zinc	Oysters, herring, meat, liver, fish, milk, whole grains, nuts, legumes

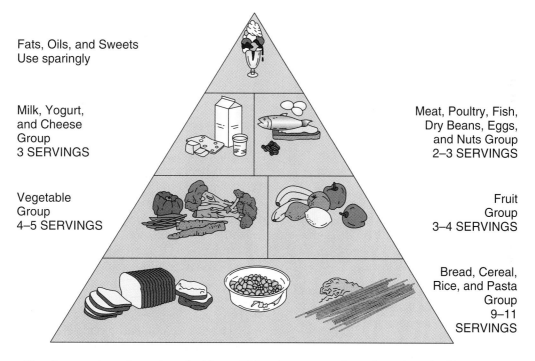

Fats, Oils, and Sweets
Use sparingly

Milk, Yogurt,
and Cheese
Group
3 SERVINGS

Meat, Poultry, Fish,
Dry Beans, Eggs,
and Nuts Group
2–3 SERVINGS

Vegetable
Group
4–5 SERVINGS

Fruit
Group
3–4 SERVINGS

Bread, Cereal,
Rice, and Pasta
Group
9–11
SERVINGS

Smaller number of servings for Teen Girls—Larger number of servings for Teen Boys

What Counts as 1 Serving? ▶ The amount you eat may be more than one serving.
For example, a dinner portion of spaghetti would count as 2 or 3 servings.

Bread, Cereal, Rice & Pasta Group	Vegetable Group	Fruit Group	Mild, Yogurt & Cheese Group	Meat, Poultry, Fish, Dry Beans, Eggs & Nuts Group	Fats & Sweets
1 slice of bread ½ cup of cooked rice or pasta ½ cup of cooked cereal 1 ounce of ready-to-eat cereal	½ cup of chopped raw or cooked vegetables 1 cup of leafy raw vegetables	1 piece of fruit or melon wedge ¾ cup of juice ½ cup cup of canned fruit ¼ cup of dried fruit	1 cup of milk or yogurt 1½ ounces of natural cheese 2 ounces of processed cheese	2½ to 3 ounces of cooked lean meat, poultry, or fish Count ½ cup of cooked beans, or 1 egg, or 2 tablespoons of peanut butter as 1 ounce of lean meat	LIMIT CALORIES FROM THESE especially if you need to lose weight

● *Figure 18.4* Food guide pyramid adapted for adolescent girls and boys. (From United States Department of Agriculture.)

nutritious snacks can be a good weapon against snacking on empty calories.

Families with low incomes may have difficulty providing the kinds of foods that meet the requirements for a growing teen. These families need help to learn how to make low-cost, nutritious food selections and plan adequate meals and snacks. The nurse can be instrumental in helping them plan appropriate food purchases. For instance, the nurse might recommend fruit and vegetable stores or farm stands that accept food stamps.

Ethnic and Cultural Influences

Culture also influences adolescent food choices and habits. For example, many Mexican-Americans are accustomed to having their big meal at noon. When school lunches do not provide such a heavy meal, the Mexican-American adolescent may supplement the lunch with sweets or fast foods. In the Asian community, milk is not a popular drink; this can result in a calcium deficiency. Many Asians are lactose-intolerant; therefore, other products high in calcium, such as tofu (soybean curd), soybeans, and greens, should be recommended to increase calcium intake. Be alert to cultural dietary influences on the adolescent; take these into consideration when helping the adolescent and the family devise an adequate food plan.

Certain religions recommend a vegetarian diet; other persons follow a vegetarian diet for ecological or philosophical reasons. If planned with care, vegetarian diets can provide needed nutrients. The most common types of vegetarian diets are the following:

- *Semivegetarian* includes dairy products, eggs, and fish; excludes red meat and possibly poultry.
- *Lacto-ovovegetarian* includes eggs and dairy products but excludes meat, poultry, and fish.
- *Lactovegetarian* includes dairy products and excludes meat, fish, poultry, and eggs.
- *Vegan* excludes all food of animal origin including dairy products, eggs, fish, meat, and poultry.

Vegan diets may not provide adequate nutrients without careful planning. All vegetarians should include whole-grain products, legumes, nuts, seeds, and fortified soy substitutes if low-fat dairy products are unacceptable.

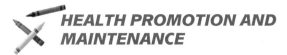

HEALTH PROMOTION AND MAINTENANCE

Adolescents have much the same need for regular health checkups, protection against infection, and prevention of accidents as do younger children.

They also have special needs that can best be met by health professionals with in-depth knowledge and understanding of adolescent concerns. The number of adolescent clinics and health centers has increased along with innovative health services such as school-based clinics, crisis hotlines, homes for runaways, and rehabilitation centers for adolescents who have been involved with alcohol or other drugs or with prostitution. Staff members in these programs provide teens with services needed for healthy growth.

Routine Checkups

A routine physical examination is recommended at least twice during the teen years, although annual physical examinations are encouraged. At this time, a complete history of developmental milestones, school problems, behavioral problems, family relationships, and immunizations should be completed. Immunization for measles, mumps, and rubella (MMR) is given if the second dose of the MMR vaccine was not administered between 4 and 6 years of age. A urine pregnancy screening is advisable before the rubella vaccine is administered to a girl of childbearing age because administration of the vaccine during pregnancy can cause serious risks to the developing fetus. A booster of Tetanus toxoid and diphtheria (Td) is given around 14 to 16 years of age (about 10 years after the last booster). If the teen has not been immunized with hepatitis B vaccine series, immunization also is recommended at this time. Any other immunizations that are incomplete should be updated. Tuberculin testing is included in at least one visit and, depending on the community, may be recommended at both visits if there is an interval of several years between visits.

Height, weight, and blood pressure are measured and recorded. Vision and hearing screening are done if they have not been part of a regular school-screening program. Adolescents up to the age of 16 years need to be screened for scoliosis. Thyroid enlargement should be checked through age 14. Sexually active girls must have a pelvic examination, screening for sexually transmitted diseases (STDs), and a Pap smear (Fig. 18–5). Urinalysis is performed on all female adolescents, and a urine culture is performed if the girl has any symptoms of a urinary tract infection such as urgency or burning and pain on urination. A routine physical is an excellent time for the nurse to counsel the adolescent about sexual activity, STDs, and human immunodeficiency virus (HIV) infection.

Body piercing and tattoos are becoming more common in the adolescent population. Piercings are seen in ears, eyebrows, noses, lips, chins, breasts, navels—in almost every part of the body. Tattoos of

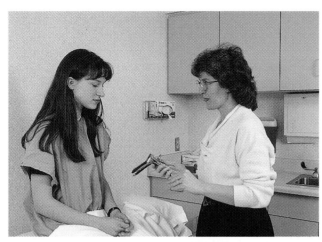

● *Figure 18.5* The adolescent is usually nervous about her first pelvic examination and Pap smear. Careful explanation by the nurse regarding these procedures may ease some of these fears.

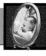

A PERSONAL GLIMPSE

Every year around our birthdays, my little brother and I always go to our pediatrician's office. After being called by the nurse, we both go down to a tiny room with bright walls, baby pictures, and the kind of mobiles hung over a crib, the same kind of decorations that cover the entire office. I suppose the room itself is comforting, but then I have to strip down to my underwear right in front of my 6-year-old brother. To make matters worse, I have to put on a skimpy little gown that hardly covers my underwear and wait in a room with huge windows and blinds that don't close, overlooking the next building's parking lot. It's so embarrassing, having to climb up onto the examining table with a gown falling down underneath me. Why can't the gowns be longer? It isn't just 6-year-olds who have to wear them!

Jessica, age 12

▶ **LEARNING OPPORTUNITY:** What do nurses and health care providers need to take into consideration regarding the privacy needs of adolescents? What specific things would you do in this situation to acknowledge and respect the needs of this adolescent girl?

all designs are seen in the adolescent. The adolescent with piercing and tattoos needs to be aware of the signs and symptoms of infection (redness, swelling, warmness, drainage, discomfort) and that these must be reported immediately if they occur. Sharing needles for piercing or tattooing needs to be discussed and the adolescent needs to be taught that sharing needles carries the same risks as sharing needles with IV drug use.

Adolescents must be given privacy, individualized attention, confidentiality, and the right to participate in decisions about their health care. They may feel uncomfortable and out of place in a pediatrician's waiting room where most of the patients are 3 feet tall or in a waiting room filled with adults. Some clinics and providers specialize in adolescent health care, but many adolescents do not have these facilities available to them.

Continuity of care helps build the adolescent's confidence in the service and the caregivers. Professionals dealing with teens should recognize that the physical symptoms offered as the reason for seeking care are often not the most significant problem about which the adolescent is concerned. An attitude of nonjudgmental acceptance on the part of health care personnel can often encourage the adolescent to ask questions and share feelings and concerns about a troubling matter. Adolescents may be accompanied to the health care facility by a family caregiver, but they need to have an opportunity to be interviewed alone. Questions must be asked in a way that is concrete and specific so that the adolescent will give direct answers. The interviewer must be alert to verbal and nonverbal clues.

Dental Checkups

Adolescents need continued regular dental checkups every 6 months. Dental **malocclusion** (improper alignment of the teeth) is a common condition that affects the way the teeth and jaws function. Correction of the malocclusion with dental braces improves chewing ability and appearance. The treatment of the malocclusion with dental braces is called **orthodontia.** Braces have become very common among adolescents because about half of them have malocclusions that can be corrected. Orthodontic treatment is usually started in early adolescence or late school age. Braces have become very widespread and are readily accepted among teens, although many teens still feel awkward and self-conscious during their orthodontic treatment. Tongue piercing among adolescents has increased and during dental checkups is a good time to discuss concerns of possible infections and teeth damage that can occur when an adolescent has a pierced tongue.

Family Teaching

The adolescent years are difficult for the maturing young person and often are just as difficult for the family caregiver. Caregivers must allow the independent teen to flourish while continuing to safeguard him or her from risky and immature behavior. Caregivers and adolescents struggle with issues related to sexuality, substance abuse, accidents, discipline, poor nutrition, and volatile emotions.

Learning about adolescent physical and psychosocial developments can help caregivers struggling to understand their teen. Caregivers will find information on sexuality and substance abuse enlightening and useful. Attending workshops or consulting counselors, teachers, religious leaders, or health care workers may enhance the caregiver's communication skills. Good communication between adolescents and their caregivers is essential to fostering healthy relationships between them. Caregivers may need both guidance in preparing their teen for adulthood and emotional support to feel successful in this difficult period. Take every opportunity to provide the family caregiver with information and support.

Health Education and Counseling

Before adolescents can take an active role in their own health care, they need information and guidance on the need for health care and how to meet that need most effectively. Education and counseling about sexuality, STDs, contraception, substance abuse, and mental health are a vital part of adolescent health care. Some of this teaching should and sometimes does come from family caregivers but often their lack of information or discomfort discussing these topics means that the job will have to be done by health professionals.

Sexuality

A good foundation in sex education can help the adolescent take pride in having reached sexual maturity; otherwise, puberty can be a frightening, shameful experience. Girls who have not been taught about menstruation until it occurs are understandably alarmed. Those who have been taught to regard it as "the curse" rather than an entrance into womanhood will not have positive feelings about this part of their sexuality.

Boys who are unprepared for nocturnal emissions may feel guilty, believing that they have caused these "wet dreams" by sexual fantasies or masturbation. They need to understand that this is a normal occurrence and simply the body's method of getting rid of surplus semen.

Assuming that adolescents are adequately prepared for the events of puberty, sex education during adolescence can deal with the important issues of responsible sexuality, contraception, and venereal disease. More adolescents today are sexually active than ever, resulting in an alarmingly rapid increase in teenage pregnancies and STDs. The

incidence of HIV infection is particularly increasing among adolescents.

Girls need to learn the importance of regular pelvic examinations and Pap smears and the technique for the monthly self-care procedure of breast self-examination (Fig. 18–6). Boys need to learn that testicular cancer is one of the most common cancers in young men between the ages of 15 and 34 and must be taught how and when to perform testicular self-examination (see Family Teaching Tips: Testicular Self-Examination) (Fig. 18–7).

Masturbation. Adolescents' growing awareness of their sexuality, sexually provocative material in the media, and lack of acceptable means to gratify sexual desires make masturbation a common practice during adolescence. Unlike young children's genital exploration, adolescent masturbation can produce orgasm in the female and ejaculation in the male. Generally it is a private and solitary activity, but occasionally it occurs with other members of the peer group. Health professionals recognize masturbation as a positive way to release sexual tension and increase one's knowledge of body sensations. The nurse can reassure adolescents that masturbation is common in both males and females and is a normal outlet for sexual urges.

Sexual Responsibility

Not all adolescents are sexually active, but the number of those who are increases with each year of age. Although abstinence is the only completely

---

FAMILY TEACHING TIPS

Testicular Self-Examination

1. Perform the examination once a month after a warm bath or shower. The scrotum is relaxed from the warmth. Select a day that is easy to remember such as the first or last day of the month.
2. Stand in front of a mirror, if possible, and look for any swelling on the skin of the scrotum.
3. Examine each testicle, one at a time, using both hands.
4. Place the index and middle fingers under the testicle and the thumbs on top. Roll each testicle gently between the thumbs and fingers. One testicle is normally larger than the other (see Fig. 18–7A).
5. The epididymis is the soft, tubelike structure located at the back of the testicle that collects and carries sperm. This must not be mistaken for an abnormal lump (see Fig. 18–7B).
6. Most lumps are found on the sides of the testicle, although they may also appear on the front. Report any lump to your health care provider at once.
7. Testicular cancer is highly curable when treated promptly.

How to Do Breast Self-Exam

1. Lie down. Flatten your left breast by placing a pillow under your left shoulder. Place your left arm behind your head.
2. Use the sensitive finger pads (where your fingerprints are, not the tips) of the middle three fingers on your left hand. Feel for lumps using a circular, rubbing motion in small, dime-sized circles without lifting the fingers. Powder, oil or lotion can be applied to the breast to make it easier for the fingers to glide over the surface and feel changes.
3. Press firmly enough to feel different breast tissues, using three different pressures. First, light pressure to just move the skin without jostling the tissue beneath, then medium pressure pressing midway into the tissue, and finally deep pressure to probe more deeply down to the ribs or to the point just short of discomfort.
4. Completely feel all of the breast and chest area up under your armpit, and up to the collarbone and all the way over to your shoulder to cover breast tissue that extends toward the shoulder.
5. Use the same pattern to feel every part of the breast tissue. Choose the method easiest for you:
   ○ Lines: start in the underarm area and move your fingers downward little by little until they are below the breast. Then move your fingers slightly toward the middle, and slowly move back up. Go up and down until you cover the whole area.
   ○ Circles: Beginning at the outer edge of your breast, move your fingers slowly around the breast in a circle. Move around the breast in smaller and smaller circles, gradually working toward the nipple. Don't forget to check the underarm and upper chest areas, too.
   ○ Wedges: Starting at the outer edge of the breast, move your fingers toward the nipple and back to the edge. Check your whole breast, covering one small wedge-shaped section at a time. Be sure to check the underarm area and the upper chest.
6. After you have completely examined your left breast, then examine your right breast using the same method and your left hand, with a pillow under your right shoulder.
7. You may want to examine your breasts or do an extra exam while showering. It's easy to slide soapy hands over your skin, and to feel anything unusual.
8. You should also check your breasts in a mirror looking for any change in size or contour, dimpling of the skin or spontaneous nipple discharge.

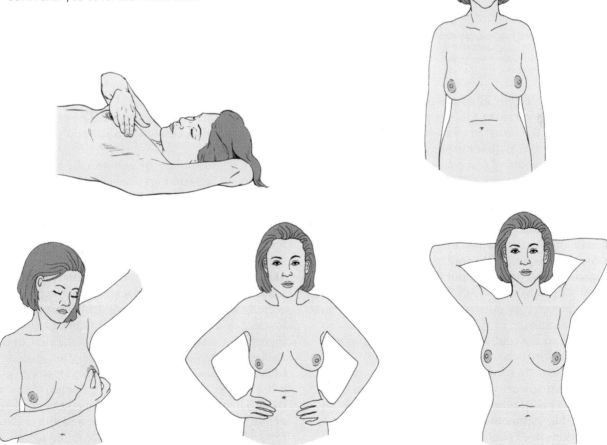

● *Figure 18.6* Breast self-examination as presented by the American Cancer Society.

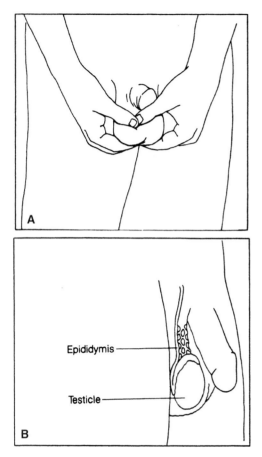

Epididymis

Testicle

B

● *Figure 18.7* **(A)** Examine each testicle with index and middle fingers under testicle and thumbs on top; **(B)** cross section of scrotum showing position of the epididymis and the testicle.

successful protection, all adolescents need to have information concerning safe sex practices to be prepared for the occasion when they wish to be sexually intimate with someone. Adolescents do not have a good record of using contraceptives to prevent pregnancy. Many teens give excuses such as "sex shouldn't be planned," because if it is planned, it is wrong or they feel guilty. They need to feel that it "just happened" in the heat of the moment, not because they really wanted or planned it. Many adolescents are beginning to realize that much more than pregnancy may be at risk, but their attitude of "it won't happen to me," which is typical of their developmental age, continues to contribute to their increasing sexual activity.

Some adults continue to resist providing contraceptive information to adolescents in school, believing that such information encourages teens to become sexually active. However, as HIV infection becomes a greater threat to every sexually active person, this argument becomes harder to defend. Adolescents need contraceptive information to prevent pregnancy, but more importantly they need

straightforward information about using condoms to protect them against HIV infection. Both male and female adolescents need this information, and girls must be advised to carry their own condoms if they believe that there is any possibility of having sexual intercourse.

Condoms have been claimed to have an 85% effectiveness rate. Condoms with spermicidal foam have an effective rate of 95%, but when users are taught how to use them correctly, the rate of effectiveness increases to 99%. The effectiveness of protection from HIV and other STDs should follow the same percentages. The safest condom is one made of latex with a prelubricated tip or reservoir and pretreated with nonoxynol-9 spermicide. Family Teaching Tips: Safe Condom Use and Figure 18–8 provide guidelines for use.

Other STDs that sexually active adolescents need to know about are syphilis, gonorrhea, genital herpes, genital warts, and chlamydial and trichomonal infections. Prevention of STDs is the primary aim of education for adolescents. If prevention proves ineffective, however, the most important factor is referral for treatment. Many adolescents are reluctant to seek treatment, fearing that their family caregivers will discover their activity. Crisis hotlines are valuable resources to assure adolescents that treatment is vital for them and their partners and that confidentiality is ensured.

Health care personnel who work with adolescents seeking treatment for an STD must be nonjudgmental, supportive, and understanding. The adolescents need treatment and information about preventing spread of the STD to others as well as how to prevent contracting another STD. See Chapter 19 for a thorough discussion of STDs and related nursing care.

Many adolescents are not sexually active, but most spend time dating or socializing with peers. In recent years the use of Rohypnol, also known as the "date rape drug," has become a concern for the adolescent. Rohypnol is not sold legally in the United States but is brought in from countries where it is sold legally. The drug, especially in combination with alcohol, causes memory loss, blackouts, and an inability to resist sexual attacks. Often the drug is secretly slipped into a person's drink. The drug has no taste or odor but within a few minutes after ingestion, the person feels dizzy, disoriented, and nauseated, then rapidly passes out. After several hours, the person awakens and has no memories of what happened while under the influence of the drug. The adolescent needs to be encouraged to stay aware and alert to avoid becoming a victim of date rape. He or she should be taught to avoid using alcohol and never to leave any drink unattended.

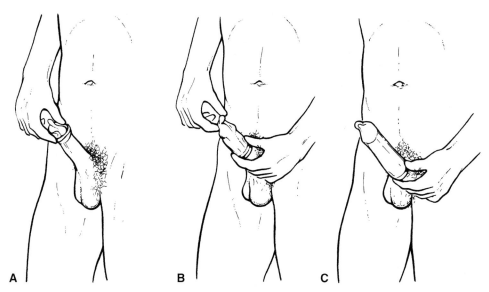

● **Figure 18.8** Putting on a condom: **(A)** Press the air out ½ inch at the tip of the condom; **(B)** holding the tip of the condom, carefully roll it down the shaft of the erect penis; **(C)** be certain that the condom covers the full length of the penis, with the rim of the condom at the base of the penis.

FAMILY TEACHING TIPS

Safe Condom Use

1. Use a new condom each time.
2. The safest type of condom is prelubricated latex with a tip or reservoir pretreated with nonoxynol-9 spermicide.
3. If the condom is not pretreated, you may lubricate it with water or water-based lubricant such as K-Y Jelly *and* a spermicidal jelly or foam containing nonoxynol-9.
4. Do not use oil-based products such as mineral oil, cold cream, or petroleum jelly for lubrication; they may weaken the latex.
5. Put the condom on as soon as the penis is erect. Retract the foreskin if not circumcised, and unroll the condom over the entire length of the penis.
6. Leave a ½ inch space at the end. Press out the tip of the condom to remove air bubbles.
7. The outside of the condom may be lubricated as much as desired with a water-soluble lubricant.
8. If the condom starts to slip during intercourse, hold it on. Do not let it slip off. Condoms come in sizes; so if there is a problem with slipping, look for a smaller size.
9. After ejaculation, hold the rim of the condom at the base of the penis and withdraw before losing the erection.
10. Remove the condom and tie a knot in the open end. Dispose of it so that no one can come in contact with semen.
11. Heat can damage condoms. Store them in a cool, dry place.
12. Immediately after intercourse, both partners should wash off any semen or vaginal secretions with soap and water.

Substance Abuse

As adolescents search for identity and independence, they are susceptible to many pressures from society and their peers. Adolescents may experiment with substances that may be habit-forming or addictive and ultimately will harm them. This may be done "just for kicks," to "go along with the crowd" (peer group), or to rebel against the authority of family caregivers or other adults. Some substances abused by adolescents also are abused by many adults; so to some adolescents, using these substances may appear sophisticated.

Alcohol and certain other drugs provide an escape, however brief, from pressures the adolescent may feel. Alcohol is the mind-altering substance most commonly abused by adolescents. Other substances that adolescents may abuse are tobacco (including smokeless tobacco), marijuana, cocaine or "crack," heroin, other street drugs, and prescription drugs. Adolescents can often obtain tobacco products despite recent federal legislation to enforce strict age limitations on their sale.

Programs developed to educate students about substance abuse meet with varying success. Health care personnel must stress to adolescents that use of alcohol or mind-altering chemicals is often accompanied by irresponsible sexual behavior that could further complicate their lives. Chapter 19 discusses these problems in more detail.

Mental Health

The turmoil that adolescents experience while searching for self-esteem and self-confidence can

FAMILY TEACHING TIPS

Internet Safety

Signs that might indicate on-line risks in a child or adolescent:

1. Spends large amounts of time on-line, especially at night
2. Has pornography on computer
3. Receives phone calls from adults you don't know
4. Makes calls, especially long distance, to numbers you don't recognize
5. Receives mail, gifts, packages from someone you don't know
6. Turns computer monitor off or changes screen when you enter room
7. Becomes withdrawn from family

To minimize on-line concerns:

1. Communicate and talk with child; openly discuss concerns and dangers.
2. Spend time with child on-line.
3. Use blocking software and devices.
4. Use caller ID to determine who is calling your child.
5. Maintain access to child's on-line account and monitor activity.

Adapted from FBI Publication, "A Parent's Guide to Internet Safety,"
http://www.fbi.gov/publications/pguide/pguidee.htm

INTERNET EXERCISE 18.1

http://www.teenhealthnet.com

Click on the area that reads "Enter teenhealthnet."

1. List six areas available that you might use when working with adolescents.

Click on the section entitled "Mental."

Click on the section entitled "Knowledge."

1. What are the three areas covered in this section?

Click on the section entitled "managing stress."

Read through this section listing methods for relaxing and reducing tension and stress.

2. List 15 areas that you might suggest to adolescents as appropriate ways to manage stress.

Accident Prevention

In every part of society, increasing numbers of adolescents are dying as a result of violence; this includes motor vehicle accidents, homicide, suicide, and other causes. Homicide ranks as the leading cause of death for 15-to 19-year-old minority youth regardless of gender.[1] Statistics regarding adolescents are difficult to interpret, but death among adolescents is often related to risky behaviors (Fig. 18–9). These behaviors include the unintentional (motor vehicles, fires) as well as the intentional (violence, suicide) injuries, alcohol and other drug use, sexual behaviors, tobacco use, and dietary behaviors. Alcohol and other drugs are often involved in fatal accidents. Death is not the only negative outcome of violence: many adolescents are injured and hospitalized or treated in emergency departments, and many suffer psychological injury from being victims of violence.

Violence is also on the rise in schools, not just inner-city schools. Weapons are detected on students in schools all over the country. Guns and knives are the weapons most often found. The problem has become so serious that some schools have installed metal detectors to protect students.

Adolescents also are victims of violence in their own homes in greater numbers than any other age group of children. Date rape and other violence in a dating relationship have become common.

Students have formed groups such as Students Against Drunk Driving to promote safety in driving (web site: *http:// www.saddonline.com*). Many schools provide support groups that help students to work through their grief after schoolmates have met with violent death.

---

cause stress that may lead to depression, suicide, and conduct disorders. Academic and social pressures add to that stress. The family also may be under stress due to unemployment or economic difficulties, separation, divorce, or death of a caregiver. Health care personnel must be sensitive to signs that the adolescent is having problems. Adolescents need the opportunity to ventilate their fears, concerns, and frustrations. The rapport between family caregivers and teens may not be such that the adolescent can express these feelings to the family. Many schools have mental health personnel on staff that can provide counseling when needed. Adolescents need counseling to work through troublesome situations and to avoid chronic mental health problems. Mental health assessment is an important part of the adolescent's total health assessment. With the increased use of computers and internet sites, internet safety is an important aspect of adolescent mental health. Parents need to be aware of their adolescent's computer activities and the sites they access, especially communication sites such as chat rooms. Discussions with adolescents regarding safety concerns on internet sites help to increase their awareness and decrease potential dangers. See Family Teaching Tips: Internet Safety.

Youth Ages 10 – 24

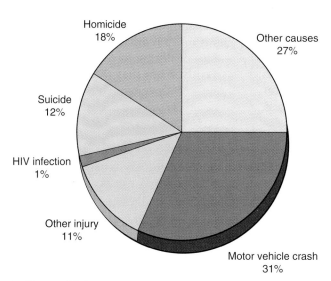

● **Figure 18.9** Leading causes of death for adolescents, many of which result from risk behaviors.

Much work needs to be done to understand the reason for this increasing violence. One factor in adolescents is that they often act recklessly without benefit of mature judgment. Adolescents have relatively easy access to guns and often use them as a means to solve problems. Efforts to control and regulate gun sales are nationally discussed topics. Acts of terror and violence in our world increase the confusion and anxiety that adolescents have regarding conflicts and conflict resolution.

Nurses who have any contact with adolescents must make every effort to help them work through their problems in nonviolent ways. The nurse can become involved at the school or community level by becoming an advocate for adolescents and an educator to promote safe driving as well as helmet wear and safety practices when using a motorcycle, all-terrain vehicle, bicycle, skateboard, or in-line skates. Nurses also can work with support groups that offer counseling to adolescents involved in date violence. As a community member and a health care worker, the nurse can provide a positive role model for adolescents.

THE ADOLESCENT IN THE HEALTH CARE FACILITY

When adolescents are hospitalized, it is usually because of a major health problem such as an injury from violence or from a motor vehicle accident,

substance abuse, attempted suicide, or a chronic health problem intensified by the physiologic changes of adolescence. Adolescents must cope with the stress of hospitalization, possibly dramatic alterations in body image, partial or total inability to conform to peer group norms, and an interrupted search for identity.

Adolescents fear loss of control and loss of privacy. Provide opportunities for the adolescent to make choices whenever possible. Protect the adolescent's privacy by providing screening and adequate covering during procedures.

Adolescents may react with anger and refuse to cooperate when their privacy or feelings of control are threatened. Be aware of this possible reaction, and avoid labeling such an adolescent as a difficult patient.

The admission interview for an adolescent may be more successful if the family caregiver and the adolescent are interviewed separately. This provides the opportunity to gain information that the adolescent may not want to reveal in the presence of the family caregiver. Thoroughly explore the adolescent's developmental level, listen carefully with empathy to his or her concerns, encourage maximum participation in self-care, and provide sufficient information to make this participation possible. As with all patients, clear, honest explanations about treatments and procedures are essential.

During the admission interview, advise the adolescent of the unit's rules. Adolescents need to know what limits are set for their behavior while hospitalized. To share feelings and gain information, many find it helpful to discuss their health problem with a peer who has had the same or a related problem.

Adolescents need access to a telephone to contact peers and keep up social contacts. Recreation areas are important. In settings specifically designed for adolescents, recreation rooms can provide an area where teens can gather to do schoolwork, play games and cards, and socialize. In many hospitals with adolescent units, video games as well as television are provided in each patient room. Access to a computer and electronic mail might also help the teen stay connected to peers. Supervision is important to decrease misuse of computer privileges. Teens are encouraged to wear their own clothes. They can be encouraged to shampoo and style their hair, and girls can wear their usual makeup.

The adolescent's health problem may require a lengthy hospitalization and intense rehabilitation efforts. Adequate preparation and guidance can help make that difficult experience easier and less damaging to normal growth and development.

KEY POINTS

- Adolescence is a turbulent time when adolescents often feel confused.
- Beginning in the preadolescent years, children go through many physical and emotional changes on their way to adulthood.
- Adolescents have many struggles in their search for identity and independence.
- Adolescents face many pressures and temptations that often are difficult to resist.
- A warm and accepting family environment, positive school experiences, and good health give the adolescent the best chance of reaching adulthood with a positive sense of self, the ability to form close relationships, and the capacity to make sound decisions about life.
- Adolescents are trying to identify their career options and determine what they want to do with their lives. Many more career opportunities are available to them than at any previous time. This abundance of choices can place more pressure on the teen making decisions.
- Only after adolescents complete the task of establishing their identity are they ready to establish an intimate relationship, the next task of development according to Erikson. Developing intimate relationships brings an additional set of problems.
- Nutritional needs are increased during adolescence because of the rapid physical growth occurring during this period.
- Many factors influence an adolescent's nutritional needs and food intake. Caregivers must be alert to nutritional deficiencies and make an effort to provide sound nutritional guidance.
- Adolescents need a strong support system to help them through this stressful stage of development.
- Adolescents need a program of health maintenance in a setting that meets their needs for privacy, individualized attention, confidentiality, and the right to participate in decisions about their health care.
- Substance abuse, sexual activity, sexual and physical abuse, and accidents can further complicate an adolescent's life. Peer pressure may be extremely influential in affecting the adolescent's attitudes and behaviors related to these issues.
- Adolescents may need to deal with violence in school, which is a widespread problem.
- In the health care facility, the adolescent fears loss of control and loss of privacy. The nurse caring for the hospitalized adolescent must be sensitive to the adolescent's needs and provide supportive care and encourages as much participation by the adolescent as possible. Health problems that threaten the adolescent's body image may threaten the satisfactory completion of developmental tasks.

REFERENCES

1. Joffe A. (1999) Introduction to adolescent medicine. In *Oski's pediatrics: Principles and practice* (3rd ed). Philadelphia: Lippincott Williams & Wilkins.

BIBLIOGRAPHY

Berger KS. (2001) *The developing person through the life span* (5th ed). New York: Worth Publishers.
Brazelton TB, Greenspan S. (2001) *The irreducible needs of children: What every child must have to grow, learn, and flourish.* Cambridge, MA: Perseus Publishing.
Craven RF, Hirnle CJ. (1999) *Fundamentals of nursing* (3rd ed). Philadelphia: Lippincott Williams & Wilkins.
Deering CG, Jennings CD. (2002) Communicating with children and adolescents. *American Journal of Nursing,* 102(3) 34–42.
Dudek SG. (2000) *Nutrition essentials for nursing practice* (4th ed). Philadelphia: Lippincott Williams & Wilkins.
Dworkin P. (2000) *Pediatrics* (4th ed). Philadelphia: Lippincott Williams & Wilkins.
Fehrenbach MJ. (2002) Tongue piercing. Retrieved from *http://dentaldirectory.virtual ave.net.*
Nagai A, Siktberg L. (2001) Osteoporosis prevention in female adolescents: Calcium intake and exercise participation. *Pediatric Nursing,* 27(2), 132.
Nicoll L. (2001) *Nurse's guide to the internet* (3rd ed). Philadelphia: Lippincott Williams & Wilkins.
Pillitteri A. (2003) *Maternal and child health nursing* (4th ed). Philadelphia: Lippincott Williams & Wilkins.
Spock B, et al. (1998) *Dr. Spock's baby and child care.* New York: Pocket Books.
Wong DL. (1998) *Whaley and Wong's nursing care of infants and children* (6th ed). St. Louis: Mosby.
Wong DL, Perry S, Hockenberry, M. (2002) *Maternal child nursing care* (2nd ed). St. Louis: Mosby.

Websites
Testicular Exam/Cancer: *http://www.cancerlinksusa.com*
Breast Self-Exam: *www.teensandbc.net*
Drug-Resistance Activities: *www.health.org/features/kidsarea*

Workbook

NCLEX-STYLE REVIEW QUESTIONS

1. The nurse is assisting with a physical exam on a 12-year-old female. Her record indicates that at age 9 she was 51 inches tall and weighed 72 pounds. Which of the following would the nurse MOST LIKELY find if the child were following a normal pattern of growth and development? The adolescent

   a. weighs 94 pounds

   b. measures 53 inches in height

   c. has a small amount of pubic hair

   d. has well-developed breasts

2. The nurse is working with a group of caregivers of adolescents who are discussing normal adolescent growth and development. Which of the following statements made by a caregiver would indicate a need for follow-up?

   a. "He wants to be a nurse after he finishes college."

   b. "She has her own money to spend now because she has a job."

   c. "My son has been spending at least ½ to 1 hour in front of the mirror the last 3 months getting ready for school."

   d. "My daughter is so slim and trim, she has lost 10 pounds in the last 6 weeks."

3. The nurse is teaching a group of adolescent girls about good nutrition habits and eating foods that will help to increase the deficient nutrients in the adolescent diet. Which of the following statements made by the girls in the group is correct?

   a. "Eating lots of broccoli will help increase the iron in my diet."

   b. "If I drink three glasses of milk each day, I will get plenty of vitamin C."

   c. "Even though I don't like eggs, if I eat four eggs a week I will get enough calcium."

   d. "I am sure I get enough vitamin A since I eat bread at every meal."

4. In working with adolescent children, the nurse would know that if the adolescents were following normal development patterns, this age child would be MOST likely be involved in which of the following activities?

   a. Working to establish a career

   b. Playing a board game with siblings

   c. Participating in a activities with peers

   d. Volunteering in community projects

5. The nurse is discussing teenage substance abuse with a group of caregivers of adolescent children. If the caregivers make the following statements, which statement is the MOST accurate regarding substance abuse in teens?

   a. "Every teenager experiments with substances."

   b. "The most common drugs used by teenagers is alcohol."

   c. "It won't really hurt teenagers if they try tobacco."

   d. "Even teenagers need a release from the pressures they face."

STUDY ACTIVITIES

1. List and compare the 15-year-old female and the 15-year-old male in regard to physical development, psychosocial development, personality development, and their feelings about body image.

Area of Development	15-Year-Old Female	15-Year-Old Male
Physical development		
Psychosocial development		
Personality development		
Body image		

2. Mattie is the mother of 13-year-old Chantal. Chantal has decided she will not eat meat or poultry because animals had to be killed to obtain it. Mattie is concerned about Chantal's nutrition. Develop a teaching plan, including a menu for a day for Mattie. Be sure your plan provides nutrients often deficient in adolescents and that supports Chantal in her choice to not eat meat and poultry.

3. You are working with a group of adolescents in a school-based clinic and plan to have a discussion about substance abuse and sexually transmitted

diseases. Make a list of questions that you think the adolescents might want to ask but are uncomfortable asking. Discuss with your peers the answers you could give to each of these questions.

CRITICAL THINKING

1. You have the opportunity to talk with a group of 16-year-old girls. Describe the guidance you will give them about breast self-examination and Pap smears.

2. Jamal is an adolescent athlete. He has told you he is planning to use a carbohydrate-loading diet before a big track meet. Using your knowledge about carbohydrate loading, detail the guidance you will give him.

3. Fifteen-year-old Caitlin is in a group discussing condom use. She scornfully tells you that girls don't need to know anything about condoms. How would you respond to Caitlin? Discuss with your peers your ideas regarding what you think should and should not be part of health education in high school settings. Give the rationales for your answers.

Health Problems of the Adolescent

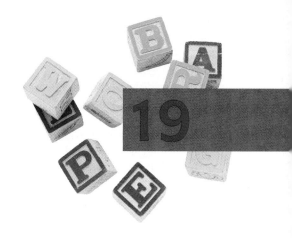

19

STUDENT OBJECTIVES

On completion of this chapter, the student will be able to

1. Define key terms.
2. Discuss the goal of health care professionals who work with obese adolescents.
3. State two goals of treatment for the hospitalized anorexic patient.
4. Discuss the factors that cause acne vulgaris.
5. List the drugs commonly used for (a) mild acne, (b) inflammatory acne, and (c) severe acne.
6. Describe infectious mononucleosis.
7. Discuss how tuberculosis is detected.
8. List the organisms that cause (a) gonorrhea, (b) chlamydia, (c) genital herpes, and (d) syphilis.
9. Identify the only certain way to prevent sexually transmitted diseases.
10. Identify the drug of choice to treat (a) gonorrhea, (b) chlamydia, (c) genital herpes, and (d) syphilis.
11. Identify how the human immunodeficiency virus is transmitted.
12. Discuss how the developmental tasks of adolescence conflict with the developmental tasks of pregnancy.
13. Discuss alcohol abuse and its impact on adolescents.
14. List nine types of substances commonly abused by adolescents and state at least one negative effect of each.
15. Discuss the warning signs seen in adolescents who are considering committing suicide.

KEY TERMS

alcohol abuse
alcoholism
amenorrhea
anorexia nervosa
bulimia
chancre
comedones
dependence
dysmenorrhea
gynecomastia
impunity
menarche
mittelschmerz
obesity
overweight
polyphagia
premenstrual syndrome
sebum
substance abuse
tolerance
vaginitis
withdrawal symptoms

Many adolescent health problems result from the rapid physiologic changes taking place, the adolescent's reaction to those changes, and the stress, conflict, and confusion that characterize adolescence. As adolescents struggle with questions about identity, independence, career, sexuality, morality, and emotions, alterations in their size and physical appearance make them uncomfortable and even unfamiliar with themselves. Coping with these changes and uncertainties is difficult for every adolescent, but for some it is impossible. Lacking adequate coping mechanisms, many adolescents feel there is no solution but escape and they seek that escape through alcohol or drugs, running away, committing suicide, or other self-destructive behavior. Motor vehicle accidents, homicide, and suicide are common causes of death in the adolescent age group.

The complex interrelationship between psychological well-being and physical health, although not completely understood, is evident throughout life but particularly during adolescence. Emotions and attitudes affect nutrition and other health behaviors and can result in general or systemic disorders, which in turn can lead to further psychological stress. The high number of adolescent pregnancies also is believed to be a result of inappropriate responses to the stresses of adolescence.

Nurses are assuming an increasingly important role in helping adolescents understand, manage, and prevent health problems. Fulfillment of this role demands an understanding of adolescent growth and development and the ability to listen, observe carefully, and project a sensitive, nonjudgmental attitude.

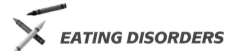 **EATING DISORDERS**

Eating disorders, especially obesity, anorexia nervosa, and bulimia, are among the most common health problems of adolescents. Food represents nurturing and security and as a result may be consumed inappropriately to try to solve problems. This misuse can result in health problems that have long-term or permanent effects.

Obesity

Obesity is a national problem in the United States largely as a result of an overabundance of food and too little exercise. The thin figure, particularly for women, has become so idealized that being fat can handicap a person socially and professionally and severely damage self-esteem. **Obesity** generally is defined as an excessive accumulation of fat that increases body weight by 20% or more over ideal weight (see Appendix A). **Overweight,** although not necessarily signifying obesity, means that a person's weight is more than average for height and body build.

Obesity often begins in childhood and, if not treated successfully, leads to chronic obesity in adult life. The obese adolescent often feels isolated from the peer group that is normally a source of support during this period. Because of the obesity, the adolescent often is embarrassed to participate in sports, thus eliminating one method of burning excess calories. Many adolescents use food as a means of satisfying emotional needs, which establishes a vicious cycle. Adolescents' eating habits include skipping meals, especially breakfast, and indulging in late-night eating. This behavior compounds the problem because calories consumed before a person goes to bed are not used for energy but are stored as fat. Snacking while watching television also contributes to the overindulgence in caloric intake.

Some adolescents suffer from **polyphagia** (compulsive overeating). They lack control of their food intake, cannot postpone their urge to eat, hide food for later secret consumption, eat when not hungry or to escape from worries, and expend a great deal of energy thinking about securing and eating food. Not all compulsive eaters are overweight, however, and in some ways this disorder resembles anorexia nervosa.

Many factors, including genetic, social, cultural, metabolic, and psychological, contribute to the development of obesity. Children of obese parents are likely to share this problem not only because of some inherited predisposition toward obesity but also because of family eating patterns and the emotional climate surrounding food. Certain cultures equate obesity with being loved and being prosperous. If these values carry over into a modern family, the adolescent is torn between the standards of the peer group and those of the family.

Obesity is difficult to treat in any age group but especially difficult in adolescence. Much of teenage life centers on food: after-school snacks, the ice cream shop, late-night diners, the pizza parlor, and fast-food restaurants serving high-fat, high-calorie foods with little nutritional value. Diets that emphasize nutritionally sound meals and reduced caloric intake produce results too slowly for impatient teenagers. Thus the many quick-weight-loss programs, diet pills, and diet books find a ready market among adolescents.

Treatment must include a thorough exploration of the obese adolescent's food attitudes. A team approach using the skills of a psychiatrist or psychologist, nutritionist, nurse, or other counselor is often useful in developing a complete treatment plan.

Summer camps that center on weight reduction with nutritious, calorie-controlled food, exercise, and activity are successful for some adolescents but are too costly for many families. In addition, many teens may fall back into old habits after summer camp is over unless there is a continuing support system.

Caregivers who work with obese adolescents should try to make them feel like worthwhile persons, stressing that obesity does not automatically make them unacceptable. Finding the support of a caring adult who will help the adolescent gain control of this aspect of his or her life can help give the necessary incentive to lose weight (see Family Teaching Tips: Tips for Caregivers of Obese Teens).

Anorexia Nervosa

Preoccupation with reducing diets and the quest for the "perfect" (i.e., thin) figure sometimes leads to **anorexia nervosa,** or self-inflicted starvation. This disorder occurs most commonly in adolescent white females although there are reported cases among males and among African-American, Hispanic, and Asian adolescents. First described more than 100 years ago, anorexia has increased in incidence in recent years and is currently estimated to affect as many as 1% of adolescent girls. Anorexia is found in all the developed countries. Two age ranges are identified as the usual age of onset: 11 to 13 years and 19 to 20 years. Although considered a psychiatric problem, it causes severe physiologic damage and even death.

Characteristics

These adolescents often are described as successful students who tend to be perfectionists and are always trying to please parents, teachers, and other adults. The families of anorexic adolescents characteristically show little emotion and display no evidence of conflict within the family. An adolescent in a controlled family environment, in which the parents do not freely express emotions, may try to establish independence and identity by controlling his or her own appetite and body weight. Depression is common in these adolescents. Anorexic persons deny weight loss and actually see themselves as fat, even when they look skeletal to others. They often adhere to a rigid program of exercise to further their efforts in weight reduction. They may make demands on themselves for cleanliness and order in their environment or they may engage in rigid schedules for studying and other ritualistic behavior. These adolescents deny hunger but often suffer from fatigue.

Clinical Manifestations and Diagnosis

Persons with anorexia are visibly emaciated and almost skeletal. They appear sexually immature, have

FAMILY TEACHING TIPS

Tips for Caregivers of Obese Teens

1. Have teen keep a food diary for a week. Include food eaten, time eaten, what teen was doing, and how teen felt before and after eating; identify what stimulates urge to eat.
2. Study diary with teen to look for eating triggers.
3. Set a reasonable goal of no more than 1 or 2 lbs a week or perhaps maintaining weight with no gain.
4. Advise teen to eat only at specific, regular mealtimes.
5. Recommend that teen eat only at dining or kitchen table (not in front of TV or on the run).
6. Have teen use small plates to make amount of food seem larger.
7. Teach teen to eat slowly: count and chew each bite (25 to 30 is a good goal).
8. Suggest that the teen try to leave a little on the plate when done.
9. Have teen survey home and get rid of tempting high-calorie foods.
10. Stock up on low-calorie snacks: carrot sticks, celery sticks, and other raw vegetables.
11. Help teen get involved in an active project that occupies time and also helps burn calories: any active team sport, bicycling, walking, hiking, swimming, skating.
12. Promote walking instead of riding whenever possible.
13. Encourage the teen to attend a support group or develop a buddy system for support.
14. Weigh only once a week on the same scale at the same time of day in the same clothing.
15. Make a chart to keep track of teen's weight.
16. Help teen to focus on a positive asset and make the most of it to help build self-concept.
17. Encourage good grooming. A group could put on a "mini" fashion show, choosing with guidance clothes that help maximize best features, or simply using magazine illustrations if actual clothing is not available.
18. Reward each small success with positive reinforcement.
19. Enlist cooperation of all family members to support the teen with encouragement and a positive atmosphere.

dry skin and brittle nails, and often have lanugo (downy hair) over their backs and extremities. Other symptoms include amenorrhea (absence of menstruation), constipation, hypothermia, bradycardia, low blood pressure, and anemia.

The American Psychiatric Association identifies the following criteria for the diagnosis of anorexia nervosa:[1]

• Weight loss leading to maintenance of body weight less than 85% of that expected for age and height; or failure to make expected weight gain during a period of growth, leading to body weight less than 85% of that expected

- Intense fear of gaining weight or becoming fat even though underweight
- Disturbance in how one's body weight or shape is experienced; undue influence of body weight or shape on self-evaluation; denial of seriousness of the current low body weight (e.g., feeling fat even when emaciated or, although underweight, perceiving one part of the body to be too fat)
- Amenorrhea as evidenced by absence of three consecutive menstrual cycles.

Treatment

Adolescents diagnosed with anorexia nervosa may be hospitalized to achieve the two goals of treatment: correction of malnutrition and identification and treatment of the psychological cause. An approach involving several disciplines is necessary. Therapy is required to help the adolescent gain insight into the problem. In addition, family therapy, nutritional therapy, and behavior modification are used. Affected adolescents fear they will gain too much weight; therefore, a compromise between what the physician prefers and what the adolescent desires may be necessary.

Adolescents with anorexia have become experts in manipulating others and their environment. Once treatment begins, they may try to avoid gaining weight by ordering only low-calorie foods; by disposing of their meals in plants, trash, toilets, or dirty linen; or by exercising in the hall or jogging in place in their rooms. In some instances, nasogastric tube feedings or total parenteral nutrition (TPN) is necessary to provide nutritional support.

Treatment based on behavior modification may deprive the patient of all privileges, such as visitors, television, and telephone, until she begins to gain weight. Privileges are then gradually restored. These techniques are effective only when the patient and the caregivers understand the program and its purpose and have agreed on individualized goals and rewards.

Group therapy may be used to rely on peer support and provide the opportunity to associate with other patients with the same diagnosis in a non-threatening setting.

The long-term outlook for the adolescent with anorexia is unclear. Death may occur from suicide, infection, or the effects of starvation. Some adolescents recover completely; others have eating problems into adulthood; still others have problems with social adjustment that are not related to eating. Predicting the outcome is difficult, and more studies are needed before a definitive answer is available (Fig. 19–1).

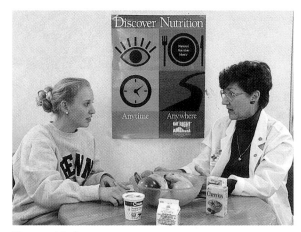

● **Figure 19.1** This anorexic teen, who is in the later stages of treatment, continues to meet with the counselor to discuss her food choices, exercise program, and overall well-being.

Bulimia

Bulimia nervosa (usually referred to simply as bulimia) is characterized by binge eating followed by purging. The typical bulimic person is a white female in late adolescence. Most often, the bulimic person is of normal weight or slightly overweight. Those who are underweight usually fulfill the criteria for anorexia nervosa, although some anorexic persons periodically practice binging and purging. Bulimia is seen increasingly in young adult women as well.

The binging often occurs late in the day when the adolescent is alone. Secrecy is an important aspect of the process. The adolescent eats large quantities of food within 1 or 2 hours. This binging is followed by guilt, fear, shame, and self-condemnation. To avoid weight gain from the food eaten, the adolescent follows the binging with purging by means of self-induced vomiting, laxatives, diuretics, and excessive exercise.

Clinical Manifestations and Diagnosis

The clues to bulimia may be few but include dental caries and erosion from frequent exposure to stomach acid, throat irritation, and endocrine and electrolyte imbalances that may cause cardiac irregularities and menstrual problems. Calluses or abrasions may be noted on the back of the hand from frequent contact with the teeth while inducing vomiting. Possible complications are esophageal tears and acute gastric dilatation. Hypokalemia also may occur especially if the adolescent abuses diuretics to prevent weight gain. Other behavior problems seen in many bulimic persons include drug abuse, alcoholism, stealing (especially food), promiscuity, and other impulsive activities.

According to the American Psychiatric Association, the diagnostic criteria for bulimia include

- Recurrent episodes of binge eating
- A feeling of lack of control over behavior during binges
- Self-induced purging; use of laxatives or diuretics; enemas or other medications; and strict dieting, fasting, or vigorous exercise to prevent weight gain
- Average of at least two binge-eating episodes a week over a 3-month period
- Obsessiveness regarding body weight and shape

Treatment

Treatment of bulimia is varied. Many aspects of the treatment are similar to treatment of the adolescent with anorexia. Food diaries often are used as a tool to assess the adolescent's eating patterns. In some instances, antidepressant drugs may be useful. The nurse can refer the adolescent to a support group that may prove helpful.

● Nursing Process for the Adolescent With Anorexia Nervosa or Bulimia

ASSESSMENT

Data collection of the adolescent with an eating disorder begins with a complete interview and history including previous illnesses, allergies, a dietary history, and a description of eating habits. The adolescent may not give an accurate dietary history or description of eating habits. Question the family caregiver in a separate interview to gain added information. In the physical exam include height, weight, blood pressure, temperature, pulse, and respirations. Carefully inspect and observe the skin, mucous membranes, state of nutrition, and state of alertness and cooperation. Complete documentation of what is found is necessary.

NURSING DIAGNOSES

Nursing diagnoses vary with the specific eating disorder, the physical condition of the adolescent, the length of time the adolescent has had the condition, and other accompanying conditions. The following diagnoses may be useful in planning care:

- Imbalanced Nutrition: Less Than Body Requirements related to self-induced vomiting and use of laxatives or diuretics
- Disturbed Body Image related to fear of obesity and potential rejection

- Risk for Activity Intolerance related to fatigue secondary to malnutrition
- Risk for Constipation related to decreased food and fluid intake
- Risk for Diarrhea related to use of laxatives
- Risk for Impaired Skin Integrity related to loss of subcutaneous fat and dry skin secondary to malnutrition
- Noncompliance with treatment regimen related to unresolved conflicts over food and eating
- Compromised Family Coping related to eating disorders, treatment regimen, and dangers associated with an eating disorder

OUTCOME IDENTIFICATION AND PLANNING

The major goals for the adolescent with an eating disorder relate to meeting nutritional needs and improving self-concept and self-esteem. Other goals include establishing appropriate activity levels, maintaining normal bowel activity, maintaining skin integrity, and complying with the treatment program. The goals for the family include understanding the condition, learning how to manage the condition and its treatment, and reinforcing the adolescent's self-esteem.

IMPLEMENTATION

Improving Nutrition. The adolescent with bulimia or anorexia nervosa does not receive the nutrients needed to achieve adequate growth during this period of development. Supervise food intake. Weigh the adolescent at the same time each day, but do not make an issue of weight fluctuation. Be observant when weighing the patient: the adolescent may try to add weight by putting heavy objects in pockets, shoes, or other hiding places. While being weighed, the patient should wear minimal clothing (preferably a patient gown with no pockets) and have bare feet.

The care provider and a dietitian work with the adolescent to devise a food plan to meet the adolescent's nutrition requirements. The goal of the food plan is not a sudden weight gain, but a slow, steady gain with an established goal that has been agreed on by the health care team and the adolescent. Often the adolescent keeps a food diary that is reviewed daily with the health team.

Patients with eating disorders are often manipulative and deceptive. Observe the patient during and after eating to make certain the teen eats the required food and does not get rid of it after apparently consuming it.

Contract agreements are often recommended for patients with eating disorders. These agreements, which are usually part of a behavioral modification plan, specify the adolescent's and the staff's responsibilities for the diet, activity expectations for the teen, and other aspects of the adolescent's behavior. The contract also may spell out specific privileges that can be gained by meeting the contract goals. This places the teen in greater control of the outcome.

In addition to daily weights, test urine for ketones and regularly evaluate the skin turgor and mucous membranes to gather further information about nutritional status. Report and document immediately any evidence of deteriorating physical condition. If weight loss continues, nasogastric tube feedings may need to be implemented. This possibility also can be included in the contract.

If the adolescent's condition is at a critical stage with fluid and electrolyte deficiencies, parenteral fluids are necessary immediately to hydrate the patient before further treatment can be implemented. Observe the adolescent continuously to prevent any attempt to remove intravenous lines or otherwise disrupt the treatment. Closely monitor serum electrolytes, cardiac and respiratory status, and renal complications. During administration of parenteral fluids, continue to encourage the adolescent to maintain an oral intake.

Reinforcing Positive Self-Concept. The nurse must function as an active, nonjudgmental listener to the adolescent. Consistent assignment of the same nursing personnel to care for the adolescent helps to establish a climate in which the adolescent can relate to the nurse and begin to build a positive self-concept. Report and document without delay any signs of depression. Also report and document any negative feelings expressed by the adolescent. Do not minimize or ignore these feelings. Reinforce positive behavior. Psychotherapy and counseling groups are necessary to help the adolescent work through feelings of negative self-worth. Encourage the adolescent to express fears, anger, and frustrations and help the patient recognize that everyone has these feelings from time to time. Never ridicule or belittle these feelings. Encourage the adolescent

to explore ways in which destructive feelings may be changed. These are feelings that can be dealt with in counseling sessions; therefore, report and document them carefully.

Balancing Rest and Activity. Exercise and activity are important parts of the contract negotiated with the adolescent. Explain to the adolescent that fatigue is a result of the extreme depletion of energy reserves related to nutritional deficits. Encourage the adolescent to become involved in all activities of daily living. Provide ample rest periods when the adolescent's energy reserves are depleted. Discourage the adolescent from pushing beyond endurance and closely observe for secretive excessive activity.

Monitoring Bowel Habits. Make a careful record of bowel movements. The adolescent may not be reliable as a reporter of bowel habits, so devise methods to prevent the teen from using the bathroom without supervision. Report at once and document constipation or diarrhea. Watch carefully to prevent the teen from obtaining and taking a laxative. These patients are devious and may go to great lengths to obtain a laxative to purge themselves of food. Report immediately any evidence or suspicions of this type of behavior.

Maintaining Skin Integrity. Good skin care is essential in the care of the adolescent with a severely restricted nutritional intake. The skin may be dry and tend to break down easily because of the lack of a subcutaneous fat cushion. Inspect daily for redness, irritation, or signs of decubitus ulcer formation. Observe specifically the bony prominences. Encourage the adolescent to be out of bed most of the day. When the teen is in bed, encourage regular position changes so that no pressure areas develop.

Improving Compliance. The long-term outcome for adolescents with eating disorders is precarious. Adolescents with severe eating disorders often have multiple inpatient admissions. During inpatient treatment, goals should be set and plans made for discharge. Specific consequences must be established for noncompliance. Counseling must continue after discharge. A support group referral may be helpful in encouraging compliance. Family involvement is necessary. The adolescent must recognize that discharge from the health care facility does not mean that he or she is "cured."

Improving Family Coping. The family of the adolescent needs counseling along with the adolescent. Some families may deny that the teen has a problem or that the problem is as severe as health care team members perceive it to be. Family therapy meets with varied success. Usually the earlier family therapy is initiated, the better the results. Family members must be able to identify behaviors of their own that contribute to the adolescent's problem. Family members also must learn to cooperate with behavior modification programs and with guidance carry them out at home when necessary. Ongoing contact between the family, the adolescent, and consistent health team members is essential (see Nursing Care Plan for the Adolescent With Anorexia Nervosa).

EVALUATION: GOALS AND OUTCOME CRITERIA

The evaluation of an adolescent with an eating disorder is an ongoing process that continues throughout the hospital stay as well as in outpatient settings. Goals and outcome criteria include

- *Goal:* The adolescent will gain a predetermined amount of weight per week.
  Criteria: The adolescent eats at least 80% of each meal, gains 1 to 2 lb (450 to 900 g) a week, keeps a food diary, and signs a contract agreement.
- *Goal:* The adolescent will show evidence of improved self-esteem.
  Criteria: The adolescent verbally expresses positive attitudes, maintains peer relationships, and improves grooming.
- *Goal:* The adolescent will pace activity to avoid fatigue.
  Criteria: The adolescent is involved in activity as prescribed in a contract; no excessive activity is detected.
- *Goal:* The adolescent's bowel elimination will be normal.
  Criteria: The adolescent experiences no episodes of diarrhea or constipation. The adolescent will not attempt deceit to obtain laxatives.
- *Goal:* The adolescent's skin will show no evidence of breakdown.
  Criteria: The adolescent's skin is intact with no signs of redness, irritation, or excessive pressure; skin turgor is good.
- *Goal:* The adolescent will show signs of compliance.
  Criteria: The adolescent agrees to, signs, and adheres to a contract agreement; keeps coun-

seling appointments; joins a support group; and continues to gain or maintain weight as per contract agreement.
- *Goal:* The family will show evidence of improved coping.
  Criteria: The family attends counseling sessions and identifies behaviors that aggravate the adolescent's condition.

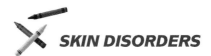

SKIN DISORDERS

Acne Vulgaris

Acne, one of the most common health problems of adolescence, may be only a mild case of oily skin and a few blackheads or it may be a severe type with ropelike cystic lesions that leave deep scars, both physical and emotional. To adolescents who want to be attractive and popular, however, even a mild case of acne (often called "zits") can cause great anxiety, shyness, and social withdrawal.

Characterized by the appearance of **comedones** (blackheads and whiteheads), papules, and pustules on the face and the back and chest to some extent, acne is caused by a variety of factors, including

- Increased hormonal levels, especially androgens
- Hereditary factors
- Irritation and irritating substances such as vigorous scrubbing and cosmetics with a greasy base
- Growth of anaerobic bacteria

Each hair follicle has an associated sebaceous gland that in adolescents produces increased **sebum** (oily secretion). The sebum is blocked by epithelial cells and becomes trapped in the follicle. When anaerobic organisms infect this collection, inflammation occurs, which causes papules, pustules, and nodules (Fig. 19–2). Several types of acne lesions are often present at one time.

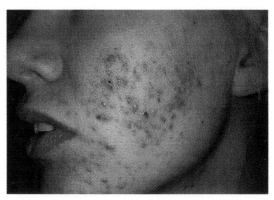

● *Figure 19.2* Facial acne in an adolescent.

NURSING CARE PLAN

for the Adolescent With Anorexia Nervosa

FW is a 15-year-old female who has had a complete physical examination to determine why she has lost weight. After her examination and testing was completed, a diagnosis of anorexia nervosa was made. The adolescent denies that she is underweight. She has been hospitalized to initiate treatment because her weight has dropped to 87 pounds (39.5 kg).

NURSING DIAGNOSIS
Imbalanced Nutrition: Less Than Body Requirements related to self-induced vomiting and use of laxatives or diuretics

GOAL: The adolescent's nutritional status will improve, reaching a goal weight of 100 pounds, and an adequate fluid intake will be maintained.

OUTCOME CRITERIA
• The adolescent gains at least 1.5 pounds (680 grams) per week.
• The adolescent eats 80% of her meals.
• The adolescent is involved in plans to improve her nutrition.
• The adolescent does not interrupt parenteral fluid administration.
• The adolescent's mucous membranes are moist; her skin turgor is good.
• The adolescent's electrolytes, cardiac and respiratory status, and renal function are within normal limits.

NURSING INTERVENTIONS	*RATIONALE*
Supervise intake by observing her during and after meals.	An adolescent with an eating disorder may go to any length to avoid eating.
Weigh daily at the same time wearing the same type of clothes. Make certain nothing can be secreted in pockets or other hiding places that could add to her weight.	An adolescent can be very innovative in finding ways to hide heavy objects on her to increase her weight gain.
Include the adolescent with other health care providers to establish a mutually agreed upon, long-term weight goal and food plan that provide her with a slow, steady, weekly weight gain. Make a contract agreement to clearly state expectations and privileges that she can gain or lose.	The adolescent is central to the planning process and cannot be made to meet goals set by others. Her participation and agreement to specific plans give her a feeling of more control of the overall outcome and encouraging her to stick to the plan.
Observe continuously when parenteral fluids are being administered to prevent any attempts to disrupt the IV line. Also encourage her to take oral fluids at the same time.	The anorectic adolescent may deprive herself so much that the fluid and electrolyte deficiencies become life-threatening. A balance must be restored before any further treatment can begin.
Test urine for ketones and regularly evaluate her skin turgor and mucous membranes.	These tests provide further indication of nutritional status.

NURSING DIAGNOSIS
Disturbed Body Image related to fear of obesity and potential rejection

GOAL: The adolescent will express positive feelings about self.

OUTCOME CRITERIA
• The adolescent verbally expresses positive attitudes about herself.
• The adolescent expresses insight into reasons behind eating patterns and self-destructive behavior.
• The adolescent expresses feelings about food, exercise, weight loss, and medical condition.

NURSING INTERVENTIONS	*RATIONALE*
Be a nonjudgmental, active listener; never minimize or ignore feelings expressed.	This is a first step in establishing and maintaining a climate of trust.
Report any negative feelings or any signs of depression expressed.	The adolescent's negative feelings and expression of depression are important to the therapeutic treatment plan. All health care providers need to know about signs of depression to alert them to take appropriate precautions.
Maintain continuity of care throughout treatment.	The same person working with the adolescent will help foster trust and a relationship will be developed.

NURSING CARE PLAN continued

for the Adolescent With Anorexia Nervosa

NURSING DIAGNOSIS
Risk for Activity Intolerance related to fatigue secondary to malnutrition

GOAL: The adolescent will balance rest and activity.

OUTCOME CRITERIA
- The adolescent follows her contract for activity.
- The adolescent is not excessively active.
- The adolescent paces her activity to avoid fatigue.

NURSING INTERVENTIONS	*RATIONALE*
Teach adolescent that a nutritional deficit depletes energy reserves and results in fatigue; encourage her to engage in activities of daily living, but provide for rest periods when her energy is low.	The adolescent needs to understand that activity and rest are related to her nutritional status and that a healthy balance is crucial to overall health.
Discourage the adolescent from pushing herself beyond her physical limits, and observe closely for secretive excessive exercise.	The adolescent with an eating disorder may attempt to burn off excess calories with exercise.

NURSING DIAGNOSIS
Risk for Constipation related to decreased food and fluid intake
Risk for Diarrhea related to use of laxatives

GOAL: The adolescent will maintain normal bowel habits.

OUTCOME CRITERIA
- The adolescent has bowel movements every day or every other day.
- The adolescent's stools are soft-formed.
- The adolescent's fluid and electrolyte balances are maintained.

NURSING INTERVENTIONS	*RATIONALE*
Observe the adolescent's trips to the bathroom and keep a careful record of bowel habits; report and document any occurrence of diarrhea or constipation at once.	Typically the adolescent may not be a reliable reporter of her bowel habits. A nurse observer is necessary to validate her stools.
Observe carefully to be certain that she does not have opportunity for purging or taking a laxative.	These adolescents can be devious and will go to almost any length to prevent weight gain.
Monitor fluid intake and output and electrolyte levels.	Loss of fluids and electrolytes can cause long-term health conditions.

NURSING DIAGNOSIS
Risk for Impaired Skin Integrity related to loss of subcutaneous fat and dry skin secondary to malnutrition.

GOAL: The adolescent's skin integrity will be maintained.

OUTCOME CRITERIA
- The adolescent has no areas of red, dry, irritated skin.
- The adolescent has no decubitus ulcer formations.
- The adolescent expresses feelings about body image and skin changes.

NURSING INTERVENTIONS	*RATIONALE*
Inspect skin daily for redness, irritation, or dryness. Provide good skin care.	Signs of redness, irritation, and dryness are preliminary signs for skin breakdown and formation of decubitus ulcers.

(nursing care plan continues on page 440)

NURSING CARE PLAN continued

for the Adolescent With Anorexia Nervosa

NURSING INTERVENTIONS	RATIONALE
Protect any bony prominences that may break down. Encourage position changes for adolescent in bed to prevent decubiti formation.	Protection of pressure on bony surfaces and frequent changes of position improve circulation and prevent formation of decubitus ulcers.

NURSING DIAGNOSIS
Noncompliance with treatment regimen related to unresolved conflicts over food and eating

GOAL: The adolescent will comply with treatment regimen.

OUTCOME CRITERIA
• The adolescent keeps counseling appointments.
• The adolescent joins a support group.
• The adolescent continues to gain weight as per her contract agreement.
• The adolescent participates in decisions about care and treatment.

NURSING INTERVENTIONS	RATIONALE
Make plans for discharge while she is still in the hospital. Include counseling plans in the contract.	Eating disorders are not cured with one hospitalization. Counseling is necessary to continue after discharge.
Encourage the adolescent to make and maintain contact with a support group after discharge.	A support group may strengthen her desire to comply with the treatment regimen.
Make clear the established consequences for noncompliance with the program.	Consequences for noncompliance are important to reinforce the need to follow the program. Consequences set out a disciplinary action that will occur if the adolescent fails to follow the program.
Encourage adolescent to make decisions about care.	When the adolescent makes decisions about care and treatment and complies with those plans, appropriate decision-making skills are fostered.

NURSING DIAGNOSIS
Compromised Family Coping related to eating disorders, treatment regimen, and dangers associated with an eating disorder

GOAL: The family's understanding of illness and treatment goals will improve.

OUTCOME CRITERIA
• The family attends counseling sessions.
• The family identifies behaviors that impact negatively on adolescent's behavior.

NURSING INTERVENTIONS	RATIONALE
Provide for family counseling as well as counseling for the adolescent.	It is important for the family to understand the dynamics of the problem and to face their possible contributions to the disorder.
Teach family members about the behavior modification program the adolescent is using. Provide guidance on how to carry out the program at home.	Eating disorders are not cured simply because the adolescent is discharged. Counseling, a continuation of the treatment program, and adherence to the signed contact agreement are essential. For these reasons, the family must become involved.

Treatment and Nursing Care

The topical medications benzoyl peroxide (Clearasil, Benoxyl) and tretinoin (Retin-A) come in a variety of forms such as topical cleansers, lotions, creams, sticks, pads, gels, and bars. The usual treatment plan for mild acne is topical application of one of these medications once or twice a day. These medications should not be applied to normal skin or allowed to get into the eyes or nose or on other mucous membranes. Antibiotics such as erythromycin and tetracycline may be administered for inflammatory acne. Antibiotic therapy requires an extended treatment course of at least 6 to 12 months followed by tapering of the dosage.

Isotretinoin (Accutane) may be used for severe inflammatory acne. This potent, effective oral medication is used for hard-to-treat cystic acne. Side effects are common but often diminish when the drug dosage is reduced. Warn the adolescent about some of the side effects including dry lips and skin, eye irritation, temporary worsening of acne, epistaxis (nosebleed), bleeding and inflammation of the gums, itching, photosensitivity (sensitivity to the sun), and joint and muscle pain. Isotretinoin is a pregnancy category X drug: it must not be used at all during pregnancy because of serious risk of fetal abnormalities. To rule out pregnancy, a urine test is done prior to beginning treatment. For the sexually active adolescent girl, an effective form of contraception must be used for a month before beginning and during isotretinoin therapy. The risk to the fetus should pregnancy occur, should be discussed with the girl, whether she is sexually active or not.

Even though the adolescent's perception of the disfigurement caused by acne may seem out of proportion to the actual severity of the condition, acknowledge and accept his or her feelings. Teach the adolescent and the family caregiver to wash the lesions gently with soap and water; do not scrub vigorously. Comedones should be removed gently by following the physician's recommendations and using careful aseptic techniques. Careful removal produces no scarring—a goal for every teen.

Understanding and support by the nurse and family caregiver are the most important aspects of caring for the adolescent with acne. Reassure the teen that eating chocolate and fatty foods does not cause acne, but a well-balanced, nutritious diet does promote healing.

MENSTRUAL DISORDERS

The beginning of menstruation, called **menarche,** normally occurs between the ages of 9 and 16 years.

For many girls this is a joyous affirmation of their womanhood, but others may have negative feelings about the event depending on how they have been prepared for menarche and for their roles as women. Irregular menstruation is common during the first year until a regular cycle is established.

Some adolescent girls experience **mittelschmerz,** a dull, aching abdominal pain at the time of ovulation (hence the name, which means "midcycle"). The cause is not completely understood but the discomfort usually lasts only a few hours and is relieved by analgesics, a heating pad, or a warm bath.

Premenstrual Syndrome

Women of all ages are subject to the discomfort of **premenstrual syndrome** (PMS) but the symptoms may be alarming to the adolescent. Symptoms include edema (resulting in weight gain), headache, increased anxiety, mild depression, and mood swings. The major cause of PMS is thought to be water retention following progesterone production after ovulation (Fig. 19–3).

Generally the discomforts of PMS are minor and can be relieved by reducing salt intake during the week before menstruation, taking mild analgesics, and applying local heat. When symptoms are more severe, the physician may prescribe a mild diuretic to be taken the week before menstruation to relieve edema; occasionally oral contraceptive pills are prescribed to prevent ovulation.

Dysmenorrhea

Dysmenorrhea (painful menstruation) is classified as primary or secondary. Many adolescent girls experience pain associated with menstruation including cramping abdominal pain, leg pain, and backache. *Primary dysmenorrhea* occurs as part of the normal menstrual cycle without any associated pelvic disease. The increased secretion of prostaglandins, which occurs in the last few days of the menstrual cycle, is thought to be a contributing factor in primary dysmenorrhea. Nonsteroidal anti-inflammatory drugs (NSAIDs), such as ibuprofen (Advil, Motrin), inhibit prostaglandins and are the treatment of choice for primary dysmenorrhea. These drugs are most effective when taken before cramps become too severe. Because NSAIDs are irritating to the gastric mucosa, they always should be taken with food and discontinued if epigastric burning occurs.

Secondary dysmenorrhea is the result of pelvic pathologic changes, most often pelvic inflammatory disease (PID) or endometriosis. The adolescent girl who has severe menstrual pain

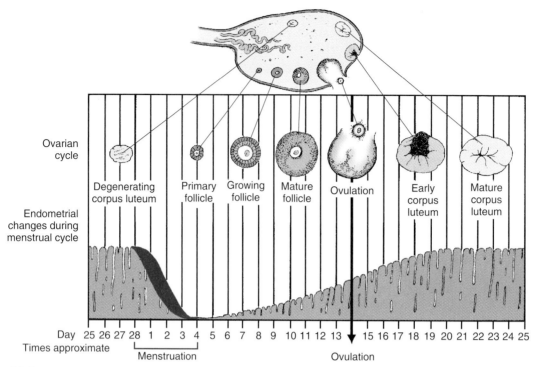

● *Figure 19.3* Schematic representation of a 28-day ovarian cycle. Menstruation occurs with shedding of the endometrium. The follicular phase is associated with the rapidly growing ovarian follicle and the production of estrogen. Ovulation occurs midcycle, and mittelschmerz may occur. The secretory phase follows in preparation for the fertilized ovum. If fertilization does not occur, the corpus luteum begins to degenerate, estrogen and progesterone levels decline, and menstruation again occurs.

should be examined by a physician to determine if any pelvic pathologic changes are present. Treatment of the underlying condition helps relieve severe dysmenorrhea.

Amenorrhea

The absence of menstruation, or **amenorrhea,** can be primary (no previous menstruation) or secondary (missing three or more periods after menstrual flow has begun). Primary amenorrhea after 16 years of age warrants a diagnostic survey for genetic abnormalities, tumors, or other problems. Secondary amenorrhea can be the result of discontinuing contraceptives, a sign of pregnancy, the result of physical or emotional stressors, or a symptom of an underlying medical condition. A complete physical examination including gynecologic screening is necessary to help determine the cause.

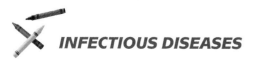

INFECTIOUS DISEASES

Some infectious diseases are common in the adolescent population. Mononucleosis is seen frequently in

this age group. The adolescent should also be evaluated for tuberculosis.

Infectious Mononucleosis

Sometimes called the "kissing disease," infectious mononucleosis ("mono") is caused by the Epstein-Barr virus, one of the herpes virus groups. The organism is transmitted through saliva. No immunization is available, and treatment is symptomatic. Adolescents and young adults seem to be most susceptible to this disorder although sometimes it also is seen in younger children.

Clinical Manifestations

Infectious mononucleosis can present a variety of symptoms ranging from mild to severe and including symptoms that mimic hepatitis. Symptoms include fever; sore throat with enlarged tonsils; thick, white membrane covering the tonsils; palatine petechiae (red spots on the soft palate) (Fig 19–4); swollen lymph nodes; and enlargement of the spleen accompanied by extreme fatigue and lack of energy. In some instances, headache, abdominal pain, and epistaxis are also present.

Diagnosis

Diagnosis of infectious mononucleosis is based on clinical symptoms, laboratory evidence of lympho-

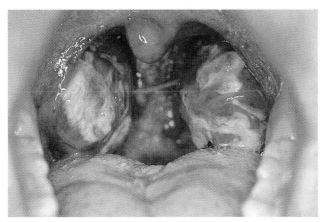

● *Figure 19.4* Tonsils of an adolescent who has infectious mononucleosis; note the red, enlarged tonsils with the thick white covering.

cytes in the peripheral blood (with 10% or more abnormal lymphocytes present in a peripheral blood smear), and a positive heterophil agglutination test. Monospot is a valuable diagnostic test—rapid, sensitive, inexpensive, and simple to perform. Monospot can detect significant agglutinins at lower levels thus allowing earlier diagnosis. Infectious mononucleosis often is confused with streptococcal infections because of the fever and the appearance of the throat and tonsils.

Treatment and Nursing Care

No cure exists for infectious mononucleosis; treatment is based on symptoms. An analgesic-antipyretic, such as acetaminophen, usually is recommended for the fever and headaches. Fluids and a soft, bland diet are encouraged to reduce throat irritation. Corticosteroids sometimes are used to relieve the severe sore throat and fever. Bed rest is suggested to relieve fatigue but is not imposed for a specific amount of time. If the spleen is enlarged, the adolescent is cautioned to avoid contact sports that might cause a ruptured spleen. Because the immune system is weakened, the adolescent must take precautions to avoid secondary infections.

The course of mononucleosis is usually uncomplicated. Fever and sore throat may last from 1 week to 10 days. Fatigue generally disappears 2 to 4 weeks after the appearance of acute symptoms but may last as long as 1 year. The limitations that this disorder imposes on the teenager's school and social life may cause depression. In most instances, however, the adolescent can resume normal activities within 1 month after symptoms present. Nursing care includes encouraging the adolescent to express feelings about the interruptions the illness is causing in school, social, and work plans. Long-term effects rarely are seen.

Pulmonary Tuberculosis

Tuberculosis is present in all parts of the world and is the most important chronic infectious disease in terms of illness, death, and cost.[2] The incidence of tuberculosis in the United States had declined steadily until about 1985. In the years since, there has been an increase in the number of cases reported in the United States. Several factors contribute to this increase; one factor is the number of people who are HIV-positive and have become infected with tuberculosis.

Tuberculosis is caused by *Mycobacterium tuberculosis*, a bacillus spread by droplets of infected mucus that become airborne when the infected person sneezes, coughs, or laughs. The bacilli, when airborne, are inhaled into the respiratory tract of the unsuspecting person and become implanted in lung tissue. This process is the beginning of the formation of a primary lesion.

Clinical Manifestations

Primary tuberculosis is the original infection that goes through various stages and ends with calcification. Primary lesions in children generally are unrecognized. The most common site of a primary lesion is the alveoli of the respiratory tract. Most cases arrest with the calcification of the primary infection. However, in children with poor nutrition or health, the primary infection may invade other tissues of the body including the bones, joints, kidneys, lymph nodes, and meninges. This is called miliary tuberculosis. In the small number of children with miliary tuberculosis, general symptoms of chronic infection such as fatigue, loss of weight, and low-grade fever may occur accompanied by night sweats.

Secondary tuberculosis is a reactivation of a healed primary lesion. It often occurs in adults and contributes to the exposure of children to the organism. Although secondary lesions are more common in adults, they may occur in adolescents. Symptoms resemble those in an adult including cough with expectoration, fever, weight loss, malaise, and night sweats.

Diagnosis

The tuberculin skin test is the primary means by which tuberculosis is detected. A skin test can be performed using a multipuncture device that deposits purified protein derivative (PPD) intradermally (tine test) or by intradermal injection of 0.1 mL of PPD. Either test is administered on the inner aspect of the forearm. The site is marked and read at 48 and 72 hours. Redness, swelling, induration, and itching of the site indicate a positive reaction. Persons with a positive reaction are further examined by radiographic evaluation. Sputum tests of young children are rarely helpful because children do not produce a good specimen. Screening by means of skin testing is recommended for all children at 12 months, before entering school, and in adolescence. Screening is recommended annually for children in high-risk situations or communities including children in whose family there is an active case, Native Americans, and children who recently immigrated from Central or South America, the Caribbean, Africa, Asia, or the Middle East. Other high-risk children are those infected with HIV, those who are homeless or live in overcrowded conditions, and those immunosuppressed from any cause.

Treatment

Drug therapy for tuberculosis includes administration of isoniazid (INH) often in combination with rifampin. Although INH has been known to cause peripheral neuritis in children with poor nutrition, few problems occur in children whose diets are well balanced. Rifampin is tolerated well by children but causes body fluids such as urine, sweat, tears, and feces to turn orange-red. A possible disadvantage for adolescents is that it may permanently stain contact lenses. Rifamate is a combination of rifampin and INH. Other drugs that may be used are ethambutol, streptomycin, and pyrazinamide.

Drug therapy is continued for 9 to 18 months. After chemotherapy has begun, the child or adolescent may return to school and normal activities unless clinical symptoms are evident. An annual chest radiograph is necessary from that time on.

Prevention

Prevention requires improvements in social conditions such as overcrowding, poverty, and poor health care. Also needed are health education, medical, laboratory, and radiographic facilities for examination and control of contacts and persons suspected of infection.

A vaccine called bacilli Calmette-Guérin (BCG) is used in countries with a high incidence of tuberculosis. It is given to tuberculin-negative persons and is said to be effective for 12 years or longer. Mass vaccination is not considered necessary in parts of the world where the incidence of tuberculosis is low. After administration of BCG vaccine, the skin test will be positive so screening is no longer an effective tool. The use of BCG vaccine remains controversial because of the effect it has on screening for the disease as well as the questionable effectiveness of the vaccine.

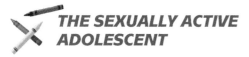

THE SEXUALLY ACTIVE ADOLESCENT

The age when adolescents become sexually active has been decreasing in recent years; with that decrease has come an increase in the complications resulting from sexual activity. Problems that result from sexual activity of adolescents include sexually transmitted diseases (STDs), genital infections, and adolescent pregnancy.

Vaginitis

Vaginitis (inflammation of the vagina) can result from a number of causes such as diaphragms or tampons left in place too long, irritating douches or sprays, estrogen changes caused by birth-control pills, and antibiotic therapy. Actually these causes are precursors that provide an opportunity for the organisms to become active. The most common causes of vaginitis are *Candida albicans,* bacterial vaginosis (caused by *Gardnerella vaginalis* and other organisms), and *Trichomonas. Trichomonas* is the only one of these organisms transmitted solely by sexual contact (Table 19–1).

Sexually Transmitted Diseases

The incidence of STDs is higher in adolescents than in any other age group. The diseases range from infections that can be easily treated to life-threatening diseases such as HIV infection (Table 19–2). Infants infected with STDs usually are infected prenatally or during birth. Children infected after the neonatal period must be considered victims of sexual abuse until disproved. Severe or repeated cases of pelvic inflammatory disease (PID) or severe genital warts are warning signs that the girl should be tested for HIV.

Prevention is the most effective tool in the campaign against STDs. The only certain way to avoid contracting an STD is sexual abstinence. However, sexual activity in adolescents indicates that this is often not a practical solution. Condoms with spermicide (discussed in Chapter 18) provide protection, although they are not fail-safe. Adolescents must be educated about all aspects of the consequences of sexual activity.

Gonorrhea

An estimated 800,000 cases of gonorrhea are reported annually, and an equal number of cases are believed to be undiagnosed. It is one of the most commonly reported communicable diseases in the United States. Also called "the clap," "the drips," or "the dose," gonorrhea has mild primary symptoms particularly in females and often goes undetected and thus untreated until it progresses to a serious pelvic disorder. This disease can cause sterility in males.

Several drugs may be used to treat gonorrhea, but the current drug of choice is ceftriaxone (Rocephin) followed by a week of oral doxycycline

TABLE 19.1	Infectious Causes of Vaginitis		
Organism/Incidence	Symptoms	Sexual Transmission	Treatment
Candida albicans First episodes occur in adolescence, especially in sexually active girls	Severe itching, exacerbated just before menstruation Odor not present Milky "cottage cheese"– like discharge may be noted on examination	Normally present in vagina; most often results from glycosuria, antibiotic therapy, birth-control pills, steroid therapy, or other factor that alters normal pH of vagina May result from oral–genital sex	Nystatin, miconazole (Monistat), or clotrimazole (Gyne-Lo-trimin) vaginal suppositories or creams
Bacterial Vaginosis (multiple organisms) Common among adolescent girls; sexual partner will probably also be infected	About half of patients have no symptoms Fishy odor after intercourse Discharge, if present, grayish and thin	Sexually transmitted	Metronidazole (Flagyl)* or ampicillin; sexual partners may be treated
Trichomonas Most frequently diagnosed STD	Itching with severe infection, especially after menstruation Discharge has foul odor and may be frothy, gray or green	Sexually transmitted	Metronidazole (Flagyl)*, sexual partners also should be treated

*Flagyl is not ordered for the pregnant patient due to possible danger to fetus.

(Vibramycin) to prevent an accompanying chlamydial infection. Adolescents are asked to name their sexual contacts so that they also may be treated. Penicillin-resistant strains of the organism have developed, so penicillin is no longer an effective method of treatment. Adolescents must learn that their bodies will not develop immunity to the organism and they might become infected again if they continue to expose themselves by engaging in sexual activity, especially high-risk sexual behavior.

Chlamydial Infection

Chlamydial infections have replaced gonorrhea as *the* most common and fasting spreading STD in the United States. Symptoms may be mild, causing a delay in diagnosis and treatment until serious complications and transmission to others have occurred.

Adolescents must be made aware of the seriousness of PID, a common result of a chlamydial infection. Pelvic inflammatory disease can cause sterility in the female primarily by causing scarring in the fallopian tubes that prohibits the passage of the fertilized ovum into the uterus. A tubal pregnancy may be the consequence of a chlamydial infection. In the male, sterility may result from epididymitis caused by a chlamydial infection.

Doxycycline or azithromycin is used to treat chlamydial infection. In the pregnant adolescent, erythromycin or amoxicillin can be used to avoid the teratogenic effects of these drugs. All sexual partners must be treated.

Genital Herpes

Genital herpes has reached epidemic proportions in the United States. The disease begins as a vesicle that ruptures to form a painful ulcer on the genitalia. The initial ulcer lasts 10 to 12 days. Recurrent episodes occur intermittently and last 4 to 5 days. No cure is available, but acyclovir (Zovirax) is useful in relieving or suppressing the symptoms. Genital herpes is associated with a much higher than average risk for cervical cancer; therefore, the female who has genital herpes should have an annual Pap smear. Genital herpes is not transmitted to the fetus in utero; for an active case of genital herpes at the time of delivery though, the infant should be delivered by cesarean birth to avoid infection during passage through the vagina. In newborns, the infection can become systemic and cause death.

Syphilis

Caused by the spirochete *Treponema pallidum*, syphilis is a destructive disease that can involve every part of the body. Untreated, it can have devastating long-term effects. Infected mothers are highly likely to transmit the infection to their unborn infants.

TABLE 19.2	Major Sexually Transmitted Diseases

Infection and Agent	Transmission	Symptoms	Possible Complications	Prevention
Gonorrhea—gonococcus: *Neisseria gonorrhoeae*	Sexual contact; mother to fetus during vaginal delivery	Yellow mucopurulent discharge of the genital area, painful or frequent urination, pain in the genital area; may be asymptomatic. Frequent cause of pelvic inflammatory disease	Sterility, cystitis, arthritis, endocarditis	Public should be educated on safe sex practices; mother should be tested before delivery. Newborn's eyes should be treated with tetracycline ointment, erythromycin ointment, or silver nitrate. All contacts should be treated with antibiotics.
Chlamydia—bacteria: *Chlamydia trachomatis*	Sexual contact; mother to fetus during vaginal delivery	Mucopurulent genital discharge, genital pain, dysuria. Frequent cause of pelvic inflammatory disease, often in combination with gonorrhea	Sterility	Public should be educated about safe sex practices. Sexual contact should be avoided when lesions are present. Infected mothers should have a cesarean delivery.
Genital herpes virus: herpes simplex type 2	Sexual contact; mother to fetus during vaginal delivery	Genital soreness, pruritus, and erythema; vesicles appear that usually last for about 10 days during which time transmission of virus is likely		Public should be educated about safe sex practices. Sexual contact should be avoided when lesions are present. Infected mother should have a cesarean delivery.
Syphillis—spirochete: *Treponema pallidum*	Sexual contact; mother to fetus via placenta; blood transfusions if undiagnosed donor is in early stage of disease	Primary stage: genital lesion, enlarged lymph nodes. Secondary stage (6 weeks later): lesions of skin and mucous membrane with generalized symptoms of headache and fever	Tertiary stage: central nervous system and cardiovascular damage, paralysis, psychosis	Public should be educated about safe sex practices. Screen blood donors; do serologic testing before and during pregnancy. Avoid contact with body secretions from infected patients.
Acquired immunodeficiency syndrome (AIDS)—virus: human immunodeficiency virus	Sexual contact; exposure to blood or blood products; mother to fetus	Active phase: rash, cough, malaise, night sweats, lymphadenopathy. Asymptomatic phase: no symptoms, but test is positive for HIV antigens. AIDS-related complex: lymphadenopathy, diarrhea, oral candidiasis, weight loss, fatigue, skin rash, recurrent infections, fever. AIDS: rare infections such as *Pneumocystis carinii* pneumonia or rare cancers such as Kaposi sarcoma or B-cell lymphomas	Neurologic impairment	Public, especially high-risk groups, should be educated about safe sex practices. Blood or blood products used for transfusion should be carefully screened. Intravenous drug abusers should not share needles. Universal precautions should be used consistently in all health care settings. Institute measures to avoid needlesticks among health care workers.

Syphilis is spread primarily by sexual contact. Symptoms of the primary stage usually appear about 3 weeks after exposure. If allowed to progress without treatment, syphilis has a secondary stage, a latent stage, and a tertiary stage.

The cardinal sign of the primary stage is the **chancre,** which is a hard, red, painless lesion at the point of entry of the spirochete. This can appear on the penis, the vulva, or the cervix. It also can appear on the mouth, the lips, or the rectal area as a result of oral-genital or anal-genital contact. The secondary stage, marked by rash, sore throat, and fever, appears 2 to 6 months after the original infection. Signs of both the first and second stages disappear without treatment, but the spirochete remains in the body. The latent period can persist for as long as 20 years without symptoms; however, blood tests are still positive. In the tertiary stage, syphilis causes severe neurologic and cardiovascular damage, mental illness, and gastrointestinal disorders.

Syphilis responds to one intramuscular injection of penicillin G benzathine; if the adolescent is sensitive to penicillin, oral doxycyline, tetracycline or erythromycin can be administered as alternative treatment. If treatment is not obtained before the tertiary stage, the neurologic and cardiovascular complications can lead to death.

Acquired Immunodeficiency Syndrome

Acquired immunodeficiency syndrome (AIDS) is caused by human immunodeficiency virus (HIV), which attacks and destroys the T-helper lymphocytes (CD4+). The T-helper lymphocytes are cells that direct the immune response to viral, bacterial, and fungal infections and remove some malignant cells from the body. AIDS has four distinct stages:

1. Early stage (acute phase): symptoms similar to those of influenza; the virus reproduces rapidly.
2. Middle period (asymptomatic phase): may last for years with vague symptoms; reproduction of the virus and loss of CD4+ T cells is slow.
3. Early symptomatic phase: period of transition with increasing symptoms; CD4+ T cell count drops.
4. AIDS: CD4+ T cell count continues to drop; opportunistic, often life-threatening diseases develop.

Transmission of HIV is by contact with infected blood or sexual contact with an infected person. The virus cannot be transmitted through casual contact. The diagnosis of any STD increases the statistical risk of HIV infection by 300%.

Because not all persons who test positive for HIV develop AIDS immediately, the U.S. Centers for Disease Control and Prevention have established criteria for a classification system for HIV Infection and AIDS surveillance. The most significant of these

criteria for adolescents and adults is a CD4+ T-lymphocyte count of fewer than 200 cells/μL (the normal count is 600–1,200 cells/μL), or less than 14% of total lymphocytes.

Infants usually are infected through the placenta during prenatal life, in the birth process when contaminated by the mother's blood, or through breastfeeding. Children and teens also can be infected through sexual abuse. Adolescents are most often infected through intimate heterosexual or homosexual relations and through intravenous drug use. Some hemophiliacs who received blood products before 1985 were infected, but safeguards are now in place and the blood supply has become much safer.

Although most children with AIDS are between the ages of 1 and 4 years, the alarming increase occurring among adolescents is causing great concern in those who work with adolescents. African-American adolescents have a disproportionately high rate of AIDS. The numbers of adolescent girls with HIV continues to rise.

Teenagers' attitude of **impunity** (the belief that nothing can hurt them) and the increasing rate of sexual activity in this age group, often involving multiple partners, contribute to the fear that this group will experience widespread illness from HIV. The incubation period for HIV can vary from 3 to 10 years; thus many who contract the disease in adolescence will not have symptoms until they are in their 20s, when they are at their reproductive peak. The proper use of a condom with spermicide (see Chap. 18) during any type of sexual contact is essential to prevent the spread of HIV. Adolescent girls may have sexual experiences with older men who have had many previous sexual partners. This increases the risk for the girl and, in turn, can increase the risk for any adolescent boy with whom she is sexually intimate. Adolescent boys also are at increased risk if they engage in unprotected homosexual relations, use intravenous drugs, have multiple partners, or have sex with a prostitute.

Cultural influences may play an important role in the spread of HIV. The adolescent girl often finds it difficult to insist that her partner use a condom. If the partner refuses and claims to be "safe" (uninfected) or protests that the condom decreases his pleasure, she might give in for fear of breaking up the relationship. In addition, in some cultures the more sexual conquests a boy has, the more manly he is considered.

About 20% to 30% of the infants born to HIV-infected mothers develop AIDS. Although the infants may test positive in the first year of life, testing is not reliable until 18 months of age because the infant may retain antibodies from the mother for this length of time. However, for affected infants younger than 1 year of age, the disease can move rapidly to AIDS and serious complications. Failure to thrive, *Pneumocystis carinii* pneumonia, recurrent bacterial infections, progressive encephalopathy, and malignancy often develop in affected infants. Some of these children progress quickly to terminal illness and death, but with aggressive chemotherapy some of them are living long enough to enter school.

Adolescents manifest the symptoms of HIV in much the same way as adults. Females rarely have Kaposi sarcoma, a cancer often seen in homosexual men. Many women including adolescents present with a chronic infection of vaginitis caused by *C albicans* that has not responded to local antifungal treatments. These infections may be controlled by oral systemic medications. The female who tests positive for HIV should have a pelvic examination every 6 months to detect early STDs and institute vigorous treatment as needed.

● Nursing Process for the Adolescent With AIDS

ASSESSMENT

When seeking data from the adolescent with AIDS, gather a complete history including chief complaint, presenting symptoms, past medical history, immunization status, family history, and social history. Interview the family caregiver if present, but be certain to provide the adolescent with a private interview. The teen may be extremely reluctant to reveal either social or sexual history, especially in the presence of a family member. Review carefully the teen girl's history of vaginal candidiasis, PID, and sexual activity. Review the teen boy's sexual activity including partners who are of the same sex or who are drug users. The adolescent may have various emotions, including anger, denial, guilt, and rebelliousness; the nurse should accept all these emotions as legitimate reactions to the illness.

During the physical exam, maintain strict standard precautions. Include vital signs and especially observe for fever, which may indicate infection, and perform a thorough survey of all body systems. Observe for poor skin turgor, rashes or lesions, alopecia, mucous membrane lesions or thrush, weight loss, mental or neurologic changes, respiratory infections or signs of tuberculosis, diarrhea or abdominal pain, vaginal discharge, perineal lesions, or genital warts. Help prepare the adolescent for diagnostic tests that must be performed.

NURSING DIAGNOSES

Following careful data collection of the adolescent, the information is reviewed and the healthcare team decides on actual or potential problems of the adolescent. Nursing diagnoses may include

- Risk for Infection related to increased susceptibility secondary to a compromised immune system
- Risk for Injury related to the possible transmission of the virus
- Risk for Impaired Skin Integrity related to perineal and anal tissue excoriation secondary to genital candidiasis or genital warts
- Acute Pain related to symptoms of the disease
- Imbalanced Nutrition: Less Than Body Requirements related to anorexia, oral or esophageal lesions, or diarrhea
- Social Isolation related to rejection by others secondary to the diagnosis of AIDS
- Hopelessness related to the diagnosis and prognosis
- Compromised Family Coping related to the diagnosis of AIDS

OUTCOME IDENTIFICATION AND PLANNING

Planning the nursing care of an adolescent with AIDS can be challenging. The adolescent needs support to accept the diagnosis and move in a positive direction to follow the treatment plan to the best of his or her ability. The nurse can play a critical role in helping the teen understand the treatment and prognosis and their impact on his or her life. Major goals for the adolescent include maintaining the highest level of wellness possible by preventing infection and the spread of the infection, maintaining skin integrity, minimizing pain, improving nutrition, alleviating social isolation, and diminishing a feeling of hopelessness. The primary goal for the family is improving coping skills and helping the teen cope with the illness.

IMPLEMENTATION

Preventing Infection. In the health care facility, strict adherence to appropriate infection control measures is extremely important. A primary goal is to teach the adolescent to prevent infections. Teach good handwashing technique; the patient should take care to wash between the fingers and under rings and should use a pump-type soap. He or she should keep nails trimmed to avoid harboring microorganisms under the nails. Teach the teen that skin care includes showering (not a tub bath) with a mild soap (no strong, perfumed soaps), using an emollient cream, and patting the skin dry while avoiding vigorous rubbing.

Raw fruits and vegetables should be washed and peeled or cooked to avoid the danger of bacteria, and meats must be well cooked. The teen must avoid unpasteurized dairy products and foods grown in organic fertilizer.

Instruct the teen to brush the teeth at least three times a day using a soft toothbrush and nonabrasive toothpaste. Routine dental care is vital.

The household where the adolescent lives must be cleaned carefully and regularly. A household bleach solution of one part bleach to 10 parts of water is a good solution to use. Particular attention should be paid to the refrigerator, the stove, the oven, and the microwave to prevent contamination of foods during preparation or storage. Household items that may be contaminated should be discarded in double plastic bags to prevent spread to others. Laundry bleach should be used when washing the adolescent's clothing especially underwear.

Teach the adolescent that someone else should care for pets. Cleaning an aquarium or birdcage or emptying a cat's litter box can expose the adolescent to opportunistic organisms that will attack the compromised immune system. Help the adolescent learn to avoid persons who have any infectious disease. Advise him or her that prompt attention to an apparently minor infection helps avoid more serious illness. The adolescent with AIDS should not receive any live vaccine immunizations but should continue to receive other immunizations as indicated.

Preventing Transmission. The good hygienic practices necessary to protect the teen from an acquired or opportunistic infection also help to prevent transmission of the virus to others. The adolescent needs counseling about sexual practices. One of the most emotionally difficult tasks for the adolescent may be to list sexual contacts. This is a delicate matter that must be approached in a nonjudgmental, sympathetic manner, but the teen needs to understand that anyone with whom he or she has been sexually intimate may be infected and must be identified.

The teen may find that the sexual partner from whom he or she contracted the virus already knew that he or she was infected. Infection with HIV does not necessarily mean that the teen was promiscuous. The adolescent may have been sexually intimate with only one person, and that person may have assured the teen that he or she was not infected. The adolescent may be extremely angry about exposure by a trusted person.

Teach the adolescent about safe sex practices. The adolescent needs to understand that he or she is protecting not only future sexual partners from contracting the disease but also himself or herself from contracting other strains of the virus. Both boys and girls need to have complete instructions on the use of condoms and spermicide (see Chap. 18). The adolescent must not be sexually intimate with anyone without using a condom, no matter what kind of argument the other person uses. Also the teen needs to learn that HIV is transmitted through vaginal intercourse, oral-genital contact, anal intercourse, or any contact with blood or body fluids including menstrual discharge. The teen that practices oral-genital sex must learn to use a dental dam (a square of latex worn in the mouth to prevent contact of body fluids with mucous membranes of the mouth).

The adolescent girl needs counseling about pregnancy. The probability of transmitting the virus to her unborn child may be as high as 30%, and no way currently exists to determine if she will pass the virus to her child. She must consider that even if her infant is not infected, there is a possibility that she may not live to see the child reach adulthood. All these considerations are overwhelming, and the adolescent needs continuous support to understand, accept, and deal with them.

A discussion of the teen's use of illicit, injectable drugs is important. Counsel the adolescent about the importance of stopping drug use. However, the reality is that he or she may not quit, so explain how to sterilize needles using chlorine bleach. A mixture of one part bleach to five parts water should be drawn through the needle into the syringe, flushed two or three times, and finally rinsed with water. Remember that the adolescent has the right to decide how to conduct his or her life, and remain nonjudgmental through all contacts with the teen.

Protecting Skin Integrity. Skin lesions are common symptoms of many STDs. The adolescent must report any new skin lesion to the health care provider for diagnosis and immediate treatment. The best preventive measure is to follow careful infection control measures including careful handwashing and to protect skin integrity by using skin emollients to guard against dryness; avoiding harsh, perfumed soaps; and guarding against injury to the skin. In advanced disease, nursing measures are implemented to protect and pad pressure points and improve peripheral circulation.

Relieving Pain. Pain is caused by several manifestations of AIDS. Skin and mucous membrane lesions may be very painful. Topical anesthetic solutions, such as viscous lidocaine, and meticulous mouth care can relieve pain caused by oral mucous membrane infections. Smoking, alcohol, and spicy or acidic foods irritate the oral mucous membranes and often cause additional pain. Pelvic inflammatory disease, a common complication of STDs, is usually accompanied by abdominal pain. The adolescent with respiratory complications also has bouts of chest pain. Administer analgesics to relieve pain and use all appropriate nursing measures to help the adolescent feel more comfortable. As the disease develops, the pain may be greater so every effort must be made to provide comfort.

Improving Nutrition. Anorexia, or a poor appetite, is a common problem of the patient with AIDS. Dehydration, diarrhea, infection, malabsorption, oral candidiasis, and some drugs also can contribute to the adolescent's poor state of nutrition. Malnutrition can cause additional problems with increased and more serious infections. The adolescent's diet must be more nutritious and higher in calories than normal. Several small meals supplemented by high-calorie, high-protein snacks may be desirable. Dietary supplements, such as Ensure and Isocal, also may be useful. Explore the adolescent's food likes and dislikes and develop a meal plan using this information. If malnutrition becomes severe, the adolescent may need tube feedings or parenteral nutrition.

Easing Social Isolation and Hopelessness. The adolescent may fear having others know about the illness because he or she anticipates a negative reaction from peers and family. Provide the teen with supportive counseling and guidance to help him or her deal with these fears. The teen may not feel that he or she can tell the family for fear of rejection. In fact, many families have rejected their children who have AIDS. Many others have risen to the challenge; although family members may tell the teenager they do not like his or her behavior, they continue to offer love and support. The adolescent may need support to help tell social acquaintances as well. Refer the teen to an adolescent HIV support group if one is available through the hospital or community. Adolescents often find that adult support groups are not as helpful because the adults' needs are different from those of adolescents.

Because the adolescent is facing life with a serious, chronic illness that requires frequent treatment and lifelong medication and has an unknown outcome, the adolescent maybe feel a special sense of purpose to "spread the word" to others. The adolescent needs support and guidance to set priorities. School officials may need to be told, but families have the legal right to decide whether or not they share the diagnosis with others. If the family is not supportive, the adolescent needs even more support from health care providers.

Helping the Family to Cope. The adolescent must be involved in telling family members about the diagnosis if they do not already know. The sexual activity of adolescent children is a topic that many families find difficult to deal with, especially if the activity is homosexual or promiscuous. The family caregivers usually need support as much as the adolescent does. They often are devastated by the prospect of their child's illness. If the adolescent is pregnant or has a child, the family also must consider the future of that child. For the family who plays a supportive role in the adolescent's life, the period after diagnosis is a difficult one. Teach the family as much about the disease as possible. They must learn how to prevent the spread of the virus among family members as well as how to prevent opportunistic infections in the adolescent who is HIV positive. It is important to teach the family about treatments, medications, nutrition guidelines, and signs and symptoms of opportunistic infections. Stress the importance of reporting even minor complications to the health care provider, and suggest ways to help support the adolescent (Table 19–3).

Although teaching the adolescent and the family all this information is necessary,

TABLE 19.3	Counseling Patients at Different Stages of HIV Infection
Stage	**Focus**
Immediately after learning of positive HIV test (regardless of disease stage)	Assist patient in accepting diagnosis and encourage him or her to verbalize feelings (anger, fear, hopelessness, etc.).
	Explain the difference between being HIV positive and having AIDS.
	Explain how HIV is spread (by direct contact with infected body fluids usually through sex, sharing needles, or blood transfusion).
	Counsel the patient on how to avoid transmitting the virus to others or contracting yet another strain.
	Teach the patient some safer sex strategies such as using condoms, dental dams; use role-playing to demonstrate how to negotiate the use of these barriers.
	Explain the pros and cons of contraceptives such as intrauterine devices, oral contraceptives, and nonoxynol-9 in women with HIV.
	Discuss why and how to notify sex partners of infection; explain that partners need counseling, testing, and, if HIV positive, referral for treatment; offer to help with the notification process if necessary.
	Discuss pregnancy and childbearing, as appropriate; explain rates of transmission from mother to newborn; suggest early prenatal care if patient is or becomes pregnant.
	If patient uses illicit, injectable drugs, explain how to sterilize needles with chlorine bleach: use a 5-to-1 ratio of water to bleach, draw up the mixture into the syringe two or three times, then flush with plain water.
	Discuss the importance of primary health care, and provide appropriate referrals.
	Provide educational literature on HIV, and refer patient to local support services and rehabilitation programs.
Asymptomatic, CD4 cells > 500 cells/μL blood	Review health maintenance activities: the need for regular gynecologic examinations and Pap smears, adequate diet, regular exercise, 8 to 10 hours sleep/night, cutting back on alcohol, tobacco, and use of recreational drugs (if not ready to stop use).
	Stress the importance of health care followup.
	Assess the patient's support systems: Does he or she have friends or relatives who can help out when symptoms develop? Does he or she have physical and economic access to health care? Refer to support groups, financial assistance programs.
Asymptomatic, CD4 cells >500 cells/μL blood, on antiretroviral medicines	Discuss prescribed drugs: indications, schedules doses, how to recognize and manage side effects.
	Discuss long-term family plans, especially arrangements for child (or children) at the parent's incapacity or death.
Visible symptoms: weight loss, thinning hair, darkening nails, skin rashes	Encourage small, frequent meals or suggest nutritional supplements, such as Ensure, to prevent weight loss.
	Offer strategies for masking signs of illness such as bright nail polish and attractive scarves or wigs.
	Explore ways for the patient to initiate age-appropriate discussion of HIV status with family.
	Counsel patient to specify guardianship for any child he or she has in a legal will.
	Discuss advanced directive alternatives available in your state such as do-not-resuscitate status and health care proxy options.
After hospitalization for opportunistic infection	Reassess home support, e.g., the need to call in a visiting nurse or volunteer buddy.
	Counsel patient to finalize do-not-resuscitate status or health care proxy arrangements per state.
End stage	Provide physical comfort through frequent turning on an air mattress, hydration therapy, lubricating skin massages.
	Acknowledge the anticipatory grief of family members and friends.

Kelly PJ, Holman S. (1993). The new face of AIDS. *AJN, 93*(3), 26–34. Used with permission. All rights reserved.

remember that a person can absorb only so much detail at one time. To teach them successfully and to be sure they understand the information, do not present too much information at one time. Give the family and the adolescent written materials that repeat the information, and review it verbally with them by asking questions and clarifying material until they show evidence of clear understanding of the concepts they need to know. While teaching, be sensitive to unspoken feelings and questions and carefully bring them into the discussion to provide the entire family with the best possible support and information.

EVALUATION: GOALS AND OUTCOME CRITERIA

- *Goal:* The adolescent will experience minimal risk of infection.
  Criteria: The adolescent practices good hygiene measures and identifies ways to prevent infection and ways to protect his or her health at home.
- *Goal:* The adolescent will not spread the disease to others.
  Criteria: The adolescent practices infection control measures and identifies sexual partners and safer sexual practices.
- *Goal:* The adolescent's skin integrity will remain intact.
  Criteria: The adolescent protects the skin and mucous membranes and promptly reports skin lesions or infections.
- *Goal:* The adolescent will experience minimal pain from complications of the disease.
  Criteria: The adolescent learns to manage pain and rests comfortably with minimal discomfort.
- *Goal:* The adolescent's food intake will meet his or her nutritional needs.
  Criteria: The adolescent eats nutritionally sound meals, includes frequent small meals in the food plan, and maintains his or her weight.
- *Goal:* The adolescent will not experience social isolation.
  Criteria: The adolescent voices fears about social isolation and makes and carries out plans to maintain relationships.
- *Goal:* The adolescent will make adjustments to his or her future expectations.
  Criteria: The adolescent expresses feelings about his or her future, seeks support from others, and begins to make realistic future plans.
- *Goal:* The family will show evidence of coping with the illness and supporting the teen.
  Criteria: The family expresses anxieties, voices understanding of the illness, and supports the adolescent in future plans.

Adolescent Pregnancy

The rate of adolescent pregnancy is about one in eight girls, resulting in 1 million adolescent pregnancies each year. About half of these result in live births; the remainder are aborted spontaneously or electively. The rate of adolescent pregnancy is higher in the United States than in any other country that keeps accurate statistics. The facts that a large number of the infants born to teenagers who are single mothers and that single-parent children are more likely to live in poverty increase the magnitude of the problem.

Many factors may contribute to the high rate of teen sexual activity and pregnancy. Adolescents are continuously bombarded with sex-oriented media. Teenagers have easy access to cars. They have less parental supervision including after school when many parents are still at work. Society is mobile and few people know their neighbors or feel responsible for them, so neighbors do not report a teen's activity as they might in closely-knit neighborhoods. Many teenagers have sex with no concern about the potential outcome. A lack of knowledge regarding fertility and contraception contribute to adolescent pregnancy. On the other hand, a girl may want to become pregnant to prove she is "grown up," to prove her femininity, to show self-assertion or hostility toward her family, or to fulfill a desire to have a baby who will love her and whom she can love. Adolescents may see motherhood as a form of economic survival with allotments of money, food stamps, and medical and dental care. They may see this as a way to escape economic oppression. Unfortunately they believe this will provide economic and personal independence. More than one of these reasons or other reasons may be involved in any teenage pregnancy.

The pregnant adolescent may have a poor record of success in school, a low self-image, poor family relationships, and inadequate financial means. She commonly receives inadequate prenatal care. These factors place her future and the future of her unborn infant in jeopardy.

Pregnancy is associated with its own developmental tasks that collide with the normal developmental tasks of adolescence often with unsatisfactory results. As an adolescent, the young woman is seeking independence; as an expectant mother with inadequate resources, she remains dependent. She is seeking identity, but the only identity she gains is that of a young, confused, at-risk mother-to-be. Her acute awareness of body image must accept the silhouette of pregnancy, which certainly is not in keeping with the slim figure desired by most adolescent girls. Pregnancy brings about many hormonal changes besides those that occur during adolescence. The adolescent's lack of knowledge about pregnancy and parenthood may cause her to have increased, unrealistic fears about herself and her pregnancy. As an adolescent, she is still trying to clarify her values and develop a positive self-concept, but the pregnancy will have a negative impact on her self-concept, especially if the father of the infant or her parents rejects her or her pregnancy.

Once pregnancy has been confirmed, the adolescent must decide whether to terminate the pregnancy by elective abortion or to carry it to term. If she chooses to have the baby, she must then decide whether to keep it or relinquish it for adoption. These are difficult choices particularly for a frightened, often unsupported, immature girl. Health professionals must provide the facts and guidance that will enable the girl to make an informed choice. School nurses, social workers, teachers, and counselors may be her only resources. Most pregnant adolescents choose to keep their babies, whether they marry the father or not. In many instances, the grandmother or grandparents of the newborn help raise the infant.

In most schools, the pregnant adolescent is encouraged to stay in school rather than drop out (Fig. 19–5). If this is not the case, the girl should be encouraged to continue her education elsewhere, even if it means relocation. Some urban schools sponsor prenatal classes and child care programs intended to encourage, support, and provide assistance to the girl in continuing her education throughout her pregnancy and parenthood.

Adolescent clinics are beginning to play a particularly important role in the management of teenage pregnancy. Many of these clinics use a team approach to work with the girl, her parents, and perhaps the young father; the physician, nurse practitioner or nurse midwife, nutritionist, and social worker offer understanding, supportive care, teaching, and counseling during the prenatal period and follow-up care after delivery. These clinics help reduce some of the risk factors common in a teen pregnancy by providing prenatal care in a comfortable, non-threatening atmosphere. If the adolescent has chosen abortion, these clinics also can provide follow-up care

and contraceptive counseling. Adolescent clinics offer care for STDs, HIV, substance abuse, and other adolescent health problems.

The adolescent has a higher incidence of pregnancy-induced hypertension, which places the infant at risk for inadequate circulation and the mother at risk for convulsions and death. The infant is more likely to be of low birth weight with possibly fatal complications. Nutrition of the mother and the fetus may be severely compromised, and social problems such as poverty and inadequate healthcare may occur that can affect the mother and infant for their entire lives.

Nurses who work with pregnant adolescents must resolve their own feelings to maintain a helpful, nonjudgmental attitude. These teenagers are fragile emotionally and mentally during this crisis. The nurse must develop a trusting relationship with the adolescent. Knowledge and understanding of adolescent psychosocial development are essential. Never fall into the habit of stereotyping adolescent mothers. As nurses work with the adolescent and develop a trusting relationship, they can help the girl look to the future and guide her in making realistic plans. The pregnant adolescent has many problems to face and needs strong support; with good prenatal and postnatal care and planning, the experience can become an opportunity for growth.

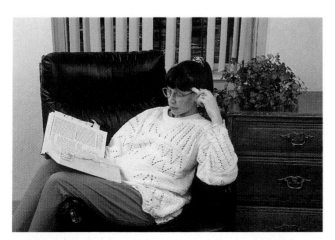

● **Figure 19.5** Although many adolescent mothers do not complete high school, some are able to continue and complete their education.

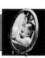

A PERSONAL GLIMPSE

Easter vacation of my junior year, I told my mom that I hadn't gotten my period for a long time. She asked me if there was any chance of me being pregnant. I said, "I don't know. Maybe." So we went to the store to get a pregnancy test. I took it and it turned dark pink immediately. When Mom told me I was pregnant, an immediate fear went through me and I started to cry. She gave me a hug and told me that I had to tell Brian (the father).

When I told him, I began to cry, because I thought for sure he was going to leave me. We sat down to talk about what we were going to do. I don't believe in abortion, but I just thought to myself, "I'm only 16! I didn't even get a chance to run around!"

But I decided to have the baby and not give it up for adoption. I kept thinking about getting fat and whether I'd be heavy after I had the baby. I cut way back on what I was eating so I wouldn't gain any weight. But when I went for a checkup they told me I had to start eating because the baby wouldn't develop right if I didn't.

(a personal glimpse continues on page 454)

A PERSONAL GLIMPSE continued

I was too scared to tell my dad, so I got Mom to call and tell him. He was so mad at me, and he just wanted to grab hold of Brian and put him in jail since he was 18. He didn't want me around him and said I was just following in my mother's footsteps and that I'd probably quit school. But then after a couple of months, Dad talked to Brian and me and he was excited about the baby. I told my dad I wasn't quitting school and that I was planning to go to nursing school.

My mom and grandparents were happy but they wished it wouldn't have happened to me, being so young. They all got pregnant young, too, so they knew what it was like.

I didn't want anyone at school to know because I thought everyone would just look down on me or just talk about me and call me a slut. I hid it the rest of my junior year, but by senior year needless to say I couldn't hide it anymore. The teachers were great. They didn't treat me any differently. I felt funny, though, because I was the only pregnant girl in school.

My girlfriends didn't care. In fact, they were excited and made bets on whether it would be a boy or a girl. Some of the guys didn't really care and still talked to me, but most of them just ignored me. I think that bugged me the most, because before I got pregnant the guys would be around me all the time. One guy who had been like a brother to me didn't even talk to me—maybe a "hi" now and then, but that was it.

Before I had my baby, I was scared of the unknown, but everything went great. Brian was even with me in the delivery room. And after I had her, I was so excited because I could still fit into my old jeans and I didn't even get stretch marks. Must have been the cocoa butter I rubbed on my stomach and butt all the time.

Sarah, age 19

> ▶ **LEARNING OPPORTUNITY:** What are some reactions that you might see in a teenager who finds herself pregnant? In the above situation, what do you think were the thoughts and feelings of the girl's boyfriend, mother, father, grandparents, and friends? As a nurse, what would be an appropriate response to each of these people in this situation?

Adolescent Fatherhood

Adolescent fathers are often overlooked in discussions about adolescent pregnancy. Recently, however, more emphasis has been placed on the adolescent father's role. Several factors affect the father's role in the pregnancy. The adolescent girl who has had multiple partners may not be sure who the father is or she may not care enough for the father to want to involve him in her pregnancy and her future. Many boys deny their role in the pregnancy or lose interest in the girl when she announces her pregnancy. All these factors help to determine the degree of responsibility that the teenage father takes. When a cooperative, interested father is involved in education about the pregnancy, parenthood, and future contraception, a better outlook for the couple can be expected. The adolescent couple commonly has serious financial problems and unrealistic expectations and may look forward to years of struggle. Support from the families of both adolescents can help improve the couple's future. The newborn that has two well-informed parents with a good support system clearly has a greater advantage than one who does not.

MALADAPTIVE RESPONSES TO THE STRESSES OF ADOLESCENCE

Adolescence is a time when the young person feels a sense of pressure and stress. Often the adolescent turns to maladaptive or unhealthy behaviors in an effort to find relief from stress. Substance abuse and suicide are two behaviors adolescents sometimes resort to in an attempt to decrease pressure.

Substance Abuse

Substance abuse is the misuse of an addictive substance that changes the user's mental state. The addictive substances commonly abused are tobacco, alcohol, and controlled or illicit drugs. Adolescents influenced by peers and in some instances adults in their family use drugs and alcohol to avoid facing their problems, escape and forget the pain of life as they see it, add excitement to social events, or bow to peer pressure. Throughout history, people have used alcohol and other mood-altering drugs as a means of relieving the tensions and pressures of their lives. Many cultures still sanction use of some of these substances but object to their *abuse* (excessive use or use in a way that is medically, socially, or culturally unacceptable).

Unfortunately frequent use or abuse of these substances can lead to addiction or **dependence** (a compulsive need to use a substance for its satisfying or pleasurable effects). Dependence may be psychological, physical, or both. Psychological dependence

COMMUNICATIONS BOX 19.1

Jenna, a 14-year-old, has come to the family planning clinic. She is in the exam room. Minimal information has been collected. She is picking at her clothes and seems very nervous.

LESS EFFECTIVE COMMUNICATION	*MORE EFFECTIVE COMMUNICATION*
Nurse: Hello, Jenna. I need to get some more information from you.	**Nurse:** Hello, Jenna. My name is Mrs. Kelley. Can you tell me how I can help you today?
Jenna: (Becoming somewhat defiant) Why do you have to ask so many questions?	**Jenna:** (Hesitantly) Well, I think I might be pregnant.
Nurse: You have to give us background information so we can take care of you.	**Nurse:** Tell me what makes you suspect that.
Jenna: Well, I don't want my family to know that I was here.	**Jenna:** I haven't had my period for 2 months.
Nurse: Oh, but we have to contact your parent or caregiver.	**Nurse:** Can you remember when you had your first period?
Jenna: (Loudly, with determination) Oh, no, you won't. I'll just not stay here if that's what happens.	**Jenna:** I was 10 years old, I think.
Nurse: You'll have to cooperate with us, Jenna.	**Nurse:** (Warmly) Good, you do remember. Jenna, can you tell me how sexually active you've been? I mean, how many sexual partners, and how often.
Jenna: (Very loud) Oh, no, I don't! I'm getting out of here.	**Jenna:** I only have had one boyfriend. We maybe have sex a couple times a month.
	Nurse: How does thinking that you may be pregnant make you feel?
	Jenna: Scared. And excited, too.
	Nurse: I can understand that. I would like to do an examination and take some tests, so we know just whether you are pregnant or if there is some other reason for your delayed period. We can deal with it one step at a time.
	Jenna: Okay.

▶ *The nurse has lost in this episode. Jenna will not be cooperative with him/her. Jenna gave many clues to her level of anxiety at the beginning by picking at her clothes and showing general signs of nervousness. The nurse did not read or at least did not respond to the signals. As Jenna showed more signs of anxiety by openly becoming defiant, the nurse simply dug in and plodded on. By not being sensitive to Jenna's signals, the nurse never even found out what the teen wanted.*

▶ *Throughout this interview, the nurse treated Jenna with respect and concern, starting by simply telling Jenna her name. This gives Jenna the feeling of value. Because Mrs. Kelley read Jenna's nervousness and showed her concern with gentle, open-ended questions, Jenna responded by giving the information and cooperation that were needed. Mrs. Kelley in no way was accusing Jenna of anything and carefully stated her questions to convey that message.*

---

means that the substance is desired for the effects or sensations it produces: alertness, euphoria, relaxation, a sense of well-being, and a false sense of control over problems. Physical dependence results from drug-induced changes in body tissue function that require the drug for normal activity. The magnitude of physical dependence determines the severity of **withdrawal symptoms** (physical and psychological symptoms that occur when the drug is no longer being used) such as vomiting, chills, tremors, and hallucinations. The symptoms vary with the amount, type, frequency, and duration of drug use. Continued use of an addictive substance can result in **tolerance** (the ability of body tissues to endure and adapt to continued or increased use of a substance); this dynamic means the drug user requires larger doses of the drug to produce the desired effect.

Four stages of use have been identified that help describe the progression of substance abuse (Table 19–4). Using the clues from these stages, the nurse who works in any capacity with adolescents can be more alert to signs of possible substance abuse.

TABLE 19.4	Progression of Substance Abuse in Adolescents		
Stage	**Predisposition**	**Behavior**	**Family Reaction**
Stage 1. Experimentation, Learning the Mood Swing			
Infrequent use of alcohol/ marijuana	Curiosity	Learning the mood	Often unaware
No consequences	Peer pressure	Feels good	Denial
Some fear of use	Attempt to assume adult role	Positive reinforcement	
Low tolerance		Can return to normal	
Stage 2. Seeking the Mood Swing			
Increasing frequency in use of various drugs	Impress others	Using to get high	Attempts at elimination
Minimal defensiveness	Social function	Pride in amount consumed	Blaming others
Tolerance	Modeling adult behavior	Used to relieve feelings (i.e., anxieties of dating)	
		Denial of problem	
Stage 3. Preoccupation with the Mood Swing			
Peer group activities revolve around use	Using to get loaded, not just high	Begins to violate values and rules	Conspiracy of silence
Steady supply		Use before and during school	Confrontation
Possible dealing			Reorganization with or without affected person
Few or no straight friends		Use despite consequences	
Consequences frequent		Solitary use	
		Trouble with school	
		Overdoses, "bad trips," blackouts	
		Promises to cut down or attempts to quit	
		Protection of supply, hides use from peers	
		Deterioration in physical condition	
Stage 4. Using to Feel Normal			
Continue to use despite adverse outcomes	Use to feel normal	Daily use	Frustration
Loss of control		Failure to meet expectations	Anger
Inability to stop		Loss of control	May give up
Compulsion		Paranoia	
		Suicide gestures, self-hate	
		Physical deterioration (poor eating and sleep habits)	

Adgar H. (1999) Adolescent drug abuse. In Oski FA (ed). *Principles and practice of pediatrics* (3rd ed). Philadelphia: Lippincott Williams & Wilkins.

The adolescents at greatest risk of becoming substance abusers are those who

- Have families where alcohol or drug abuse is or has been present
- Suffer from abuse, neglect, loss, or have no close relationships as a result of a dysfunctional family
- Have behavior problems such as aggressiveness or are excessively rebellious
- Are slow learners or have learning disabilities or attention deficit disorder
- Have problems with depression and low self-esteem

In some instances, early identification of these factors by family, teachers, counselors, or other care-givers and prompt referral for treatment can help avoid the potential tragedy of substance abuse.

The most effective and least expensive treatment for substance abuse is prevention beginning with education in the early school years. Information about drugs and about how to cope with problems without using drugs should be provided. "Scare" techniques are completely ineffective because they arouse disbelief and often add the tempting thrill of danger. The impact of educational programs may be diluted if the child comes from a home where alcohol or other drugs are used by family caregivers.

Alcohol Abuse

In many parts of American culture, drinking alcoholic beverages is considered acceptable and desirable social behavior. Although the purchase of alcohol is legally restricted to adults 21 years of age and older in all states and the District of Columbia, it is available in many homes and consequently is the first drug most adolescents try. It is also the most commonly abused drug among adolescents. **Alcohol abuse** occurs when a person ingests a quantity sufficient to cause intoxication (drunkenness). **Alcoholism** (chronic alcohol abuse or dependence) has reached epidemic proportions in America.

Drinking often begins in the late school-age years and increases in frequency throughout adolescence. Some adolescents use alcohol in combination with marijuana and other drugs, potentiating the effects of both substances and increasing the probability of intoxication.

Alcoholism is costly in dollars and in damage to the lives of alcohol abusers and their families. During adolescence, alcohol abuse is closely linked to automobile accidents. A car is another symbol of adult status and a means to escape adult supervision. Drinking with friends before or while driving often has tragic results. Most states determine charges of driving under the influence using a standard of 0.1% blood alcohol content, but many states have lowered the limit to 0.08%. Many adolescents do not realize that fine motor control and judgment are affected at even lower levels, and driving ability may be decreased. The number of fatal alcohol-related accidents involving adolescents has decreased because all states have set 21 years as the legal age for drinking, but the fatality rate still remains high.

Adolescents who receive treatment and counseling for problem drinking are more likely to recover than adults who have been problem drinkers over a long period. However, adolescents are difficult to treat due to their feelings of immortality and the rapid progression of the disease in adolescents.

Treatment. Alcoholism is not a weakness of character but a major chronic, progressive, and potentially fatal disease process that affects every organ of the body, mental health, and social competence. Alcoholism tendencies appear to be inherited, so children with a family history of alcoholism may be prone to alcohol problems. Treatment is lengthy and expensive and has no chance of success until the alcoholic acknowledges the problem and his or her helplessness to deal with it.

Treatment begins with detoxification ("drying out") and management of withdrawal symptoms. After that, a well-balanced diet, high-potency vitamins (especially vitamin B), and plenty of rest help to eliminate the disease's harmful side effects.

Counseling to identify and address the problems that led to compulsive drinking is an essential part of treatment. Many counselors who work with alcoholic patients are people who are recovering from a drinking problem themselves. This experience gives the counselor additional insight and empathy for the problem and the victim and adds credibility to the counseling offered.

Alcoholics Anonymous (AA), the best known of all self-help groups, offers fellowship and understanding to the compulsive drinker (website: http://www.alcoholics-anonymous.org). Chapters are available in every sizable community, and many have special programs for adolescents as well as for families of alcoholics (Alateen, Al-Anon, ACOA-Adult Children of Alcoholics). Anyone who has a desire to stop drinking is welcomed into AA and is helped to stay sober by taking it "one day at a time." Recovery from alcoholism is a lifetime matter. The earlier the problem is diagnosed, the better the person's chances to respond to treatment. Ongoing support from health professionals, peers, family, and community is essential to successful treatment.

Tobacco Abuse

Tobacco is a commonly abused drug among adolescents. *Any* use of tobacco is abuse. A high percentage of young people try tobacco, by either smoking or chewing. Many adolescents smoke because it gives them a feeling of maturity. Threats of long-term physical illnesses are far enough in the future that adolescents tend to ignore them. Many elementary and secondary schools have developed programs that warn children of the dangers of smoking, but the danger seems distant and children believe that they can quit any time they want to. The more immediate result of smoking that may stir interest in adolescents is the fact that their hair, breath, and clothes smell bad. Adolescents also have strong feelings of fairness and justice, so they may respond to the fact that children who are around persons who smoke are at increased risk for respiratory illness and cancer.

The use of "smokeless tobacco" (snuff or chewing tobacco) has increased steadily among adolescent males in the last several years. These teenagers believe that they are not damaging their lungs, but this type of tobacco use can cause mouth, lip, and throat cancers that are disfiguring and life-threatening.

Adolescents whose family caregivers smoke are especially prone to become smokers, and they have difficulty accepting the fact that they are seriously endangering themselves by smoking. Most hospitals, schools, and public buildings have adopted no-smoking policies. Perhaps the pressure of society will help deter smoking in the future. There is an effort at the federal level to discourage adolescents from beginning to smoke, but adolescents do not seem to be responding to the warnings. This may be due in part to the above-mentioned attitude among adolescents that nothing can hurt them.

Marijuana Abuse

The most frequently used illicit drug among adolescents is marijuana. The reported use of marijuana among adolescents has decreased somewhat, but smoking marijuana at a younger age appears to be a current trend. Many adolescents believe that marijuana smoking is not risky.

The effects of marijuana are mostly behavioral. It affects judgment, sense of time, and motivation. These effects make driving hazardous and may even cause hallucinations at higher doses. In addition, marijuana smoke is three to five times more carcinogenic than cigarette smoke. The marijuana available today may be three to five times more potent than that smoked in the 1960s. Because marijuana is illegal, no manufacturing control over it exists and the user has no idea where it came from or what additives may have been used. Nurses must make every effort to inform adolescents about the dangers of marijuana and to discourage them from using it.

Cocaine Abuse

Although cocaine may not rank among the first three drugs most commonly used by adolescents, it is an extremely dangerous drug. Use of cocaine and its derivative, "crack," had decreased among adolescents, but statistics indicate that cocaine use is no longer decreasing. Cocaine and crack use can be found everywhere from inner cities to rural neighborhoods.

Cocaine is a fine, white, powdery substance that directly affects the brain cells and causes physical and psychological effects. It usually is inhaled or smoked and is absorbed through the mucous membranes into the bloodstream. The physical results are an increase in pulse, respirations, blood pressure, and temperature. The psychological effect is a feeling of euphoria and increased sociability. The high is reached in about 20 minutes and lasts 20 to 30 minutes. In contrast, crack enters the bloodstream in about 30 seconds with a fast, powerful but short high that lasts only about 5 minutes. As a result of the rapid, short high from crack, users tend to seek repeated highs over a short period, decreasing the time it takes to become addicted. Because of the rapid absorption of crack, immediate cardiac arrest can occur from its use. After smoking crack, the user may experience a "crash" that causes depression. To relieve this depression, crack users turn to alcohol and marijuana. This multiple use further complicates the drug's effects. Some cocaine users inject cocaine to obtain a faster high, which adds to their risk of contracting HIV from contaminated needles.

Nurses must stress to adolescents the danger of using cocaine and crack. School education programs should start at the elementary level. Nurses can perform a community service by volunteering to present programs to local schoolchildren. Children and adolescents must be alerted to the dangers of these drugs and taught ways to refuse offers of drugs. A complete drug-education program also should include activities that help the students increase their feeling of self-worth.

Narcotics

The most commonly abused narcotics are morphine and heroin. These drugs decrease anger, sex drive, and hunger by producing a dreamlike, euphoric state. Highly addictive and extremely expensive, narcotics result in teenage prostitution, pushing (selling) drugs, and robbery as a means to support the drug habit. As mentioned earlier, any drugs that are injected subject adolescents to the added risk of contracting HIV from using contaminated needles.

Although heroin use in actual numbers is lower than that of other illicit drugs, adolescents' use of heroin has increased due to several factors. In general, there is a decrease among teens in the perceived danger of drug use. This trend seems to be evident across the entire scope of illicit drug use. Because heroin is now available in forms that can be smoked or snorted, the threat of HIV infection is no longer a deterrent.

Other Abused Drugs

Other mood-altering drugs commonly abused by adolescents include hallucinogens (psychedelic drugs), depressants, amphetamines, and analgesics. Anabolic steroids, although not mood-altering, are also abused by adolescents.

Hallucinogens (psychedelic drugs), although not addictive in a physical sense, can create a psychological dependence from the resulting hallucinations. This category of drugs includes LSD, PCP ("angel dust"), psilocybin (derived from mushrooms), mescaline, DMT (derived from plants), and airplane glue. These drugs cause distortions in vision, smell or hearing. Effects can include intoxication, "bad trips," flashbacks and overdosage. The drug known as Ecstasy is similar to amphetamines in chemical makeup, but it has the effect of elevating mood and increasing tactile sensations like the hallucinogens. Use of Ecstasy has increased dramatically in the adolescent population. The drug releases large amounts of serotonin, the neurotransmitter that regulates mood and emotion, and does not have the unpredictable effects of the other psychedelics. The drug is used in party and club settings where the users dance and party for extended periods of time; the drug suppresses their needs to eat, drink, or sleep.

Depressants, sometimes referred to as hypnotics, are as addictive as narcotics, and withdrawal from them must be carefully controlled to prevent delirium, seizures, or death. Barbiturates, glutethimide (Doriden), ethchlorvynol (Placidyl), and methaqualone (Quaalude) are the most commonly abused drugs in this group; they are sometimes used with alcohol, which increases the intoxicating effects such as sleepiness, slurred speech, and impaired cognitive and motor functions.

Amphetamines ("uppers" or "speed") produce increased alertness, wakefulness, reduced awareness of fatigue, and increased confidence and energy. Although not physically addicting, they encourage psychological dependence and are abused by millions of Americans, many of whom become trapped in a destructive cycle of uppers and "downers" (barbiturates). The amphetamines are often manufactured in "meth labs" in people's homes, which increases the potential dangers to the adolescent who uses these substances.

Adolescents abuse analgesics, particularly those that are combinations of narcotic and non-narcotics such as Percocet and Darvon. Chronic abuse can result in blood and kidney disorders. These drugs may be prescribed to a family member, which makes them easy for the adolescent to obtain.

Anabolic steroids are not mood-altering drugs, but their abuse among athletes is a cause for great concern. Adolescent athletes take the anabolic steroids to build up muscle mass in the belief that the drug will increase their athletic ability. These athletes take megadoses of illegally obtained drugs. Other adolescents may take them to build muscles and to achieve a "manly" appearance that they believe will make them more attractive. The side effects of euphoria and decreased fatigue make these drugs even more inviting to adolescents. Some use also has been reported in high school female athletes.

The use of excessively large doses of steroids may cause **gynecomastia** (excessive development of mammary glands in the male) or premature fusion of the long bones, which stunts growth in the adolescent who has not yet completed growth. Liver damage, predisposition to atherosclerosis, acne, hypertension, aggressiveness, and psychotic and manic symptoms also may result.[3] School programs about drug abuse should include the topic of anabolic steroid abuse.

Treatment. The best treatment for the abuse of all of these drugs is prevention. When prevention is ineffective, emergency care and long-term treatment become necessary. An overdose or a "bad trip" may force the adolescent to seek treatment. Emergency measures may even require artificial ventilation and oxygenation to restore normal respiration.

Long-term treatment involves many health professionals such as psychiatric nurses, psychologists or psychiatrists, social workers, drug rehabilitation counselors, and community health nurses. The teen is an important member of the treatment team and must admit the problem and the need for help and be willing to take an active part in treatment. Both outpatient and inpatient treatment programs are available. Many of these programs are geared specifically to adolescents. The human services section of the local telephone directory provides specific listings.

INTERNET EXERCISE 19.1

http://www.dancesafe.org/parents

Click on the section entitled "Communicating with your teenagers about drugs."
Read down to and including the section called "Communication Approaches."

1. What are four important communication methods suggested for parents to use in communicating with their teens?

2. List seven barriers that parents should be aware of when communicating with their teenage children.

Suicide

Suicide is one of the leading cause of death in adolescents 10 to 19 years of age; this falls just short of the homicide rate (see Fig. 18–9 in Chap. 18). Because some deaths reported as accidents, particularly one-car accidents, are thought to be suicides, the rate actually may be higher. Adolescent males commit suicide four times more often than girls, but girls attempt suicide five times more often than boys. Boys use more violent means of committing suicide than girls do and, therefore, are successful more often.

Adolescents who have attempted suicide once have a high risk of attempting it again, perhaps more effectively. Attempted suicide rarely occurs without warning and usually is preceded by a long history of emotional problems, difficulty forming relationships, feelings of rejection, and low self-esteem. Loss of one or both parents through death or divorce, a family history that includes suicide of one or more members, and lack of success in academic or athletic performance are other common contributing factors. To this history is added one or more of the normal developmental crises of adolescence: difficulty establishing independence, identity crisis, lack of intimate relationships, breakdown in family communication, a sense of alienation, or a conflict that interferes with problem solving. The adolescent's situation may be further complicated by an unwanted or unplanned pregnancy, alcohol or drug addiction, or physical or sexual abuse that lead to depression and a feeling of total hopelessness.

Health professionals involved with adolescents and family caregivers must be aware of factors that place a teen at risk for suicide as well as hints that signal an impending suicide attempt (see Family Teaching Tips: Adolescent Suicide Warning Signs for Caregivers). Some of these desperate young people will verbalize their hopelessness with statements such as "I won't be around much longer" or "After Monday, it won't matter anyhow." They may begin giving away prized possessions or appear suddenly elated after a long period of acting dejected. Never ignore these behaviors, and make an effort to ensure the teen's safety until counseling and treatment resources are in place. Strive to help the teen under-

stand that although suicide is an option in problem solving, it is a final option and other options exist that are not so final. Be aware of the community resources such as hotlines and counselors that specialize in working with persons who are contemplating or have attempted suicide.

During the initial interview with the adolescent, include questions that draw out feelings of alienation, depression, and hopelessness. If any of these indications are present, report and document these findings immediately. Question the family caregiver about any such signs and follow through with seeking additional help for the adolescent.

FAMILY TEACHING TIPS

Adolescent Suicide Warning Signs for Caregivers

WARNING SIGNS IN TEEN'S BEHAVIOR
1. Previous suicide attempt
2. Thoughts of wishing to kill self
3. Plans for self-destructive acts
4. Feeling "down in the dumps"
5. Withdrawal from social activities
6. Loss of pleasure in daily activities
7. Change in activity—increase or decrease
8. Poor concentration
9. Complaints of headaches, upset stomach, joint pains, frequent colds
10. Change in eating or sleeping patterns
11. Strong feelings of guilt, inadequacy, hopelessness
12. Preoccupation with thoughts of people dying, getting sick, or being injured
13. Substance abuse
14. Violence, truancy, stealing, or lying
15. Lack of judgment
16. Poor impulse control
17. Rapid swing in appropriateness of expressed emotions, sudden lift in mood
18. Pessimistic view of self and world
19. Saying goodbye
20. Giving things away

CHANGES IN TEEN'S INTERPERSONAL RELATIONSHIPS
1. Conflicts with peers
2. Loss of boyfriend or girlfriend
3. School problems—behavioral or academic
4. Feelings of great frustration, being misunderstood, or not being part of the group
5. Lack of positive support from family, peers, or other
6. Earlier suicide of family member, friend, or classmate
7. Separations, deaths, births, moves, or serious illnesses in the family

KEY POINTS

▸ For many teens, adolescence is filled with a multitude of problems. Minor problems can seem major and major ones seem insurmountable.

▸ Teens with a positive self-esteem and a supportive family environment are more likely to weather this turbulent time with fewer problems than those with a poor self-image, fewer successes, and an unfavorable home environment.

▸ The choices that adolescents make related to nutrition, friends and associates, alcohol and other drugs, sexuality, and school and career plans can affect their entire adult life.

▸ The primary objective in adolescent health care is prevention of health problems. Providing competent, compassionate care for adolescents with physiologic and psychological problems is the second objective; the third is to restore health as quickly and completely as possible.

▸ Motor vehicle accidents, homicide, and suicide are the leading causes of death among adolescents. Nurses play an important part in promoting adolescent safety.

▸ Health problems of adolescents include poor nutrition, sexually transmitted diseases, substance abuse, and suicide. Nurses must identify these problems and refer the adolescent and family for help.

REFERENCES

1. American Psychiatric Association. (2000) *Diagnostic and statistical manual of mental disorders, text revision* (4th ed). Washington, DC: APA.
2. Starke JR. (1999) Tuberculosis. In *Oski's pediatrics: Principles and practice* (3rd ed). Philadelphia: Lippincott Williams & Wilkins.
3. (2002) *Anabolic steroids: A threat to mind and body*. National

Institute of Drug Abuse research report, National Institutes of Health, retrieved from
http://www.thebody.com/nih/steroids

BIBLIOGRAPHY

Adger H. (1999) Adolescent drug abuse. In *Oski's pediatrics: Principles and practice* (3rd ed). Philadelphia: Lippincott Williams & Wilkins.

Adger H. (1999) Sexually transmitted diseases. In *Oski's pediatrics: Principles and practice* (3rd ed). Philadelphia: Lippincott Williams & Wilkins.

American Psychiatric Association. (2000) *Diagnostic and statistical manual of mental disorders, text revision* (4th ed). Washington, DC: APA.

Berger KS. (2001) *The developing person through the life span* (5th ed). New York: Worth Publishers.

Butensky EA. (2001) The role of nutrition in pediatric HIV/AIDS: A review of micronutrient research. *Journal of Pediatric Nursing*, 16(6), 402.

Craven RF. (2002) *Fundamentals of nursing: Human health and function*. Philadelphia: Lippincott Williams & Wilkins.

Hess D, DeBoer S. (2002) Emergency: Ecstasy. *American Journal of Nursing*, 102(4), 45.

Holzemer WL. (2002) HIV and AIDS: The symptom experience. *American Journal of Nursing*, 102(4), 48.

Joffe A. (1999) Eating disorders. In *Oski's pediatrics: Principles and practice* (3rd ed). Philadelphia: Lippincott Williams & Wilkins.

North American Nursing Diagnosis Association. (2001) *NANDA nursing diagnoses: Definitions and classification 2001–2001*. Philadelphia: NANDA.

Norris AE, Beaton MM. (2002) Who knows more about condoms? A comparison between nursing students, education students and at-risk adolescents. *American Journal of Maternal/Child Nursing*, 27(2), 103

Pillitteri A. (2003) *Maternal and child health nursing* (4th ed). Philadelphia: Lippincott Williams & Wilkins.

Renker PR. (2002) "Keep a blank face. I need to tell you what has been happening to me." Teens stories of abuse and violence before and during pregnancy. *American Journal of Maternal/Child Nursing*, 27(2), 109.

Rew L et al. (2001) Sexual abuse, alcohol and other drug use, and suicidal behaviors in homeless adolescents. *Issues in Comprehensive Pediatric Nursing*, 24(4), 225–40.

(2000) *Springhouse nurse's drug guide* (3rd ed). Springhouse, PA: Springhouse Corporation.

Sparks S, Taylor C. (2001) *Nursing diagnosis reference manual* (5th ed). Springhouse, PA: Springhouse Corporation.

Starke JR. (1999) Tuberculosis. In *Oski's pediatrics: Principles and practice* (3rd ed). Philadelphia: Lippincott Williams & Wilkins.

Story M, Strong J. (2000) *Nutrition and the pregnant adolescent a practical reference guide*. Minneapolis, MN: Centers for Leadership, Education and Training in Maternal and Child Nutrition.

Wong DL. (1998) *Whaley and Wong's nursing care of infants and children* (6th ed). St. Louis: Mosby.

Wong DL, Perry S, Hockenberry M . (2002) *Maternal child nursing care* (2nd ed). St. Louis: Mosby.

Wong DL, Hess C. (2000) *Wong and Whaley's clinical manual of pediatric nursing* (5th ed). St. Louis: Mosby.

Websites
Tobacco: *www.tobaccofreekids.org*
Alcohol: *www.ncadd.org*
STDs: *www.ashastd.org*
Pregnancy: *www.advocatesforyouth.*
Suicide: *www.suicidology.org*
www.dancesafe.org
www.clubdrugs.org

Workbook

NCLEX-STYLE REVIEW QUESTIONS

1. A nurse admits an adolescent girl with a diagnosis of possible anorexia nervosa. Of the following characteristics, which would MOST likely be seen in the adolescent with anorexia? The adolescent

   a. gets low grades in school

   b. has a sedentary life style

   c. freely express emotions

   d. follows a strict routine

2. The nurse is assisting with a physical exam on an adolescent diagnosed with bulimia. Of the following signs and symptoms, which would MOST likely be seen in the adolescent with bulimia?

   a. Dry skin

   b. Dental caries

   c. Low body weight

   d. Amenorrhea

3. In planning care for an adolescent with an eating disorder, which of the following goals would be MOST important for the adolescent? The adolescent will

   a. verbally express positive attitudes and feelings

   b. plan and participate in age appropriate activities

   c. maintain a fluid and electrolyte balance

   d. have normal bowel and bladder patterns

4. The nurse is discussing sexually transmitted diseases with a group of adolescents. If the adolescents make the following statements, which statement indicates a need for further teaching?

   a. "Even though guys don't like to use condoms, at least they protect a person from most STDs."

   b. "My girlfriend has never had sex with anyone except me, so I don't have to worry about STDs."

   c. "It is a relief to know that other than HIV, most STDs can be treated with antibiotics."

   d. "My girlfriend is pregnant but since she does not have an STD, our baby most likely won't either."

5. The nurse is discussing teenage depression and suicide with a group of caregivers of adolescent age children. If the caregivers made the following statements, which statement would require further data collection?

   a. "My child has so many ideas about how she can fix all the problems in the world."

   b. "She told me she is happy that she broke up with her long-time boyfriend."

   c. "My son enjoys spending all his time playing his CD player alone in his room."

   d. "My child eats all the time but never seems to want to go to sleep."

STUDY ACTIVITIES

1. Using the table below, compare the five most common sexually transmitted diseases (STDs) seen in adolescents. Describe the symptoms, treatment and complications or long-term concerns seen with these diseases.

2. Explore the options available in your community for a pregnant 10th-grade girl. Answer these questions: (a) Can she continue school? (b) What sources for maternity care are available if she has no health insurance? (c) Will child care be available to her after she has the baby so she can return to school?

3. Tanya, 16 years old, is 65 inches (165 cm) tall and weighs 98 lb (44.5 kg). She moans about how fat her thighs are. You believe she is anorexic. List the symptoms you will observe for in addition to her weight loss. A diagnosis of anorexia nervosa is confirmed for Tanya and she is hospitalized for treatment. Develop a nursing care plan for her.

Sexually Transmitted Disease (STD)	Symptoms	Treatment	Complications or Long-Term Concerns

CRITICAL THINKING

1. Brian is HIV positive and lives with his family. The family is frightened that other members may get the virus. Describe how you can reassure the family and help to prevent spread of the virus in the home. Identify the guidelines that you will give the family caregivers to help them protect Brian from infectious or opportunistic diseases.

2. Identify factors that put adolescents at greatest risk of becoming substance abusers. Make a list of these factors; for each factor describe what you think could be helpful in reducing this risk for adolescents.

3. Explain the most likely reasons why alcohol is the most commonly abused drug among adolescents.

Discuss your reasons with your peers and share ideas about what could be done to decrease alcohol use in adolescents in your community.

4. *Dosage Calculation:* An adolescent with a diagnosis of gonorrhea is being treated with Rocephin. The dose to be given is 250 mg IM. The medication is available in a preparation of 1 gram/10 ml. Answer the following:
   a. How many mg (milligrams) are in 1 gram?
   b. How many ml will be given to this adolescent?
   Following the administration of the Rocephin, the adolescent will be given doxycycline 100 mg bid by mouth for 7 days. Answer the following:
   a. How many mg will be given in a 24-hour period?
   b. How many total mg will be given in the 7 days?

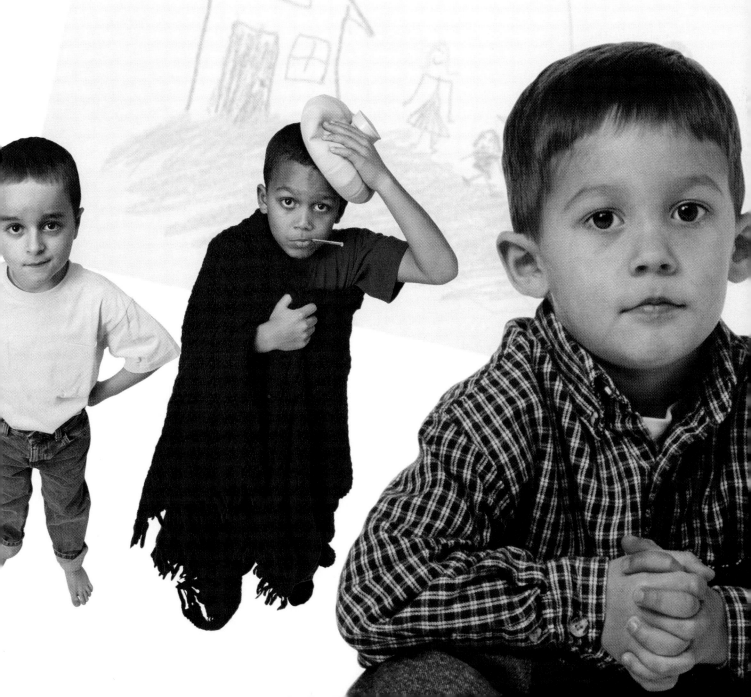

Care of the At-Risk Child

UNIT **4**

The Child in a Stressed Family

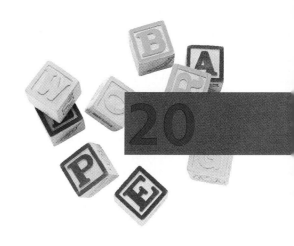

20

THE INFANT OF A SUBSTANCE-ABUSING MOTHER
  The Effects of Cocaine on the Neonate
  The Effects of Heroin and Other Opiates on the Neonate
  The Neonate With Fetal Alcohol Syndrome
PARENTS ADDICTED TO DRUGS OR ALCOHOL
  The Effect of Parental Substance Abuse on the Family
  Children Coping With Parental Addiction

CHILD ABUSE
  Physical Abuse
  Munchausen by Proxy Syndrome
  Emotional Abuse and Neglect
  Sexual Abuse
  Nursing Process in the Care of an Abused Child
THE RUNAWAY CHILD
THE LATCHKEY CHILD
DIVORCE AND THE CHILD
THE HOMELESS FAMILY

STUDENT OBJECTIVES

On completion of this chapter, the student will be able to

1. Identify the behaviors of the pregnant drug abuser that put her fetus in danger.
2. Describe the effects that cocaine abuse during pregnancy may have on the fetus.
3. Identify nursing care that may be helpful when caring for crack cocaine infants.
4. Describe characteristics of the infant with fetal alcohol syndrome.
5. Describe the unpredictable behavior of an addicted parent and its effect on the child.
6. List six behaviors that suggest there is an addiction problem in the child's family.
7. Identify how poor parenting skills may lead to child abuse.
8. State the amount of time that a health care facility can hold a child while investigating for possible child abuse.
9. Identify the circumstances under which physical punishment can be classified as abusive.
10. Describe the differences between bruises that occur accidentally to a young child and those that have been inflicted in an abusive manner.
11. Define Munchausen syndrome by proxy.
12. Identify ways that a child may be emotionally abused.
13. List the services offered by the National Runaway Switchboard.
14. Describe emotional reactions that a child may have to divorce.
15. Describe the effects of homelessness on the health care of children.

KEY TERMS

child neglect
co-dependent parent
dysfunctional family
fetal alcohol syndrome
incest
latchkey child
microcephaly
micrognathia
neonatal abstinence syndrome
palpebral fissures
philtrum
sexual abuse
sexual assault
teratogen

ubstance abuse is a family problem. If one member of the family abuses cigarettes, alcohol, or drugs, every member of that family is affected. The problem has grown to alarming proportions since the early 1980s. The number of infants born to substance-abusing mothers has grown consistently during this time, resulting in a large number of babies who face great physical and emotional challenges with few or limited family resources. In addition, children who have at least one parent who is a substance abuser are at risk for a variety of problems that researchers relate to substance abuse in the family. Behavior problems, school failures, and child abuse are just a few of the negative results that can occur.

THE INFANT OF A SUBSTANCE-ABUSING MOTHER

Maternal substance abuse takes an enormous toll on the unborn child. Most illicit drugs cross the placenta easily, and the concentration of these drugs in the fetus is estimated to be as high as 50% of that in the mother. Use of more than one drug at a time (polydrug use), including alcohol and cigarettes, is common among women. The compounded effect of these drugs further compromises the well-being of the fetus. Cigarette smoking, the most common form of substance abuse, impairs fetal development as severely as illicit drugs and alcohol. Even with an increase in available information and more prenatal teaching regarding nicotine and alcohol use, a large number of pregnant women continue to use nicotine and many continue to use alcohol, putting themselves at risk for alcohol-related prenatal problems.

Substance abuse occurs among women of all economic and social backgrounds. The pregnant substance abuser may have no prenatal care or may receive irregular care. Substance abuse is very difficult to overcome even for well-motivated pregnant women. Drug treatment programs tailored for pregnant and parenting women are cost-effective and have been proven to help them overcome their addiction problems and greatly improve birth outcomes. Unfortunately programs of this type are very difficult to find and are often overburdened when found.

The first trimester is the most dangerous time for fetal exposure to **teratogens.** In some cases the pregnant woman who is dependent on illicit drugs may be more interested to get her next supply of drugs than to keep an appointment. If the woman's financial status does not provide enough money for food, health care, and drugs, she may use her limited resources to get more drugs. As a result, the unborn child suffers not only from the effects of the drugs but from nutritional deprivation and inadequate care as well. In addition, the illicit drug abuser may be sexually promiscuous, perhaps practicing prostitution to obtain money to support her habit. Thus she puts herself and her unborn child at risk of sexually transmitted diseases. If she injects drugs, she also may be at great risk for HIV infection or hepatitis. Many women with a substance abuse problem deny or try to hide their drug dependence and avoid contact with health care workers for fear of detection.

The Effects of Cocaine on the Neonate

During pregnancy, cocaine (often used in the form of "crack" because it is cheaper) causes vasoconstriction of the placental blood vessels, which results in a variety of problems. Spontaneous abortion, premature birth, and premature separation of the placenta are common. The decrease in circulation to the fetus can cause intrauterine growth retardation. In addition, disorganized behavioral states may be detected both prenatally and postnatally. Serious congenital anomalies, which may include permanent neurologic damage, can occur as a result of polydrug use. Many cocaine users also use other drugs, specifically alcohol, marijuana, and cigarettes, and these further endanger the health of the fetus.

At birth, newborns who have been exposed to cocaine often are irritable, hyperactive, easily startled, and cry at any sound or even the softest touch. Most newborns of drug-dependent women show signs of withdrawal, also called **neonatal abstinence syndrome** (NAS). This syndrome is characterized by central nervous system hyperirritability, poor feeding, vomiting, diarrhea, respiratory distress, disturbed sleep patterns, shrill high-pitched cry, and convulsions. Also characteristic are vague autonomic symptoms including yawning, sneezing, sweating, stuffy nose, mottling, increased tearing, and fever. At birth, these infants commonly have a low birth weight and poor Apgar scores. The infant may not be able to take nutrition normally and may need gavage feeding. Breast-feeding is not attempted because cocaine can stay in breast milk for 60 hours after drug use.

Many of these newborns are admitted to the neonatal intensive care unit because of prematurity, very low birth weight, and other birth problems. At times, the mother may abandon the infant in the hospital, so the infant may be sent to a foster home when ready for discharge.

Nursing Care of the Cocaine-Exposed Infant

Caring for cocaine-exposed infants is challenging. They often suffer from poor sleep patterns, diarrhea, and dehydration. They commonly do not respond to the usual means of quieting infants such as swaddling, offering pacifiers, and rocking. Wrapping the infant securely with arms brought to the midline and holding him or her snugly against the body in an upright position may help. When the infant is rocked, the movement should be vertical (up and down) rather than the usual back-and-forth method. Reducing stimuli such as noise, bright lights, and sudden movements helps quiet the infant. Soft music also may help. These infants seem to take nourishment better when held upright and fed slowly. They may need to have smaller, more frequent feedings because they tire so quickly.

If the mother plans to take the baby home, intensive teaching is required. The mother should be drug-free and enrolled in a program to support her resolve to quit using drugs. The mother needs to learn basic parenting skills. In addition, the infant may show many signs that can be interpreted as rejection of the caregiver; the caregiver must understand that these behaviors are general reactions and not specifically directed at him or her. Provide caregivers with complete instructions including written materials. Be certain that the teaching materials are presented at a level and in language that the caregiver can understand.

Close home contact should be planned to follow up on the infant after discharge. The Brazelton Neonatal Assessment Scale (see Fig. 8–14 in Chap. 8) can be used to determine the progress of the infant's development. Encourage the caregiver to phone for help if there is a problem with the infant. Ongoing support for these families is essential.

The demand for foster care has risen with the increased use of crack cocaine. The children of families in which alcohol and other substances are abused tend to enter foster care at a younger age than children in the general population.[1]

The Effects of Heroin and Other Opiates on the Neonate

Crack cocaine has become the most commonly abused illicit drug since its appearance in the 1980s. However, heroin and other opiates continue to be used, and in some parts of the country heroin use is increasing. The death rate for neonates of heroin-addicted mothers is greater than that for babies of non-addicted mothers.

The effects of maternal abuse of these drugs are similar to those of crack cocaine. Hypoxia during labor may cause meconium staining and aspiration pneumonia in the newborn, contributing to increased illness and possible death. These infants often have jaundice, aspiration pneumonia, transient tachypnea, respiratory distress syndrome, and congenital malformations. Prenatal care is commonly poor. The infant may have a high-pitched cry and increased muscle tone and may be irritable. Infants of mothers who have been taking methadone have similar withdrawal symptoms. However, these infants may have a higher birth weight because, while in the methadone treatment program, the mother is required to have consistent prenatal care.

Withdrawal symptoms apparently are related to the mother's drug habit. Newborns whose mothers took large doses over a long period have the most severe withdrawal. Timing of withdrawal symptoms is related to how close to delivery the mother took heroin. The closer to delivery the last dose occurred, the later the withdrawal symptoms appear. These symptoms may continue for 2 months or more.

Nursing care of the infant of a heroin or opiate abuser is similar to the care of the infant of a cocaine-addicted mother. Paregoric is used to treat infants with opiate-induced NAS to manage the symptoms. Phenobarbital is used in infants with non-opiate NAS. Some physicians may prescribe the two drugs in combination.

The Neonate With Fetal Alcohol Syndrome

Alcohol is second only to nicotine as the substance most commonly abused by pregnant women. Any ingestion of alcohol during pregnancy is considered unwise. Even moderate maternal drinking has been demonstrated to produce infants with poor intrauterine growth and congenital anomalies, and heavy maternal drinking produces even greater abnormalities. The abnormalities characteristically seen in the infant whose mother consumed alcohol during pregnancy are commonly referred to as fetal alcohol effects (FAE) or **fetal alcohol syndrome** (FAS). Infants with FAS are shorter, weigh less, and may have **microcephaly** (small head), facial deformities, hearing disorders, poor coordination, minor joint and limb abnormalities, heart defects, delayed development, and mental retardation. The facial deformities are characteristic and include short **palpebral fissures** (opening between the eyes); a flat **philtrum** (vertical groove in the middle of the upper lip); a thin upper lip; a short, upturned nose; and **micrognathia** (a small lower jaw). Infants may have a few or many of these abnormalities. These neonates are jittery and may evidence failure to thrive (Fig. 20–1).

The fetus may be affected by a number of factors related to the mother's drinking. The alcoholic mother may be malnourished. She may have an alcohol-induced illness such as gastric hemorrhage or cirrhosis of the liver. Alcohol crosses the placenta

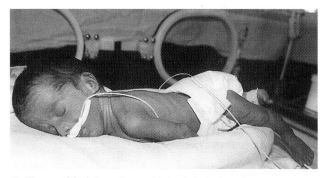

● *Figure 20.1* A newborn with fetal alcohol syndrome.

easily, directly affecting the fetus as well as being present in the amniotic fluid that the fetus ingests.

At birth, the infant may be hypoglycemic from the effect of the alcohol. All infants at risk should be screened with a reagent strip in the nursery within the first few hours after birth. Symptoms of neonatal hypoglycemia for which the nurse should be alert include tremors, lethargy, seizures, irregular respirations, and apnea. These neonates also may have respiratory distress syndrome.

Newborns with FAS need a quiet, non-stimulating environment. Intravenous fluids are administered as needed to avoid dehydration, and anticonvulsant drugs are administered if the infant is having seizures.

The number of infants believed to have FAE may be twice the number of those with FAS. Many of the infants with FAE are not clearly identified. The effects of FAE include alcohol-related physical features, growth retardation, and various cognitive deficits. They are believed to be, at least in part, the result of the mother's consuming lower levels of alcohol as well as possible genetic differences in susceptibility.

Infants and toddlers with FAS often have difficulty with feedings. They also may be hyperactive or have attention deficit disorders, intellectual slowness, poor fine-motor control, and developmental delay of gross motor skills. Children with FAS and FAE need a supportive educational environment throughout their school years.

✏ PARENTS ADDICTED TO DRUGS OR ALCOHOL

More than 10% of children come from a home affected by the alcoholism of one or both parents. Alcoholism exacts a terrible toll on the functioning of the family. Children of alcoholics are four times more likely to become alcoholics. When other substances are included, the number of affected homes increases substantially. Many women who abuse drugs and alcohol were themselves victims of physical, emotional, or sexual abuse as children.[2]

The Effect of Parental Substance Abuse on the Family

Developmental delays occur in young children of substance abusers. Infants of cocaine abusers avoid the caregiver's gaze, which contributes further to bonding delays. The parent who is addicted may be so involved in procuring the drug that any pretense of good parenting is forgotten. The parent, caught in the ups and downs of addiction, is not dependable and cannot provide any stability for the child. The parent may waver between overindulgence—smothering the child with attention, leniency, and gifts—and the opposite behavior of irritability, unreasonable accusations, threats, and anger. This unpredictable behavior has a severe impact on the relationships in the family. Children of substance-abusing parents often become loners and avoid relationships with others for fear that the substance-abusing parent might do or say something to embarrass them in front of their peers.

As the parent's substance abuse worsens, the family's dysfunction and social isolation increase. The **co-dependent parent** supports, directly or indirectly, the addictive behavior of the other parent. This behavior usually involves making excuses for the addict's actions and expecting others (i.e., the children) to overlook the parent's moodiness, erratic behavior, and consumption of alcohol or drugs. Co-dependency adds to the dilemma of children living with an addicted parent.

Children Coping With Parental Addiction

Children rarely talk about the parent's problem even to the other parent. These children often suffer from guilt, anxiety, confusion, anger, depression, and addictive behavior. Children react in a variety of ways. An older child, often a girl, may take on the responsibility of running the household, taking care of the younger children, making meals, and performing the tasks that the parent normally should do. These children may become overachievers in school but remain isolated emotionally from their peers and teachers. Another child in the family may try to deflect the embarrassment and anger of the other siblings by trying to make everyone feel good. As these children become adolescents or young adults, they may have problems such as substance abuse or eating disorders. The child in the family who "acts out" and engages in delinquent behavior is most likely to come to the attention of social services and be identified as a child who needs help.

Behaviors that may alert nurses and other health care personnel to an addiction problem in the family are

- The loner child who avoids interaction with class-mates
- The child who is failing in school or has numerous episodes of unexcused absences or truancy
- The child with frequent minor physical complaints such as headaches or stomach aches
- The child who steals or commits acts of violence
- The aggressive child
- The child who abuses drugs or alcohol

Nurses and others who work with children must be alert to these signals for help. Children can benefit from programs that support them and help them understand what is happening in the home. Such a program may include group therapy sessions at school in which the child learns that others have the same problems; this reduces his or her feelings of isolation. Other programs may include the whole family perhaps as part of the program for the addicted parent who is trying to break the addiction. Professional help is necessary to prevent the child from developing more serious problems. The earlier the child can be identified and treatment begun, the better the prognosis. Box 20–1 provides a list of resources for drug and alcohol problems.

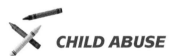

CHILD ABUSE

Every family faces many types of stress at one time or another. In addition to substance abuse, events that create stress for a family include illness, job loss, economic crisis or poverty, relocation, birth, death, and trauma. How the family handles these stresses affects greatly the emotional, social, and physical health of each member of the family. A **dysfunctional family** is one that cannot resolve these stresses and work through them in a positive, socially acceptable manner. The atmosphere in such a family creates additional stress for all family members. Because of the lack of support within the family for individual members, these members respond negatively to real or perceived problems. This may set the stage for child abuse, runaway children, substance abuse, and other unhealthy coping behaviors. Single-parent families often face multiple pressures at the same time; this dynamic creates additional stress and adds to the risk of dysfunctional coping.

Although child abuse has occurred throughout history, the evolution of cultural practices in the United States during the last few decades of the 20th century has emphasized the rights of children. Thus

---

BOX 20.1	Resources for Information and Help With Drug and Alcohol Problems

If you suspect your child may be using alcohol or drugs, you must confront the situation directly. Your doctor, local hospital, school social worker, or county mental health society may be able to refer you to a treatment facility.

A number of helpful national organizations are just a phone call away. If you have a computer and access to the internet, several groups also offer valuable information at their World Wide Web sites.

Center for Substance Abuse Treatment: For drug and alcohol information and referral, call 1-800-662-HELP. Web site: *www.samhsa.gov/centers/csat2002*

The National Clearinghouse for Alcohol and Drug Information: For pamphlets, publications, and materials for schools, call 1-800-SAY-NOTO. Web site: *www.health.org*

American Council for Drug Education: Call 1-800-488-DRUG.

National Families in Action: Call 404-248-9676. Web site: *www.emory.edu/NFIA*

National Family Partnership: Call 1-800-705-8897. Web site: *www.nfp.org*

PRIDE (Parents' Resource Institute for Drug Education): Call 770-458-9900. Web site: *www.prideusa.org*

Community Anti-Drug Coalitions of America: For information on current issues or legislation, call 1-800-54 CADCA. Web site: *www.cadca.org*

Al-Anon/Alateen Family Group Headquarters, Inc.: Call 1-800-356-9996. Web site: *www.al-anon.org*

Alcoholics Anonymous World Services: Check the phone directory for your local AA chapter or call 212-870-3400. Web site: *www.aa.org*

Nar-Anon Family Group Headquarters, Inc.: Call 310-547-5800. Web site: *www.naranon.com*

Partnership for a Drug-Free America: Web site: *www.drugfreeamerica.org*

U.S. Department of Education: Call 1-800-624-0010. Web site: *www.ed.gov*

National Criminal Justice Reference Service: Web site: *www.ncjrs.org*

Drug Free Kids *www.drugfreeusa.net*

---

any sort of mistreatment and abuse of children is regarded as unacceptable. The term *child abuse* has come to mean any intentional act of physical, emotional, or sexual abuse including acts of negligence committed by a person responsible for the care of the child.

Each year, increasing numbers of child abuse cases are brought to the attention of authorities. Estimates of the number of children treated in emergency departments following an episode of abuse range from 500,000 to 1 million annually. However, the actual number of abused children may be much higher, because many more cases may go undetected.

Child abuse is not limited to one age group and can be detected at any age. The courts have even viewed fetal exposure to drugs and alcohol as child abuse. Surprisingly, adolescents have the greatest incidence of abuse. For children younger than 2 years of age, the rate is estimated at six per 1,000; the rate for children 15 to 17 years of age escalates to more than 14 per 1,000.[3]

Child abuse has long-term as well as immediate effects. The abused child may be hyperactive, may exhibit angry, antisocial behavior, or may be especially withdrawn. Abusive parents often were abused themselves as children; thus the problem of child abuse continues in a cyclical fashion from generation to generation. Abusive parents can be found at all socioeconomic levels, but families with greater financial means may be able to evade detection more easily. Low-income families show greater evidence of violence, neglect, and sexual abuse according to some studies. Commonly, abusive parents have inadequate parenting skills; therefore, they have unrealistic expectations of the child and do not respond appropriately to the child's behavior.

State laws require health care personnel to report suspected child abuse. This requirement overrides the concern for confidentiality. Laws have been enacted that protect the nurse who reports suspected child abuse from reprisal by a caregiver (e.g., being sued for slander) even if it is found that the child's situation is not a result of abuse. If the nurse does not report suspected child abuse, the penalty for the nurse can be loss of the nursing license. Usually the health care facility can hold a child for 72 hours after suspected abuse has been reported so that a caseworker can investigate the charge. After this 72-hour period, a hearing is held to determine if the charges are true and to decide where the child should be placed.

Physical Abuse

Physical abuse often occurs when the caregiver is unfamiliar with normal child behavior. Inexperienced caregivers do not know what is normal behavior for a child and become frustrated when the child does not respond in the way they expect. Some young women become pregnant to have a child to love, and they expect that love to be returned in full measure. When the child resists the mother's control or seems to do the opposite of what she expects, the mother takes it as a personal affront and becomes angry, possibly responding with physical punishment. Some cultures support physical punishment for children, citing the old principle "Spare the rod, spoil the child." Despite evidence that physical punishment often results in negative behavior and that other forms of punishment are more effective, corporal punishment continues to be approved occasionally, even in some schools. However, physical punishment that leaves marks, causes injury, or threatens the child's physical or emotional well-being is considered abusive.

An important role of the health care team is to identify abusive or potentially abusive situations as early as possible. When a child is brought to a physician or hospital because of physical injuries, family caregivers may attribute the injury to some action of the child's that is not in keeping with the child's age or level of development. The caregiver may also attribute the injury to an action of a sibling. Whenever the child's symptoms do not match the injury the caregiver describes, be alert for possible abuse. However, do not accuse the caregiver before a complete investigation takes place.

Young, active children often have a number of bruises that occur from their usual activities. Most of these bruises occur over bony areas such as the knees, elbows, shins, and forehead. Bruises that occur in areas of soft tissue, such as the abdomen, buttocks, genitalia, thighs, and mouth, may be suspect (Fig. 20–2). Bruises in the inner aspect of the upper arms may indicate that the child raised the arms to protect the face and head from blows. Bruises may be distinctive in outline, clearly indicating the instrument that was used. Hangers, belt buckles, electrical cords, handprints, teeth (from biting), and sticks leave identifiable marks (Fig. 20–3). Bruises may be in varying stages of healing, which indicate that not all the injuries occurred during one episode

Signs or possible evidence of child abuse can be further evaluated by the use of technology. On a radiograph, bone fractures in various stages of healing may be noted. Spiral fractures of the long bones of a young child are not common, and their presence might indicate possible abuse. Infants who have been harshly shaken may not show a clear picture of abuse, but computed tomography scanning may demonstrate cerebral edema or cerebral hemorrhage.

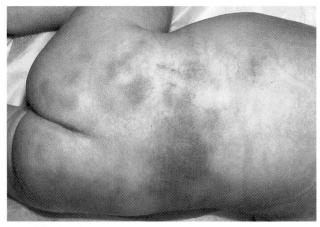

● **Figure 20.2** Bruises on a child's body may be caused by physical abuse.

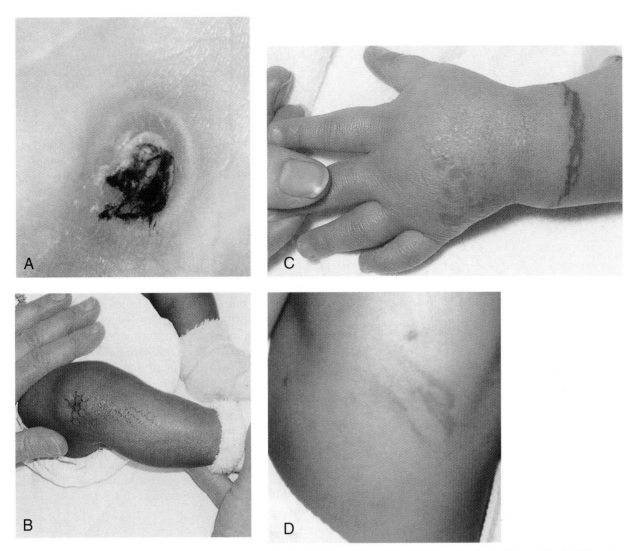

● **Figure 20.3 (A)** Cigarette burn on child's foot. **(B)** Imprint from a radiator cover. **(C)** Rope burn from being tied to crib rail. **(D)** Imprint from a looped electrical cord.

Burns are another common type of injury seen in the abused child (Fig. 20–4). Although burns may be accidental in young children, certain types of burns are highly suspicious. Cigarette burns, for example, are common abuse injuries. Burns from immersion of a hand in hot liquid, a hot register (as evidenced by the grid pattern), a steam iron, or a curling iron are not uncommon. Caregivers have been known to immerse the buttocks of a child in hot water if they thought the child was uncooperative in toilet training. Caregivers are often unaware of how quickly a child can be seriously burned. A burn that is neglected or not reported immediately must be considered suspicious until all the facts can be gathered and examined.

Munchausen by Proxy Syndrome

In Munchausen by proxy syndrome, one person either fabricates or induces illness in another to get attention. The child is frequently brought to a health care facility reporting symptoms of illness when the child is actually well. When injury to a child is involved, the mother is most often the person who has the syndrome. Often the mother injures the child to get the attention of medical personnel. She may slowly poison the child with prescription drugs, alcohol, or other drugs, or she may suffocate the child to cause apnea. Many times the symptoms are not easy to find on physical exam but are reported as history such as seizures or abdominal pain. The mother appears very attentive to the child and often is familiar with medical terminology. This situation is frustrating for health care personnel because it is difficult to catch the suspect in the act of endangering the child. Close observation of the caregiver's interactions with the child is necessary. For instance, if episodes of apnea occur only in the presence of the caregiver, be alert for this syndrome. The caregiver who suffers from this syndrome must receive psychiatric help.

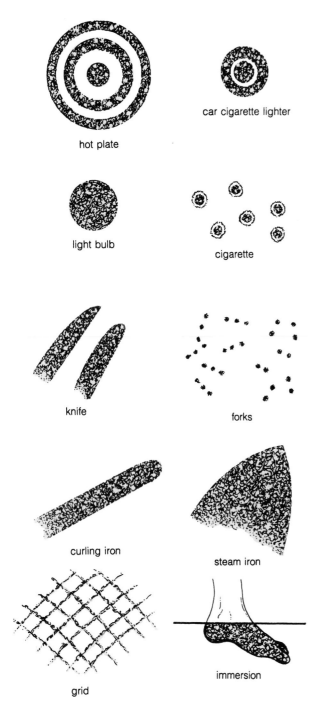

● *Figure 20.4* Burn patterns from objects used for inflicting burns in child abuse.

Emotional Abuse and Neglect

Injury from emotional abuse can be just as serious and lasting as that from physical abuse, but it is much more difficult to identify. Several types of emotional abuse can occur, including

- Verbal abuse such as humiliation, scapegoating, unrealistic expectations with belittling, and erratic discipline

- Emotional unavailability when caregivers are absorbed in their own problems
- Insufficient or poor nurturing or threatening to leave the child or otherwise end the relationship
- Role reversal in which the child must take on the role of parenting the parent and is blamed for the parent's problems

Children may show evidence of emotional abuse by appearing worried or fearful or having vague complaints of illness or nightmares. Caregivers may display signs of inappropriate expectations of the child when in the health care facility by sometimes mocking or belittling the child for age-appropriate behavior. In young children, failure to thrive may be a sign of emotional abuse. In the older child, poor school performance and attendance, poor self-esteem, and poor peer relationships may be clues.

Child neglect is failure to provide adequate hygiene, health care, nutrition, love, nurturing, and supervision needed for growth and development. If a child is not given adequate care for a serious medical condition, the caregivers are considered neglectful. For example, if a child is seriously burned, even accidentally, and the caregivers do not take the child for evaluation and treatment until several days later, they may be judged to be neglectful. Often the child with failure to thrive as a result of being underfed, deprived of love, or constantly criticized can be classified as neglected; however, be careful not to make an unsubstantiated accusation of neglect.

Sexual Abuse

Sexual abuse of children has existed in all ages and cultures, but it seldom has been admitted when perpetrated by parents or other relatives in the home. **Incest** (sexually arousing physical contact between family members not married to each other) occurs in an estimated 240,000 to 1 million American families annually, and that number is growing each year. As with other types of child abuse, sexual abuse knows no socioeconomic, racial, religious, or ethnic boundaries. However, substance abuse, job loss, and poverty are contributing factors. Like other forms of child abuse, sexual abuse is being recognized and reported more often. The National Center on Child Abuse and Neglect defines **sexual abuse** as contacts or interactions between a child and an adult when the child is being used for sexual stimulation of the perpetrator or other person. When a person has power or control over a child, that person, even if a child, can be a sexual abuser. For example, someone who is the same age but bigger or stronger could sexually abuse a child his or her own age.

Several terms are commonly used when sexual abuse is discussed. From a legal viewpoint, sexual contact between a child and another person in a care-taking position, such as a parent, babysitter, or teacher, is classified as sexual abuse. A sexual contact made by someone who is not functioning in a caretaker role is classified as **sexual assault.** Incest includes fondling of breasts or genitalia, intercourse (vaginal or anal), oral-genital contact, exhibitionism, and voyeurism.

Regardless of the relationship of the perpetrator to the child, the outcome of the abuse is devastating. Episodes of sexual abuse that involve a person whom the child trusts seem to be the most damaging. Incest often goes unreported because the person committing the act uses intimidation by means of threats, appeals to the child's desire to be loved and to please, and convinces the child of the importance of keeping the act secret.

When a child is sexually assaulted by a stranger, the caregivers usually become aware of the incident, promptly report it, and take the child for a physical examination. However, in the case of incest, the child rarely tells another person what is happening. The child may exhibit physical complaints such as various aches and pains, gastrointestinal upsets, changes in bowel and bladder habits (including enuresis), nightmares, and acts of aggression or hostility. Some of these complaints or behaviors may be the presenting problem when a health care provider sees the child.

● Nursing Process in the Care of an Abused Child

ASSESSMENT

When assessing a child who may have been abused or neglected, the healthcare provider must be thorough and complete in observation and documentation. The child should have a complete physical exam; all bruises, blemishes, lacerations, areas of redness and irritation, and marks of any kind on the child's body must be carefully described and accurately documented. It may be necessary to request that photographs be taken. Observe the interaction between the child and the caregiver, and carefully document your observations using nonjudgmental terms. The child's body language may be revealing, so be alert for significant information. For example, if the child shrinks away from contact by the caregiver or health care practitioner or, on the other hand, is especially clinging to the caregiver, watch for other signs of inappropriate behavior. These assessments vary with the child's age (Table 20–1).

Perhaps the most difficult part may be to maintain a nonjudgmental attitude throughout the interview and examination. Be calm and reassuring with the child; let the child lead the way when possible.

NURSING DIAGNOSES

The nursing diagnoses vary with the type of abuse or neglect that the child may have experienced. Appropriate nursing diagnoses for a child with a fracture, for example, include care before and after the fracture has been set and cast. Various nursing diagnoses are appropriate for the care of a child with burns based on the care needed for the burns. A child who is nutritionally deprived needs diagnoses that address nutritional needs. Additional nursing diagnoses that may be used are

- Anxiety/Fear by child related to history of abuse and fear of abuse from others
- Ineffective Individual Coping by the nonabusive parent related to fear of violence from abusive partner or feelings of powerlessness
- Impaired Parenting related to situational stressors or poor coping skills
- Disabled Family Coping related to unrealistic expectations of child by parent

OUTCOME IDENTIFICATION AND PLANNING

Major goals for the abused child include caring for any injuries the child has sustained as well as relieving anxiety and fear. An important family goal is to improve coping skills of the caregiver or family.

IMPLEMENTATION

Relieving the Child's Anxiety and Fear. Observe the child for behavior that indicates anxiety or fear such as withdrawal, ducking or shying away from the nurse or caregivers, and avoiding eye contact. Assign one nurse to care for the child so that the child can relate to one person consistently. Provide physical contact such as hugging, rocking, and caressing only if the child accepts it. Identify nursing actions that seem to comfort the child, and use them consistently. Use a calm, reassuring, and kind manner, and provide a safe atmosphere in which the child has an opportunity to express feelings and fears. Use play to help the child express some of these emotions. Be careful not to do anything that might alarm or upset the

TABLE 20.1	Signs of Abuse in Children
Physical Signs	**Behavioral Signs**

Physical Signs	Behavioral Signs
Physical Abuse	
Bruises and welts: may be on multiple body surfaces or soft tissue; may form regular pattern (e.g., belt buckle)	Less compliant than average
	Signs of negativism, unhappiness
Burns: cigar or cigarette, immersion (stocking/glovelike on extremities or doughnut-shaped on buttocks or genitals), or patterned as an electrical appliance (e.g., iron)	Anger, isolation
	Destructive
	Abusive toward others
Fractures: single or multiple; may be in various stages of healing	Difficulty developing relationships
	Either excessive or absent separation anxiety
Lacerations or abrasions: rope burns; tears in and around mouth, eyes, ears, genitalia	Inappropriate caretaking concern for parent
	Constantly in search of attention, favors, food, etc.
Abdominal injuries: ruptured or injured internal organs	Various developmental delays (cognitive, language, motor)
Central nervous system injuries: subdural hematoma, retinal or subarachnoid hemorrhage	
Physical Neglect	
Malnutrition	Lack of appropriate adult supervision
Repeated episodes of pica	Repeated ingestions of harmful substances
Constant fatigue of listlessness	Poor school attendance
Poor hygiene	Exploitation (forced to beg or steal; excessive household work)
Inadequate clothing for circumstances	Role reversal with parent
Inadequate medical or dental care	Drug or alcohol use
Sexual Abuse	
Difficulty walking or sitting	Direct or indirect disclosure to relative, friend, or teacher
Thickening or hyperpigmentation of labial skin	Withdrawal with excessive dependency
Vaginal opening measures >4 mm horizontally in preadolescence	Poor peer relationships
	Poor self-esteem
Torn, stained, or bloody underclothing	Frightened or phobic of adults
Bruises or bleeding of genitalia or perianal area	Sudden decline in academic performance
Lax rectal tone	Pseudomature personality development
Vaginal discharge	Suicide attempts
Recurrent urinary tract infections	Regressive behavior
Nonspecific vaginitis	Enuresis or encopresis
Venereal disease	Excessive masturbation
Sperm or acid phosphatase on body or clothes	Highly sexualized play
Pregnancy	Sexual promiscuity
Emotional Abuse	
Delays in physical development	Distinct emotional symptoms or functional limitations
Failure to thrive	Deteriorating conduct
	Increased anxiety
	Apathy or depression
	Developmental lags

child. Psychological support is provided through social services or an abuse team.

Supporting the Nonabusive Caregiver. In some cases, one caregiver in the family may be an abuser while the other is not. The nonabusive caregiver is a victim as well as the child. Give the nonabusive caregiver an opportunity to express fears and anxieties. He or she may feel powerless in the situation. Help the passive caregiver decide whether to continue the

relationship or leave it. Try to preserve the caregiver's self-esteem as this is not an easy decision to make. Remember that confidentiality is essential when discussing such problems.

Observing Interaction Between the Caregiver and Child. While caring for the abused child when the caregiver is present, take the opportunity to observe how the caregiver relates to the child and how the child reacts to the caregiver. Give the caregiver the same courtesy extended to all caregivers. Offer a compliment when the caregiver does something well in caring for the child. Give the caregiver an opportunity to discuss in private any concerns; during this time, you may be able to gain his or her confidence.

Promoting Parenting Skills. Often abuse occurs when a caregiver is unfamiliar with normal growth and development and the behaviors common to a particular stage of development. Help the caregiver develop realistic expectations of the child. To help accomplish this goal, design a teaching plan and include the caregiver in caring for the child. Teach the caregiver the child's expected responses and help him or her learn about normal development. Praise the caregiver for displaying positive behaviors. Point out specific behaviors of the child and explain them to the caregiver. Explore the reasons for the caregiver's absence when he or she does not visit regularly. Discuss specific behaviors of the child that are upsetting to the caregiver and explain that these are common for the child's age.

The caregiver may be facing temporary or permanent placement of the child in another home. Help the caregiver and the child accept this change. Emotions that a caregiver has had over a long period cannot be easily switched off. The assistance of social services and a child life specialist is beneficial in these situations. Act as a member of the team to aid in the transition. The foster parents may need support from the nursing staff to help ease the child's transition to the new home. Abused children must be followed carefully after discharge from the health care facility to ensure that their well-being is protected.

EVALUATION: GOALS AND OUTCOME CRITERIA

- *Goal:* The child will exhibit decreased signs of anxiety and fear.
  Criteria: The child's play, facial expressions, and posture are relaxed; the child displays no withdrawal or guarding during contacts with the nursing staff.
- *Goal:* The nonabusive caregiver will begin to cope with fears and feelings of powerlessness.
  Criteria: The nonabusive caregiver expresses fears and concerns and makes plans to resolve problems.

- *Goal:* The caregiver will exhibit positive interaction with the child.
  Criteria: The caregiver talks with the child, is sensitive to his or her needs, and refrains from making unreasonable demands on the child.
- *Goal:* The caregiver will be involved in the child's care and will verbalize examples of normal growth and development and ways to handle the child's misbehavior.
  Criteria: The caregiver states age-appropriate behavior for the child, discusses ways to handle the child's irritating behavior, and is involved in counseling or other discharge plans.

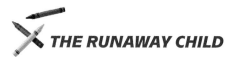

THE RUNAWAY CHILD

In the United States, as many as 750,000 to 2 million adolescents run away from home each year. A child can be considered a runaway after being absent from home overnight or longer without permission from a family caregiver. Most children who run away from home are 10 to 17 years of age.

A child may run away from home in response to circumstances that he or she views as too difficult to tolerate. Physical or sexual abuse, alcohol or drug abuse, divorce, stepfamilies, pregnancy, school failure, and truancy may contribute to a child's desire to escape. However, some adolescents are not runaways but rather "throwaways" who have been forced to leave home and are not wanted by the adults in the home. Often the throwaways have been forced out of the home because their behavior is unacceptable to family caregivers or because of other family stresses such as divorce, remarriage, and job loss.

Runaway or throwaway adolescents often turn to stealing, drug dealing, and prostitution to provide money for alcohol, drugs, food, and, possibly, shelter. Many of these adolescents live on the streets because they cannot pay for shelter; they avoid going to public shelters for fear of being found by police. They may become victims of pimps or drug dealers who use the adolescents for their own gain.

There are numerous programs to help runaways, especially in urban areas. A 24-hour National Runaway Switchboard (1-800-621-4000) is available to give runaways information and referral (website: *http:// www.nrscrisisline.org*). This service may help the runaway to find a safe place to stay and may provide counseling, shelter, health care, legal aid, message relay to the family, and transportation home if desired. Runaways are not forced to go home but may be encouraged to inform their family that they are all right. Other free hotline numbers are also available.

A sexually transmitted disease, pregnancy, AIDS, or drug overdose are the usual reasons that runaways are seen at a health care facility. When caring for such a child, be nonjudgmental. Any indication of being disturbed or disgusted by the adolescent's lifestyle may end any chance of cooperation and cause the adolescent to refuse to give any additional information. Try to build a trusting relationship with the child. Remember that the runaway viewed his or her problems as so great that escaping was the only way to resolve them. Counseling is necessary to begin to resolve the problems.

Health teaching for the runaway must be suited to his or her lifestyle and must be at a level the child can understand. Without prying excessively, try to find out the runaway's living circumstances and adjust the teaching plans accordingly. Remember that the child's problems did not come about overnight, nor will they be resolved quickly. Caring for a runaway can be frustrating, challenging, and sometimes rewarding for the health care staff.

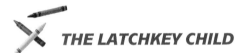

THE LATCHKEY CHILD

As a result of the increased number of families in which both parents work and the increase in single-parent families in which the parent must work, many children need after-school care and supervision; unfortunately, adequate or appropriate child care may not be readily available. A **latchkey child** is one who comes home to an empty house after school each day because the family caregivers are at work. The term was coined because this child often wears the house key around her or his neck. These children usually spend several hours alone before an adult comes home from work. The number of latchkey children may be as high as 10 million in the United States.

Latchkey children often have fears about being at home alone. When more than one child is involved and the older child is responsible for the younger one, conflicts can arise. The older child may have to assume responsibility that is beyond the normal expectations for the child's age. This can be a difficult situation for the caregivers and the children. The caregivers must carefully outline permissible activities and safety rules (Fig. 20–5). A plan should be in place to help the older child solve any arising problems that involve both children. The older child should not feel that the complete responsibility is on his or her shoulders but rather that it is a shared responsibility

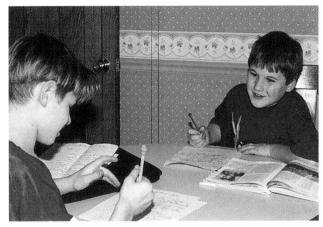

● *Figure 20.5* A 12-year-old boy and his 9-year-old brother come home to an empty house after school with specific rules about activities to be done as they wait the arrival of their caregiver.

with the caregiver. Some schools have after-school latchkey programs that provide safe activities for children. In addition, some communities have programs in which an adult telephones the child regularly every day after school or there is a telephone hotline that the child can call (see Family Teaching Tips: Tips for Latchkey Children).

Despite concerns that latchkey children are more likely to become involved with smoking, stealing, or taking drugs, researchers have not found sufficient data to support this fear. Children who are given responsibility of this kind and who are recognized for their dependability usually live up to the expectations of the adults in their social environment.

INTERNET EXERCISE 20.1

www.missingkids.org

On the left hand side of screen, click on the area that says, "Education and Resources."
Scroll down.
Click on "Know the Rules: After-school safety tips for children who are home alone."
Read section entitled "Maturity . . . not age . . . should be determining factor."

1. List two questions that parents should ask themselves when considering leaving a child at home alone.

2. List six factors that a parent should consider before allowing a child to stay home alone.

Nurses must recognize the need for after-school services for these children and take an active role in the community to plan and support such services. Maintain a list of the facilities available to support families with latchkey children. The nurse can give caregivers guidance in planning children's after-

FAMILY TEACHING TIPS

Tips for Latchkey Children

1. Teach the child to keep the key hidden and not show it to anyone.
2. Plan with the child the routine to follow when arriving home; plan something special each day.
3. Plan a telephone contact on the child's arrival home; either have the child call you or you call the child.
4. Always let the child know if you are going to be delayed.
5. Review safety rules with the child. Post them on the refrigerator as a reminder.
6. Use a refrigerator chart to spell out daily responsibilities, and have the child check off tasks as they are completed.
7. Let the child know how much you appreciate his or her responsible behavior.
8. Have a trusted neighbor for backup if the child needs help; be sure the child knows the telephone number, and post it by the phone.
9. Post telephone emergency numbers that the child can use; practice when to use them.
10. Teach the child to tell telephone callers that the caregiver is busy but never to say that the caregiver is not home.
11. Teach the child not to open the door to anyone.
12. Be specific about activities allowed and not allowed.
13. Carefully survey your home for any hazards or dangerous temptations (e.g., guns, motorcycle, ATV, swimming pool). Eliminate them, if possible, or ensure that rules about them are clear.
14. See if your community has a telephone friend program available for latchkey children.
15. A pet can relieve loneliness, but give the child clear guidelines about care of the pet during your absence.

school activities and offer support to the caregivers in their attempts to provide for their children.

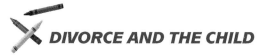

DIVORCE AND THE CHILD

Divorce has increased to the point where one in two marriages ends in divorce. About 50% of children experience the separation or divorce of their parents before they complete high school. Some children may experience more than one divorce because many of those who remarry divorce a second time. Divorce can be traumatic for children but may be better than the constant tension and turmoil that they have lived through in their home.

Children often feel responsible for the breakup and believe that it would not have occurred if they had just done the right thing or been good. On the other hand, children may blame one of the parents for deciding to end the marriage and causing the children grief and unhappiness. Children commonly feel unloved and, in a sense, feel that they too are being divorced. Counseling can help children to acknowledge and understand their anger and their need to blame one or the other parent. This process may take a considerable amount of time to resolve. Both parents should make every effort to eliminate the child's feeling of guilt and should avoid using the child as a spy or go-between with the estranged spouse. Parents must avoid trying to buy the affection of the children. This is especially true for the noncustodial parent, who must not shower the children with special gifts, trips, and privileges when the children are visiting.

Children should be encouraged to ask questions about the separation and divorce. A child who does not ask questions may be afraid to ask for fear of retaliation by one of the parents. Children should be discouraged from thinking that they might be able to do something that would get the parents back together again. They must be helped to recognize the finality of the divorce. Plans for the children should be made (e.g., where and with whom the children will live, where they will go to school) and shared with the children as soon as possible. This can give the children a sense of security in their chaotic personal world. Each child's confidence and self-esteem must be strengthened through careful handling of the transition (Fig. 20–6).

When a child of a divorce is hospitalized, the nurse must be certain to have clear information about who is the custodial parent as well as who may visit or otherwise contact the child. The custodial parent's instructions and wishes should be honored.

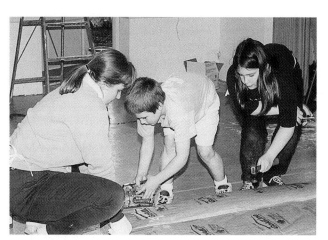

● *Figure 20.6* These school-age children feel more secure and build their confidence as they do a project together with their newly divorced mother.

The nurse may encourage the child to express feelings of fear and guilt. The nurse also can help the child understand that other children have divorced parents. The school nurse may function as an advocate for a counseling program in the school setting that brings together children of divorces. During counseling, children can voice their fears and concerns and begin to work through them with the help of an objective counselor in a protected environment. One of the most important aspects of such groups is the reassurance the children get that they are not alone in this crisis.

When the custodial parent begins to date and plans to remarry, the child may again have strong emotions that must be worked through. If the remar-

riage brings together a blended family of children from the previous marriages of both adults, the children may need extra support in accepting the new stepparent and stepsiblings. Adults who seek preventive counseling when planning to form a stepfamily have greater success than those who seek help only after problems are overwhelming.

Children react in various ways to a parent's new marriage, depending in part on age. The new marriage may introduce additional problems of a new home, a new neighborhood, and a new school that can cause anxiety for any child. Although children should not be permitted to veto the parent's choice of a new partner, every effort should be made to help them adjust to this new family member and view the change in a non-threatening way.

A PERSONAL GLIMPSE

When I was 15, my dad told me that he and my mom were getting a divorce. I think he expected me to be sad or surprised, but really I was relieved. I hated living in a house with parents fighting all the time or just not talking to each other. Also I didn't think it was good for my younger brother.

Though I was happy that the era of fighting was over, the time after the divorce was difficult. Both my parents were very mean to one another, while trying to get me to take sides. I felt they were too concerned with their own lives. I was mad at them for the way they were acting and I didn't think they were being good parents. I figured that I could take care of myself and my brother better than they could; so I changed a lot. I had parties while I was babysitting, stayed out past curfew, skipped classes and studied less, and contradicted my parents' rules for my brother. I thought I was acting like an adult by making my own decisions and not caring about what my parents thought, but really I was acting more childish than ever before. The worst part was that I put myself and my brother in a lot of danger.

It would have been better for me to work with my parents than against them. I just didn't realize how hard it was for them; after all, I thought the divorce was a great idea. I wish they had confided in me. I think I would have understood. I also wish I had told them how I felt. I think they assumed I wasn't angry because I was okay with them getting a divorce.

Joelle, age 24

> ▶ **LEARNING OPPORTUNITY:** What are some ways in which children deal with their parents' divorce? Describe the ways in which you think divorce is different for the adolescent child than for the younger child.

THE HOMELESS FAMILY

A growing number of families are homeless in the United States. The causes of homelessness include job loss, loss of housing, drug addiction of adult caregivers, insufficient income, domestic turmoil, and separation or divorce. Single mothers with children make up an increasing number of these families. Many of these homeless single mothers and their families have multiple problems. Often there are higher rates of abuse, drug use, and mental health problems in homeless families. Many of these families lived with relatives for a time before being reduced to living in a car, an empty building, a welfare hotel, or perhaps a cardboard box. These families sometimes seek temporary housing in a shelter for the homeless. They often move from one living situation to another, living in a shelter for the time allowed and then moving elsewhere, only to return after a while to repeat the cycle.

Homelessness creates additional stresses for the family. Many homeless families have young children but have problems gaining entry into the health care system, even though these children are at high risk for developing an acute or chronic condition. Health care for these families commonly occurs as crisis intervention instead of the more effective preventive intervention. Pregnant homeless women with their attendant problems receive little if any prenatal care, are poorly nourished, and bear low-birth-weight infants. Most of the children of homeless families do not have adequate immunizations. Homeless children often suffer from chronic illnesses at a higher rate than that of the general population. These chronic conditions may include anemia, heart disease, peripheral vascular disease, and neurologic disorders. Many homeless children have developmental delays, perform poorly when they attend school, and suffer from anxiety and depression in addition to having behavioral problems.

Many shelters available to the homeless are over-crowded, lack privacy (the bathroom facilities are used by many people), and have no personal bedding, no cribs for infants, and no facilities for cooking or refrigerating food. Because of limits to the length of stay, many families must move from one shelter to another. This adds to the problems these families face by contributing to a lack of consistency in the services and programs available to them.

Nurses can set the tone of the interaction between the homeless family and the health care facility. Establishing an environment in which the caregiver feels respected and comfortable is important. Focusing initially on the positive factors in the caregiver's relationship with the children alleviates some of the caregiver's guilt and fear of being criticized. Make every effort to offer down-to-earth suggestions and help the family in the most practical manner.

On the child's admission to the health care facility, the healthcare team performs a complete admission assessment. Ask the caregiver about the family's living arrangements; such information will help in the care and planning for the child. During this interview, the nurse may become aware of problems of other family members that need attention. When giving assistance and guidance, be careful to supplement, not take over, the family's functioning. For instance, tell the family how to go about getting a particular benefit and be certain they have complete and accurate information but do not take the steps for them. These families need to feel self-reliant and in control, and they need realistic solutions to their problems.

Outreach programs for the homeless have been established in many major cities. These programs conduct screening, treat acute illnesses, and help families contact local health care services when needed. Provide information to the family about any assistance that is available.

KEY POINTS

▶ Many stresses, such as job loss, financial crisis, illness, injury, loss of home, and death, cause families to respond in a dysfunctional way.

▶ A growing number of families cannot handle these kinds of stresses.

▶ Child abuse can be physical, emotional, or sexual and often is complicated by the use of drugs and alcohol.

▶ The nurse must serve as an advocate for children in abusive homes.

▶ Older children often try to escape home situations that they find unacceptable by running away, but they find life in the outside world even more traumatic.

▶ The caregivers of latchkey children must plan ahead to help the children accept the responsibilities they must assume when home alone.

▶ The nurse may help alleviate some burdens of divorce and homelessness on the family through counseling and education.

▶ The nurse must be sensitive to the underlying needs of children in dysfunctional families and help by providing guidance for the whole family.

REFERENCES

1. Walker C, Zangrillo P, Smith J. (1991) *Parental drug abuse and African American children in foster care: Issues and study findings.* Washington, DC: U.S. Department of Health and Human Services, National Black Child Development Institute.
2. Hall JM. (2000) Core issues for female child abuse survivors in recovery from substance misuse. *Qualitative Health Research,* 10(5), 612–31.
3. Wissow L. (1999) Child maltreatment. In *Oski's pediatrics: Principles and practice* (3rd ed). Philadelphia: Lippincott Williams & Wilkins.

BIBLIOGRAPHY

Berger KS. (2001) *The developing person through the life span* (5th ed). New York: Worth Publishers.

Bishop V, Rankin W. (2001) Children affected by violence. *Journal of Pediatric Nursing,* 16(5, 377.

Blackmore CA. (2001) Munchausen syndrome by proxy: A complex problem. *Community Practitioner,* 74(7), 259–62.

Bolland JM, et. al. (2001) Hopelessness and violence among inner-city youths. *American Journal of Maternal/Child Nursing,* 5(4), 237–44.

Brazelton TB, Greenspan S. (2001) *The irreducible needs of children: What every child must have to grow, learn, and flourish.* Cambridge, MA: Perseus Publishing.

Clements P. (2001) Kids in chaos. *Nursing Spectrum,* 2(7), 20.

Gottesman MM. (2001) Children in foster care: A nursing perspective on research, policy, and child health issues. *Journal of the Society of Pediatric Nurses,* 6(2), 55–64.

Huang C. (2001) School-aged homeless sheltered children's stressors and coping behaviors. *Journal of Pediatric Nursing,* 16(2), 102–9.

Jackson PL, Vessey JA. (2000) *Primary care of the child with a chronic condition* (3rd ed). St. Louis: Mosby.

McClain N, et. al. (2000) Evaluation of sexual abuse in the pediatric patient. *Journal of Pediatric Health Care,* 14(3), 93.

Marinko CA. (2000) Breaking the cycle of abuse. *Nursing Spectrum,* 9(18), 14.

Nelms BC. (2001) Emotional abuse: Helping prevent the problem. *Journal of Pediatric Health Care,* 15(3), 103.

Pillitteri A. (2003) *Maternal and child health nursing* (4th ed). Philadelphia: Lippincott Williams & Wilkins.

Price J. (2001) Current debates in child sexual abuse. *Current Paediatrics,* 11(3), 202–206.

Salvage J. (2000) Confronting child abuse: It's an uncomfortable truth, but child sex abuse begins at home. *Nursing Times,* 96(34), 26.

Wissow L. (1999) Child maltreatment. In *Oski's pediatrics:* *Principles and practice* (3rd ed). Philadelphia: Lippincott Williams & Wilkins.

Wong DL. (1998) *Whaley and Wong's nursing care of infants and children* (6th ed). St. Louis: Mosby.

Websites

Runaways: *www.saferchild.org*

Homeless Children: *www.standupforkids.org*

www.yourfamilyshealth.com

Workbook

NCLEX-STYLE REVIEW QUESTIONS

1. The nurse is caring for an infant born to a mother who abused cocaine during her pregnancy. Which of the following characteristics would the nurse likely see in this infant? The infant

   a. sleeps for long periods of time

   b. weighed above average when born

   c. cries when touched

   d. has facial deformities

2. The nurse is assisting with a physical exam on a child who has been admitted with a diagnosis of possible child abuse. Which of the following findings might alert the nurse to this possibility that the child has been abused? The child

   a. has a fractured bone

   b. has bruises on the knees and elbows

   c. is hyperactive and angry

   d. has a burn that has not been treated

3. The nurse is interviewing the caregiver of a 5-year-old child who has been admitted with bruises on the abdomen and thighs as well as additional bruises in various stages of healing. Which of the following statements made by the caregiver might alert the health care team to the possibility of child abuse?

   a. "His brother just plays too rough with him."

   b. "My child goes to the day care after school."

   c. "He just learned to ride his bicycle."

   d. "When he is in trouble, I make him go to his room."

4. In caring for a child who has been admitted after being sexually abused, which of the following interventions would be included in the child's plan of care?

   a. Observe for signs of anxiety.

   b. Weigh on the same scale each day.

   c. Encourage frequent family visits.

   d. Test the urine for glucose upon admission.

5. The nurse is discussing divorce with a group of children whose parents have been recently divorced. If children in the group made the following statements, which statement would require follow-up?

   a. "I know my parents both care about me and love me."

   b. "My aunt and uncle are not married anymore either."

   c. "They told me they wouldn't ever get back together again."

   d. "If I hadn't been in trouble at school, things would be okay."

STUDY ACTIVITIES

1. You are on duty in the emergency department when an infant is admitted with injuries that cause you to suspect abuse. The mother says her boyfriend was babysitting for her. State how you feel about this. Describe the observations that you will make when assessing the infant. What are your plans to approach the mother? Write out an effective communication you might have with the mother.

2. Children react differently to living with a family caregiver who is addicted. Make a list of the behaviors you might see that would cause you to be alert to a child with such a family problem. Research your community for resources available to children from families where addiction is a problem. Share the information you find with your classmates.

3. You have an opportunity to talk to a youth group about the hazards of becoming a runaway. Explain some of the points that you will make. Create a poster that might be helpful in encouraging a runaway child to seek help; include a phone number you have found that offers help to runaway children.

CRITICAL THINKING

1. Maria, a pregnant teen, has been bragging about the "partying" she has been doing. Discuss your feelings about this. Explain what you would tell her about the use of alcohol during pregnancy and the symptoms of fetal alcohol syndrome.

2. Your neighbor, 17-year-old Holly, has an active 18-month-old toddler named Jason. You overhear Holly screaming at him and saying, "I'm going to beat you if you don't listen to me!" Describe your feelings about this. Discuss with your peers what you would say and do regarding this situation.

3. You have an 8-year-old daughter who must stay alone every day until you get home from work. How will you prepare her? What plans will you make?

The Child With a Chronic Health Problem

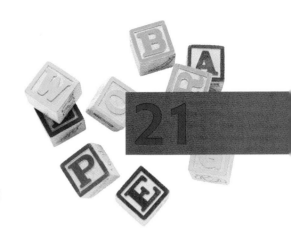

21

COMMON PROBLEMS IN CHRONIC
ILLNESS
EFFECTS OF CHRONIC ILLNESS ON
THE FAMILY
  Parents and Chronic Illness

The Child and Chronic Illness
Siblings and Chronic Illness
Nursing Process in Caring for a Child
  With a Chronic Illness

STUDENT OBJECTIVES

On completion of this chapter, the student will be able to

1. Define the key terms.
2. Identify 10 conditions that cause chronic illness.
3. Identify 10 concerns common to many families of a child with a chronic illness.
4. Describe economic pressures that can overwhelm families of chronically ill children.
5. Discuss the importance of respite care.
6. Discuss the effect that a developmental stage may have on the child's needs.
7. Identify positive and negative responses that well siblings may manifest in response to an ill sibling.
8. Describe how the nurse can help the family adjust to the child's condition.
9. Identify several ways the nurse may encourage self-care by the child.
10. Discuss general guidelines for preparing the family for home care of the child.

KEY TERMS

chronic illness
denial
gradual acceptance
overprotection
rejection
respite care
stigma

Chronic illness is a leading health problem in the United States. The numbers of chronically ill children are growing as more infants and children survive prematurity, difficult births, congenital anomalies, accidents, and illnesses that once were fatal. Most children experience only brief, acute episodes of illness; however, a significant number are affected by chronic health problems. Diseases that cause chronic illness in children include congenital heart disease, cystic fibrosis, juvenile arthritis, asthma, hemophilia, muscular dystrophy, leukemia and other malignancies, spina bifida, and immunodeficiency syndromes. When a family member has a chronic illness, the entire family is affected in many ways. Chronic illness may affect the child's physical, psychosocial, and cognitive development. Because nurses are usually involved from the early stages of diagnosis and the child and family have ongoing and long-term needs, the nurse can play a vital role in helping the family adjust to the condition.

COMMON PROBLEMS IN CHRONIC ILLNESS

Chronic illness is a condition of long duration or one that progresses slowly, shows little change, and often interferes with daily functioning. Specific chronic health problems of children were discussed in earlier chapters. Each requires individualized management based on the disease process and the abilities of the patient and family to understand and comply with the treatment regimen. All chronic health problems, however, create some common difficulties for patients and families; these are the focus of this chapter. Some of these concerns are

- Financial concerns such as payment for treatment, living expenses at a distant health care facility, caregiver's job loss because of time not at work
- Administration of treatments and medications at home
- Disruption of family life such as vacations, family goals, careers
- Educational opportunities for the child
- Social isolation due to the child's condition
- Family adjustments due to the disease's changing course
- Reaction of well siblings
- Stress among caregivers
- Guilt about and acceptance of the chronic condition
- Care of the child when family caregivers can no longer provide care

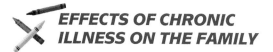

EFFECTS OF CHRONIC ILLNESS ON THE FAMILY

The diagnosis of a chronic health problem causes a crisis in the family, whether it happens during the first few hours or days of the child's life or much later. How families cope with chronic illness varies greatly from one family to another, but they all face many of the same problems.

Parents and Chronic Illness

When family caregivers learn of the child's diagnosis, their first reactions may be shock, disbelief, and denial. These reactions may last for a varied amount of time from days to months. The initial response may be one of mourning for the "perfect" child they lost combined with guilt, blame, and rationalization. The caregivers may seek advice from other professionals and actually may go "shopping" for another physician, hoping to find the diagnosis is incorrect or not as serious as they have been told. They may refuse to accept the diagnosis or talk about it, or they may delay seeking or agreeing to treatment. Gradually, however, they adjust to the diagnosis. They may enter a period of chronic sorrow when they adapt to the child's state of chronic illness but do not necessarily accept it. They often waver between the stages and they experience emotional highs and lows as they care for the child and meet the challenges of daily life. Families who have a strong support system usually are better able to meet these challenges.

Economic pressures can become overwhelming to the families of chronically ill children. If the family does not have adequate health insurance, the costs of treatment may be enormous. Away-from-home living costs may become a problem if the child must go to a distant hospital for further diagnosis or treatment. To keep health insurance benefits, a family caregiver may feel tied to a job, which creates additional stress. The time required to take the child to medical appointments can be excessive and may cause an additional threat to job security because of the time lost from the job.

Families must make many adjustments to care for the chronically ill child. The family caregivers may have to learn to perform treatments and give medications. Family life is often disrupted. Vacations may be nonexistent, and the family may be limited in how they can spend their leisure time. Families may have difficulty finding babysitters and have little opportunity for a break from the routine. Some families become isolated from customary social activities because of the responsibilities of caring for their child. **Respite care** (care of the ill child so that the caregivers can have a period of rest and refreshment) is often desperately needed but is not readily available in many communities. Families where both parents work may have to forgo a second income so that one adult can stay home with the child.

As the child grows, concerns about education may become foremost among the caregivers' worries. These concerns include the availability of appropriate education, early learning opportunities, physical accessibility of the facilities, acceptance of the child by school personnel and classmates, inclusion versus segregated classes, availability and quality of homebound teaching, and general flexibility of the school's teachers and administrators. Few schools are prepared to accommodate treatments at school that would otherwise require the child to leave during the school day. Family caregivers often must become the child's advocate to preserve as much normalcy as possible in the child's educational experience.

As the child's condition changes, the family must make additional changes. All these stresses may strain a marriage, and couples may have little time left for each other when caring for a chronically ill child. Sometimes partners in relationships blame each other for the child's problems, which further strains the relationship. Single-parent families have significant needs to which health care personnel must be especially sensitive.

The Child and Chronic Illness

The child with a chronic illness may face many problems that interfere with normal growth and development. For example, the child who must be immobilized during school age while in the stage of industry versus inferiority cannot complete the tasks of industry such as helping with household chores or working on special projects with siblings or peers. These problems

---

COMMUNICATIONS BOX 21.1

The nurse is completing a home visit to see 14-year-old Anna, who has had a severe exacerbation of her cystic fibrosis. Her mother, Marie, cares for her. The nurse notices that Marie appears exhausted.

LESS EFFECTIVE COMMUNICATION

Nurse: Marie, you look exhausted. Are you getting enough sleep?

Marie: Oh, I'm okay.

Nurse: Well, you mustn't let yourself get overtired or you won't be able to take care of Anna.

Marie: I'll be all right. I can take care of her just fine.

Nurse: If you need help, I could see if I can find someone to help you out. You know you can't do everything yourself.

Marie: Really, I'll be okay. You just caught me at a bad time.

Nurse: Well, all right, but I worry about you.

▶ *The nurse's first comment put Marie on the defensive. Marie felt she had to defend herself and protest that she was doing everything she should to take care of her daughter. Unfortunately, the nurse did nothing to boost Marie's self-image, so Marie continued to defend herself. The nurse ended up without helping to solve the problem.*

MORE EFFECTIVE COMMUNICATION

Nurse: Marie, I know that caring for Anna is very wearing. Perhaps we can plan together to give you some respite from caring for her 24 hours a day.

Marie: Oh, I don't know. I'm doing all right, I think.

Nurse: You are doing a great job. However, I am concerned about the long term. I don't want you to run the risk of tiring yourself so much you won't be able to care for her.

Marie: Well, yes, but I am strong, I think I can handle it.

Nurse: Yes, I know you are strong and I have such admiration for the job you are doing. But let's just sit down and look at some ways we can plan together to ease things a little for you and perhaps give you some free time.

Marie: Okay. I guess that sounds like a good idea.

▶ *By opening the subject with a positive, noncritical statement, the nurse begins to establish a good connection with Marie. Immediately Marie feels the nurse's recognition of her hard work. The nurse continues by telling her what a good job she is doing. By suggesting they work on solving the problem together, the nurse gains Marie's cooperation.*

A PERSONAL GLIMPSE

I am 16 years old and I was diagnosed with cystic fibrosis at birth. Every morning I wake up and have many things that I have to accomplish; taking a breathing treatment, having percussion done, and taking many pills. I guess it isn't so bad if you are used to doing it every day, but it is a bit annoying having the same routine all the time. I have been doing all of this for 16 years. I sometimes feel that I am very different from other people. My friends don't feel it is weird having me as a friend, but they know that I have this disease and they are afraid of what can happen to me. My friends don't treat me any different. I think that is the most important thing. It is good that I have friends who can care so much that they don't let it bother them.

I don't like it when I have to cough all the time; every one stares at me. When I am in school, at lunch I have to take pills before I eat. Everyone is always asking me why I am taking the pills. Even when I go to a friend's house, I have to take my medication and get my percussions done. My friends usually help out with the percussions.

A lot of times I feel very lonely because I am the only one in my family that has this disease. No one knows what I am feeling, and that sometimes makes me very lonely and afraid. I have a twin brother who really cares for me a lot. When anyone asks about my illness, he is usually the person to explain it to them. He has always been there for me when I needed him. When I have to go in the hospital, he gets my work for me. We are very close. I am glad to have a brother like him.

I am very lucky to have a family that cares for me and loves me like they do. They are always helping me when I need percussions done and they are very supportive. I don't know what I would do without their help. They all took care of me when I couldn't. They still do now. I owe them a lot of credit. I love them very much and always will.

Gretchen, age 16

> ► **LEARNING OPPORTUNITY:** Do you think this adolescent has accepted her disease? What are the things she shared that you think show that she has or has not accepted her condition? What are your thoughts about her family and friends?

Several typical responses have been identified: **overprotection, rejection, denial,** and **gradual acceptance.** Overprotective caregivers try to protect the child at all costs: they hover, which prevents the child from learning new skills; they fail to use discipline; and they use any means to prevent the child from experiencing any frustration. Rejecting caregivers distance themselves emotionally from the child: although they provide physical care, they tend to scold and correct the child continuously. Caregivers in denial behave as though the condition does not exist and they encourage the child to overcompensate for any disabilities. Caregivers who respond with gradual acceptance take a common-sense approach to the child's condition; they help the child to set realistic goals for self-care and independence and encourage the child to achieve social and physical skills within his or her capability (Fig. 21–1).

Children often perceive any illness as punishment for a bad thought or action. The child's perception of chronic illness is subject to this magical thinking as well depending on the child's developmental stage at the time of diagnosis. This perception also is influenced by the attitudes of parents and peers and by whether or not the dysfunctional body part is visible. Problems such as asthma, allergies, and epilepsy are difficult for children to understand because "what's wrong" is inside, not outside.

The child's family, peers, and school personnel comprise the support system that can affect the child's adaptation. Sometimes the efforts necessary to meet the child's physical needs are so great that finding time and energy to meet the child's emotional needs can be difficult for members of the support team. The older child with a chronic illness also has developing sexual needs that should not be ignored but must be acknowledged and provided for.

Additional stresses continue to occur as the disease progresses. For instance, Hodgkin's disease

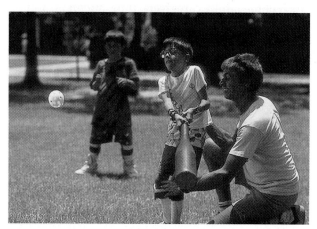

● *Figure 21.1* This father and brother encourage a child with a disability to participate in outdoor activities.

vary with the diagnosis and condition. The child's attitude toward the condition is a critical element in its long-term management and the family's adjustment.

The child's response to the chronic condition is influenced by the response of family caregivers.

can be successfully treated for a time with chemotherapy and radiation therapy, but this requires adding the side effects of treatment (steroid-induced acne, edema, and alopecia) to the disease manifestations of night sweats, chronic fatigue, pruritus, and gastrointestinal bleeding. The child with Duchenne's muscular dystrophy gradually weakens, so that in adolescence he or she is wheelchair-bound when peers are actively involved in sports and exploring sexual relationships. These stresses can add up to more than one young person can cope with for long.

Discrimination continues to be present in the life of the chronically ill child and the family. Discrimination can occur in relationships among children, and social exclusion of the chronically ill child is common. Physical barriers may present problems that families must struggle to help their child overcome. Sometimes hurtful discrimination is as simple as being stared at in public places.

INTERNET EXERCISE 21.1

www.faculty.fairfield.edu/fleitas/contents.html

Bandaides and Blackboards
Click on "Kids."
Click on star next to section, "To tell or not to tell."
Read this section.

1. List five reasons kids choose **NOT** to tell others that they have a chronic health condition.

2. List five reasons kids choose **TO TELL** others that they have a chronic health condition.

Siblings and Chronic Illness

Some degree of sibling rivalry can be found in most families with healthy children, so it is not surprising that a child with a chronic health problem can seriously disrupt the lives of brothers and sisters. Much of the family caregivers' time, attention, and money are directed toward management of the ill child's problem. This can cause anger, resentment, and jealousy in the well siblings. The caregivers' failure to set limits for the ill child's behavior while maintaining discipline for the healthy siblings can cause further resentment. Some family caregivers unknowingly create feelings of guilt in the healthy children by overemphasizing the ill child's needs.

Siblings may feel **stigma** (embarrassment or shame) because of a brother or sister with a chronic illness, especially if the ill child has a physical disfigurement or apparent cognitive deficit. Siblings may choose not to tell others about the ill child or may be selective in whom they tell, choosing to tell only persons they can trust. An older sibling is more likely to tell others than a younger one, perhaps because the older child tends to understand more about the illness and its effect.

Both positive and negative influences can be found in the behaviors of well siblings. Some siblings react with anger, hostility, jealousy, increased competition for attention, social withdrawal, and poor school performance. On the other hand, many siblings demonstrate positive behaviors such as caring and concern for the ill sibling, cooperating with family caregivers in helping care for the ill child, protecting the ill child from negative reaction of others, and including the ill child in activities with peers.

How well siblings react to a chronically ill sibling may ultimately depend on how the family copes with stress and how its members feel about one another. Families that seem to adapt most successfully to the presence of a child with chronic illness are those in which the caregivers

- Find time for special activities with the healthy children
- Explain the ill child's condition as simply as possible
- Involve the healthy siblings in the care of the ill child according to his or her developmental ability
- Set behavioral limits for all children in the family

This delicate balance is challenging and takes great effort and caring for a family to sustain, but the results are well worth it.

● Nursing Process in Caring for a Child With a Chronic Illness

ASSESSMENT

The assessment of the family and the child with a disability or chronic illness is an ongoing process by the health care team. The information and data collected are reviewed and updated with each visit the child makes to the health care facility. Include the child in the admission and ongoing interview processes if he or she is old enough and able to participate. The child may have had many visits and treatments in the past that have left negative memories, so approach the child in a low-key, kind, gentle manner to gain cooperation. Unless the child is newly diagnosed, the family caregivers may have a good understanding of the condition. Observe for evidence of the family's knowledge and understanding so that plans can be made to supplement it as needed.

During any interview with the child or family caregivers, determine how the family is coping with the child's condition and observe for the family's strengths, weaknesses, and acceptance of the diagnosis. Identify the needs that change with the child's condition and include them in planning care. Also consider needs that change with the child's growth and development.

Adjust the physical exam to correspond with the child's illness and current condition. Throughout the physical exam, make every effort to gain the child's cooperation and explain what is being done in terms that the child can understand. Offer praise for cooperation throughout the process to gain the child's (and the family caregivers') goodwill.

NURSING DIAGNOSES

The nursing diagnoses vary depending on the illness or disability, but certain developmental diagnoses are appropriate regardless of the medical diagnosis, such as

- Delayed Growth and Development related to impaired ability to achieve developmental tasks or family caregivers' reactions to the child's condition
- Self-Care Deficit related to limitations of illness or disability
- Anxiety related to procedures, tests, or hospitalization
- Risk for Social Isolation of the child or family related to the child's condition
- Anticipatory Grieving of family caregiver related to possible losses secondary to condition
- Interrupted Family Processes related to adjustment requirements for the child with chronic illness or disability
- Health-Seeking Behaviors by caregivers related to home care of the child

OUTCOME IDENTIFICATION AND PLANNING

Major goals for the chronically ill child are to accomplish growth and development milestones, perform self-care tasks, decrease anxiety, and experience more social interaction. Goals for the caregiver or family are to increase their social interaction; decrease their feelings of grief, anger, and guilt; increase their adjustment to living with a chronically ill child; and teach them about caring for the chronically ill or disabled child.

IMPLEMENTATION

Encouraging Optimal Growth and Development. The family caregivers may become overprotective and prevent the ill child from exhibiting growth and development appropriate for his or her age and disability. Help the caregivers recognize the child's potential and set realistic growth and development goals. Consistent care by the same staff helps to provide a sense of routine in which the child can be encouraged to have some control and perform age-appropriate tasks within the limitations of the disability. Set age-appropriate limits and enforce appropriate discipline. Accomplish this gradually by displaying a kind and caring attitude. Give the child choices within the limits of treatments and other aspects of required care. Encourage the child to wear regular clothes rather than stay in pajamas to reduce feelings of being an invalid. Encourage the child to learn about the condition. Introducing the child to other children with the same or a similar condition can help dispel feelings that he or she is the only person with such a condition. An older child or adolescent benefits from social interaction with peers with and without disabilities (Fig. 21–2). Encourage family caregivers to help the adolescent join in age-appropriate activities. The adolescent also may need some help dressing or using makeup to improve his or her appearance and minimize any physical disability.

Promoting Self-Care. To encourage the child to assist in self-care, devise aids to ease tasks.

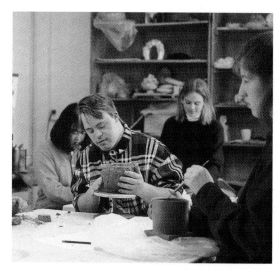

● *Figure 21.2* The adolescent with disabilities benefits from social interaction.

When appropriate, integrate play and toys into the care to help encourage cooperation. Praise the child genuinely and generously for tasks attempted even if they are not totally completed. Do not expect the child to perform tasks beyond his or her capabilities. Make certain that the child is well rested before attempting any energy-taxing tasks. Use a chart or other visual aid with listed tasks as a tool to help the child reach a desired goal. Stickers can record the child's progress. School-age children often respond well to contracts: for instance, a special privilege or other incentive is awarded when a set number of stickers is earned. Remember that these tasks often are hard work for the child.

Reducing Anxiety About Procedures and Treatments. Periodically the child may need to undergo procedures, tests, and treatments. The child may also be hospitalized frequently. Many of the procedures may be painful or at least uncomfortable. Explain the tests, treatments, and procedures to the child ahead of time and encourage the child to ask questions. Acknowledge to the child that a particular procedure is painful and help him or her to plan ways to cope with the pain. Advise family caregivers that they should also help the child to prepare for hospitalization ahead of time whenever possible.

Preventing Social Isolation. The chronically ill child may feel isolated from peers. When the child is hospitalized, consider arranging for contact with peers by phone, in writing, or through visits. Many pediatric units have special programs that help children deal with chronic conditions and the hospitalizations that occur with these conditions (Fig. 21–3). Encourage regular school attendance as soon as the child is physically able. If the child is a member of an inclusive classroom, suggest that the caregiver make arrangements with the school for rest periods as needed. Ask the child about interests; these may give some clues about suitable after-school activities that will increase the child's interactions with peers. Make suggestions and confer with family caregivers to ensure that proposed plans are carried out. Listen carefully to the child's discussions about social activities to gain insight into his or her feelings about socialization.

A child who requires constant or frequent attention often can be exhausting for the family

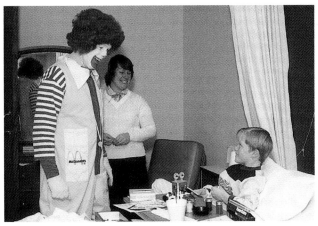

● *Figure 21.3* Ronald McDonald, a familiar face to many children, visits a hospitalized child who has a long-term illness.

caregivers. The family with no close extended family and few close friends may find getting away for rest and relaxation, even for an evening, almost impossible. Help the family caregivers find resources for respite care. Any caregiver, no matter how devoted, needs to have a break from everyday cares and concerns. Refer the family to social services where they can get help. Sometimes a caregiver may feel that another person cannot care for the child adequately. Encourage this caregiver to express fears and anxieties about leaving the child. This helps the caregiver to work through some of these anxieties and feel more confident about getting away for a period of rest.

Aiding Caregivers' Acceptance of the Condition. When anyone suffers a serious loss, a grief reaction occurs. This is true of family caregivers when they first learn that their child has a chronic or disabling illness. Encourage family caregivers to express these feelings and help them to understand that this reaction is common and acceptable.

Denial is usually the first reaction that family caregivers have to the diagnosis. This is a time when they say, "How could this be?" or "Why my child?" Let them express their emotions, and respond in a nonjudgmental way. Staying with them and offering quiet, accepting support may be helpful. Statements such as "It will seem better in time" are inappropriate. Acknowledge the caregivers' feelings as acceptable and reasonable.

During the next stage called guilt, listen to the caregivers express their feelings of guilt and remorse. Again, acknowledging their feelings is useful. Accept expressions of anger by family caregivers without viewing them as a personal attack. Using active listening techniques that reflect the caregivers' feelings, such as "You sound very angry," is a helpful method of handling these emotions.

Grief reactions also may occur when the family caregivers are informed that their child is deteriorating or has had a setback. Although caregivers usually cycle through these reactions much more quickly by this time, the same methods are useful.

Helping the Family Adjust to the Child's Condition. The family's adjustment to the condition is assessed during initial and ongoing interviews. Adjustment may depend on how recently the child has been diagnosed. After determining the family's needs, provide an opportunity for the family members to express their feelings and anxieties. Help them explore any feelings of guilt or blame about the child's condition. Encourage them to express doubts they may have about their ability to cope with the child's future. Help the caregivers look realistically at their resources, and give them suggestions about ways to cope. Serve as a role model when caring for the child, expressing a positive attitude toward the child and the illness or disability.

Question the family to determine the resources and support systems available to them. Remind them that these support systems may include immediate family members, extended family, friends, community services, and health care providers.

Encourage the caregivers to discuss the needs of the well siblings and their adjustment to the ill child's condition. Help the family meet the needs of the well siblings, and help the siblings feel comfortable with the ill child's problems and needs. Assist the family in setting reasonable expectations for all their children.

Planning for Home Care. Home care planning begins when the child is admitted to the health care facility and continues until discharge. Focus plans for care at home on the continuing care, medications, and treatments the child will need. During a health care visit or hospitalization, include family caregivers when caring for the child so that they become comfortable with the care. Children are often sent home with sophisticated equipment and treatments; therefore, demonstrate the use of the equipment and treatments and give the family caregivers a chance to perform the treatments under guidance and supervision. A discussion of the home's facilities may be appropriate to help the family accommodate any special needs the child may have. Give the caregivers a list of community services and organizations that they can turn to for help and support including appropriate disease- or disability-specific organizations.

Teach the caregivers about growth and development guidelines so that they have a realistic concept of what to expect as the child develops. Throughout the child's stay, encourage caregivers to express their concerns to help solve whatever problems the family anticipates having while caring for the child at home. Give the family the name and telephone number of a contact person they can call for support. Families face many hurdles while caring for a chronically ill child but they are more likely to feel that they can competently face the future with the reassurance that help is just a telephone call away.

Caring for a chronically ill child can be an overwhelming task that requires cooperation by all involved with the child and the family. Family caregivers deserve all the help they can get (see Nursing Care Plan for the Chronically Ill Child and Family).

EVALUATION: GOALS AND OUTCOME CRITERIA

- *Goal:* The child will achieve highest level of growth and development within constraints of illness and the family caregivers will acknowledge appropriate growth and development expectations.
  Criteria: The child attains growth and development milestones within her or his capabilities; the family caregivers acknowledge the child's capabilities, encourage the child, and set realistic goals for the child.
- *Goal:* The child will become involved in self-care activities.
  Criteria: The child participates in self-care as appropriate for age and capabilities.
- *Goal:* The child's anxiety will be decreased.
  Criteria: The child's anxiety is minimized as evidenced by cooperation with care and treatments.
- *Goal:* The child and the family will actively socialize with others.

NURSING CARE PLAN

for the Chronically Ill Child and Family

BT is a 10-year-old who has Duchenne muscular dystrophy. His condition has worsened and he has recently begun to use a walker. He has gradually begun to need more assistance in his activities of daily living. He has a sister who is 8 years old and a 5-year-old brother. Both parents live at home.

NURSING DIAGNOSIS
Delayed Growth and Development related to impaired ability to achieve developmental tasks or family caregivers' reactions to the child's condition

GOAL: The child will achieve the highest levels of growth and development within constraints of illness and the family caregivers will acknowledge appropriate growth and development expectations.

OUTCOME CRITERIA
• The child attains growth and development milestones within his capabilities.
• The family encourages the child to reach his potential.
• The family sets realistic developmental goals for the child.

NURSING INTERVENTIONS	*RATIONALE*
Encourage the child to participate in growth and development activities to the best of his abilities	Milestones of growth and development are attained when activities are offered to help child develop those skills.
Discuss with the child's family the effects of overprotectiveness on his development.	Many families react to a child's long-term illness by shielding the child from challenges that the child could cope with if allowed to do so.
Help the child's family recognize his potential and help them to set realistic goals; encourage them to set age-appropriate limits for activities with appropriate discipline for violations.	Family caregivers may not know what to expect in terms of their child's development and may tend to overprotect the child, which prevents him from reaching his potential; it is important to allow him to reach for his potential without overprotection.

NURSING DIAGNOSIS
Self-Care Deficit related to limitations of illness or disability

GOAL: The child will become involved in self-care activities.

OUTCOME CRITERIA
• The child participates in self-care as appropriate for his age and capabilities.
• The child demonstrates evidence of using creative problem-solving techniques.
• The child demonstrates a positive outlook about his achievements.

NURSING INTERVENTIONS	*RATIONALE*
Generously praise any self-care the child performs; carefully avoid expecting him to do tasks beyond his capabilities.	Positive reinforcement gives the child self-confidence and pride in his accomplishments.
When the child finds a task difficult to accomplish, assist him by devising aids to help him with the task rather than doing it for him.	Difficult accomplishments reinforce the importance of self-care and independence; demonstrating creative problem-solving techniques provides skills that the child can use in the future.
Encourage the child to carry out self-care appropriate for his age and stage of mobility; allow him to make as many choices as possible.	The child will have a better feeling of control and self-worth; he will be encouraged to try new things and not let his illness unnecessarily stop him.

NURSING DIAGNOSIS
Risk for Social Isolation of the child or family related to the child's condition

GOAL: The child and the family will actively socialize with others.

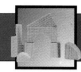

NURSING CARE PLAN continued

for the Chronically Ill Child and Family

OUTCOME CRITERIA
- The child participates in activities with his peers.
- The child's family finds adequate respite care for Billy.
- The child's family gets away for a break with minimal anxieties.

NURSING INTERVENTIONS	**RATIONALE**
Encourage the family to establish and maintain the child's contacts with his peers. Advise the family that it may take advance planning and creative solutions for him to participate in activities such as team sports.	The child needs to feel that he is part of the world in which his schoolmates and friends are involved; he needs activities to look forward to.
Help family caregivers find resources for respite care by making referrals to social services or other resources as necessary.	Family caregivers who periodically get away from the responsibilities of caring for the child will be re-energized and return with a refreshed spirit.
Encourage the family caregivers to express anxieties about leaving the child with someone else.	Talking with the family about such fears helps them to work through anxieties, dismiss unrealistic fears, and make specific plans for legitimate ones. This helps the family to have a more restful time when away.

NURSING DIAGNOSIS
Interrupted Family Processes related to adjustment requirements for the child with chronic illness or disability

GOAL: The family caregivers will deal with their feelings of anger, grief, guilt, and loss.

OUTCOME CRITERIA
- The family members express fears and anxieties about the child's weakening condition.
- The family verbalizes a positive attitude to the child about his adaptations to his growing weakness.
- The child's family expresses feelings of guilt about his illness and deals with them positively.

NURSING INTERVENTIONS	**RATIONALE**
Provide opportunities for family members to express feelings including fears about his or her weakening condition.	The family may need encouragement to talk about some of their fears and anxieties.
Maintain a positive but realistic attitude about the child's growing disabilities both when providing care and when discussing the impact of the child's illness on the family.	The nurse serves as a role model for the family; modeling a positive attitude will help family caregivers take the same approach.
Explore with the child's family their feelings of guilt.	The family needs to resolve their feelings of guilt.
Provide the family with resources and support systems. Encourage them to talk with their younger children about their feelings concerning the child's illness.	The family needs to use community resources and support systems to help them with the long-term needs of the entire family.

NURSING DIAGNOSIS
Health Seeking Behaviors by caregivers related to home care of the child

GOAL: The family caregivers will actively participate in the child's home care.

OUTCOME CRITERIA
- The family members ask appropriate questions about the child's care.
- The family members demonstrate the ability to perform the child's care and treatment.
- The family members make contact with support groups and community services.

(nursing care plan continues on page 494)

NURSING CARE PLAN continued

for the Chronically Ill Child and Family

NURSING INTERVENTIONS	RATIONALE
Explain and demonstrate any equipment used in the child's care; demonstrate treatments or therapy that the family will need to do at home; provide opportunities for practice under the guidance of a nurse or therapist. Provide the family with a list of community services and organizations where they can turn for help and support; include the name and telephone number of a contact person at the health care facility whom the family can call with questions or concerns.	Watching someone who knows how to perform a technique well and performing that technique yourself are very different matters. Practice and opportunities for questions are essential. Knowing whom to contact and how to reach that person gives the family reassurance that help is close by and increases their self-confidence about being able to handle their child's care.

Criteria: The child and family use opportunities to socialize with others; the family seeks and finds adequate respite care for the child.

- *Goal:* The family will deal with their feelings of anger, grief, guilt, and loss.
  Criteria: The family caregivers express their feelings of guilt, fears, and anxieties and they receive support while working toward accepting the child's condition.
- *Goal:* The family caregivers will adjust to the requirements of caring for the child with chronic illness or disability.
  Criteria: The family caregivers express ways they can cope with their child's condition and list the resources and support systems available to them.
- *Goal:* The family caregivers will actively participate in the child's home care.
  Criteria: The family caregivers ask pertinent questions, contact support groups and community agencies for help, and demonstrate their ability to perform care and treatments.

KEY POINTS

- Advances in medical technology have increased the number of families who must care for a child with a chronic illness or disability.
- Caring for such a child over a long period can create much stress in the family.

- Family caregivers often react with denial, guilt, and anger when they first realize that they have a child with serious, long-term problems.
- Caregivers sometimes focus on the ill child while losing sight of the needs of the well siblings.
- Volunteer and community agencies provide support and guidance for families that is often specific to the child's condition.
- Families must set realistic goals for all family members and use all support systems available to them.

BIBLIOGRAPHY

Balling K, McCubbin M. (2001) Hospitalized children with chronic illness: Parental caregiving needs and valuing parental expertise. *Journal of Pediatric Nursing*, 16(2).

Berger KS. (2001) *The developing person through the life span* (5th ed). New York: Worth Publishers.

Brazelton TB, Greenspan S. (2001) *The irreducible needs of children: What every child must have to grow, learn, and flourish.* Cambridge, MA: Perseus Publishing.

Hutton N. (1999) Special needs of children with chronic illnesses. In *Oski's pediatrics: Principles and practice* (3rd ed). Philadelphia: Lippincott Williams & Wilkins.

Keefe S. (2002) Caring for children with disabilities. *Nursing Spectrum*, 3(5), 26–27.

Perry DF, Ireys HT. (2001) Maternal perceptions of pediatric providers for children with chronic illnesses. *American Journal of Maternal/Child Nursing*, 5(1), 15–20.

Pillitteri A. (2003) *Maternal and child health nursing* (4th ed). Philadelphia: Lippincott Williams & Wilkins.

Sein EP. (2001) Chronic Illness: The child and the family. *Current Paediatrics*, 11(1), 46–50.

Smucker JMR. (2001) Managed care and children with special health care needs. *Journal of Pediatric Health Care,* 15(1), 3.

Wong DL. (1998) *Whaley and Wong's nursing care of infants and children* (6th ed). St. Louis: Mosby.

Websites
www.wish.org
www.fathersnetwork.org
www.coachart.org
www.kcdream.org

Workbook

NCLEX-STYLE REVIEW QUESTIONS

1. In planning care for a child diagnosed with a chronic illness, which of the following goals would be MOST LIKELY be part of this child's plan of care? The child will

   a. achieve the highest levels of growth and development

   b. participate in age appropriate activities

   c. eat at least 75% of each meal

   d. share feelings about changes in body image

2. The nurse is working with the caregivers of a child who has a chronic illness. Of the following statements made by the child's caregivers, which statement is an example of the common response called overprotection?

   a. "My child was born with this and it will always be part of our lives."

   b. "She should be punished when she breaks things because she knows better."

   c. "I know I should let her try new activities, but she just gets frustrated."

   d. "My child just isn't what I expected when I decided to become a parent."

3. The nurse is working with the caregivers of a child who has a chronic illness. Of the following statements made by the child's caregivers, which statement is an example of the common response called acceptance?

   a. "My child was born with this and it will always be part of our lives."

   b. "She should be punished when she breaks things because she knows better."

   c. "I know I should let her try new activities, but she just gets frustrated."

   d. "My child just isn't what I expected when I decided to become a parent."

4. In working with families of children who have chronic illnesses, an important nursing intervention would be which of the following? The nurse would encourage the family members to

   a. refrain from talking about the condition

   b. openly express their feelings

   c. prevent the child from overhearing conversations

   d. tell stories about themselves

5. In working with siblings of children who have chronic illnesses, it is important for the nurse to recognize that in many cases the siblings

   a. may feel embarrassed about their brother or sister's condition

   b. are the primary caregiver for the sick child

   c. excel in school in an effort to decrease the family stress

   d. get jobs at a young age to help support the family

STUDY ACTIVITIES

1. Lena and Josh are the young parents of Nina, a 12-month-old with meningomyelocele (spina bifida). Nina must be catheterized at least four times a day and also has mobility problems. Explore some of the economic and other stresses that this young couple faces.

2. Using your local phone book, make a list of agencies to which you could refer families for assistance and support in the care of a chronically ill child.

3. Eight-year-old Jason, a patient in your pediatric unit, is undergoing chemotherapy. He seems very lonely and sad, although his family visits him regularly. You decide he may need contact with children his own age. Describe plans that you will make to provide contact with peers.

CRITICAL THINKING

1. You are caring for 5-year-old Abby, a bright girl with cystic fibrosis. Her mother, Mattie, has been overprotective and has always done everything for her. Describe how you will involve Abby in self-care. Explain what you can say or do to help Mattie encourage Abby to do more of her own care.

2. Nine-year-old Tyson is angry. He tells you that he hates his 6-year-old brother, Josh, who has Down's syndrome. Relate how you would discuss this with Tyson. If you had the opportunity to talk to his family caregiver, what would you say?

3. Cassie is a 16-year-old with cerebral palsy. She wants to go to the school prom, but her family caregivers are very resistant to the idea. Cassie pleads with you to talk to them. How will you approach this problem? What are your responses to Cassie and to her caregivers?

The Dying Child

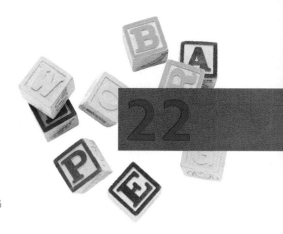

22

STUDENT OBJECTIVES

On completion of this chapter, the student will be able to

1. Describe the role of anticipatory grief in the grieving process.
2. Identify reasons why nurses may have difficulty working effectively with dying children.
3. Identify how a nurse can personally prepare to care for a dying child.
4. List the factors that affect the child's understanding of death.
5. Describe how a child's understanding of death changes at each developmental level.
6. State the importance of encouraging families to complete unfinished business.
7. Describe why a family may suffer excessive grief and guilt when a child dies suddenly.
8. Describe possible reactions in a child when a sibling dies.
9. Identify settings for caring for the dying child and the advantages and disadvantages of each.

KEY TERMS

anticipatory grief
hospice
thanatologist
unfinished business

The most difficult death to accept is the death of a child. We can accept that elderly patients have lived a full life and that life must end, but the life of a child still holds the hopes, dreams, and promises of the future. When a child's life ends early, whether abruptly as the result of an accident or after a prolonged illness, we ask ourselves, "Why? What's the justice of this?" Caring for a dying child and his or her family is stressful but can also be extremely rewarding.

Caring for a family facing the death of their child calls on all the nurse's personal and professional skills. It means offering sensitive, gentle, physical care and comfort measures for the child and continuing emotional support for the child, the family caregivers, and the siblings. This kind of caring demands an understanding of the nurse's own feelings about death and dying, knowledge of the grieving process that terminally ill patients and their families experience, and a willingness to become involved.

Like chronic illness, terminal illness creates a family crisis that can either destroy or strengthen the family as a unit and as individuals. Nurses and other health professionals who can offer knowledgeable, sensitive care to these families help to make the remainder of the child's life more meaningful and the family's mourning experience more healing. Helping a family struggle through this crisis and emerge stronger and closer can yield deep satisfaction.

Diagnosis of a fatal illness initiates the grieving process in the child and the family: denial and isolation, anger, bargaining, depression and acute grief, and, finally, acceptance. Not every child or family will complete the process because each family, as well as each death, is personal and unique.

When death is expected, the family begins to mourn, a phenomenon called **anticipatory grief.** For some people, this shortens the period of acute grief and loss after the child's death. Unexpected death offers no chance for preparation, and grief may last longer and be more difficult to resolve.

Death is a tragic reality for thousands of children each year. Accidents are the leading cause of death in children between the ages of 1 and 14 years; cancer is the number one fatal disease in this age group. Nearly all these children leave behind at least one grieving family caregiver and perhaps brothers, sisters, and grandparents. Nurses who care for children and families must be prepared for encounters with the dying and the bereaved.

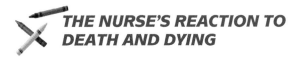

THE NURSE'S REACTION TO DEATH AND DYING

I am a student nurse. I am dying. I write this to you who are and will become nurses in the hope that

by my sharing my feelings with you, you may someday be better able to help those who share my experience. . . . You slip in and out of my room, give me medications and check my blood pressure. Is it because I am a student nurse, myself, or just a human being, that I sense your fright? And your fears enhance mine. Why are you afraid? I am the one who is dying!

I know you feel insecure, don't know what to say, don't know what to do. But please believe me, if you care, you can't go wrong. Just admit that you care . . . Don't run away—wait—all I want to know is that there will be someone to hold my hand when I need it. . . . If only we could be honest, both admit our fears, touch one another. If you really care, would you lose so much of your valuable professionalism if you even cried with me? Just person to person? Then it might not be so hard to die in a hospital—with friends close by.[1]

The feelings expressed by this young student nurse are not uncommon. Health care workers often are uncomfortable with dying patients, so they avoid them and are afraid that the patients will ask questions they cannot or should not answer. These caregivers signal by their behavior that the patient should avoid the fact of his or her impending death and should keep up a show of bravery. In effect, they are asking the patient to meet their needs instead of trying to meet the patient's needs.

Death reminds us of our own mortality, a thought with which many of us are uncomfortable. The thought that someone even younger than we are is about to die makes us feel more vulnerable. Every nurse needs to examine his or her own feelings about death and the reasons for these feelings. How have you reacted to the death of a friend or a family member? When growing up, was talking and thinking about death avoided because of your family's attitudes? Admitting that death is a part of life and that patients should be helped to live each day to the fullest until death are steps toward understanding and being able to communicate with those who are dying. A workshop, conference, or seminar in which one's own feelings about life and death are explored is useful in preparing the nurse to care for the dying child and family (Box 22–1).

Learning to care for the dying patient requires talking with other professionals, sharing concerns, and comforting each other in stressful times. It calls for reading studies about death to discover how dying patients feel about their care, their illness, their families, and how they want to spend the rest of their lives. It also requires being a sensitive, empathic, nonjudgmental listener to patients and families who need to express their feelings even if they may not be able to express them to each other. Caring for the dying is usually a team effort that may involve a nurse, a

<table>
<tr><td>BOX 22.1</td><td>Questions to Cover in a Self-Examination About Death</td></tr>
</table>

Some Considerations in the Resolution of Death and Dying
1. What was your first conscious memory of death? What were your feelings and reactions?
2. What is your most recent memory of death? How was it the same or different from your first memory?
3. What experience of death had the most effect on you? Why?

Get Comfortable and Imagine Now
You have just been told you have 6 months to live. What is your *first* reaction to that news?

3 months later—What relationships might require you to tie up loose ends? What unfinished business do you have to deal with? You and your significant other are trying to cope with the news.

What changes occur in your relationship?

1 month remains—What do you need to have happen in the remaining time? What hopes, dreams, and plans can or need to be fulfilled?

1 week remains—You are very weak and barely have enough energy to talk. You don't even want to look at yourself. Nausea and vomiting are constant companions. Write a letter to the one person you feel would be the most affected by your dying.

24 hours remain—You are dying. Breathing is difficult; you feel very hot inside; overwhelming fatigue is ever-present. How would you like to spend this last day? These questions can be used in a group with a hospice or other facilitator. They can be used to help heighten your awareness of yourself: who are you; how you have gotten to where you are today; what you are doing with your life and why; how you would change the way you live; your feelings about death in general, in relation to your friends and family, and in regard to your own death.

With permission from Ruth Anne Sieber, Hospice: The Bridge, Lewistown, PA.

A PERSONAL GLIMPSE

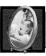

I sat in silence rocking the baby, reflecting upon life and death. And as I felt the small bundle of warmth stir within my arms, I realized that while life's essence had died within one it had been born anew within another, continuing and completing the cycle. And that there is never really death, only passing from this world into another; that the spiritual flame is never extinguished, only shared and passed on. And as I held the baby closer still I felt how young and innocent she was, how very much she had to experience and learn. And I felt her vulnerability as my own, realizing that the child in my arms was me, just as she was a symbol of all humanity—and the child within each one of us.

Karen Wapner, age 17 (written while working through her grief after the death of a very close friend)

▶ **LEARNING OPPORTUNITY:** What are your feelings and beliefs regarding death? Discuss with your peers your concept of death and dying.

deals with the death has a great impact on the child's understanding of death, but children usually do not have a realistic comprehension of the finality of death until they near preadolescence. Although the dying child may be unable to understand death, the emotions of family caregivers and others alert the child that something is threatening his or her secure world. Dealing with the child's anxieties with openness and honesty restores the child's trust and comfort.

Developmental Stage

Infants and toddlers have little if any understanding of death. The toddler may fear separation from beloved caregivers but have no recognition of the fact that death is nearing and irreversible. A toddler may say, "Nana's gone bye-bye to be with God" or "Grampy went to heaven" and a few moments later ask to go visit the deceased person. This is an opportunity to explain to the child that Nana or Grampy is in a special place and cannot be visited, but the family has many memories of him or her that they will always treasure. The child should not be scolded for not understanding. Questions are best answered simply and honestly.

If the infant's or toddler's own death is approaching, family caregivers can be encouraged to stay with the child to provide comfort, love, and security.

physician, a chaplain, a social worker, a psychiatrist, a hospice nurse, or a **thanatologist** (a person [sometimes a nurse] trained especially to work with the dying and their families), but the nurse often is the person who coordinates the care.

THE CHILD'S UNDERSTANDING OF DEATH

Stage of development, cognitive ability, and experiences all influence children's understanding of death. The death of a pet or a family member may be a child's first experience with death. How the family

Maintaining routines as much as possible helps to give the toddler a greater sense of security. The ego-centric thinking of preschool children contributes to the belief that they may have caused a person or pet to die by thinking angry thoughts. Magical thinking also plays an important part in the preschooler's beliefs about death. It is not unusual for a preschool child to insist on burying a dead pet or bird, then in a few hours or a day or two dig up the corpse to see if it is still there. This may be especially true if the child has been told that it will "go to heaven." Many preschoolers think of death as a kind of sleep; they do not understand that the dead person will not wake up. They may fear going to sleep after the death of a close family member because they fear that *they* may not wake up. Family caregivers must watch for this kind of reaction then encourage children to talk about their fears while reassuring them that they need not fear dying while sleeping. The child's feelings must be acknowledged as real, and the child must be helped to resolve them. The feelings must never be ridiculed.

A preschool child may view personal illness as punishment for thoughts or actions. Because preschoolers do not have an accurate concept of death, they fear separation from family caregivers. Caregivers can provide security and comfort by staying with the child as much as possible.

The child who is 6 or 7 years old is still in the magical thinking stage and continues to think of death in the same way as the preschool child does. At about 8 or 9 years of age, children gain the concept that death is universal and irreversible. Around this age, death is personified—that is, it is given characteristics of a person and may be called the devil, God, a monster, or the bogeyman. Children of this age often believe they can protect themselves from death by running past a cemetery while holding their breath, keeping doors locked, staying out of dark rooms, staying away from funeral homes and dead people, or avoiding stepping on cracks in the sidewalk.

When faced with the prospect of their own death, school-age children usually are sad that they will be leaving their family and the people they love (Fig. 22–1). They may be apprehensive about how they will manage when they no longer have their parents around to help them. Often they view death as another new experience like going to school, leaving for camp, or flying in an airplane for the first time. They may fear the loss of control that death represents to them and express this fear through vocal aggres-sion. Family caregivers and nurses must recognize this as an expression of their fear and avoid scolding or disciplining them for this behavior. This is a time when the people close to the child can help him or her voice anxieties about the future and provide an outlet

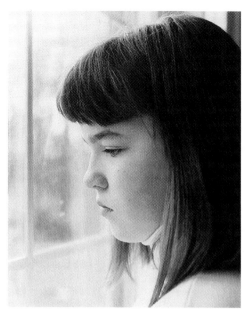

● *Figure 22.1* School-age children are often sad when faced with their own death and leaving their family.

for these aggressive feelings. The presence of family members and maintenance of relatively normal routines help to give the child a sense of security.

Adolescents have an adult understanding of death but feel that they are immortal—that is, death will happen to others but not to them. This belief con-tributes to adolescents' sometimes dangerous, life-threatening behavior. This denial of the possibility of serious personal danger may contribute to an adoles-cent's delay in reporting symptoms or seeking help. Diagnosis of a life-threatening or terminal illness creates a crisis for the adolescent. To cope with the illness, the adolescent must draw on cognitive func-tioning, past experiences, family support, and problem-solving ability. The adolescent with a terminal illness may express helplessness, anger, fear of pain, hopelessness, and depression. Adolescents often try to live the fullest lives they can in the time they have.

Adolescents may be upset by the results of treat-ments that make them feel weak and alter their appearance such as alopecia, edema resulting from steroid therapy, and pallor. They may need assistance in presenting themselves as attractively as possible to their peers. Adolescents need opportunities to acknowledge their impending death and can be encouraged to express fears and anxieties and ask questions about death. Participating in their usual activities helps adolescents feel in control.

Experience With Death and Loss

Every death that touches the life of a child makes an impression that affects the way the child thinks about every other death, including his or her own. Attitudes of family members are powerful influences. Family caregivers must be able to discuss death with children when a grandparent or other family member dies, even though the discussion may be painful. Otherwise the child thinks that death is a forbidden topic; avoiding the subject leaves room for fantasy and distortion in the child's imagination.

Many books are available to help a child deal with loss and death. *A Balloon Story,* a simply produced 13-page coloring storybook by hospice nurse Ruth Anne Sieber, is an introduction to loss appropriate for the young child. This story of two children who go to a fair with their mothers is illustrated with large line drawings to color. The children each select and purchase a helium balloon of which they are quite proud. Unfortunately, Nathan's balloon slips from his hand and floats away forever. Nathan displays typical grief reactions of protest, anger, and finally acceptance (Fig. 22–2). Reading the story to a child provides the adult with the perfect opening to discuss loss. A small booklet for caregivers accompanies *A Balloon Story* and contains excellent guidelines for discussing death and loss with a child. *A Balloon Story* can be obtained from Hospice: The Bridge, Lewistown Hospital, Lewistown, PA 17044.

Another small booklet that is excellent to use with any age group is *Water Bugs and Dragonflies.* This story approaches life and death as stages of existence by illustrating that after a water bug turns into a dragonfly, he can no longer go back and tell the other curious water bugs what life is like in this beautiful new world to which he has gone. This story can serve as the foundation for further discussion about death (Fig. 22–3).

Available books on death vary in their approaches. A number of books focus on the death of an animal or pet. Many stories deal with death as a result of old age. Several books have an accident as the cause of death. Most of the books are fiction, but several nonfiction ones are available for older children (Box 22–2). There is no discussion of one's own death in these books, which is consistent with the Western philosophy of handling death as

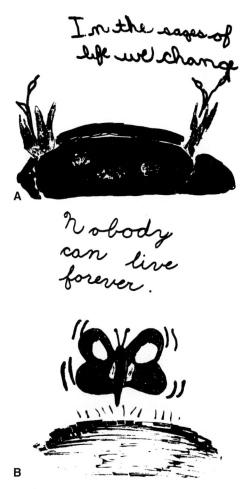

● *Figure 22.3* Drawings done by fourth-grade students after a presentation about death that included a reading of *Water Bugs and Butterflies.* **(A)** In the s[t]ages of life we change. At the center of the drawing is a pond with three lily pads. The stems at the end represent plants that waterbugs crawl up on before turning into dragonflies. **(B)** Nobody lives forever. (Courtesy of Ruth Anne Sieber.)

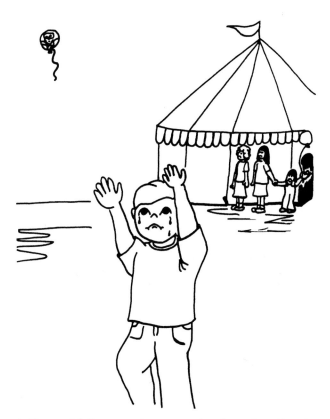

● *Figure 22.2* Nathan cried and kept jumping and reaching after everyone else had given up. (Courtesy of Ruth Anne Sieber.)

BOX 22.2 | Books About Death for Children

Author	Book	Publisher	Who Died	Age Appropriate
Blume, Judy	Tiger Eyes	Scarsdale, NY: Bradbury Press	Father	11–15
Bunting, E.	The Happy Funeral	New York: Harper and Row	Grandfather	3–7
Carrick, C.	The Accident	New York: Houghton Mifflin, Clarion Books	Dog	6–11
Claudy, A.F.	Dusty Was My Friend	Human Sciences Press	Friend	6–11
Edleman, Hope	Motherless Daughters	Dell Publishing Company	Mother	14 and up
Graeber, C.	Mustard	New York: MacMillian Publishing Co.	Cat	6–10
Hemery, Kathleen	The Brightest Star	Omaha, NE: Centering Corporation	Mother	4–8
Henkes, Kevin	Sun & Spoon	New York: Greenwillow Books	Grandmother	9–13
Hermes, P.	You Shouldn't Have to Say Goodbye	New York: Harcourt Brace Jovanovich	Mother	9–13
Hesse, K.	Poppy's Chair	New York: MacMillian Publishing Co.	Grandfather	6–11
Hickman, M.W.	Last Week My Brother Anthony Died	Abington Press	Brother	3–7
Holmes, Margaret Mudlaff, Sasha	Molly's Mom Died	Omaha, NE: Centering Corporation	Mother	5–9
Lorenzen, K.	Lanky Longlegs	New York: Atheneum. A Margaret K. McElderry Book	Brother	9–13
Lowden, Stephanie Golightly	Emily's Sadhappy Season	Omaha, NE: Centering Corporation	Father	4–8
Schotter, R.	A Matter of Time	New York: Collins Press	Mother	14 and up
Scrivani, Mark	I Heard Your Mommy Died	Omaha, NE: Centering Corporation	Mother	3–7
Scrivani, Mark	I Heard Your Daddy Died	Omaha, NE: Centering Corporation	Father	3–7
Scrivani, Mark	When Death Walks In: For Teens Facing Grief	Omaha, NE: Centering Corporation		13 and up
Shook-Hazen, B.	Why Did Grandpa Die	Racine, WI: Western Publishing Co.	Grandfather	3–7
Smith, D.B.	A Taste of Blackberries	Boston: Thomas Crowell Company	Friend	6–11
Thomas, J.R.	Saying Goodbye to Grandma	New York: Clarion Books	Grandmother	6–11
Tiffault, Benette	A Quilt for Elizabeth	Omaha, NE: Centering Corporation	Father	4–8
Vigna, Judith	Saying Goodbye to Daddy	Morton Grove, IL: Albert Whitman & Co.	Father	6–9

something that happens to others but not to oneself.[2]

Awareness of Impending Death

Children know when they are dying. They sense and fear what is going to happen even if they cannot identify it by name. Their play activities, artwork, dreams, and symbolic language demonstrate this knowledge.

Family caregivers who insist that a child not learn the truth about his or her illness place health care professionals at a disadvantage because they are not free to help the child deal with fears and concerns. If caregivers permit openness and honesty in communication with a dying child, the health care staff can meet the child's needs more effectively, dispel misunderstandings, and see that the child and the family are able to resolve any problems or **unfinished business.** Completing unfinished business may mean spending more time with the child, helping siblings to understand the child's illness and

impending death, and giving family members a chance to share their love with the child. Allowing openness does not mean that nurses and other personnel offer information not requested by the child but means simply that the child be given the information desired gently and directly in words the child can understand. The truth can be kind as well as cruel. Honest, specific answers leave less room for misinterpretation and distortion.

Adolescents usually are sensitive to what is happening to them and may need the nurse to be an advocate for them if they have wishes they want to fulfill before dying. An adolescent who senses the nurse's willingness and ability may discuss feelings that he or she is uncomfortable discussing with family members. The nurse can talk with the adolescent and work with the family to help them understand the adolescent's desires and needs. The nurse can call on hospice workers, social or psychiatric services, or a member of the clergy to help the family express and resolve their concerns and recognize the adolescent's needs.

THE FAMILY'S REACTION TO DYING AND DEATH

Diagnosis of a potentially fatal disease, such as AIDS, cystic fibrosis, or cancer, sends feelings of shock, disbelief, and guilt through every family member. Anticipatory grief begins then and continues until remission or death. When the disease rapidly advances, anticipatory grief may be short-lived as the child's death nears.

Family Caregivers

The family caregivers of children in the final stages of a terminal illness may have had to cope with many hospital admissions between periods at home. During this time, the family may face decisions about the child's physical care as well as learning to live with a dying child (Fig. 22–4). As the child's condition deteriorates, the family can be encouraged to talk to their child about dying. This is a task they may find very difficult. Support from a religious counselor, hospice nurse, or social service or psychiatric worker can help them through this difficult task. Family caregivers can be encouraged to provide as much normalcy as possible in the child's schedule. School attendance and special trips can be encouraged within the child's capabilities and desires.

During this time, family caregivers may find themselves going through a grieving process of anger, depression, ambivalence, and bargaining over and over again. The caregivers may direct anger at the hospital staff, themselves (because of guilt), at

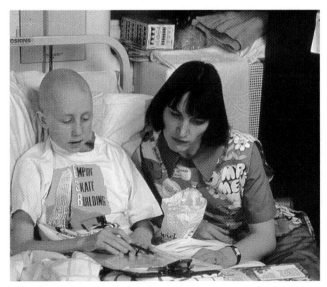

● **Figure 22.4** Caregivers experience and deal with grief in many different ways. This mom finds comfort in spending quiet moments with her dying child.

each other, or at the child. Reassure the caregivers that this is a normal reaction, but avoid taking sides.

If the child improves enough to go home again, parents may find that they tend to be overprotective of the child. As in chronic illness, this overprotective attitude reinforces the child's sick behavior and dependency and is usually accompanied by a lack of discipline. Failure to set limits accentuates the child's feelings of being different and creates problems with siblings. The child learns to manipulate family members, only to find that this kind of behavior does not bring positive results when attempted with peers or health care personnel.

When the child has to return to the hospital because of increasing symptoms, family caregivers may reexperience all stages of the grieving process. The family members dread the child's approaching death and fear that the child will be in great pain or may die when they are not present. Nurses can help relieve these fears by keeping the family informed about the child's condition, making the child as comfortable as possible, and reassuring the family members that they will be summoned if death appears to be near.

When death comes, it is perfectly appropriate to share the family's grief, crying with them then giving them privacy to express their sorrow. The nurse can stay with the family for a while, remaining quietly supportive with an attitude of a comforting listener. An appropriate comment may be, "I am so sorry" or "This is a very sad time." The nurse needs to keep the focus on the family's grief and what the nurse can do to support them. This is not an appropriate time for the nurse to share personal experiences of loss.

The family may want to hold the child to say a final good-bye, and the nurse can encourage and assist them in this. Intravenous lines and other equipment can be removed to make holding the child easier. The family may be left alone during this time if they desire. The nurse must be sensitive to the family's needs and desires to provide them with comfort.

During anticipatory grief, the family of a child with a terminal illness has an opportunity to complete any unfinished business. This can help them prepare for the child's death. However, when a child dies suddenly and unexpectedly, the family has not had the opportunity to go through anticipatory grief. Such a family may have excessive guilt and remorse for something they felt they left unsaid or undone. Even if a child has had a traumatic death with disfigurement, the family must be given the opportunity to be with, see, and hold the child to help with closure of the child's life. The nurse can prepare the family for seeing the child, explaining why parts of the body may be covered. Viewing the child, even if severely mutilated, helps the family to have a realistic view of the child and aids in the grief process.

The family may face a number of decisions that must be made rather quickly, especially when the child's death is unexpected. Families of terminally ill children usually have made some plans for the child's death and may know exactly what they want done. However, when the child dies unexpectedly, decisions may be necessary concerning organ donation, funeral arrangements, and an autopsy. If the death has been the result of violence or is unexplained, law requires an autopsy, but there may be other reasons that an autopsy is desired. An autopsy might be helpful in finding causes and treatments for other children diagnosed with the same disease, especially if it is a diagnosis about which little research is available. Organ donation can be discussed with the family by the hospital's organ donor coordinator or other designated person. The family needs to be well informed and must be supported throughout these difficult decisions.

Grief for the death of a child is not limited in time but may continue for years. Sometimes professional counseling is necessary to help family members work through grief. The support of others who have experienced the same sort of loss can be helpful. Two national organizations founded to offer support are the Candlelighters Childhood Cancer Foundation (P.O. Box 498 Kensington, MD 20895-0498, 800-366-2223, *http://www.candlelighters.org*) and The Compassionate Friends (PO Box 3696, Oak Brook, IL 60522-3696; 877-969-0010, *http://www.compassionate-friends.org*). These organizations have many local chapters.

The Child

The dying child may have a decreased level of consciousness, although hearing remains intact. Family members at the bedside and health care personnel may need to be reminded to avoid saying anything that would not be said if the child were fully conscious. Gentle touching and caressing may provide comfort to the child. Excellent nursing care is required. Medications for pain are given intravenously because they are poorly absorbed from muscle due to poor circulation. Mucous membranes are kept clean, and petroleum jelly (Vaseline) can be applied to the lips to prevent drying and cracking. The conjunctiva of the eyes can be moistened with normal saline eye drops, such as Artificial Tears, if drying occurs. The skin is kept clean and dry, and the child is turned and positioned regularly to provide comfort and to prevent skin breakdown. While caring for the child, the nurse should talk to the child and explain everything that is being done.

As death approaches, the internal body temperature increases; thus, dying patients seem to be unaware of cold even though their skin feels cool. Explain this to family members so they do not think the child needs additional covering. Just before death, the child who has remained conscious may become restless, followed by a time of peace and calm. The nurse and family members should be aware of these reactions and know that death is near.

Siblings

Just as in the case of chronic illness, siblings resent the attention given to the ill child and are angry about the disruption in the family. Reaction varies according to the sibling's developmental age and parental attitudes and actions. Younger children find it almost impossible to understand what is happening; it is difficult even for older children to grasp. Reaction to the illness and its accompanying stresses can cause classroom problems for school-age siblings; these may be incorrectly labeled as learning disabilities or behavioral disorders unless school personnel are aware of the family situation.

When the child dies, young siblings who are still prone to magical thinking may feel guilty, particularly if a strong degree of rivalry existed before the illness. These children need continued reassurance that they did not cause or help to cause their sibling's death.

The decision of whether or not a sibling should attend funeral services for the child may be difficult. Although there has been little research, the current thinking among many health professionals supports

---

INTERNET EXERCISE 22.1

http://dying.about.com

Click on "Grieving Child."
Click on section entitled "How children deal with the death of a sibling."

1. List some statements that well-meaning friends and relatives often say to children who are grieving.

2. List four ideas of ways that adults can help a child who has lost a sibling.

Click on section entitled, "Talking to children about death."
Read this section.

1. List the normal children's reactions to death for each stage of growth and development.

2. State suggestions of ways to help a child deal with the death of a sibling.

BOX 22.3	Guidelines for Helping Children Cope With Death

DO
1. Know your own beliefs.
2. Begin where the child is.
3. Be there.
4. Confront reality.
5. Encourage expression of feelings.
6. Be truthful.
7. Include the child in family rituals.
8. Encourage remembrance.
9. Admit when you don't know the answer.
10. Use touch to communicate.
11. Start death education early, simply, using naturally occurring events.
12. Recognize symptoms of grief, and deal with the grief.
13. Accept differing reactions to death.

DON'T
1. Praise stoicism (detached, unemotional behavior).
2. Use euphemisms (mild expressions substituted for ones that might be offensive).
3. Be nonchalant.
4. Glamorize death.
5. Tell fairy tales or half-truths.
6. Close the door to questions.
7. Be judgmental of feelings and behaviors.
8. Protect the child from exposure to experiences with death.
9. Encourage forgetting the deceased.
10. Encourage the child to be like the deceased.

Courtesy of Alice Demi, President, Grief Education Institute, PO Box 623, Englewood, CO 80151.

the presence of the sibling. The sibling may be encouraged to leave a token of love and good-bye with the child—a drawing, note, toy, or another special memento. Siblings can visit the dead child in privacy with few other mourners present. Dealing with the realities of the brother's or sister's death openly is likely to be more beneficial than avoiding the issue and allowing the sibling to use his or her imagination about death (Box 22–3).

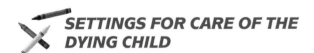

SETTINGS FOR CARE OF THE DYING CHILD

The family's response to and acceptance of a child's death can be greatly influenced by where the child dies. In a hospital, the child may receive the most professional care and the most technologically advanced treatment, but having a child in the hospital can contribute to family separation, a feeling of loss of control, and a sense of isolation. An increasing number of families are choosing to keep the child at home to die.

Hospice Care

In medieval times, a **hospice** was a refuge for various travelers: not only those traveling through the countryside but the terminally ill who were leaving this life for another. Hospices often were operated by religious orders and became havens for the dying. The current hospice movement in health care began in England, when Dr. Cicely Saunders founded St. Christopher's Hospice in London in 1967. This institution has become the model for others in the United States and Canada, with an emphasis on sensitive, humane care for the dying. Hospice principles of care include relief of pain, attention to the needs of the total person, and absence of heroic life-saving measures.

The first hospice in the United States was the New Haven Hospice in Connecticut. Many communities now have hospice programs that may or may not be affiliated with a hospital. Some programs offer a hospice setting to which patients go in terminal stages of illness; others provide support and guidance for the patient and family while the patient remains in the hospital or is cared for at home. Most of these hospice programs are established primarily for adults, but some programs also accept children as patients.

Children's Hospice International, founded in 1983, is an organization dedicated to hospice support of children. Through an individualized plan of care, Children's Hospice addresses the physical, developmental, psychological, social, and spiritual needs of children and families in a comprehensive and consistent way. It serves as a resource and advocacy center, providing education for parents and professionals. The organization conducts seminars and conferences, publishes training manuals, and supports a clearinghouse of information available through a national hotline (1-800-24-CHILD). Its Internet Web page (*http://www.chionline.org*) provides information for adults and games, books, and an excellent list of Web sites for children.

Home Care

Caring for the dying patient, young or old, at home has become increasingly common in recent years. More families are choosing to keep their child at home during the terminal stage of illness. Factors that contribute to the decision to care for a child at home include

- Concerns about costs for hospitalization and non-medical expenses such as the family's travel, housing, and food
- Stress from repeated family separations
- Loss of control over the care of the child and family life

Families feel that the more loving, caring environment of the home draws the family closer and helps to reduce the guilt that often is a part of bereavement. All family members can be involved to some extent in the child's care and in this way gain a feeling of usefulness. Family caregivers feel that they remain in control.

There are disadvantages, however. Costs that would have been covered by health insurance if the child were hospitalized may not be covered if the child is cared for at home. Caring for a dying child can be extremely difficult emotionally and physically. Not every family has someone who can carry out the procedures that may need to be performed regularly. In some instances, home nursing assistance is available, but this varies from community to community. Usually the home care nurse visits several days a week and may be on call the rest of the time. In some communities, hospice nurses may provide the teaching and support that families need.

Deciding whether or not to care for a dying child at home is an extremely difficult decision for a family. Family members need support and guidance from health care personnel when they are trying to make the decision, after the decision is made, and even after the child dies.

Hospital Care

Dying in a hospital has limitations and advantages. The child and the family may find support from others in the same situation. Family members may not have the physical or emotional strength to cope with total care of the child at home, but they can participate in care supported by the hospital staff (Fig. 22–5). Hospital care is much more expensive, but this may not be important to some families especially those with health insurance. The hospital is still the culturally accepted place to die, and this is important to some persons. Patients and families who choose hospital care need to know that they have rights and can exert some control over what happens to them.

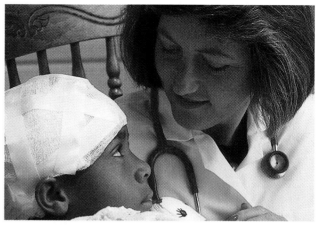

● **Figure 22.5** The nurse helps support the dying child in the hospital setting.

● Nursing Process for the Dying Child

ASSESSMENT

The assessment of the terminally ill child and family is an ongoing process developed over a period of time by the healthcare team. The healthcare team assessment covers the child's developmental level, the influence of cultural and spiritual concerns, the family's support system, present indications of grieving (e.g., anticipatory grief), interactions among family members, and unfinished business. To understand the child's view of death, consider the child's previous experiences, developmental level, and cognitive ability.

NURSING DIAGNOSES

Nursing diagnoses for the dying child include those appropriate for the child's illness as well as the following, which are specific to the dying process:

- Acute Pain related to illness and weakened condition
- Risk for Social Isolation related to terminal illness
- Anxiety related to condition and prognosis
- Compromised Family Coping related to approaching death
- Powerlessness of family caregivers related to inability to control child's condition

OUTCOME IDENTIFICATION AND PLANNING

The goals set and the planning done to meet those goals depend on the stage of the illness, the child's and the family's acceptance of the illness, and their attitudes and beliefs about death and dying. Major goals for the child include minimizing pain, diminishing feelings of abandonment by peers and friends, and relieving anxiety about the future. Goals for the family include helping coping with the impending death and identifying feelings of powerlessness.

IMPLEMENTATION

Relieving Pain and Discomfort. The child may be in pain for many reasons such as chemotherapy; nausea, vomiting, and gastrointestinal cramping; pressure caused by positioning; or constipation. Until the child is comfortable and relatively pain-free, all other nursing interventions are fruitless: pain becomes the child's primary focus until relief is provided. Nursing measures to relieve pain may include positioning, using pillows as needed; changing linens; providing conscientious skin and mouth care; protecting skin surfaces from rubbing together; offering backrubs and massages; and administering antiemetics, analgesics, and stool softeners as appropriate.

Providing Appropriate Social Interactions. Encourage the child's siblings and friends to maintain contact. Provide opportunities for peers to visit, write, or telephone, as the child is able. Read to the child and engage in other activities that he or she finds interesting and physically tolerable. When possible, encourage the child to make decisions to foster a feeling of control. Explain all procedures and how they will affect the child. Provide the child with privacy, but do not neglect him or her. Provide ample periods of rest. Continue to talk to and tell the child what you are doing even though the child may seem unresponsive.

Easing the Child's Anxiety. Ask family caregivers about the child's understanding of death and previous experiences with death. Observe how the child exhibits fear, and ask family caregivers for any additional information. Encourage the child to use a doll, a pillow, or another special "warm fuzzy" for comfort. Use words such as "dead" or "dying" if appropriate in conversation, because this may give the child an opening to talk about death. Nighttime is especially frightening for children because they often think they will die at night. Provide company and comfort, and be alert for periods of wakefulness when the child may need someone to talk to. Be honest and straightforward, and avoid injecting your beliefs into the conversation. If appropriate, read a book about death to the child to initiate conversation (although this should have been done much earlier in the child's care).

Helping the Family Cope. Family caregivers may need encouragement to discuss their feelings about the child. Emotions and fears must be acknowledged and caregivers reassured that their reactions are normal. The support of a member of the clergy may be helpful during this time. Help family members contact their own spiritual counselor, or offer to contact the hospital chaplain if the family desires. Encourage family caregivers to eat and rest properly so they will not become ill or exhausted themselves. Explain the child's condition to the family and answer any questions. The family can be reassured that everything is being done to keep the child as comfortable and pain-free as possible. Interpret signs of approaching death for the family.

If appropriate, ask the family about the siblings: what they know, how much they understand, and if the family has discussed the approaching death. Offer to help the caregivers talk with siblings.

Helping the Family Feel Involved in the Child's Care. Respond to the family's need to feel some control over the situation by suggesting specific measures they can perform to provide comfort for the child such as positioning, moistening lips, and reading or telling a favorite story. Encourage the caregivers to talk to the child even if the child does not respond. Discourage whispered conversations in the room. Encourage and help the family to carry out cultural customs if they wish. Help the family complete any unfinished business on the agenda; this may include the need for the child to go home to die. Help family contact support persons such as hospice workers or social services. (See Nursing Care Plan for the Dying Child and the Family.)

EVALUATION: GOALS AND OUTCOME CRITERIA

- *Goal:* The child will have minimal pain. *Criteria:* The child rests quietly and denies pain when asked.
- *Goal:* The child will have social interaction with others.

NURSING CARE PLAN

for the Dying Child and Family

JR is a 7-year-old who has a terminal illness. She is not expected to live more than a few more weeks. She has a brother who is 10 and a sister who is 4. A family member is with her continuously.

NURSING DIAGNOSIS
Acute Pain related to illness and weakened condition

GOAL: The child will have minimal pain.

OUTCOME CRITERIA
- The child has uninterrupted periods of quiet rest.
- Using a pain scale, the child indicates that she experiences relief from pain.

NURSING INTERVENTIONS	*RATIONALE*
Pain relief must be the primary focus of all nursing care until the child is comfortable. Administer pain relief medication, but also include such nursing measures as positioning, providing backrubs and massages, changing linens, providing conscientious skin and mouth care, and protecting skin surfaces from rubbing together to increase child's comfort.	Pain is the child's primary focus; until pain is relieved, all other nursing interventions are fruitless. Each child's pain experience is unique, and it may vary from one time to another. Some measures may relieve pain in one situation but not another. Discover the measures that work most frequently for this child.

NURSING DIAGNOSIS
Risk for Social Isolation related to terminal illness

GOAL: The child will have social interaction with others.

OUTCOME CRITERIA
- The child engages in social interaction with her classmates and other peers.
- The family caregivers and others play games with or read to child within her physical limitations.
- The caregivers talk with child when giving care regardless of her apparent level of consciousness.

NURSING INTERVENTIONS	*RATIONALE*
Encourage child's siblings and peers (including school friends) to maintain contact; provide opportunities for such contact by arranging for convenient visiting hours, providing paper and pens for writing, and making a telephone available. Spend time with and talk to the child, even when you are not sure she is responsive.	The child needs to feel that she is not cut off from everyone and everything. This helps relieve boredom and also diverts the child's attention from her condition. Hearing is often the last sense to shut down; the child will feel reassured by your voice and presence.

NURSING DIAGNOSIS
Anxiety related to condition and prognosis

GOAL: The child will express feelings of anxiety and use available supports to cope with anxiety.

OUTCOME CRITERIA
- The child talks to her family or the nurse about death.
- The child has a "warm fuzzy" close by.
- The child freely expresses her fears about dying especially fears about nighttime.

NURSING INTERVENTIONS	*RATIONALE*
Discuss with the family the child's understanding of death, and note how she exhibits fear. Use straightforward terminology when discussing death.	The child may or may not have discussed death with the family, and it is important for the nurse to respond to the child appropriately. The nurse is able at the same time to get a sense of how family members view the child's death and what sort of help they may need to discuss the topic with their child and each other.

NURSING CARE PLAN continued

for the Dying Child and Family

NURSING INTERVENTIONS	RATIONALE
Encourage the child to keep a favorite object or "warm fuzzy" for comfort and reassurance. Provide company and comfort particularly at night. Keep a night light on to ease anxieties.	Many children think they will die at night; periods of wakefulness are common. If the child is left alone, fears may compound. A night-light provides some sense of security.

NURSING DIAGNOSIS
Compromised Family Coping related to approaching death

GOAL: The family members will develop ways to cope with the child's approaching death.

OUTCOME CRITERIA
- The family caregivers express their feelings and anxieties.
- The family caregivers contact a spiritual advisor for support.
- The family caregivers identify signs in the child that indicate approaching death.

NURSING INTERVENTIONS	RATIONALE
Encourage family caregivers to discuss their feelings about the child and to acknowledge their fears and emotions; reassure them that their reactions are normal.	It may be very difficult for family members to talk about their child's death; they may feel they need to "keep up a brave front" for the child and siblings. However, it is important for them to acknowledge the death and begin to express some of their emotions.
Help the family contact their spiritual advisor or a hospital chaplain, if they desire.	The support of a spiritual counselor, particularly one known to the family, may be helpful.
Help the family recognize and acknowledge signs of the child's impending death. Help them talk with her siblings.	Acknowledging the impending signs of death helps the family caregivers to be realistic about the approaching death. They also may need support and guidance to know how to talk with the other children.
Make sure family caregivers are resting and eating adequately.	The family caregivers must avoid exhaustion; lack of sleep and inadequate nutrition will only make it harder for them to cope.

NURSING DIAGNOSIS
Powerlessness of family caregivers related to inability to control child's condition

GOAL: The family members will be involved in child's care to decrease feelings of powerlessness.

OUTCOME CRITERIA
- The family caregivers provide comfort measures for the child.
- The family caregivers talk with child and complete unfinished business with her.

NURSING INTERVENTIONS	RATIONALE
Suggest specific care measures that family members might perform to comfort the child; encourage the family to carry out cultural practices if they desire.	Caregivers need to feel they are doing something to help their child; performing meaningful cultural customs helps the family express feelings and provides a feeling of continuity.
Explain "unfinished business" to the family and encourage them to complete any unfinished business on their agenda.	Discussion of unfinished business provides another opportunity for family members to engage in meaningful activity with their child before the child's death.
Encourage family members to talk to the child even when she seems unresponsive.	The child may be able to hear voices even when unable to respond; family caregivers will feel better when they can still communicate love and support.

Criteria: Within physical capabilities the child engages in activities with peers, family, and others.

- *Goal:* The child will express feelings of anxiety and use available supports to cope with anxiety.
  Criteria: The child keeps a "warm fuzzy" close by for comfort and talks about death to the nurse or family. When awake at night, the child is comforted by the presence of someone to talk to.
- *Goal:* The family members will develop ways to cope with the child's approaching death.
  Criteria: The family members express their feelings; identify signs that indicate approaching death; use available support systems and people. The siblings visit and talk about their feelings regarding the approaching death of their sister or brother.
- *Goal:* The family members will be involved in child's care to decrease feelings of powerlessness.
  Criteria: The family members provide comfort measures for the child, talk to the child, and complete unfinished business with the child.

KEY POINTS

- A child's death affects health care personnel as well as the family. To work with dying patients effectively, health care personnel must work through their own feelings about death.
- The child's stage of development, cognitive ability, and experiences contribute to his or her understanding of death.
- The concept of death is greatly influenced by magical thinking before the age of 8 or 9 years.
- Adolescents have an attitude of immortality and may deny the possibility that they will die.
- The grieving process is multi-step and does not

follow a predictable schedule from one person to another.

- Family experiences vary with the length of the child's illness. With a chronic illness, the family experiences anticipatory grief, which gives them an opportunity to complete unfinished business and helps them to resolve their grief when death occurs. However, if a child dies suddenly or unexpectedly, the family has not had that resolution opportunity and may experience grief more profoundly.
- Hospital, home, and hospice care are all options during the terminal stage of the child's illness. Each type of care has advantages and disadvantages.

REFERENCES

1. (1970). *American Journal of Nursing, 70*(2), 335.
2. Bowden VR. (1993) Children's literature: The death experience. *Pediatric Nursing* 19(1), 17–21.

BIBLIOGRAPHY

Berger KS. (2001) *The developing person through the life span* (5th ed). New York: Worth Publishers.

Brazelton TB, Greenspan S. (2001) *The irreducible needs of children: What every child must have to grow, learn, and flourish.* Cambridge, MA: Perseus Publishing.

Busch T, Kimble CS. (2001) Grieving children: Are we meeting the challenge? *Pediatric Nursing,* 27(4), 414.

Pillitteri A. (2003) *Maternal and child health nursing* (4th ed). Philadelphia: Lippincott Williams & Wilkins.

Ritchie MA. (2001) Psychosocial nursing care for adolescents with cancer. *Issues in Comprehensive Pediatric Nursing,* 24(3), 165–75.

Wong DL. (1998) *Whaley and Wong's nursing care of infants and children* (6th ed). St. Louis: Mosby.

Websites
http://www.candlelighters.org
http://compassionatefriends.org
http://www.chionline.org
http://www.hospicenet.org

Workbook

NCLEX-STYLE REVIEW QUESTIONS

1. When working with the family of a child who is terminally ill, the child's siblings make the following statements to the nurse. Which statements is an example of the stage of grief referred to as bargaining?

   a. "I just want him to come to my birthday party next month."

   b. "It makes me mad that they said my brother is going to die."

   c. "I think he will get well now that he has a new medicine."

   d. "When he dies at least he won't have any more pain."

2. When working with the family of a child who is terminally ill, the child's siblings make the following statements to the nurse. Which statements is an example of the stage of grief referred to as denial?

   a. "I just want him to come to my birthday party next month."

   b. "It makes me mad that they said my brother is going to die."

   c. "I think he will get well now that he has a new medicine."

   d. "When he dies at least he won't have any more pain."

3. The nurse is working with a group of 4- and 5-year-old children who are talking about death and dying. One child in the group recently experienced the death of the family pet. Which of the following statements would the nurse expect a 5-year-old child to say about the death of the pet?

   a. "I think he was sad to leave us."

   b. "He's only a little dead."

   c. "A monster came and took him during the night."

   d. "I will be real good so I won't die."

4. The nurse is discussing the subject of death and dying with a group of adolescents. Which of the following statements made by an adolescent would be expected considering her or his stage of growth and development?

   a. "I always hold my breath and run past the cemetery to protect myself."

   b. "It would be sad to die because my girlfriend would really miss me."

   c. "Others die in car wrecks, but even if I had a wreck, I wouldn't be killed."

   d. "It makes me nervous to go to sleep. I am afraid I won't wake up."

5. The nurse is with a family whose terminally ill child has just died. Which of the following statements made by the nurse would be the MOST therapeutic statement?

   a. "It will not hurt as much as time passes."

   b. "My sister died when I was a teenager. I know how you feel."

   c. "I will leave the call light here. Call me if you need me."

   d. "This is a really sad and difficult time."

STUDY ACTIVITIES

1. List and compare thoughts and ideas a child of each of the following ages would most likely have regarding death and dying:

Pre-school	School-age	Adolescent

2. Research your community to find the procedure for organ donation. Make arrangements for a speaker from the organization to discuss organ donation with your class. If such a person is not available, research organ donation on the internet and share your findings with your class.

3. Survey your community to see if there is a hospice available. Describe how it functions. Find out if it accepts children as patients and if there are any restrictions concerning children. Discuss your findings with your peers.

CRITICAL THINKING

1. Describe your feelings about the story by the student nurse early in this chapter.
2. The Andrews family has an 8-year-old daughter with a terminal illness. Discuss the factors they need to consider when deciding if they wish to care for her at home.
3. The Andrews decide they cannot care for the child at home. Examine your feelings about this. Discuss your feelings with your peers. Talk about what you would say to this family to support them in their decision.

Glossary

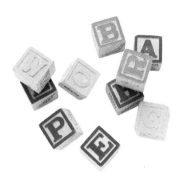

absence seizure seizure in which there is a sudden, brief loss of awareness, then a return to an alert state.

abuse misuse, excessive use, rough or bad treatment; used to refer to misuse of alcohol or drugs (substance abuse) and mistreatment of children or family members (child abuse, domestic abuse).

achylia absence of pancreatic enzymes in gastric secretions.

acid-base balance state of equilibrium between the acidity and the alkalinity of body fluids.

acidosis excessive acidity of body fluids

acrocyanosis cyanosis of the hands and feet seen periodically in the newborn.

actual nursing diagnoses diagnoses that identify existing health problems.

adenoids mass of lymphoid tissue in the nasal pharynx; extends from the roof of the nasal pharynx to the free edge of the soft palate.

adenopathy enlarged lymph glands.

akinetic seizure that causes a sudden, momentary loss of consciousness and muscle tone; also called atonic.

alcohol abuse drinking sufficient alcoholic beverages to induce intoxication.

alcoholism chronic alcohol abuse.

alkalosis excessive alkalinity of body fluids.

allergen antigen that causes an allergic reaction.

allograft skin graft taken from a genetically different person for temporary coverage during burn healing. Skin from a cadaver sometimes is used.

alopecia loss of hair.

amblyopia dimness of vision from disuse of the eye; sometimes called "lazy eye."

amenorrhea absence of menstruation.

ankylosis immobility of a joint.

anorexia nervosa eating disorder characterized by loss of appetite due to emotional causes, e.g., usually excessive fear of becoming (or being) fat.

anthelmintic medication that expels intestinal worms; vermifuge.

anticipatory grief preparatory grieving that often helps caregivers mourn the loss of their child when death actually comes.

antigen protein substance found on the surface of red blood cells capable of inducing a specific immune response and reacting with the products of that response.

antigen-antibody response response of the body to an antigen causing the formation of antibodies that protect the body from an invading antigen.

anuria absence of urine.

apnea temporary interruption of the breathing impulse.

archetypes predetermined patterns of human development, which according to Carl Jung, replace instinctive behavior of other animals; prototype.

areola darkened area around the nipple.

arthralgia painful joints.

ascites edema in the peritoneal cavity.

associative play being engaged in a common activity without any sense of belonging or fixed rules.

astigmatism error in light refraction on the retina caused by unequal curvature in the eye's cornea; light rays bend in different directions to produce a blurred image.

ataxia lack of coordination caused by disturbances in the kinesthetic and balance senses.

atonic seizure that causes a sudden, momentary loss of consciousness and muscle tone; also called akinetic.

atresia absence of a normal body opening or the abnormal closure of a body passage.

aura a sensation that signals an impending epileptic attack; may be visual, aromatic, or other sensation.

autistic totally self-centered and unable to relate to others, often exhibiting bizarre behaviors. Autistic children can sometimes be destructive to themselves and others.

autograft skin taken from an individual's own body. Except for the skin of an identical twin, autograft is the only kind of skin accepted permanently by recipient tissues.

autonomy ability to function in an independent manner.

autosomal dominant trait trait or condition appearing in a heterozygous person resulting from a dominant gene within a pair.

autosomal recessive trait trait or condition that is not expressed unless both parents carry the gene for that trait.

autosomes 22 pairs of chromosomes that are alike in the male and female. The sex chromosomes are not autosomes.

azotemia nitrogen-containing compounds in the blood.

Babinski reflex the flaring open of the infant's toes when the lateral plantar surface is stroked. Also called the plantar reflex, this reaction usually disappears by the end of the first year.

bilateral pertaining to both sides; e.g., bilateral cleft lip involves both sides of the lip.

binocular vision normal vision maintained through the muscular coordination of eye movements of both eyes. A single vision results.

blended family both partners in a marriage bring children from a previous marriage into the household: his, hers, and theirs.

body surface area (BSA) most reliable formula to calculate dosages. Using a West nomogram, the child's weight is marked on the right scale and the height is marked on the left scale. A straightedge is used to draw a line between the two marks. The point at which line crosses the column labeled SA (surface area) is the BSA expressed in square meters (m^2).

bonding development of a close emotional tie between the newborn and the parent or parents.

bottle mouth (nursing bottle) caries condition caused by the erosion of enamel on the infant's deciduous teeth from sugar in formula or sweetened juice that coats the teeth for long periods. This condition also can occur in infants who sleep with their mothers and nurse intermittently throughout the night.

brachycephaly shortness of the head.

bulimia eating disorder characterized by episodes of binge eating followed by purging by self-induced vomiting or use of laxatives.

caput succedaneum edematous swelling of the soft tissues of the scalp caused by prolonged pressure of the occiput against the cervix during labor and delivery. The edema disappears within a few days.

carditis inflammation of the heart.

case management a systematic process to ensure that a client's health and service needs are meet.

cataract development of opacity in the crystalline lens that prevents light rays from entering the eye.

cavernous hemangiomas congenital malformations that are subcutaneous collections of blood vessels with bluish overlying skin. Although these lesions are benign tumors, they may become so extensive as to interfere with the functions of the body part on which they appear.

celiac syndrome term used to designate the complex of malabsorptive disorders.

cephalhematoma collection of blood between the periosteum and the skull caused by excessive pressure on the head during birth.

chancre hard, red, painless primary lesion of syphilis at the point of entry of the spirochete.

chelating agent agent that binds with metal.

child advocacy speaking or acting on behalf of a child to ensure that her or his needs are recognized.

child neglect failing to provide adequate hygiene, health care, nutrition, love, nurturing, and supervision as needed for a child's growth and development.

child-life program program to make hospitalization less threatening for children and their parents. These programs are usually under the direction of a child-life specialist whose background is in psychology and early childhood development.

chordee chordlike anomaly that extends from the scrotum to the penis; pulls the penis downward in an arc.

chorea continuous, rapid, jerky involuntary movements

chromosomes threadlike structures that occur in pairs and carry genetic information.

chronic illness condition that interferes with daily functioning, progresses slowing, and shows little change over a long duration of time.

circumcision surgical removal of all or part of the foreskin (prepuce) of the penis.

circumoral pallor a white area around the mouth.

classification ability to group objects by rank, grade, or class.

clonus rapid involuntary muscle contraction and relaxation.

clove hitch restraints restraints used to secure an arm or leg; used most often when a child is receiving an intravenous infusion. The restraint is made of soft cloth formed in a figure eight.

co-dependent parent parent who supports, directly or indirectly, the other parent's addictive behavior.

cognitive development progressive change in the intellectual process including perception, memory, and judgment.

cohabitation family a living situation where a man and woman live together but are not legally married.

colic recurrent paroxysmal bouts of abdominal pain that are fairly common among young infants and that usually disappear around the age of 3 months.

colostomy a surgical procedure in which a part of the colon is brought through the abdominal wall to create an outlet for elimination of fecal material.

colostrum thin, yellowish, milky fluid secreted by the mother's breasts during pregnancy or just after delivery (before the secretion of milk).

comedones collection of keratin and sebum in the hair follicle; blackhead; whitehead.

communal family alternative family in which members share responsibility for homemaking and childrearing. All children are the collective responsibility of adult members.

community-based nursing a type of nursing practice focused on wellness and a holistic approach to caring for the child in a community setting.

congenital hip dysplasia abnormal fetal development of the acetabulum that may or may not cause dislocation of the hip. If the malformed acetabulum permits dislocation, the head of the femur displaces upward and backward. This may be difficult to recognize in early infancy.

congestive heart failure (CHF) result of impaired pumping capability of the heart. It may appear in the first year of life in infants with conditions such as large ventricular septal defects, coarctation of the aorta, and other defects that place an increased workload on the ventricles.

conjunctivitis acute inflammation of the conjunctiva that may be caused by a virus, bacteria, allergy, or foreign body.

conservation ability to recognize that change in shape does not necessarily mean change in amount or mass.

contracture fibrous scarring that forms over a burned movable body part. This part of the healing process can cause serious deformities and limit movement.

cooperative play children play with each other, as in team sports.

coryza runny nose.

cradle cap accumulation of oil and dirt that often forms on an infant's scalp; seborrheic dermatitis.

craniotabes softening of the occipital bones caused by a reduction of mineralization of the skull.

critical pathways standard plans of care used to organize and monitor the care provided.

croup general term that typically includes symptoms of a barking cough, hoarseness, and inspiratory stridor.

cultural competency the capacity of the nurse to work with people by integrating their cultural needs into their nursing care.

currant jelly stools stools that consist of blood and mucus.

cyanotic heart disease congenital heart disease that causes right-to-left shunting of blood in the heart; results in a depletion of oxygen to such an extent that the oxygen saturation of the peripheral arterial blood is 85% or less. Defects that permit right-to-left shunting may occur at the atrial, ventricular, or aortic level.

dawdling wasting time; whiling away time; being idle.

débridement removal of necrotic tissue.

decentration ability to see several aspects of a problem at the same time and understand the relationships of various parts to the whole situation.

deciduous teeth primary teeth that usually erupt between 6 and 8 months of age.

deliriants inhalants that contain chemicals whose fumes can produce confusion, disorientation, excitement, and hallucinations.

denial defense mechanism in which the existence of unpleasant actions or ideas is unconsciously repressed; in the grieving process, one of the stages many people go through; also a type of response by caregivers when caring for chronically ill children in which the caregivers deny the condition's existence and encourage the child to overcompensate for any disabilities.

dependence compulsive need to use a substance for its satisfying or pleasurable effects.

dependent nursing actions nursing actions that the nurse performs as a result of a physician's orders, such as administering analgesics for pain.

development progressive change in the child's maturation.

developmental tasks basic achievements associated with each stage of development. Basic tasks must be mastered to move on the next developmental stage. To achieve maturity, a person must successfully complete developmental tasks at each stage

diabetic ketoacidosis characterized by drowsiness, dry skin, flushed cheeks, cherry-red lips, and acetone breath with a fruity smell as a result of excessive ketones in the blood in uncontrolled diabetes.

diplopia double vision.

discipline to train or instruct to produce self-control and a particular behavior pattern, especially moral or mental improvement.

ductus arteriosus prenatal blood vessel between the pulmonary artery and the aorta that closes functionally within the first 3 or 4 days of life.

ductus venosus prenatal blood vessel between the umbilical vein and the inferior vena cava; does not achieve complete closure until the end of the second month of life.

dysarthria poor speech articulation.

dysfunctional family family that cannot resolve routine stresses in a positive, socially acceptable manner.

dysmenorrhea painful menstruation.

dysphagia difficulty swallowing.

early adolescence begins at about age 10 in girls and about age 12 in boys with a dramatic growth spurt that signals the advent of puberty; preadolescence; pubescence.

echolalia "parrot speech" typical of autistic children. They echo words they hear, such as a television commercial, but do not appear to understand the words.

ego in psychoanalytic theory, the conscious self that controls the pleasure principle of the id by delaying the instincts until an appropriate time.

egocentric concerned only with one's own activities or needs; unable to put oneself in another's place or to see another's point of view.

elbow restraints restraints made of muslin with two layers. Pockets wide enough to enclose tongue depressors placed vertically along the width of the fabric. The restraints are wrapped around the arm to prevent the infant from bending the arm.

electrolytes chemical compounds (minerals) that break down into ions when placed in water.

emetic agent that causes vomiting.

en face position establishment of eye contact in the same plane between the caregiver and infant; extremely important to parent-infant bonding; also called mutual gazing.

encephalopathy degenerative disease of the brain.

encopresis chronic involuntary fecal soiling with no medical cause.

enuresis involuntary urination especially at night; bedwetting beyond the usual age of control.

epiphyses growth centers at the ends of long bones and at the wrists.

epistaxis nosebleed.

erythema toxicum fine rash of the newborn that may appear over the trunk, back, abdomen, and buttocks. It appears about 24 hours after birth and disappears in several days.

eschar hard crust or scab.

esotropia eye deviation toward the other eye.

exotropia eye deviation away from the other eye.

extended family consists of one or more nuclear families plus other relatives; often crosses generations to include grandparents, aunts, uncles, and cousins. The needs of individual members are subordinate to the needs of the group, and the children are considered an economic asset.

external hordeolum purulent infection of the follicle of an eyelash; generally caused by *Staphylococcus aureus*. Localized swelling, tenderness, and pain are present with a reddened lid edge; a stye.

extracellular fluid fluid situated outside a cell or cells.

extravasation escape of fluid into surrounding tissue.

extrusion reflex infant's way of taking food by thrusting the tongue forward as if to suck; has the effect of pushing solid food out of the mouth.

febrile seizure seizure occurring in infants and young children commonly associated with a fever of 102° to 106° (38.9° to 41.1°).

fertilization process by which the male's sperm unites with the female's ovum.

fetal alcohol syndrome (FAS) symptoms seen in an infant born to a woman who abused alcohol during pregnancy including shorter stature, lower birth weight, possible microcephaly, facial deformities, hearing disorders, poor coordination, minor joint and limb abnormalities, heart defects, delayed development, and mental retardation.

fetus term for the organism after it has reached the eighth week of life and acquires a human likeness.

fontanelle "soft spot" covered by a tough membrane at the junctures of the six bones of a newborn's skull. At birth, two fontanelles can be detected—the anterior fontanelle at the junction of the frontal and parietal bones and the posterior fontanelle at the junction of the parietal and occipital bones. They are ossified (filled in by bone) during the normal growth process.

foramen ovale opening between the left and right atria of the fetal heart that closes with the first breath.

forceps marks noticeable marks on the infant's face that may occur if delivery was assisted with forceps; usually disappear within a day or two.

gag reflex reaction to any stimulation of the posterior pharynx by food, suction, or passage of a tube that causes elevation of the soft palate and a strong involuntary effort to vomit; continues throughout life.

galactosemia recessive hereditary metabolic disorder in which the enzyme necessary for converting galactose into glucose is missing. The infant generally appears normal at birth but experiences difficulties after the ingestion of milk.

gastroenteritis infectious diarrhea caused by infectious organisms including salmonella, *Escherichia coli*, dysentery bacilli, and various viruses, most notably rotaviruses.

gastrostomy tube tube surgically inserted through the abdominal wall into the stomach under general anesthesia. Used in children who have obstructions or surgical repairs in the mouth, pharynx, esophagus, or cardiac sphincter of the stomach or who are respirator-dependent.

gavage feeding nourishment provided directly through a tube passed into the stomach.

genes units threaded along chromosomes that carry genetic instructions from one generation to another. Like chromosomes, genes also occur in pairs. There are thousands of genes in the chromosomes of each cell nucleus.

genetic counseling study of the family history and tissue analysis of both partners to determine chromosome patterns for couples concerned about transmitting a specific disease to their unborn children.

goniotomy surgical opening into Schlemm's canal that allows drainage of aqueous humor; performed to relieve intraocular pressure in glaucoma.

gradual acceptance type of response by caregivers when caring for chronically ill children in which caregivers adopt a common-sense approach to the child's condition and encourage the child to function within his or her capabilities.

granulocytes type of white blood cell; divided into eosinophils, basophils, and neutrophils.

growth result of cell division and marked by an increase in size and weight; physical increase in body size and appearance caused by increasing numbers of new cells.

gynecomastia excessive growth of the mammary glands in the male.

halo traction metal ring attached to the skull that is added to a body cast using stainless steel pins inserted into the skull and into the femurs or iliac wings.

health maintenance organizations (HMOs) professional groups of physicians, laboratory service personnel, nurse practitioners, nurses, and consultants who care for the family's health on a continuing basis and are geared to health care and disease prevention. The family pays a set fee for total care; that fee covers any necessary hospitalization. The emphasis is on health and prevention.

hemarthrosis bleeding into the joints.

hemolysis destruction of red blood cells with the release of hemoglobin into the plasma.

hernia abnormal protrusion of part of an organ through a weak spot or other abnormal opening in a body wall.

heterograft graft of tissue obtained from an animal. For burn patients, pig skin (porcine) is often used.

heterosexual relationship intimate relationship between two people of the opposite sex.

hierarchical arrangement grouping by some common system such as rank, grade, or class.

hip dysplasia see congenital hip dysplasia.

hirsutism abnormal body and facial hair growth.

homeostasis uniform state; signifies biologically the dynamic equilibrium of the healthy organism.

homograph graft of tissue, including organs, from a member of one's own species.

homosexual relationship intimate relationship between two people of the same sex.

homozygous term used to describe a particular trait of an individual when any two members of a pair of genes carry the same genetic instructions for that trait.

hospice provides comforting and supportive care to terminally ill patients and their families. There are few hospice programs for children in the United States.

hyaline membrane disease also known as respiratory distress syndrome (RDS); occurs due to immature lungs that lack sufficient surfactant to decrease the surface tension of the alveoli; affects about half of all preterm newborns.

hydrotherapy use of water in a treatment.

hyperlipidemia increase in the level of cholesterol in the blood.

hyperopia refractive condition in which the person can see objects better at a distance; farsightedness.

hyperpnea increase in depth and rate of breathing.

hyperthermia overheating.

hypervolemic increased volume of circulating plasma.

hypocholia diminished flow of pancreatic enzymes.

hyposensitization immunization therapy by injection; immunotherapy.

hypothermia low body temperature; may be a symptom of a disease or dysfunction of the temperature-regulating mechanism of the body, or it may be deliberately induced, such as during open-heart surgery, to reduce oxygen needs and provide a longer time for the surgeon to complete the operation without brain damage. When caring for the newborn, it is important to remember that heat loss can lead to hypothermia because of the infant's immature temperature-regulating system.

hypovolemia decreased volume of circulating plasma.

id in psychoanalytic theory, part of the personality that controls physical needs and instincts of the body; dominated by the pleasure principle.

ileostomy a surgical procedure in which a part of the ileum is brought through the abdominal wall to create an outlet to drain fecal material.

imperforate anus congenital disorder in which the rectal pouch ends blindly above the anus and there is no anal orifice.

impunity belief, common among adolescents, that nothing can hurt them.

incest sexually arousing physical contact between family members not married to each other.

independent nursing actions nursing actions that may be performed based on the nurse's own clinical judgment.

induration hardness.

infantile spasms a type of seizure activity that occurs in an infant between 3 and 12 months and usually indicates a cerebral defect with a poor prognosis.

inhalant substance that may be taken into the body through inhaling; substance whose volatile vapors can be abused.

insulin reaction excessively low blood sugar caused by insulin overload; results in too rapid metabolism of the body's glucose; insulin shock; hypoglycemia.

intercurrent infection infection that occurs during the course of an already existing disease.

interdependent nursing actions nursing actions that the nurse must work with other health team members to accomplish such as meal planning with a dietary therapist and teaching breathing exercises with a respiratory therapist.

intermittent infusion device a type of device that is used for administering medications by the intravenous route and can be left in place and used at intervals.

interstitial fluid also called intracellular or tissue fluid; has a composition similar to plasma but contains almost no protein. This reservoir of fluid outside the body cells decreases or increases easily in response to disease.

interstitial keratitis inflammation of the cornea; often caused by congenital syphilis and usually accompanied by lacrimation, photophobia, and opacity of the lens; may lead to blindness.

intracellular fluid fluid contained within the cell membranes; constitutes about two-thirds of total body fluids.

intrathecal administration injection into the cerebrospinal fluid by lumbar puncture.

intravascular fluid fluid situated within the blood vessels or blood plasma.

invagination telescoping; infolding of one part of a structure into another.

Kussmaul breathing abnormal increase in the depth and rate of the respiratory movements.

kwashiorkor syndrome occurring in infants and young children soon after weaning; results from severe deficiency of protein. Symptoms include a swollen abdomen, retarded growth with muscle wasting, edema, gastrointestinal changes, thin dry hair with patchy alopecia, apathy, and irritability.

kyphosis backward and lateral curvature of the spine; hunchback.

lacrimation secretion of tears.

lactose a sugar found in milk that, when hydrolyzed, yields glucose and galactose.

lactose intolerance inability to digest lactose because of an inborn deficiency of the enzyme lactase.

lanugo fine, downy hair that covers the skin of the fetus.

latchkey child child who comes home to an empty house after school each day because family caregivers are at work.

lecithin major component of surfactant.

leukemia uncontrolled reproduction of deformed white blood cells.

leukopenia leukocyte count less than 5,000 mm^3.

libido sexual drive.

lordosis forward curvature of the lumbar spine; swayback.

lymphoblast lymphocyte that has been changed by antigenic stimulation to a structurally immature lymphocyte.

lymphocytes single-nucleus, nonphagocytic leukocytes that are instrumental in the body's immune response.

magical thinking child's belief that thoughts are powerful and can cause something to happen (e.g., illness or death of a loved one occurs because the child wished it in a moment of anger).

malocclusion the improper alignment of the teeth.

marasmus deficiency in calories as well as protein. The child suffers growth retardation and wasting of subcutaneous fat and muscle.

meconium first stools of the newborn; amniotic fluid together with a sticky, greenish-black substance composed of bile, mucus, cellular waste, intestinal secretions, fat, hair, and other materials swallowed during fetal life.

menarche beginning of menstruation.

metered-dose inhaler hand-held plastic device that delivers a premeasured dose of medicine.

microcephaly small head.

micrognathia abnormal smallness of the lower jaw.

milia pearly white cysts usually seen over the bridge of the nose, chin, and cheeks of a newborn. They are usually retention cysts of sebaceous glands or hair follicles and disappear within a few weeks without treatment.

mittelschmerz pain experienced midcycle in the menstrual cycle at the time of ovulation.

mongolian spots areas of bluish-black pigmentation resembling bruises; most often seen over the sacral or gluteal regions of infants of African, Mediterranean, Native American, or Asian descent; usually fade within 1 or 2 years.

monocytes 5% to 10% of white blood cells that defend the body against infection.

Moro reflex abduction of the arms and legs and flexion of the elbows in response to a sudden loud noise, jarring, or abrupt change in equilibrium: fingers flare except the forefinger and thumb which are clenched to form a C-shape. Occurs in the normal newborn up to the end of the fourth or fifth month.

mummy restraint used to restrain an infant or small child during procedures that involve only the head or neck.

mutation fundamental change that takes place in the structure of a gene; results in the transmission of a trait different from that normally carried by that particular gene.

mutual gazing see *en face position*.

myoclonic seizure characterized by sudden jerking of a muscle or group of muscles often in the arms or legs. There is no loss of consciousness.

myopia ability to see objects clearly at close range but not at a distance; nearsightedness.

myringotomy incision of the eardrum performed to establish drainage and to insert tiny tubes into the tympanic membrane to facilitate drainage of serous or purulent fluid in the middle ear.

nebulizer tube attached to a wall unit or cylinder that delivers moist air via a face mask.

negativism opposition to suggestion or advice; associated with the toddler age group because the toddler, in search of autonomy, frequently responds "no" to almost everything.

neonatal abstinence syndrome (NAS) symptoms seen in the newborn of the woman who has abused substances during pregnancy; withdrawal symptoms.

neonate term used to describe a newborn in the first 28 days of life.

noctural emissions involuntary discharge of semen during sleep; also known as wet dreams.

noncommunicative language egocentric speech exhibited by children who talk to themselves, toys, or pets without any purpose other than the pleasure of using words.

nuchal rigidity stiff neck.

nuclear family family structure that consists of only the father, the mother, and the children living in one household.

nursing process proven form of problem solving based on the scientific method. The nursing process consists of five components: assessment, nursing diagnosis, planning, implementation, and evaluation.

nutrition history information regarding the child's eating habits and preferences.

obesity excessive accumulation of fat that increases body weight by 20% or more over ideal weight.

objective data in the nursing assessment, the data gained by the nurse's direct observation.

oliguria decreased production of urine especially in relation to fluid intake.

onlooker play interest in the observation of an activity without participation.

opisthotonos arching of the back so that the head and the heels are bent backward and the body is forward.

orchiopexy surgical procedure used to bring an undescended testis down into the scrotum and anchor it there.

orthodontia a type of dentistry dealing with prevention and correction of incorrectly positioned or aligned teeth.

orthoptics therapeutic exercises to improve the quality of vision.

outcomes goals that are specific, stated in measurable terms, and have a time frame for accomplishment.

overprotection type of response by caregivers when caring for chronically ill children in which the caregivers protect the child at all costs, prevent the child from achieving new skills by hovering, avoid the use of discipline, and use every means to prevent the child from suffering any frustration.

overriding aorta in tetralogy of Fallot; the aorta shifts to the right over the opening in the ventricular septum so that blood from both right and left ventricles is pumped into the aorta.

overweight more than 10% over ideal weight.

palmar grasp reflex phenomenon that results when pressure is placed on the palm of the hand near the base of the digits causing flexion or curling of the fingers.

palpebral fissures opening between the eyes.

papoose board commercial restraint board for use with toddlers or preschool-age children that uses canvas strips to secure the child's body and extremities. One extremity can be released to allow treatment to be performed on that extremity.

parallel play one child plays alongside another child or children involved in the same type of activity but the children do not interact with each other.

partial seizure a type of seizure with manifestations that vary depending on the area of the brain where they arise.

patient-controlled analgesia (PCA) programmed intravenous infusion of narcotic analgesia that the patient can control within set limits.

pediatric nurse practitioner (PNP) professional nurse prepared at the postbaccalaureate level to give primary health care to children and families. These nurses use pediatricians or family physicians as consultants but offer day-to-day assessment and care.

pedodontist dentist who specializes in the care and treatment of children's teeth.

personal history data collected regarding the child's habits, activities, and behaviors.

petechiae small bluish-purple spots caused by tiny broken capillaries; pinpoint hemorrhages beneath the skin.

phenylketonuria (PKU) recessive hereditary defect of metabolism that results in a congenital disease due to a defect in the enzyme that normally changes the essential amino acid, phenylalanine, into tyrosine. If untreated, PKU results in severe mental retardation.

philtrum vertical groove in the middle of the upper lip.

phimosis adherence of the foreskin to the glans penis.

photophobia intolerance to light.

photosensitivity sensitivity to sunlight.

physiologic jaundice icterus neonatorum; jaundice that occurs in a large number of newborns but has no medical significance; result of the breakdown of fetal red blood cells.

pica compulsive eating of nonfood substances.

pinna the upper, external, protruding part of the ear.

plantar grasp reflex phenomenon that results when pressure is placed on the sole of the foot at the base of the toes; causes the toes to curl downward.

play therapy technical of psychoanalysis that psychiatrists or psychiatric nurse clinicians use to uncover a disturbed child's underlying thoughts, feelings, and motivations to help understand them better.

point of maximum impulse (PMI) the point over the heart on the chest wall where the heartbeat can be heard the best using a stethoscope.

polyarthritis inflammation of several joints.

polydipsia abnormal thirst.

polyphagia increased food consumption.

polyuria dramatic increase in urinary output, often with enuresis.

premenstrual syndrome (PMS) symptoms in the period before menstruation including edema (resulting in weight gain), headache, increased anxiety, mild depression, or mood swings; premenstrual tension.

primary circular reactions a stage of development named by Piaget in which the infant explores objects by touching or putting them in their mouth; the infant is unaware of actions that he or she can cause.

priapism prolonged, abnormal erection of the penis.

primary nursing system whereby one nurse plans the total care for a child and directs the efforts of nurses on the other shifts.

primary prevention limiting the spread of illness or disease by teaching especially regarding safety, diet, rest, exercise.

pruritus itching.

pseudomenses false menstruation; a slight red-tinged vaginal discharge in female infants resulting from a decline in the hormonal level after birth compared with the higher concentration in the maternal hormone environment before birth.

pseudostrabismus the cross-eyed look found in infants due to incomplete development of the nerves and muscles that control focusing and coordination; begins to disappear in the sixth month.

puberty period during which secondary sexual characteristics begin to develop and reproductive maturity is attained.

pulmonary stenosis narrowing of the opening between the right ventricle and the pulmonary artery that decreases blood flow to the lungs.

pulse oximeter photoelectric device used to measure oxygen saturation in an artery; can be attached to an infant's finger, toe, or heel.

punishment penalty given for wrongdoing.

purpura hemorrhages into the skin or mucous membranes.

purpuric rash rash consisting of ecchymoses (bruises) and petechiae caused by bleeding under the skin.

recessive gene gene carrying different information for a trait within a pair that is not expressed (e.g., blue eyes versus brown eyes). A recessive gene is detectable only when present on both chromosomes.

refraction the way light rays bend as they pass through the lens of the eye to the retina.

regurgitation spitting up of small quantities of milk; occurs rather easily in the young infant.

rejection type of response by caregivers when caring for chronically ill children in which the caregivers distance themselves emotionally from the child and, although they provide physical care, tend to scold and correct the child continuously.

respiratory distress syndrome (RDS) see *hyaline membrane disease*.

respite care care of the child by someone other than the usual caregiver so that the caregiver can get temporary relief and rest.

reversibility ability to think in either direction.

right ventricular hypertrophy increase in thickness of the myocardium of the right ventricle.

risk nursing diagnoses category of diagnoses that identifies health problems to which the patient is especially vulnerable.

ritualism practice employed by the young child to help develop security; consists of following a certain routine; makes rituals of simple tasks.

rooming-in arrangement in which the health care facility permits a family caregiver to stay with a child. A cot or sleeping chair is provided for the caregiver.

rooting reflex infant's response of turning the head when the cheek is stroked toward the stroked side.

rumination voluntary regurgitation.

runaway child child who is absent from home for overnight or longer without the permission of the caregiver.

school history information regarding the child's grade level in school and his or her academic performance.

school phobia child's fear resulting in dread of a school situation or fear of leaving home; can be a combination of both.

scoliosis lateral curvature of the spine.

seborrhea a scalp condition characterized by yellow, crusty patches; also called cradle cap.

sebum oily secretion of the sebaceous glands.

secondary circular reactions a stage of development named by Piaget in which the infant realizes that his or her actions cause pleasurable sensations.

secondary prevention limiting the impact or reoccurrence of disease by focusing on early diagnosis and treatment.

seizure series of involuntary contractions of voluntary muscles; convulsion.

sexual abuse sexual contact between a child and someone in a caretaking position such as a parent, babysitter, or teacher.

sexual assault sexual contact made by someone who is not functioning in the role of the child's caretaker.

single-parent family household headed by one adult of either sex. There may be one or more children in the family.

skeletal traction pull exerted directly on skeletal structures by means of pins, wire, tongs, or another device surgically inserted through the bone.

skin traction pull on tape, rubber, or plastic materials attached to the skin that indirectly exerts pull on the musculoskeletal system.

smegma the cheeselike secretion of the sebaceous glands found under the foreskin.

social history information about the environment in which the child lives.

socialization process by which a child learns the rules of the society and culture in which the family lives; its language, values, ethics, and acceptable behaviors.

solitary independent play playing apart from others without making an effort to be part of the group or group activity.

spina bifida failure of the posterior lamina of the vertebrae to close; leaves an opening through which the spinal meninges and spinal cord may protrude.

startle reflex follows any loud noise; similar to the Moro reflex, but the hands remain clenched. This reflex is never lost.

steatorrhea fatty stools.

step reflex also called the dance reflex; tendency of infants to make stepping movements when held upright.

stepfamily consists of custodial parent, children, and a new spouse.

stigma negative perception of a person because he or she is believed to be different from the general population; may cause embarrassment or shame in the person being stigmatized.

strabismus failure of the two eyes to direct their gaze at the same object simultaneously; squint; crossed eyes.

striae stretch marks.

stridor shrill, harsh respiratory sound, usually on inspiration.

subjective data in the nursing assessment, data spoken by the child or family.

sublimation process of directing a desire or impulse into more acceptable behaviors.

substance abuse the misuse of an addictive substance, such as alcohol or drugs, that changes the user's mental state.

sucking reflex infant's response of strong, vigorous sucking when a nipple, finger, or tongue blade is put in his or her mouth.

superego in psychoanalytic theory, the conscience or parental value system; acts primarily as a monitor over the ego.

supernumerary excessive in number (e.g., more than the usual number of teeth).

suture narrow band of connective tissue that divides the six nonunited bones of a newborn's skull.

symmetry a balance in shape, size, and position from one side of the body to the other; a mirror image.

sympathetic ophthalmia inflammatory reaction of the uninjured eye. Symptoms can include photophobia, lacrimation, and some dimness of vision.

synovitis inflammation of a joint; most commonly the hip in children.

talipes equinovarus clubfoot with plantar flexion.

temper tantrum behavior in children that springs from frustrations caused by their urge for independence; a violent display of temper. The child reacts with enthusiastic rebellion against the wishes of the caregiver.

teratogens from the Greek *terato*, meaning monster, and *genesis*, meaning birth; an agent or influence that causes a defect or disruption in the prenatal growth process. The effect of a teratogen depends on when it enters the fetal system and the stage of differentiation of the organs or organ systems at that time. Generally the fetus is most vulnerable to teratogens during the first trimester.

tertiary prevention a focus on rehabilitation and teaching to prevent further injury or illness.

thanatologist person, sometimes a nurse, trained especially to work with the dying and their families.

therapeutic play play technique that may be used by play therapists, nurses, child-life specialists, and trained volunteers.

thermoregulation regulation of temperature.

throwaway child child (often a teenager) who has been forced to leave home and is not wanted back by the adults in the home.

tinea ringworm.

tissue perfusion circulation of blood through the capillaries carrying nutrients and oxygen to the cells.

tolerance in substance abuse, ability of body tissues to endure and adapt to continued or increased use of a substance.

tonic neck reflex also called the fencing reflex; seen when the infant lies on the back with the head turned to one side, the arm and leg on that side extended, and the opposite arm flexed as if in a fencing position.

tonic-clonic a type of seizure characterized by muscular contractions and rigidity changing to generalized jerking movements of the muscles followed by a state of relaxation.

tonsils two oval masses attached to the side walls of the back of the mouth between the anterior and posterior pillars (folds of mucous membranes at the sides of the passage from the mouth to the pharynx).

total parenteral nutrition (TPN) the administration of dextrose, lipids, amino acids, electrolytes, vitamins, minerals, and trace elements into the circulatory system to meet the nutritional needs of the child whose needs cannot be met through the gastrointestinal tract.

tracheostomy surgical opening into the trachea to provide an open airway in emergency situations or when there is a blocked airway.

traction force applied to an extremity or other part of the body to maintain proper alignment and to facilitate healing of a fractured bone or dislocated joint.

tympanic membrane sensor device used to determine the temperature of the tympanic membrane by rapidly sensing infrared radiation from the membrane. The tympanic thermometer offers the advantage of recording the temperature rapidly with little disturbance to the child.

unfinished business completing matters that will help ease the death of a loved one; saying the unsaid and doing the undone acts of love and caring that may seem difficult to express; recognizing time is limited and filling that time with the important issues that need to be taken care of.

unilateral one side (e.g., in cleft lip, only one side of the lip is cleft).

unoccupied behavior daydreaming; fingering clothing or a toy without any apparent purpose.

urostomy a surgical opening created to help with the elimination of urine.

urticaria hives.

vaginitis inflammation of the vagina.

vascular nevus commonly known as a strawberry mark; a slightly raised, bright-red collection of hypertrophied skin capillaries that does not blanch completely on pressure.

ventricular septal defect abnormal opening in the septum of the heart between the ventricles; allows blood to pass directly from the left to the right side of the heart; the most common intracardiac defect.

ventriculoatrial shunting plastic tubing implanted into the cerebral ventricle passing under the skin to the cardiac atrium; provides drainage for excessive cerebrospinal fluid.

ventriculoperitoneal shunting plastic tubing implanted into the cerebral ventricle passing under the skin to the peritoneal cavity, providing drainage for excessive cerebrospinal fluid. Excessive tubing can be inserted to accommodate the child's growth.

vernix caseosa greasy, cheeselike substance that protects the skin during fetal life; consists of sebum and desquamated epithelial cells.

wellness nursing diagnoses diagnoses that identify the potential of an individual, family, or community to move to a higher level of wellness.

West nomogram graph with several scales arranged so that when two values are known, the third can be plotted by drawing a line with a straightedge; commonly used to calculate BSA.

wheezing sound of expired air being pushed through obstructed bronchioles.

withdrawal symptoms in substance abuse, physical and psychological symptoms that occur when the drug is no longer being used.

Answers to NCLEX-Style Review Questions

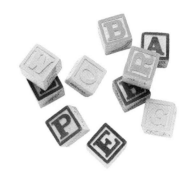

Chapter 1
1. b
2. a
3. c
4. b
5. c

Chapter 2
1. a
2. b
3. c
4. d
5. d

Chapter 3
1. b
2. a
3. d
4. b
5. d

Chapter 4
1. a
2. d
3. c
4. c
5. b

Chapter 5
1. c
2. b
3. b
4. d
5. b

Chapter 6
1. c
2. a
3. b
4. b
5. d

Chapter 7
1. b
2. c
3. c
4. a
5. a

Chapter 8
1. a
2. a
3. a
4. c
5. c

Chapter 9
1. d
2. b
3. b
4. b
5. a

Chapter 10
1. b
2. a
3. a
4. c
5. a

Chapter 11
1. d
2. b
3. d
4. c
5. c

Chapter 12
1. c
2. a
3. b
4. c
5. d

Chapter 13
1. b
2. c
3. a
4. b
5. a

Chapter 14
1. c
2. a
3. c
4. d
5. d

Chapter 15
1. a
2. a
3. b
4. b
5. c

Chapter 16
1. a
2. c
3. b
4. d
5. a

Chapter 17
1. c
2. d
3. b
4. c
5. b

Chapter 18
1. c
2. d
3. a
4. c
5. b

Chapter 19
1. d
2. b
3. c
4. b
5. c

Chapter 20
1. c
2. d
3. a
4. a
5. d

Chapter 21
1. a
2. c
3. a
4. b
5. a

Chapter 22
1. a
2. c
3. d
4. c
5. d

Appendix A
Growth Charts

Birth to 36 months: Boys
Length-for-age and Weight-for-age percentiles

NAME _____

RECORD # _____

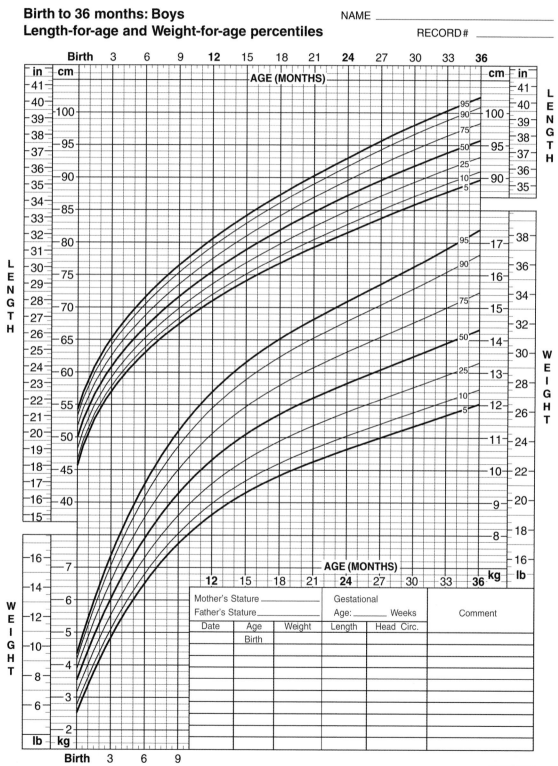

Published May 30, 2000 (modified 4/20/01).
SOURCE: Developed by the National Center for Health Statistics in collaboration with
the National Center for Chronic Disease Prevention and Health Promotion (2000).
http://www.cdc.gov/growthcharts

SAFER · HEALTHIER · PEOPLE™

Birth to 36 months: Boys
Head circumference-for-age and
Weight-for-length percentiles

NAME _____

RECORD# _____

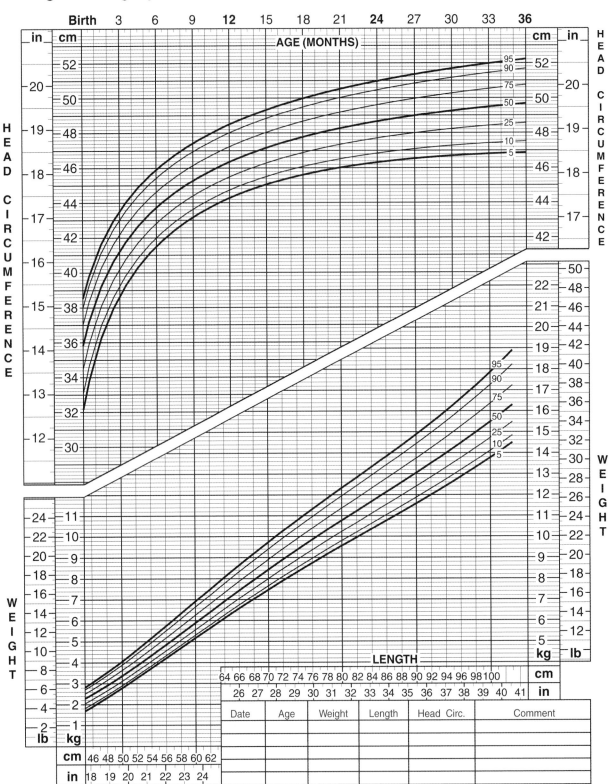

Published May 30, 2000 (modified 10/16/00).
SOURCE: Developed by the National Center for Health Statistics in collaboration with
   the National Center for Chronic Disease Prevention and Health Promotion (2000).
   http://www.cdc.gov/growthcharts

SAFER ● HEALTHIER ● PEOPLE™

Birth to 36 months: Girls
Length-for-age and Weight-for-age percentiles

NAME _____

RECORD # _____

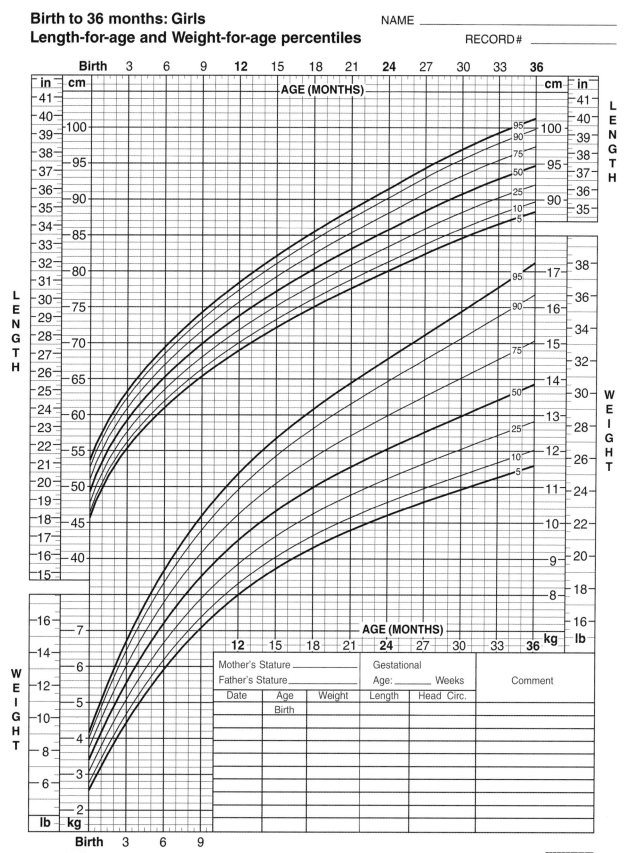

Published May 30, 2000 (modified 4/20/01).
SOURCE: Developed by the National Center for Health Statistics in collaboration with
the National Center for Chronic Disease Prevention and Health Promotion (2000).
http://www.cdc.gov/growthcharts

SAFER · HEALTHIER · PEOPLE™

Birth to 36 months: Girls
Head circumference-for-age and
Weight-for-length percentiles

NAME _____

RECORD # _____

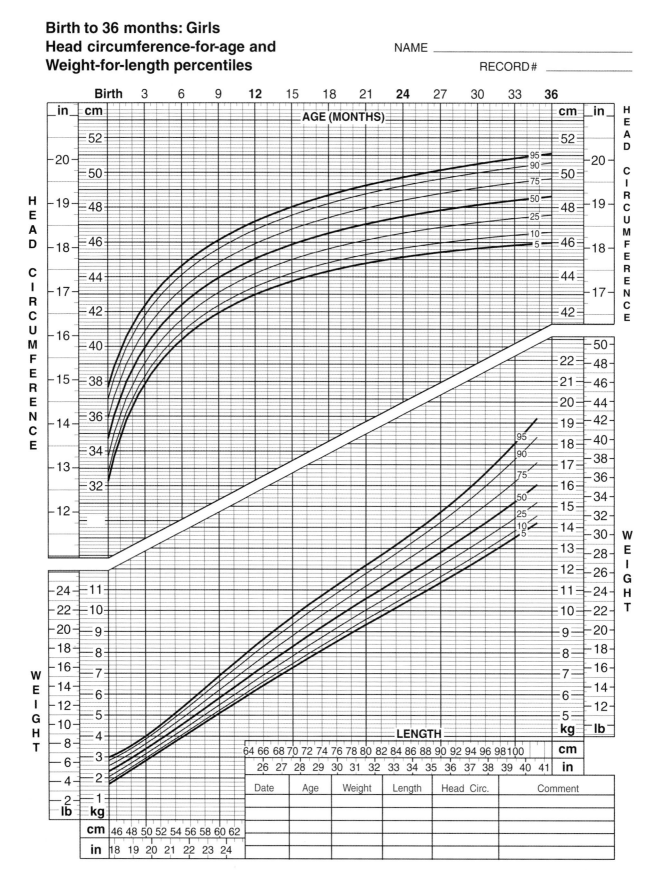

Published May 30, 2000 (modified 10/16/00).
SOURCE: Developed by the National Center for Health Statistics in collaboration with
the National Center for Chronic Disease Prevention and Health Promotion (2000).
http://www.cdc.gov/growthcharts

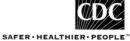

SAFER · HEALTHIER · PEOPLE™

2 to 20 years: Boys
Stature-for-age and Weight-for-age percentiles

NAME _____

RECORD# _____

Mother's Stature _____ Father's Stature _____

Date	Age	Weight	Stature	BMI*

*To Calculate BMI: Weight (kg) ÷ Stature (cm) ÷ Stature (cm) x 10,000
or Weight (lb) ÷ Stature (in) ÷ Stature (in) x 703

AGE (YEARS)

STATURE

WEIGHT

Published May 30, 2000 (modified 11/21/00).

SOURCE: Developed by the National Center for Health Statistics in collaboration with
the National Center for Chronic Disease Prevention and Health Promotion (2000).
http://www.cdc.gov/growthcharts

SAFER · HEALTHIER · PEOPLE™

2 to 20 years: Girls
Stature-for-age and Weight-for-age percentiles

NAME _____

RECORD# _____

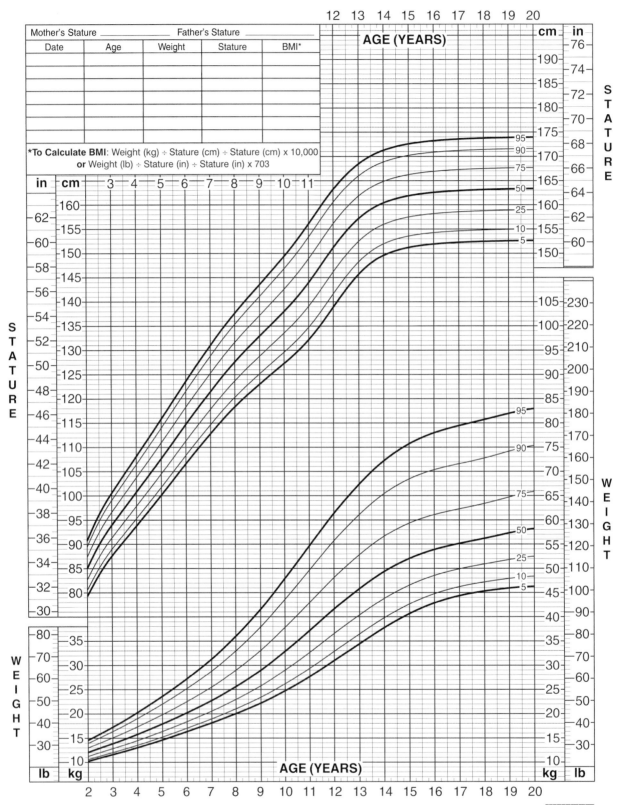

Published May 30, 2000 (modified 11/21/00).
SOURCE: Developed by the National Center for Health Statistics in collaboration with
the National Center for Chronic Disease Prevention and Health Promotion (2000).
http://www.cdc.gov/growthcharts

SAFER · HEALTHIER · PEOPLE™

Appendix B

Pulse, Respiration, and Blood Pressure Values for Children

NORMAL PULSE RANGES IN CHILDREN

Age	Normal Range	Average
0–24 hours	70–170 bpm	120 bpm
1–7 days	100–180 bpm	140 bpm
1 month	110–188 bpm	160 bpm
1 month–1 year	80–180 bpm	120–130 bpm
2 years	80–140 bpm	110 bpm
4 years	80–120 bpm	100 bpm
6 years	70–115 bpm	100 bpm
10 years	70–110 bpm	90 bpm
12–14 years	60–110 bpm	85–90 bpm
14–18 years	50–95 bpm	70–75 bpm

bpm, beats per minute.

NORMAL BLOOD PRESSURE RANGES

Age	Systolic (mm Hg)	Diastolic (mm Hg)
Newborn–12 hr (less than 1000 g)	39–59	16–36
Newborn–12 hr (3000 g)	50–70	24–45
Newborn–96 hr (3000 g)	60–90	20–60
Infant	74–100	50–70
Toddler	80–112	50–80
Preschooler	82–110	50–78
School-Age	84–120	54–80
Adolescent	94–140	62–88

VARIATIONS IN RESPIRATIONS WITH AGE

Age	Rate per Minute
Newborn	40–90
1 year	20–40
2 years	20–30
3 years	20–30
5 years	20–25
10 years	17–22
15 years	15–20
20 years	15–20

Appendix C

Conversion Chart: Fahrenheit to Celsius

Celsius	Fahrenheit
34.0	93.2
34.2	93.6
34.4	93.9
34.6	94.3
34.8	94.6
35.0	95.0
35.2	95.4
35.4	95.7
35.6	96.1
35.8	96.4
36.0	96.8
36.2	97.2
36.4	97.5
36.6	97.9
36.8	98.2
37.0	98.6
37.2	99.0
37.4	99.3
37.6	99.7
37.8	100.0
38.0	100.4
38.2	100.8
38.4	101.1
38.6	101.5
38.8	101.8
39.0	102.2
39.2	102.6
39.4	102.9
39.6	103.3
39.8	103.6
40.0	104.0
40.2	104.4
40.4	104.7
40.6	105.2
40.8	105.4
41.0	105.9
41.2	106.1
41.4	106.5
41.6	106.8
41.8	107.2
42.0	107.6
42.2	108.0
42.4	108.3
42.6	108.7
42.8	109.0
43.0	109.4

$(°C) \times (9/5) + 32 = °F.$

$(°F - 32) \times (5/9) = °C.$

Appendix D

Good Sources of Essential Nutrients

Protein	Vitamin A	Vitamin B			Vitamin C	Vitamin D	Minerals		
		Thiamine	Riboflavin	Niacin			Calcium	Iron	Iodine
Meat, poultry, fish, milk products and eggs. Whole wheat grains, nuts, peanut butter, legumes are also good sources of protein, but need to be supplemented by some animal protein, such as meat, eggs, milk, cheese, cottage cheese or yogurt.	Green leafy vegetables, deep yellow vegetables and fruits, whole milk or whole milk products, egg yolk.	Meat, fish, poultry, eggs, whole grain, legumes, potatoes, green leafy vegetables.	Milk (best source), meat, egg yolk, green vegetables.	Meat, fish, poultry, peanut butter, wheat germ, brewer's yeast. Although the amount in milk is small, children whose intake of milk is adequate do not develop pellagra.	Citrus fruits and tomatoes, fresh or frozen citrus fruit juices, strawberries, cantaloupe. Breast milk is an adequate source of vitamin C for young infants only if the mother's diet contains sufficient vitamin C.	Sunlight, fish liver oils, fortified milk and synthetic vitamin D.	Milk and milk products, squash, sweet potatoes, raisins, rhubarb, well-cooked dried beans, turnip greens, Swiss chard, mustard greens.	Green leafy vegetables, liver, meats and eggs, dried fruits, whole grain or enriched bread and cereals.	Seafoods, plants grown on soil near the sea, iodized salt.

Appendix E
Standard Precautions

Use Standard Precautions, or the equivalent, for the care of all patients. *Category IB**

A. Handwashing

(1) Wash hands after touching blood, body fluids, secretions, excretions, and contaminated items, whether or not gloves are worn. Wash hands immediately after gloves are removed, between patient contacts, and when otherwise indicated to avoid transfer of microorganisms to other patients or environments. It may be necessary to wash hands between tasks and procedures on the same patient to prevent cross-contamination of different body sites. *Category IB*

(2) Use a plain (nonantimicrobial) soap for routine handwashing. *Category IB*

(3) Use an antimicrobial agent or a waterless antiseptic agent for specific circumstances (e.g., control of outbreaks or hyperendemic infections), as defined by the infection control program. *Category IB* (See Contact Precautions for additional recommendations on using antimicrobial and antiseptic agents.)

B. Gloves

Wear gloves (clean, nonsterile gloves are adequate) when touching blood, body fluids, secretions, excretions, and contaminated items. Put on clean gloves just before touching mucous membranes and nonintact skin. Change gloves between tasks and procedures on the same patient after contact with material that may contain a high concentration of microorganisms. Remove gloves promptly after use, before touching noncontaminated items and environmental surfaces, and before going to another patient, and wash hands immediately to avoid transfer of microorganisms to other patients or environments. *Category IB*

C. Mask, Eye Protection, Face Shield

Wear a mask and eye protection or a face shield to protect mucous membranes of the eyes, nose, and mouth during procedures and patient-care activities that are likely to generate splashes or sprays of blood, body fluids, secretions, and excretions. *Category IB*

D. Gown

Wear a gown (a clean, nonsterile gown is adequate) to protect skin and to prevent soiling of clothing during procedures and patient-care activities that are likely to generate splashes or sprays of blood, body fluids, secretions, or excretions. Select a gown that is appropriate for the activity and amount of fluid likely to be encountered. Remove a soiled gown as promptly as possible, and wash hands to avoid transfer of microorganisms to other patients or environments. *Category IB*

E. Patient-Care Equipment

Handle used patient-care equipment soiled with blood, body fluids, secretions, and excretions in a manner that prevents skin and mucous membrane exposures, contamination of clothing, and transfer of microorganisms to other patients and environments. Ensure that reusable equipment is not used for the care of another patient until it has been cleaned and reprocessed appropriately. Ensure that single-use items are discarded properly. *Category IB*

F. Environmental Control

Ensure that the hospital has adequate procedures for the routine care, cleaning, and disinfection of environmental surfaces, beds, bedrails, bedside equipment, and other frequently touched surfaces, and ensure that these procedures are being followed. *Category IB*

G. Linen

Handle, transport, and process used linen soiled with blood, body fluids, secretions, and excretions in a manner that prevents skin and mucous membrane exposures and contamination of clothing, and that avoids transfer of microorganisms to other patients and environments. *Category IB*

H. Occupational Health and Bloodborne Pathogens

(1) Take care to prevent injuries when using needles, scalpels, and other sharp instruments or devices; when handling sharp instruments after procedures; when cleaning used instruments; and when disposing of used needles. Never recap used needles, or otherwise manipulate them using both hands, or use any other technique that involves directing the

---

(From Recommendations for Isolation Precautions in Hospitals developed by the Centers for Disease Control and Prevention and the Hospital Control Practices Advisory Committee [HICPAC], February 18, 1997.)

*Category IB. Strongly recommended for all hospitals and reviewed as effective by experts in the field and a consensus of HICPAC members on the basis of strong rationale and suggestive evidence, even though definitive studies have not been done.

point of a needle toward any part of the body; rather, use either a one-handed "scoop" technique or a mechanical device designed for holding the needle sheath. Do not remove used needles from disposable syringes by hand, and do not bend, break, or otherwise manipulate used needles by hand. Place used disposable syringes and needles, scalpel blades, and other sharp items in appropriate puncture-resistant containers, which are located as close as practical to the area in which the items were used, and place reusable syringes and needles in a puncture-resistant container for transport to the reprocessing area. *Category IB*

(2) Use mouthpieces, resuscitation bags, or other ventilation devices as an alternative to mouth-to-mouth resuscitation methods in areas where the need for resuscitation is predictable. *Category IB*

I. Patient Placement

Place a patient who contaminates the environment or who does not (or cannot be expected to) assist in maintaining appropriate hygiene or environmental control in a private room. If a private room is not available, consult with infection control professionals regarding patient placement or other alternatives. *Category IB*

Index

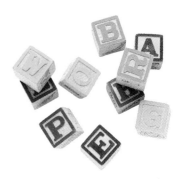

Page numbers followed by f indicate figures; those followed by t indicate tables.